Acute Rheumatic Fever and Rheumatic Heart Disease

Acute Rheumatic Fever and Rheumatic Heart Disease

Edited by

SCOTT DOUGHERTY, MBCHB, BMSC (HONS), MRCP (LOND)
Internist, Department of Internal Medicine, Belau National Hospital,
Ministry of Health, Koror, Republic of Palau

JONATHAN CARAPETIS, MBBS, BMEDSC, PHD, FRACP,
FAFPHM, FAHMS
Executive Director, Telethon Kids Institute, Perth, Western Australia
Professor, University of Western Australia, Perth, WA
Consultant, Perth Children's Hospital, Perth, WA

LIESL ZÜHLKE, MBCHB, DCH, FCPAEDS, CERT CARD, MPH,
FACC, FESC, MSC, PHD
Specialist Paediatrician and Paediatric Cardiologist, Division of Paediatric Cardiology,
Department of Paediatrics, Red Cross War Memorial Children's Hospital,
Division of Cardiology, Department of Medicine, Grotte Schuur Hospital,
Faculty of Health Sciences, University of Cape Town

NIGEL WILSON, MBCHB, DIPOBST, DCH, MRCP (UK),
FRACP, FCANZ
Paediatric Cardiologist, Green Lane Paediatric and Congenital Cardiology Department,
Starship Hospital, Auckland District Health Board, Auckland, New Zealand

Clinical Associate Professor, Department of Paediatrics,
University of Auckland, Auckland, New Zealand

ELSEVIER

Publisher: Dolores Meloni
Acquisitions Editor: Robin R. Carter
Editorial Project Manager: Megan Ashdown
Production Project Manager: Poulouse Joseph
Cover Designer: Alan Studholme

3251 Riverport Lane
St. Louis, Missouri 63043

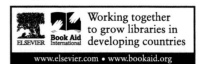

Working together
to grow libraries in
developing countries

www.elsevier.com • www.bookaid.org

List of Contributors

Sulafa K.M. Ali, FRCPCH, FACC
Professor, Pediatrics and Child Health
University of Khartoum
Khartoum, Sudan

Consultant, Pediatric Cardiologist
Pediatric Cardiology
Sudan Heart Center
Khartoum, Sudan

Manuel J. Antunes, MD, PhD DSc
Professor of Cardiothoracic Surgery
Faculty of Medicine
University of Coimbra

Clinic of Cardiothoracic Surgery
Faculty of Medicine
University of Coimbra
Portugal

**Michael G. Baker, MBChB, DCH, DObst,
   FNZCPHM, FAFPHM (RACP)**
Professor of Public Health
Department of Public Health
University of Otago
Wellington, New Zealand

Raghav Bansal, MBBS, MD, DM
Electrophysiology Fellow, Arrhythmia Associates
Holy Family Hospital
Mumbai, Maharashtra, India

Doctor, Cardiology
All India Institute of Medical Sciences
New Delhi, Delhi, India

Andrea Beaton, MD
Assistant Professor of Pediatrics
Cincinnati Children's Hospital Medical Center
University of Cincinnati College of Medicine
Cincinnati Ohio, United States

**Jonathan Carapetis, MBBS, BMedSc, PhD,
   FRACP, FAFPHM, FAHMS**
Executive Director
Telethon Kids Institute
Perth, Western Australia

Professor
University of Western Australia
Perth, WA

Consultant
Perth Children's Hospital
Perth, WA

Antoinette Cilliers, MBBCh, FCPaed
Professor of Paediatric Cardiology
Chris Hani Baragwanath Academic Hospital
University of the Witwatersrand
Johannesburg, Gauteng, South Africa

Gonçalo F. Coutinho, MD, PhD
Consultant of Cardiothoracic Surgery
University Centre and Hospital of Coimbra
Cardiothoracic Surgery Department
Coimbra, Portugal

Madeleine Cunningham, MS, PhD
George Lynn Cross Professor
Department of Microbiology and Immunology
University of Oklahoma Health Sciences Center
Oklahoma City, OK, United States

Jessica L. de Dassel, BSc, MIPH, PhD
Charles Darwin University
Darwin, NT, Australia

Global and Tropical Health
Menzies School of Health Research
Darwin, NT, Australia

Scott Dougherty, MBChB, BMSc (Hons), MRCP (Lond)
Internist
Department of Internal Medicine
Belau National Hospital
Ministry of Health
Koror, Republic of Palau

Mark E. Engel, BSc (MED) Hons, MSc, MPH, PhD
Associate Professor
Department of Medicine
Groote Schuur Hospital
Faculty of Health Sciences
University of Cape Town
Cape Town, Western Cape, South Africa

Daniel Engelman, MBBS, BMedSci, MPHTM, PhD
Paediatrician
General Medicine
Royal Children's Hospital
Melbourne, VIC, Australia

Research Fellow
Tropical Diseases
Murdoch Children's Research Institute
Melbourne, VIC, Australia

Honorary Senior Fellow
Paediatrics
University of Melbourne
Melbourne, VIC, Australia

Mohammed R. Essop, MBBCh, MRCP (UK), FCP (SA), FRCP (Lond), FACC
Professor
Division of Cardiology
University of the Witwatersrand
Johannesburg, Gauteng, South Africa

Kirsten Finucane, MBChB, FRACS, ONZM
Chief of Surgery
Paediatric and Congenital Cardiac Service
Starship and Auckland City Hospital
Auckland, New Zealand

Tom Gentles, MB ChB, FRACP, FCSANZ
Paediatric Cardiologist
Director
Green Lane Paediatric and Congenital
Cardiology Service
Auckland, New Zealand

Luiza Guilherme, MSc, PhD
Professor of Immunology
Heart Institute (InCor)
University of São Paulo
Institute for Investigation in Immunology
National Institute of Science and Technology
São Paulo, Brazil

Susan J. Jack, MBChB, Dip Paeds, MPH+TM, PhD, FNZCPHM
Public Health Physician/Medical Officer of
Health/Clinical Director
Public Health South
Southern District Health Board
Dunedin, New Zealand

Adjunct Senior Lecturer
Department of Preventive & Social Medicine
University of Otago
Dunedin, New Zealand

Joseph Kado, MBBS, DCH, MMed(Paeds)
Doctor, Group A Streptococcal & Rheumatic Heart
Disease
Telethon Kids Institute
Perth, WA, Australia

University of Western Australia
Perth, WA, Australia

Ganesan Karthikeyan, MBBS, MD, DM, MSc
Professor of Cardiology
Department of Cardiology
All India Institute of Medical Sciences
New Delhi, Delhi, India

Jerome H. Kim, MD, FACP, FIDSA
Director General, International Vaccine Institute
Seoul, South Korea

A. Sampath Kumar, MBBS, MS, MCh
Retired Professor and Head
Department of CTVS
AIIMS, New Delhi, Delhi, India

Senior Consultant
Max Super Speciality Hospital, Vaishali
Ghaziabad (NCR), Uttar Pradesh, India

Raman Krishna Kumar, MD, DM, FAHA
Department of Pediatric Cardiology
Amrita Institute of Medical Sciences and Research
Centre
Amrita Vishwavidyapeetham
Cochin, Kerala, India

Chim C. Lang, BMSc (Hons), MBChB, MD, FRCP (Lond), FRCP (Edin), FACC, FAMM, FESC
Professor of Cardiology
Division of Molecular and Clinical Medicine
University of Dundee, Dundee, United Kingdom

Professor of Cardiology and Consultant Cardiologist
University of Dundee
Dundee, United Kingdom

Diana Lennon, MBCHB, FRACP
Department of Paediatrics, Child & Youth Health
The University of Auckland, School of
    Population Health
Auckland, New Zealand

Paediatrician in Infectious Diseases
Department of Paediatrics
Starship Children's Hospital
Auckland, New Zealand

Mariana Mirabel, MD, PhD, FESC
Cardio-oncology Unit HYPAARC
Hôpital Européen Georges Pompidou
Paris, France

Institut National de la Sante et de la
Recherche Medicale Paris, France

Université Paris Descartes
Paris, France

Ana Mocumbi, MD, PhD, FESC
Associate Professor
Internal Medicine
Division of Cardiology
Universidade Eduardo Mondlane
Faculty of Medicine
Maputo, Mozambique

Instituto Nacional de Saúde
Division of Non Communicable Diseases
Maputo, Mozambique

Ari Horton, MBBS (Hons), FRACP
Consultant Paediatric Cardiologist
Monash Heart and Monash Children's Hospital
Monash Health, VIC, Australia

Monash Cardiovascular Research Centre
Melbourne, VIC, Australia

Department of Paediatrics, Monash University
Melbourne, VIC, Australia

Ify R. Mordi, MD, MBChB, MRCP (UK)
Clinical Lecturer
Division of Molecular and Clinical Medicine
University of Dundee
Dundee, United Kingdom

Specialty Registrar
Department of Cardiology, Ninewells Hospital
Dundee, United Kingdom

Cardiologist and Lecturer in Cardiology
University of Dundee, Dundee, United Kingdom

Jeremiah Mwangi, MA
Executive Director
Reach, Geneva, Switzerland

Bruno Nascimento, MD, MSC, PhD, FACC
Associate Professor of Medicine
Departamento de Clínica Médica
Faculdade de Medicina da, Universidade Federal de
    Minas Gerais
Serviço de Cardiologia e Cirurgia Cardiovascular
Hospital das Clínicas da Universidade
    Federal de Minas Gerais
Belo Horizonte, MG, Brazil

Mpiko Ntsekhe, BA, MD, MPhil, PhD, FACC
Professor of Cardiology
Division of Cardiology, Department of Medicine
University of Cape Town & Groote Schuur Hospital
Cape Town, Western Cape, South Africa

Emmy Okello, MBChB, MMed, PhD, FACC
Consultant Cardiologist and Head Division of
    Cardiology, Uganda Heart Institute
Kampala, Uganda

Joshua Osowicki, MBBS, BmedSci, FRACP
Tropical Diseases
Murdoch Children's Research Institute
Melbourne, VIC, Australia

Department of Paediatrics
University of Melbourne
Melbourne, VIC, Australia

Infectious Diseases Physician
Infectious Diseases Unit
Department of General Medicine
The Royal Children's Hospital
Melbourne, VIC, Australia

Tom Parks, BA, MB, BChir, MD, MRCP, DTM&H
Faculty of Infectious and Tropical Diseases
London School of Hygiene and Tropical Medicine
Wellcome Centre for Human Genetics
University of Oxford
Oxford, United Kingdom

Susanna Price, MBBS, BSc, FRCP, EDICM, PhD, FFICM, FESC
Professor
Consultant Cardiologist and Intensivist
Royal Brompton Hospital
National Heart and Lung Institute
Imperial College London
London, United Kingdom

Anna P. Ralph, BMEDSCI, MBBS (HONS), MPH, DTMH, FRACP, PHD
Professor and Divisional Leader
Global and Tropical Health
Menzies School of Health Research
Darwin, NT, Australia

Staff Specialist in Infectious Diseases and General Medicine
Royal Darwin Hospital
Darwin, NT, Australia

Co-Director, Rheumatic Heart Disease Australia

Bo Remenyi, MBBS, FRACP, PhD
Paediatric Cardiologist
Royal Darwin Hospital Australia

Research Fellow
Division of Child Health
Menzies School of Health Research
Darwin, Australia

Craig Sable, MD
Associate Chief
Division of Cardiology

Director
Echocardiography
Children's National Hospital

Professor of Pediatrics
George Washington University School of Medicine
Washington, DC, United States

Masood Sadiq, MBBS, MRCP (UK), FRCP (Ed), FCPS, FRCPCH
Professor of Paediatric Cardiology
Dean, The Institute of Child Health
Children's Hospital
Lahore, Punjab, Pakistan

Nagendra Boopathy Senguttuvan, MD, DM, FACC, FSCAI
Associate Professor & Senior Consultant Interventional Cardiology
Department of Cardiology
Sri Ramachandra Institute of Higher Education and Research
Chennai, Tamilnadu, India

Karen Sliwa, MD, PhD, FESC, FACC
Professor
Hatter Institute for Cardiovascular Research in Africa
Department of Cardiology & Medicine
Faculty of Health Sciences
University of Cape Town
Cape Town, Western Cape, South Africa

Mary McKillop Institute
Australian Catholic University
Melbourne, VIC, Australia

Priya Soma-Pillay, MBChB (Pret), FCOG (SA), MMed (O&G) Pret, PhD (Pret)
Professor
Obstetrics and Gynaecology
Department of Obstetrics and Gynaecology
University of Pretoria and Steve Biko Academic Hospital
Steve Biko Academic Hospital
Pretoria, Gauteng, South Africa

Andrew C. Steer, MBBS, BMedSci, FRACP, MPH, PhD
Group Leader
Tropical Diseases
Murdoch Children's Research Institute
Melbourne, VIC, Australia

Theme Director, Infection and Immunity
Murdoch Children's Research Institute
Melbourne, VIC, Australia

Professorial Research Fellow, Department of Paediatrics
University of Melbourne, Melbourne, VIC, Australia

Infectious Diseases Physician
Infectious Diseases Unit
Department of General Medicine
The Royal Children's Hospital Melbourne
Parkville, VIC, Australia

Johan Vekemans, MD, PhD
Medical Officer
Initiative for Vaccine Research
World Health Organization
Geneva, Switzerland

David Watkins, MD, MPH
Assistant Professor
Department of Medicine
Department of Global Health
University of Washington
Seattle, WA, United States

Rachel Webb, MbChB, MPH&TM, FRACP
Senior Lecturer in Paediatrics
University of Auckland
Paediatric Infectious Diseases Physician
Starship Children's Hospital
Paediatrician
Department of Paediatrics
Middlemore Hospital
Auckland, New Zealand

Nigel Wilson, MBChB, DipObst, DCH, MRCP, FRACP, FCANZ
Paediatric Cardiologist, Green Lane
    Paediatric and Congenital Cardiology
Department, Starship Hospital
Auckland District Health Board
Auckland, New Zealand

Clinical Associate Professor
Department of Paediatrics
University of Auckland
Auckland, New Zealand

Rosemary Wyber, MBChB, MPH, FRACGP
Doctoral candidate
The George Institute for Global Health
Sydney, NSW, Australia

Head of Strategy, END RHD
Telethon Kids Institute
Perth, WA, Australia

Liesl Zühlke, MBChB, DCH, FCPaeds, Cert Card, MPH, FACC, FESC, MSc, PhD
Specialist Paediatrician and Paediatric Cardiologist
Division of Paediatric Cardiology
Department of Paediatrics
Red Cross War Memorial Children's Hospital
Division of Cardiology
Department of Medicine
Grotte Schuur Hospital
Faculty of Health Sciences
University of Cape Town

Professor Diana (Dinny) Lennon

Dinny was a New Zealander and world-class researcher, inspiring teacher, mentor, and pediatric infectious diseases clinician. She was passionate for child health, especially for the Māori and Pacific children of her country. Her determination and energy to make things better for children was limitless and led to advances in clinical care, national vaccine policy change, and better rheumatic fever control.

Early in her career, Dinny developed an understanding of epidemiology and the social determinants of child health. She systematically researched preventable infectious diseases affecting New Zealand children, developing appropriate solutions accessible to children. She was an original thinker who became a translational researcher, not just describing disease but implementing practical measures to reduce the burden of disease. Her work ensured the introduction of a vaccine against Haemophilus influenzae type b, including setting up and leading clinical trials culminating in the mass MeNZB vaccination program. Dinny advocated tirelessly, both nationally and globally, for rheumatic fever prevention and control. She developed the Auckland Regional Rheumatic Fever Register, and co-led New Zealand's guidelines for the diagnosis and management of rheumatic fever. She recognized and promoted the value of nurses in primary and secondary prevention in the community.

She initiated and led a randomized controlled trial of primary prevention of rheumatic fever with a school-based sore throat program, which has been described as the most innovative rheumatic fever research for over 50 years. This led to the government's rheumatic fever prevention program in 2012.

Dinny set an example in her empowerment of women in medicine in New Zealand. She was one of the first women Professors of Pediatrics and was an inspirational role model. She was brave, tireless, and often forthright to improve child health outcomes.

At her funeral in 2018, Māori elders paid Dinny the ultimate tribute for a New Zealander: "kua hinga te totara i te wao nui a Tane" (A great totara tree has fallen in the forest of Tane).

Innes Asher and Nigel Wilson
August 2019

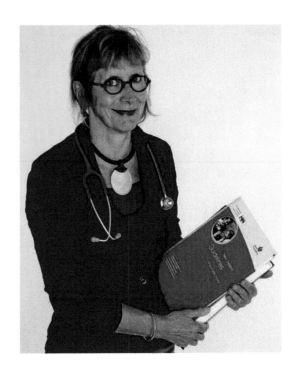

Professor Bongani Mbawethu Mayosi

Professor Bongani Mayosi has been described as the "Madiba" of Medicine in Africa. Born in Nqamakwe in the Amatole district of the Eastern Cape, he was a brilliant academic from his early student days, having completed school at just 16 years of age and going on to capture the highest honors at medical school. This period was followed by a rapid ascendency through cardiology residency and then a Nuffield Scholarship to Oxford where Bongani obtained his DPhil. He was further lauded as the youngest, and first black, Head of Department of Medicine at Groote Schuur Hospital, Cape Town, South Africa. In his term, he was able to transform the department to the largest on the continent while championing an era of enhanced research and outstanding clinical output from a diverse group of basic and clinical scientists.

Recognition of Bongani Mayosi's achievements was embodied in his many awards and positions of leadership. He was endowed with his country's highest honor, the Order of Mapungubwe (Silver), in 2009. He was an A-rated National Research Foundation researcher, a member of the Academy of Science of South Africa, and a former President of the College of Physicians of South Africa. In 2017 he was elected to the US National Academy of Medicine. He was a President of the South African Heart Association and the Pan-African Society of Cardiology (PASCAR), galvanizing colleagues to engage in collaborative activities relevant to the needs of Africa. At the time of his tragic passing, he was Dean of the Faculty of Health Sciences at the University of Cape Town.

More than all these accolades, though, he was a true son of Africa. He rejoiced in the wealth of human capital on the continent and dedicated his research to cardiovascular diseases of the poor, affecting the science relating to rheumatic heart disease (RHD) in every aspect. Other areas of research were on cardiomyopathies, TB pericarditis, and heart failure. He led the largest African studies on Rheumatic Heart Disease Genetics (RHDGen) and the Global Rheumatic Heart Disease Registry (REMEDY), and spearheaded the INVICTUS studies (INVestIgation of rheumatiC AF Treatment Using vitamin K antagonists, rivaroxaban or aspirin Studies) which will arguably be the largest trial ever conducted in RHD. He led work on primary and secondary prevention of RHD, and cost-effectiveness analyses thereof and of course the ASAP program was established by PASCAR under his leadership. His input into RHD policy through the Addis Ababa Communique, the Cairo Accord, The Cape Town declaration, and ultimately the WHO resolution against RF/RHD was monumental. The vision of "Elimination of Rheumatic Heart Disease in our lifetime" permeated through all the scientific endeavors, focusing always on the patient and outcomes of those living with, and affected by, the disease.

On the personal side, Bongani was one of the most engaging, charismatic, and enthusiastic people one could ever encounter, filling a room with his bright smile and warm personality. He saw the world "*not for what it was, but for what he would like it to be*"; he believed resolutely in lifting as one rose, and thus created opportunity for research and scholarship in many parts of Africa and the Middle East. His vision of a 1000 PhDs extended across Africa and he encouraged, mentored, and supported clinical scientists from across the continent in their aspirations and career trajectories. He believed in excellence but also in service, lived in humility and in pursuit of wisdom, and was a renowned teacher, scientist, clinician, and advocate for those living in injustice and poverty. He was known for an astoundingly rigorous work ethic, but always having the time to greet and engage with all members of the hospital, and ensured transparent, fair, and collegial relationships in his professional life, even when under personal attack. His exceptional ability to approach complex issues with clarity, provide strategic leadership, and enthuse others will be hard to find in another.

Bongani was the beloved husband to Nonhlanhla, and father to three accomplished daughters. He loved dancing, and work colleagues at conferences will not forget him often being the first on the dance floor.

He was dearly loved by all who knew him and inspired a generation (if not generations) of scientists across Africa and beyond. His loss resonated deeply and he will be sorely missed.

The passing of, unarguably, the most brilliant black academic in South Africa was marked by deep grief and introspection regarding the toll exacted on those in leadership during periods of tumultuous change. Thus, after his death, the medical, university, and academic community renewed goals for the careful consideration of self-care, well-being, and support for depression and anxiety.

Bongani believed in the need for this book and had agreed to be one of its editors. Sadly, this was not to be. This book is dedicated to his memory, and to that of Diana Lennon, and together we celebrate their incredible legacy in the field of rheumatic fever and rheumatic heart disease.

Uhambe kakuhle, nyana womgquba, Bongani. (Go well, son of the soil)

Liesl Zühlke and Mark Engel
August 2019

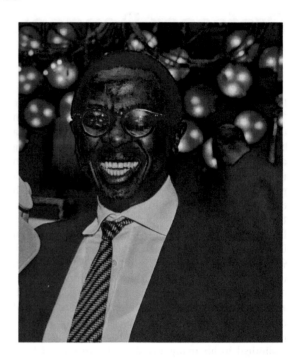

Preface

This book arose when the lead editor arrived to work in the Republic of Palau, an island nation situated in the tropical waters of the western Pacific Ocean, and realised there was no definitive modern text that covered the field of acute rheumatic fever and rheumatic heart disease. Determined to address this need, he procured a publisher and sought worldwide authorship.

Most of the knowledge base pertaining to acute rheumatic fever and rheumatic heart disease originally came from the United States and United Kingdom in the 1930s—1950s. For nearly 50 years, there was little new research as affluent countries with improved living conditions meant few new cases were occurring. In these countries, rheumatic fever was destined to be confined to the history books. However, the disease was just not being addressed, let alone counted, in low- and middle-income countries where it continued to present a major public health crisis. Acute rheumatic fever and rheumatic heart disease affect the most disadvantaged people of the poorest regions and countries throughout the world. Fortunately, in the past 3 decades, new initiatives and research have come from countries where acute rheumatic fever and rheumatic heart disease remain endemic, which in reality is most countries of the world. Despite this, there remain fewer researchers in proportion to disease burden when compared with nearly all other medical conditions.

We are all fortunate that the leading authorities and researchers we contacted to write chapters for this book accepted the challenge. They are all in demand with busy productive lives and we are very grateful and thank them for their considerable efforts and commitment to the task, as we are to their ongoing commitment to control, manage, and prevent ongoing cases across the world. Their outstanding research and clinical expertise is evident in the chapters we present.

We believe that our vision has been achieved: we have put together the planned authoritative modern text in one volume that will be useful for those new to the field, and indeed for those already experienced in the vast array of issues facing clinicians and researchers. This text also encompasses much of the recent research, which has led to a better understanding of the true complexities of acute rheumatic fever and rheumatic heart disease. Excitingly, the lived experience of those affected by this disease is being increasingly heard and encouraged.

Finally, we must give full credit to our lead editor Scott Dougherty. Not only did he have the vision for the book, but he has encouraged and cajoled the authors and at times his fellow editors to complete their tasks. He has kept his poise and sense of humour with the inevitable delays and frustrations with a project of this size. All this whilst undertaking a busy clinical workload in a country and department without the academic resources of high-income countries. How apt that this book should arise from a resource-poor environment coping with the daily challenges of acute rheumatic fever and rheumatic heart disease.

LZ JC NW SD
January 2020

Contents

CHAPTER 1

Epidemiology, Risk Factors, Burden and Cost of Acute Rheumatic Fever and Rheumatic Heart Disease

DAVID WATKINS • MICHAEL G. BAKER • RAMAN KRISHNA KUMAR • TOM PARKS

INTRODUCTION

Acute rheumatic fever (ARF) is an immune-mediated, nonsuppurative consequence of group A β-hemolytic streptococcus (GAS) infection. Although episodes of ARF can result in significant disability, the major impact of ARF at the population level is that it causes long-term, irreversible damage to heart valves—termed rheumatic heart disease (RHD)—often as a result of recurrences. For this reason, we discuss the epidemiology of two conditions together emphasizing they continue to be a major public health problem in many parts of the world, resulting in substantial disability, premature mortality, and economic losses.

This chapter summarizes four basic types of information. We first review the primary literature on the epidemiology of ARF and RHD, and then we summarize what is known about major risk factors for the conditions. We go on to discuss "global" disease burden estimates, that is, efforts to synthesize and aggregate the primary descriptive epidemiology literature to estimate levels and trends in fatal and nonfatal RHD. We conclude by highlighting what is known about the economic consequences of RHD.

EPIDEMIOLOGY OF ACUTE RHEUMATIC FEVER AND RHEUMATIC HEART DISEASE

The epidemiological model of ARF/RHD predominant in the literature suggests a clear stepwise relationship between GAS, ARF, and RHD. Although this relationship remains important, the situation is likely to be more complicated, especially in the settings where RHD is endemic today (Fig. 1.1) For example, in most low- and middle-income countries (LMICs), RHD is reported much more frequently than ARF, with most patients presenting for the first time with complications of RHD in late adolescence or early adulthood.

A variety of approaches (study types) have been used in the literature to measure ARF and RHD incidence, prevalence, and mortality. Each has limitations and advantages, so getting a complete picture of the burden of ARF/RHD in a country will often require triangulating multiple sources of data derived from different types of studies (Table 1.1).

Incidence of Acute Rheumatic Fever

Few contemporary studies have been published on the epidemiology of ARF worldwide. The most up-to-date summaries of ARF incidence data come from two systematic reviews and a recent *Lancet* Seminar.[2-4] Seckeler and Hoke also review studies conducted before 1970.[5] In addition, some regions of the world—such as Africa—remain underrepresented in the literature. Among the published estimates, rates are reported to vary from 5 to 50 per 100,000 person-years. Rates as high as 194 per 100,000 have been reported among Indigenous populations in the Northern Territory of Australia, but it is not clear whether these figures represent truly "higher" rates than the rest of the world, or whether surveillance is simply better, leading to

Acute Rheumatic Fever and Rheumatic Heart Disease. https://doi.org/10.1016/B978-0-323-63982-8.00001-5

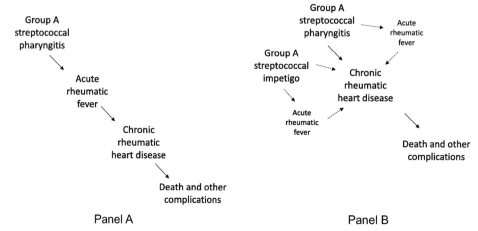

FIG. 1.1 **Epidemiological models describing the relationship between Acute Rheumatic Fever and Rheumatic Heart Disease.** Panel A: classical model. Panel B: contemporary model. (Adapted from Parks T et al.[1])

improved ascertainment.[6] Where it has been measured, the incidence of ARF appears to be declining over time (Fig. 1.2), though again, the regions of the world that are currently very poor and endemic for RHD are underrepresented in this literature.

A major inconsistency in the literature is a lack of a clear relationship between high incidence of ARF and high prevalence of RHD. For instance, one recent study of ARF epidemiology set in primary care clinics in Fiji (where RHD is known to be highly endemic) found only 25 cases per 100,000 population of definite ARF at ages 4–20 years.[7] However, relative to the number of definite ARF cases, substantially more cases of polyarthralgia and monoarthritis were observed, raising the possibility that ARF is underdiagnosed in these settings. There are several possible explanations for the scarcity of ARF in these settings including (i) a distinct clinical phenotype in which progression to RHD tends to be subclinical, (ii) the relative availability of antiinflammatories and antibiotics that may mask florid ARF, (iii) low rates of presentation to healthcare to receive a diagnosis of ARF, which can reflect both lack of awareness among the general public as well as barriers to accessing primary healthcare services, and (iv) low recognition of ARF among healthcare workers—a problem made more challenging by the 2015 Jones criteria, which require the use of echocardiography to make a diagnosis of ARF in most cases.[8]

One other challenge in interpreting the ARF literature is that many studies fail to differentiate between primary (first) attacks of ARF and recurrences, and some studies have only measured primary ARF.[5] Estimates of the

incidence of primary ARF are useful in understanding the proportion of the population affected and in tracking the success of primary prevention programs. Estimates of the incidence of recurrent ARF are useful in tracking the success of secondary prevention programs—that is, high recurrence rates suggest low levels of adherence to antimicrobial prophylaxis. Together, estimates of the incidence of both primary and recurrent ARF paint a picture of the true population exposure to GAS (which is responsible for both types of ARF) and other risk factors.

Prevalence of Rheumatic Heart Disease

A systematic review of RHD prevalence studies conducted in 2016 for the Global Burden of Disease 2015 study found data on RHD prevalence from 59 countries.[9] Most of these datasets were echocardiography-based prevalence studies conducted in LMIC settings; however, this review also included hospital administrative datasets (mostly from high- or upper-middle-income country settings) and auscultation-based prevalence studies. This review complements a 2014 systematic review by Rothenbühler and colleagues that identified 33 datasets from auscultation- or echocardiography-based RHD prevalence studies in LMICs.[10]

School-based echocardiographic surveys of asymptomatic children have become the standard means of assessing the prevalence of RHD. The 2012 World Heart Federation criteria for RHD have helped enforce some standardization in reporting, but questions remain about the epidemiological significance and clinical implications of "latent" RHD (including "borderline" and

TABLE 1.1
Epidemiological Methods for Measuring Acute Rheumatic Fever and Rheumatic Heart Disease.

Study Type	Limitations	Advantages
Clinical registries	Heavily dependent on referral pathways: Healthcare infrastructure in the area and willingness of the potential sources of referral Underreporting: Mild cases, missed diagnosis, marginalized sections of the population may be missed altogether Overreporting: Sampling from outside the study area due to referral to specialist centers Denominator: Dependent on census data, errors may result from under or over estimation of the migrant population	Wide coverage Relatively easy to organize
Community-based surveys	Logistics of selecting a representative population of a region can be challenging Regions with low prevalence require very large sample size	Better suited for high-prevalence regions Clearly defined denominator
School surveys	Focus entirely on the 5–15-year-old group Limited value in areas with poor school enrollment rates Affected children may not attend schools (absenteeism) School surveys may yield a much lower prevalence in regions where affected RHD patients are older	Clearly defined denominator Allows systematic and well-organized survey Better suited for RHD than ARF
Hospital statistics	Outpatient clinic records and inpatient admissions: Only those who are relatively sick will be represented Procedure records: Likely to miss valve lesions that do not require a procedure	Diagnosis is likely to be accurate although usually dependent on clinical coding
ARF/RHD mortality statistics	Underreporting in areas with poor health infrastructure Weak mortality statistics in some regions (e.g., Africa) Misclassification of underlying cause of deaths (e.g., coded as heart failure or stroke instead of RHD)	Premature mortality is a key measure for estimating disease burden

ARF, acute rheumatic fever; *RHD*, rheumatic heart disease

"subclinical" definite RHD).[11] Short-term follow-up studies suggest that the vast majority of subclinical RHD remains stable or regresses.[12] Subclinical RHD is associated with worse long-term outcomes than similar individuals in the population who do not have subclinical RHD, though the risk of complications is nearly 10 times higher among individuals with clinically diagnosed RHD.[13] Overall, longer-term follow-up studies are needed to understand the link between subclinical RHD in children and RHD-related disability and mortality in later life. Additionally, it remains a possibility that the current definitions of subclinical and borderline RHD

are capturing some individuals who do not actually have RHD.

Similar to ARF, RHD is experiencing a decline in many LMICs paralleled by improvements in human development. For example, Negi and colleagues conducted a study using a stratified sample in Northern India using identical survey methods in 1992–93 and 2007–08. They found a fivefold reduction in RHD prevalence in school children between 5 and 15 years together with a sharp decline in recurrent ARF among RHD patients during this period.[14] Sociodevelopmental indices in this region of India improved substantially between 1992 and

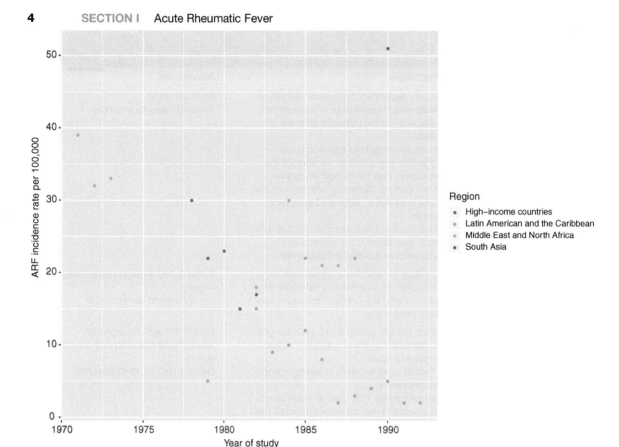

FIG. 1.2 **Estimates of Acute Rheumatic Fever incidence in the published literature.** Data from Tibazarwa KB et al.[2]

2008. Similarly, southern Indian states that have much better sociodevelopmental indices than their northern counterparts have also shown a markedly reduced prevalence of RHD in recent surveys.[15,16] This was also demonstrated in a large study across 10 districts of India conducted by the Indian Council of Medical Research.[17] The same pattern is also apparent in cross-country comparisons of RHD prevalence.[9]

At the same time, "hot spots" of RHD have been documented in middle-income countries, such as Brazil, that have high rates of economic and health inequality across subnational units.[18] These subnational hot spots could be masked by country-level estimates, which reflect the average of low- and high-risk populations. Within relatively small regions, there are consistently demonstrable gradients in RHD prevalence that point toward the influence of poverty and access to healthcare on the disease. Rural populations have consistently higher prevalence in comparison to their urban counterparts. This has been demonstrated in both clinical and echocardiographic surveys.[14,17] Some of the highest RHD prevalence estimates ever reported have come from studies involving the poorest sections of the society.[19] These studies also report aggressive disease patterns such as early onset mitral stenosis that have almost disappeared from low-prevalence regions.

At an ecological level, a strong correlation was found between increasing ARF/RHD rates and decline in access to primary care in central Asia after the breakup of the Soviet Union.[20] Conversely, some LMICs with excellent primary care such as Cuba, Thailand, and Sri Lanka have levels of ARF and RHD that are comparable to high-income countries.[9,21]

Heart Failure due to Rheumatic Heart Disease

The Global Burden of Disease study also estimated the worldwide prevalence of heart failure because of RHD over 1990–2015.[9] For 1990, the estimated prevalence of mild, moderate, and severe heart failure was 160,000, 130,000, and 350,000 cases, respectively. The corresponding prevalence for 2015 was 300,000, 240,000, and 660,000 cases. The increase in the number of prevalent cases of RHD-associated heart failure has primarily been due to population growth and aging, a trend that will probably continue over the coming decades. Heart failure carries a significant risk for death and other adverse health outcomes (discussed in detail in Chapter 16).

Excess Mortality from Rheumatic Heart Disease

Relatively little is known about mortality from RHD in some world regions, particularly in African countries without vital registration systems (i.e., standardized approaches to recording and certifying deaths, including their cause). Even in countries with complete vital registration, accurate measurement of RHD-related mortality can be challenging for a number of reasons. Perhaps the most significant of these is that the WHO International Form of Medical Certificate of Cause of Death specifies that there can only be one "underlying" cause of death.[22] Among individuals with RHD, it is likely that many deaths are being coded to sequelae such as atrial fibrillation, endocarditis, and stroke, or to nonspecific causes of death such as heart failure, rather than RHD. In the settings where RHD is endemic, clinical differentiation between the causes of heart failure or the underlying etiology of stroke is typically challenging, particularly if availability of echocardiography is limited. Consequently, if an individual with RHD dies after an ischemic stroke, there is no clear consensus on whether such a death should be assigned to RHD itself or to stroke (or to atrial fibrillation, for that matter), and it is likely that coding practices vary greatly by region.[9,11] As the global population with RHD ages and becomes increasingly exposed to risk factors for atherosclerotic coronary and cerebrovascular disease, these sorts of confusions will probably become amplified and will require better coding guidelines to track RHD mortality accurately.

Despite the challenges in assigning deaths to RHD, there is a strong consensus that in endemic settings RHD is a significant contributor to risk of mortality. For example, in one study, at least 10% of patients with RHD who were admitted to the hospital (for any reason) die from their disease.[23] However, few studies have examined rates of RHD-attributable mortality in the general population, not least because of the difficulties assigning the underlying cause of death outlined earlier. One alternative approach to this problem is to estimate how often patients with RHD die compared to individuals in the general population who have similar characteristics. (This approach is widely used in cancer epidemiology because, similar to RHD, patients with cancer often die of complications rather than cancer itself.) In Fiji, for example, excess mortality due to RHD was examined by combining multiple sources of routine data using probabilistic record linkage. The authors were able to provide the first population-based estimate of RHD-related mortality in an LMIC setting, 9.9 deaths per 100,000 population.[24] In this study, almost half of RHD-attributable deaths occurred before age 40, and there were 1.6-fold more deaths than reported through the death certification process and twofold higher rates in some age groups than estimated in the Global Burden of Disease 2013 study. Although the generalizability of this study beyond the Pacific region is limited, it is clear that RHD can be a significant contributor to mortality in endemic countries beyond what is reflected in vital registration statistics.

One important subpopulation at excess risk of mortality from RHD are pregnant females. Hemodynamic changes during pregnancy are poorly tolerated in the presence of some lesions such as severe mitral and aortic stenosis and among individuals with pulmonary hypertension (see Chapter 9).[11] In countries where there is low capacity to diagnose RHD during pregnancy and refer for specialist antenatal care and delivery, a significant proportion of pregnant women with severe RHD experience fetal loss, critical illness, or even death.[25] The most striking example is a report from Senegal that estimated a case fatality ratio of 34% for pregnant patients with structural heart disease.[26]

RISK FACTORS FOR ACUTE RHEUMATIC FEVER AND RHEUMATIC HEART DISEASE

There are considerable gaps in knowledge about the etiology, pathogenesis, and risk factors for ARF/RHD that currently limit our ability to develop and implement effective interventions for this disease.[27–30] Drawing on studies identified in prior literature reviews, we discuss the factors that have been associated with an increased or decreased risk of ARF and RHD. A variety of study designs have been used to address this issue, including case-control studies, cross-sectional studies, and cohort studies. Interpretation and generalization of study findings is difficult, because the majority of such studies have been small and frequently of poor quality. Still, broad conclusions are possible, and the wide range of potential risk factors can be organized according to a conceptual model (Fig. 1.3).[31] These factors are discussed in the following sections.

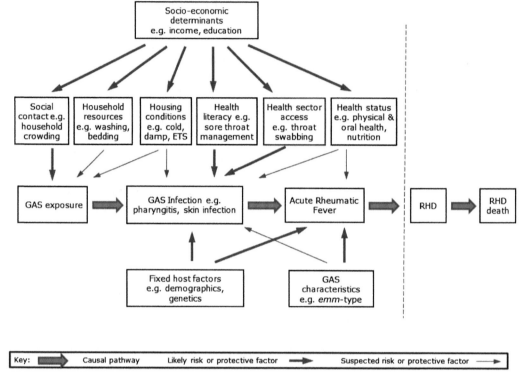

FIG. 1.3 **Major hypothesized risk and protective factors along the causal pathway from group A streptococcal exposure to Acute Rheumatic Fever and Rheumatic Heart Disease.** Information synthesized from the studies reviewed in this chapter. *ETS*, environmental tobacco smoke, *GAS*, group A streptococcus. (Adapted from Baker M et al.[31])

Pathogen and Host Factors that Lead to Acute Rheumatic Fever and Rheumatic Heart Disease

Factors specific to the streptococcal organism

Exposure to GAS is necessary for the development of ARF, and evidence of this exposure is a prerequisite for ARF diagnosis.[8] Unfortunately, only one-third to two-thirds of ARF cases report a sore throat (presumed to be caused by GAS pharyngitis) in the preceding weeks.[32–34] Contemporary studies in settings with high endemic ARF suggest a diverse array of organism-specific genetic factors are likely to play a role in the epidemiology of ARF.[32,35–37] Other infectious agents could potentially act as cofactors to influence the risk of either GAS infection or ARF.[38,39]

It is possible that GAS skin infections (impetigo) can also initiate the autoimmune processes leading to ARF either directly or via pharyngitis.[1,40] In Australian Aboriginal populations, streptococcal skin infections are far more commonly associated with ARF than streptococcal pharyngitis.[40–42] In New Zealand, genetic typing of GAS strains obtained from ARF cases showed a strong association with strains usually identified in pyoderma cases.[43] There is also evidence that scabies skin infections may be important as a site of GAS coinfection, especially in Aboriginal and Pacific Island populations that experience high rates of ARF.[44] Molecular mechanisms that may allow scabies infestations to facilitate GAS infection of skin lesions have been identified.[45]

Host demographics

Host factors include those that are largely fixed (such as demographics, ancestry, and genetics) and those that are influenced by early life exposure to other risk factors. The risk of ARF is strongly influenced by specific demographic factors, particularly age and ethnicity (discussed further later). ARF is rare in children under 4 years old; incidence rises to a peak at around 9–12 years then declines in those over 20 years old.[46] This very specific age group vulnerability to ARF suggests a strong contribution from maturation processes in the immune system.[47] Some studies report a higher risk for females, particularly for RHD in LMICs, which may be at least partially associated with healthcare seeking behaviors resulting from pregnancy.[48–50]

Host genetic factors

Inherited genetic variants are likely to be important in ARF susceptibility but are poorly understood.[51] Familial ARF has been described for more than a century.[28] Further evidence for a genetic component comes from the finding that the pooled proband-wise concordance risk for ARF is 44% in monozygotic twins and 12% in dizygotic twins, with an estimated heritability of 60%.[51] The differences in incidence in relation to ethnicity have often been taken as evidence that host genetic factors influence susceptibility. In New Zealand, for example, the elevated risk for Māori and Pacific children is marked, even after stratifying for deprivation.[52] A Hawaiian study found that risk of ARF was significantly higher for people of Pacific ethnicity compared with other ethnicities, despite similar living conditions.[53] Nonetheless, it is clear high rates of ARF were observed internationally in all ethnicities earlier in the 20th century and before.[54] Thus, while host genetic factors may play a role in determining susceptibility among individuals within a community (typically of the same ethnic group) with the same nongenetic risk factors, they are likely to contribute very little to the differences in incidence in relation to ethnicity.

Several small candidate gene studies have been published, but their results are mostly inconsistent and have been difficult to interpret.[55] A number of genetic polymorphisms have been significantly associated with ARF and RHD overlapping genes including IFN-γ, ACE, FCN, FcgammaRIIA, TLR-2, and HLA.[56–60] Different HLA class II antigen associations with ARF have been observed in several populations, which are perhaps unsurprising given the HLA class II region is strongly associated with a wide spectrum of autoimmune disorders.[55,61]

To overcome the problems of small datasets, international multicountry transethnic genome-wide association study meta-analyses are now underway to identify genetic determinants of RHD susceptibility. The first such study was based on 2852 individuals recruited in eight Oceanian countries. It identified a novel susceptibility signal in the immunoglobulin heavy chain locus.[62] A more recent study in the Australian Aboriginal population identified the HLA-DQ locus as being the strongest genetic marker associated with RHD, with the data supporting a role for cross-reactivity with GAS epitopes in etiology.[63] These findings were significant in that they have provided additional insight into how the disease develops, with potential implications for vaccine development. Nevertheless, genetic susceptibility probably remains a minor determinant of the epidemiology of RHD relative to factors that influence the acquisition of streptococcal disease in the population.

Host oral health status

Some observational studies have found an association between dental caries and ARF.[64] Both RHD and poor oral health are more prevalent in deprived populations, potentially due to common bacterial causes. GAS can live in dental plaque,[65] and dental microbiota have been linked to endocarditis[66] and a multitude of systemic diseases.[67] It has also been suggested that certain oral bacteria produce an enzyme that can weaken tissue resistance to bacterial penetration,[68–70] which could influence the risk of ARF by creating conditions that enhance bacterial spread.

One compelling hypothesis is that exposure to sugar drives the association between poor oral health and ARF.[71] A cohort study of 20,333 children in Auckland found that those with five or more primary teeth affected by caries were 57% more likely to develop ARF or RHD compared with those who were caries-free.[72] There is biological plausibility for high sugar intake being a risk factor for ARF: GAS can ferment sucrose (table sugar) and fructose (which along with glucose forms the disaccharide sucrose).[73,74] High sucrose intake may well enhance conditions that promote the growth of GAS in the oral cavity, increasing the likelihood of developing GAS pharyngitis and thus ARF.[71] A study in Bangladesh found that not brushing teeth after a meal increased the chances of developing ARF by 2.5-fold.[50] Of course, dental caries is a multifactorial condition that does not correlate perfectly with sugar intake; in many cases other socioeconomic factors may influence caries development and contribute to ARF risk through unrelated mechanisms.

Host nutritional status

Macronutrient intake and body-mass index have been proposed as factors that influence development of ARF. Low body-mass index and low birth weight were found to be significant risk factors for RHD in Congo,[75] and low body-mass index was associated with RHD in India.[76] In Bangladesh, low consumption of certain foodstuffs (eggs, milk, chicken, pulses, fruits, and bread) was associated with ARF risk, and increased consumption of soybean oil appeared to be protective.[77,78] This study also documented an increased risk of ARF in children with an upper arm circumference that was <80% of normal for their age, that is, children at past or present risk of protein-energy malnutrition. The authors postulated that malnutrition could inhibit the immune response to GAS and predisposing ARF.[78] These findings are not universal; however, a study in Fiji did not identify low weight, height, or body-mass index for age as significant risk factors for RHD.[79]

Low intake of certain micronutrients may also play a role in development of ARF. The importance of vitamin D to human immune system function is increasingly being recognized.[80] Although there have been no reported associations of low vitamin D intake with ARF, one study noted an association between low serum vitamin D levels and recurrent GAS tonsillopharyngitis.[81] Similarly, iron deficiency may predispose to repeated GAS infections. A protective association between increased serum iron and ARF was documented in a case-control study in Bangladesh.[77]

Social and Environmental Conditions

Socioeconomic status is a key determinant that influences multiple potential risk factors for ARF and RHD. ARF has been associated with low maternal education in Yugoslavia[82] and with low income in Bangladesh[83] and Australia.[84] RHD has been associated with low household income in Yemen[85] and Uganda.[86] On an ecological level, ARF is clearly associated with socioeconomic deprivation across Africa, the Americas, Asia, Europe, and the Pacific.[20,87–92] However, socioeconomic status in itself is a "distal" risk factor that influences a variety of "proximal" risk behaviors and patterns of environmental exposure (Fig. 1.3). This section reviews the specific proximal risk factors that have been implicated in the acquisition of GAS infection and in the development of ARF and RHD.

GAS is highly infectious and spread via salivary and nasal droplet transmission[93]; almost half of the siblings of cases with GAS pharyngitis become infected.[94] Hence, environmental factors that influence survival and transmission of GAS organisms are important, as are health-seeking behaviors that serve to interrupt transmission.

Household crowding, including bed sharing

Humans are the established reservoir for GAS. Being near others is a known risk factor for transmission, with outbreaks well documented in schools, daycare centers, military barracks, and crowded homes.[95] Transmission occurs rapidly in cramped living conditions. This situation has been implicated as a key factor mediating ARF outbreaks in US military camps.[96–98]

Household overcrowding is a highly plausible risk factor for ARF, as it increases the effective reproduction number for GAS infections in the home. Household crowding can manifest in a range of ways, including high household occupancy, bedroom deficits, and bed sharing. One study found a significant positive association between crowding (children per bedroom) and GAS carriage.[99] Among remote Australian communities at risk of ARF, one cohort study found a correlation between the number of cases of pyoderma per household and number of people per bedroom.[41] Another found a correlation between acquisition of pathogenic GAS strains and household size.[100]

Historically, there is evidence from the United States and New Zealand that ARF is associated with poor housing and crowding at a neighborhood level.[101,102] Among a substantial literature of small studies, four higher-quality studies in LMICs have reported associations between RHD and measures of household crowding. A cross-sectional study in Congo and a case-control study in Uganda identified significant associations between larger household size and RHD.[75,86] Similarly, a cross-sectional study in South Africa identified having more than three siblings as a risk factor for RHD.[103] Conversely, a cohort study in New Caledonia did not identify number of siblings as a risk factor for RHD, but did identify an association with more than two people sharing a bedroom.[104] Similarly, a Yugoslavian case-control study found an association with bed sharing (≥2 people per bed).[82,105,106] Two cohort studies have reported on these associations in high-income countries: a UK study found no significant association between measured household crowding as a child and death from RHD in later life,[107] while a Finnish study found that growing up in large households was associated with an increased risk of occurrence and death from RHD.[108] It should be noted that many of these studies found significant associations only on univariate analyses, suggesting that housing conditions are linked with other, more proximal, exposures and behaviors.

Household resources, including washing and laundry

GAS has been reported to survive on inanimate objects for more than 6 months.[109] Handwashing may be protective,[110,111] as is regular bathing, such as swimming in chlorinated pools.[112] Removing dust, handwashing, and disinfecting surfaces are used as control measures in hospitals affected by GAS outbreaks.[110,113,114] Lack of washing facilities and resources may contribute to an increase in bacterial load on the skin of household members or on inanimate objects, resulting in increased transmission of bacteria and associated skin and pharyngeal infections. However, it has not been definitively proven that lack of washing is a significant independent risk factor for ARF.

Housing conditions, including tenure, damp, and cold

Many housing factors, including crowding, household facilities, and the indoor air environment are influenced by housing tenure. Poor housing conditions (e.g., cold, damp, mold) could potentially contribute to an indoor environment that increases the risk of GAS transmission. GAS incidence was significantly higher in social housing compared with private housing in Singapore[115] and in households that lacked a kitchen in India.[116] In an outbreak in a UK boarding school, the attack rate was significantly higher in poorly ventilated dormitories compared with those that were well ventilated.[117] In Yugoslavia, home dampness and a change in place of residence in the last 5 years were significantly associated with ARF.[82] Substandard housing was associated with ARF in Bangladesh.[83]

Healthcare utilization and health literacy

Effective antibiotic treatment of GAS infections interrupts the development of ARF and RHD. (The epidemiological evidence for the effectiveness of primary and secondary prevention strategies is reviewed elsewhere.[11]) Widespread availability of comprehensive primary and secondary prevention measures in Baltimore,[118] Cuba,[21] and Costa Rica[119] coincided with significant reductions in ARF incidence rates documented in ecological evaluations. Other studies were successful in reducing ARF in part because they expanded access to secondary prevention measures using an active (community-based) case-finding approach.[120] Conversely, ARF remains relatively common in many populations where access to healthcare is a known public health problem.[28,121]

A key component of the success of large-scale ARF/RHD programs has been the education of the public and healthcare providers, resulting in increased use of evidence-based primary and secondary prevention measures. Low levels of maternal education were a significant risk factor for ARF in Yugoslavia,[82] and ARF and RHD were associated with maternal illiteracy in Bangladesh.[50] Enhancing awareness of ARF and its prevention was a major aspect of the Cuban intervention

program that occurred from 1986 to 96—during which period the ARF incidence declined 7.4-fold.[21] Martinique and Guadeloupe also received a 10-year ARF control and prevention intervention that included educating healthcare professionals on ARF, and emphasizing to the public the importance of primary prevention among schoolchildren.[122] Increasing awareness of the need for primary prevention in children with symptoms of pharyngitis is a major focus of the New Zealand Rheumatic Fever Prevention Programme, though the effectiveness of this program remains uncertain.[123,124]

Summary of Risk and Protective Factors for Acute Rheumatic Fever and Rheumatic Heart Disease

The literature review earlier illustrates the breadth, complexity, and gaps in current knowledge of risk factors for ARF and RHD. We can broadly conclude, however, that the major risk factors influencing ARF and RHD are well established: children have a period of vulnerability to ARF starting from about age four until about age 20. If they are exposed to GAS infection, in the throat and probably the skin also, then they have a small risk of developing the autoimmune disease ARF about 3 weeks later. Individual risk is partly influenced by genetic factors, but the most consistent distal risk factor is poverty and social deprivation, which creates the conditions for exposure to more proximal risk factors including (i) poor-quality housing and household crowding; (ii) poor nutritional status, and (iii) low utilization of and access to healthcare. The published evidence to date is based on relatively poor-quality studies, however, and it has been difficult to identify the most important mediators of ARF/RHD risk that might provide effective points of intervention.

MEASURES OF GLOBAL DISEASE BURDEN

Two groups routinely release estimates of the burden of RHD: the Institute for Health Metrics and Evaluation (IHME), which publishes the Global Burden of Disease studies,[125] and the Metrics, Measurement, & Evaluation department at the World Health Organization (WHO), which publishes the Global Health Estimates reports.[126] RHD is included among the causes of death and disability that are routinely tracked by IHME and WHO in their health estimates. Although ARF is not included in these health estimates, its contributions to health loss globally are largely reflected in the estimates of RHD mortality, as nearly all individuals who die of ARF die from rheumatic carditis. The data inputs and methods used by IHME and WHO are somewhat different, but they lead to broadly similar conclusions about the relative magnitude of the burden of RHD globally.

In 2000, there were an estimated 320,000–380,000 deaths and 12–13 million disability-adjusted life-years (DALYs) from RHD (Table 1.2). (DALYs are a summary measure of health that incorporates premature mortality and disability into a single number that can be compared across diseases and age groups. Over 80% of DALYs from RHD are due to premature mortality, with the remainder being due to nonfatal disease that causes disability.) By 2016, the number of deaths had declined to 290,000–310,000 and the number of DALYs to 9.8–10 million, indicating progress on reducing RHD at a global level.

The distribution of disease burden by income group varies remarkably. Most deaths and DALYs from RHD are in middle-income countries, particularly the two most populous countries (India and China) that together account for over half of RHD deaths globally. On the other hand, in relative terms, the number of deaths and DALYs from RHD has declined most noticeably in high-income countries and upper-middle-income countries (including China) but not in lower-middle-income countries (including India). There has been very little change in RHD burden in low-income countries as a group, though there are notable counterexamples such as Rwanda and Ethiopia. (These conclusions are based on overall numbers of deaths and DALYs across all age groups; trends in age-specific rates are discussed in the following paragraphs.)

Sustainable Development Goal 3 (SDG3) set targets for reducing premature mortality (defined as death before age 70) between 2015 and 2030. For noncommunicable diseases, the target was set as a one-third reduction in mortality over this period, or an approximately 2.6% average annual rate of decline. By this measure, progress on RHD has been relatively favorable, especially compared to other noncommunicable diseases. The annual rate of decline in premature mortality rates was 2.3%–2.9% globally (Table 1.3).

Estimates of progress on RHD across low- and middle-income countries vary somewhat between IHME and WHO; the best-performing group was upper-middle-income countries (4.4% average rate of decline annually) according to IHME and low-income countries (3.6%) according to WHO, while the worst-performing group was lower-middle-income countries in both sets of estimates (2.2%–2.5%). Both sets of estimates concur that as of 2016 the highest premature death rates were in lower-middle-income countries and were 5–10-fold higher compared to rates in high-income countries.

IHME, but not WHO, also produces estimates of RHD prevalence. The number of individuals living with RHD was estimated at 18 million in 1990, 23 million in 2000, and 30 million in 2016.[127] This increase was due mostly to demographic factors (population growth and aging) rather than to real increases in age-specific prevalence. (Using IHME's standard population, there was no detectable change in age-standardized prevalence between 1990 and 2016.)

Patterns of RHD prevalence by age and sex are shown in Fig. 1.4. Consistent with nearly all primary datasets, the prevalence of RHD is significantly higher among females than among males, with about 17 million versus 13 million cases in total, or 460 cases versus 340 cases per 100,000 population (respectively) in 2016. The increase in cases between 2000 and 2016 can also be seen in Fig. 1.4; for both sexes, the increase was concentrated in the 15–49 age group. Notably, while RHD among children tends to garner much of the attention of researchers and health advocates, nearly 80% of RHD cases in 2016 were estimated to occur among individuals over the age of 15.

Watkins and colleagues summarized the major limitations of IHME's estimates of RHD; these limitations are, broadly speaking, applicable to the WHO estimates as well.[9] As mentioned earlier, health loss from ARF is not directly reflected in these figures, but it probably adds little to overall health loss from GAS diseases and is small in relation to RHD itself. Regarding nonfatal health loss from RHD, current estimates of years lived with disability only include heart failure and do not incorporate other sequelae such as stroke and infective endocarditis. (In addition, these sequelae probably have second-order effects on overall disease burden estimates; their rates were substantially lower than heart failure rates in contemporary cohort studies.[128])

Watkins and colleagues recommended that the descriptive epidemiological research agenda for RHD focus on three priority topics. First, prevalence studies need to sample more broadly than merely among children attending schools. RHD is more common among children living in community settings than among schoolchildren, and it is also more common among adults than among children; however, data in these groups are at present quite sparse. Second, as mentioned previously in this chapter, the issue of misclassification of RHD-related deaths is of continued concern. Prospective linked data studies would prove useful in ascertaining the reliability of vital registration data in estimating RHD-related mortality. Third, better data are needed on long-term outcomes of individuals living with RHD. A quantitative understanding of

TABLE 1.2

Deaths and Disability-Adjusted Life-Years From Rheumatic Heart Disease by World Bank Income Group, All Ages, Both Sexes, 2000 and 2016.

| | GLOBAL BURDEN OF DISEASE | | | | GLOBAL HEALTH ESTIMATES | | | |
| | 2000 | | 2016 | | 2000 | | 2016 | |
	Deaths	DALYs	Deaths	DALYs	Deaths	DALYs	Deaths	DALYs
Global	380,000	13,000,000	310,000	9,800,000	320,000	12,000,000	290,000	10,000,000
High-income countries	39,000	630,000	41,000	540,000	22,000	460,000	22,000	360,000
Upper-middle-income countries	150,000	4,000,000	93,000	2,200,000	120,000	3,600,000	100,000	2,700,000
Lower-middle-income countries	170,000	7,100,000	160,000	6,100,000	160,000	7,200,000	150,000	6,400,000
Low-income countries	18,000	840,000	18,000	900,000	18,000	1,000,000	17,000	1,000,000

DALYs, disability-adjusted life-years.
Data are from GBD Causes of Death Collaborators.[125]

TABLE 1.3
Progress on Rheumatic Heart Disease Mortality Among Individuals Aged 0–69 Years by World Bank Income Group, All Ages, Both Sexes, 2000–16.

	GLOBAL BURDEN OF DISEASE					GLOBAL HEALTH ESTIMATES				
	2000		2016		AARC	2000		2016		AARC
	Deaths	Mortality rate[a]	Deaths	Mortality rate[a]		Deaths	Mortality rate[a]	Deaths	Mortality rate[a]	
Global	240,000	4.1	180,000	2.5	−2.9%	200,000	3.4	170,000	2.4	−2.3%
High-income countries	10,000	1.1	7900	0.77	−2.1%	6800	0.71	3900	0.38	−3.8%
Upper-middle-income countries	83,000	3.8	44,000	1.8	−4.4%	64,000	2.9	46,000	1.9	−2.7%
Lower-middle-income countries	130,000	5.8	110,000	3.9	−2.5%	120,000	5.1	110,000	3.6	−2.2%
Low-income countries	13,000	3.3	12,000	1.9	−3.2%	14,000	3.3	12,000	1.8	−3.6%

AARC, average annual rate of change.
Figures are authors' calculations based on data from GBD Causes of Death Collaborators.[125]
[a] Expressed per 100,000 population per year.

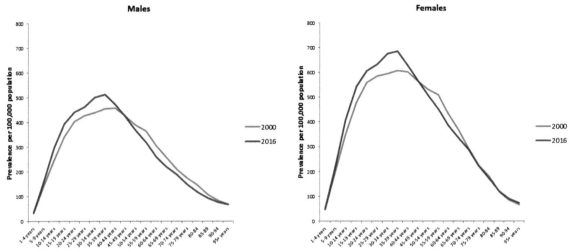

FIG. 1.4 **Global prevalence of Rheumatic Heart Disease (number of cases) by age and sex, 2000–16.** (Data from IHME.[129])

progression rates from subclinical to clinical disease and from asymptomatic to symptomatic disease is lacking and could be measured by means of cohort studies based in community settings.[11]

The question of RHD hot spots in large middle-income countries will continue to be addressed by future iterations of the Global Burden of Disease study as subnational estimates are developed for an increasing number of countries. For example, subnational estimates were released for Brazil starting with the GBD 2016 study. The all-ages prevalence of RHD at the national level is currently estimated at about 800 per 100,000, ranging from 710 per 100,000 in the state of Maranhão to 840 per 100,000 in the state of Santa Catarina.[129] Continued research on variations in RHD prevalence across subnational units will strengthen the empirical foundation for subnational estimation in future GBD studies; however, care should be taken to obtain representative samples rather than sample only high-risk groups (such as Indigenous populations), which produce biased estimates of population statistics. Scheel and colleagues recently demonstrated the utility of a rigorous sampling approach in a study conducted in northern Uganda.[130]

ECONOMIC CONSEQUENCES OF ACUTE RHEUMATIC FEVER AND RHEUMATIC HEART DISEASE

Evidence is limited on the economic impact of ARF and RHD in countries where RHD is endemic. A Brazilian study in the early 2000s found that the cost of care was about US$ 1500 (in 2012 US dollars) per patient per year in direct medical costs from the provider perspective.[131] This study also documented high rates of absenteeism from school and work, that is, "indirect costs." In South Korea, where RHD prevalence and mortality are much lower, the cost of RHD was estimated at US$ 1.4 million per million population, with about 40% of costs being indirect.[132] A recent study from Australia found that healthcare costs for GAS-related diseases were US$ 190 million over 2005–15, although ARF and RHD accounted for a very small fraction of costs and were concentrated among Indigenous persons.[133]

Preliminary work on the cost of RHD in Uganda and India estimated that costs nationally were around US$ 12 million and US$ 8.0 million per one million population, respectively, with about 80% of total costs being indirect.[134] The economic impact of ARF and RHD in Fiji was estimated at US$ 48 million over 5 years, or US$ 3643 per patient per year, with the overwhelming majority of costs related to premature mortality.[135]

Finally, a working paper for *Disease Control Priorities, Third Edition* sought to estimate the global economic impact of RHD using an economic measure of the so-called "intrinsic" value of health (instead of simply looking at the consequences of RHD on human capital). This analysis drew on data from the Global Burden of Disease 2015 study and looked at the economic benefits of reducing age-specific death rates from RHD globally to rates seen in high-income countries. Using this approach, the authors estimated that the value of avertable mortality from RHD worldwide in 2015 was about US$ 65 billion.[136] The largest share of this figure was found in the East Asia and Pacific region, which is home to most of the deaths from RHD worldwide (including China, which has lower death rates but a very large population size, and a number of Pacific Island nations that have very high death rates).

More data are needed on the economic burden of ARF and RHD to inform policy and resource allocation decisions in limited-resource settings. The data earlier, although scarce, support the notion that chronic RHD is associated with very high healthcare costs among those who are affected (especially for those who have undergone surgery), lost time off work and school, and forgone life opportunities due to premature death. Additionally, it is possible that persons living with RHD poses a high burden to their households in caregiver time and use of "coping mechanisms" (e.g., borrowing money or selling assets) to pay for healthcare—although studies need to be undertaken to better characterize the extent of these household- and community-level effects.[137]

REFERENCES

1. Parks T, Smeesters PR, Steer AC. Streptococcal skin infection and rheumatic heart disease. *Curr Opin Infect Dis.* 2012;25(2):145–153.
2. Tibazarwa KB, Volmink JA, Mayosi BM. Incidence of acute rheumatic fever in the world: a systematic review of population-based studies. *Heart.* 2008;94(12):1534–1540.
3. Jackson SJ, Steer AC, Campbell H. Systematic review: estimation of global burden of non-suppurative sequelae of upper respiratory tract infection: rheumatic fever and post-streptococcal glomerulonephritis. *Trop Med Int Health.* 2011;16(1):2–11.
4. Karthikeyan G, Guilherme L. Acute rheumatic fever. *Lancet.* 2018;392(10142):161–174.
5. Seckeler MD, Hoke TR. The worldwide epidemiology of acute rheumatic fever and rheumatic heart disease. *Clin Epidemiol.* 2011;3:67–84.
6. Lawrence JG, Carapetis JR, Griffiths K, Edwards K, Condon JR. Acute rheumatic fever and rheumatic heart disease: incidence and progression in the Northern Territory of Australia, 1997 to 2010. *Circulation.* 2013;128(5):492–501.
7. Parks T, Kado J, Colquhoun S, Carapetis J, Steer A. Underdiagnosis of acute rheumatic fever in primary care settings in a developing country. *Trop Med Int Health.* 2009;14(11):1407–1413.
8. Gewitz MH, Baltimore RS, Tani LY, et al. Revision of the Jones Criteria for the diagnosis of acute rheumatic fever in the era of Doppler echocardiography: a scientific statement from the American Heart Association. *Circulation.* 2015;131(20):1806–1818.
9. Watkins DA, Johnson CO, Colquhoun SM, et al. Global, regional, and national burden of rheumatic heart disease, 1990–2015. *N Engl J Med.* 2017;377(8):713–722.
10. Rothenbuhler M, O'Sullivan CJ, Stortecky S, et al. Active surveillance for rheumatic heart disease in endemic regions: a systematic review and meta-analysis of prevalence among children and adolescents. *Lancet Glob Health.* 2014;2(12):e717–e726.
11. Watkins DA, Beaton AZ, Carapetis JR, et al. Rheumatic heart disease worldwide: JACC scientific expert panel. *J Am Coll Cardiol.* 2018;72(12):1397–1416.
12. Beaton A, Aliku T, Dwyer A, et al. Latent rheumatic heart disease: identifying the children at highest risk of unfavorable outcome. *Circulation.* 2017;136(23):2233–2244.
13. Engelman D, Mataika RL, Ah Kee M, et al. Clinical outcomes for young people with screening-detected and clinically-diagnosed rheumatic heart disease in Fiji. *Int J Cardiol.* 2017;240:422–427.
14. Negi PC, Kanwar A, Chauhan R, Asotra S, Thakur JS, Bhardwaj AK. Epidemiological trends of RF/RHD in school children of Shimla in north India. *Indian J Med Res.* 2013;137(6):1121–1127.
15. Nair B, Viswanathan S, Koshy AG, Gupta PN, Nair N, Thakkar A. Rheumatic heart disease in Kerala: a vanishing entity? An echo Doppler study in 5-15-years-old school children. *Internet J Rheumatol.* 2015;2015:930790.
16. Kumar RK, Tandon R. Rheumatic fever & rheumatic heart disease: the last 50 years. *Indian J Med Res.* 2013;137(4):643–658.
17. Kumar R, Sharma M. *Jai Vigyan Mission Mode Project: Community Control of Rheumatic Fever/Rheumatic Heart Disease in India.* Comprehensive project report 2000-2010. New Delhi: Indian Council of Medical Research; 2015.
18. Nascimento BR, Sable C, Nunes MCP, et al. Comparison between different strategies of rheumatic heart disease echocardiographic screening in Brazil: data from the PROVAR (rheumatic valve disease screening program) study. *J Am Heart Ass.* 2018;7(4).
19. Sadiq M, Islam K, Abid R, et al. Prevalence of rheumatic heart disease in school children of urban Lahore. *Heart.* 2009;95(5):353–357.
20. Omurzakova NA, Yamano Y, Saatova GM, et al. High incidence of rheumatic fever and rheumatic heart disease in the republics of Central Asia. *Int J Rheum Dis.* 2009;12(2):79–83.
21. Nordet P, Lopez R, Duenas A, Sarmiento L. Prevention and control of rheumatic fever and rheumatic heart disease: the Cuban experience (1986-1996-2002). *Cardiovasc J Afr.* 2008;19(3):135–140.
22. WHO. *Medical Certification of Cause of Death: Instructions for Physicians on Use of International Form of Medical Certificate of Cause of Death.* 4th ed.; 1979. Geneva http://apps.who.int/iris/handle/10665/40557.
23. Steer AC, Kado J, Jenney AW, et al. Acute rheumatic fever and rheumatic heart disease in Fiji: prospective surveillance, 2005–2007. *Med J Aust.* 2009;190(3):133–135.
24. Parks T, Kado J, Miller AE, et al. Rheumatic heart disease-attributable mortality at ages 5-69 years in Fiji: a five-year, national, population-based record-linkage cohort study. *PLoS Neglected Trop Dis.* 2015;9(9):e0004033.

25. Watkins DA, Sebitloane M, Engel ME, Mayosi BM. The burden of antenatal heart disease in South Africa: a systematic review. *BMC Cardiovasc Disord.* 2012;12:23.
26. Diao M, Kane A, Ndiaye MB, et al. Pregnancy in women with heart disease in sub-Saharan Africa. *Arch Cardiovasc Dis.* 2011;104(6−7):370−374.
27. Carapetis JR, Beaton A, Cunningham MW, et al. Acute rheumatic fever and rheumatic heart disease. *Nat Rev Dis Primers.* 2016;2:15084.
28. Kerdemelidis M, Lennon DR, Arroll B, Peat B, Jarman J. The primary prevention of rheumatic fever. *J Paediatr Child Health.* 2010;46(9):534−548.
29. Bryant PA, Robins-Browne R, Carapetis JR, et al. Some of the people, some of the time: susceptibility to acute rheumatic fever. *Circulation.* 2009;119(5):742−753.
30. Azevedo PM, Pereira RR, Guilherme L. Understanding rheumatic fever. *Rheumatol Int.* 2012;32(5): 1113−1120.
31. Baker MG, Gurney J, Oliver J, et al. Risk Factors for Acute Rheumatic Fever: Literature Review and Protocol for a Case-Control Study in New Zealand. *Int J Environ Res Public Health.* 2019;16(22):4515.
32. Lennon D, Stewart J, Farrell E, Palmer A, Mason H. School-based prevention of acute rheumatic fever: a group randomized trial in New Zealand. *Pediatr Infect Dis J.* 2009;28(9):787−794.
33. Dajani AS. Current status of nonsuppurative complications of group A streptococci. *Pediatr Infect Dis J.* 1991; 10(10 Suppl):S25−S27.
34. Veasy LG, Wiedmeier SE, Orsmond GS, et al. Resurgence of acute rheumatic fever in the intermountain area of the United States. *N Engl J Med.* 1987;316(8): 421−427.
35. Carapetis JR, McDonald M, Wilson NJ. Acute rheumatic fever. *Lancet.* 2005;366(9480):155−168.
36. Erdem G, Mizumoto C, Esaki D, et al. Group A streptococcal isolates temporally associated with acute rheumatic fever in Hawaii: differences from the continental United States. *Clin Infect Dis.* 2007;45(3):e20−e24.
37. Pruksakorn S, Sittisombut N, Phornphutkul C, Pruksachatkunakorn C, Good MF, Brandt E. Epidemiological analysis of non-M-typeable group A Streptococcus isolates from a Thai population in Northern Thailand. *J Clin Microbiol.* 2000;38(3):1250−1254.
38. Pichichero ME, Casey JR. Systematic review of factors contributing to penicillin treatment failure in *Streptococcus pyogenes* pharyngitis. *Otolaryngol Head Neck Surg.* 2007;137(6):851−857.
39. Olgunturk R, Okur I, Cirak MY, et al. The role of viral agents in aetiopathogenesis of acute rheumatic fever. *Clin Rheumatol.* 2011;30(1):15−20.
40. McDonald M, Currie BJ, Carapetis JR. Acute rheumatic fever: a chink in the chain that links the heart to the throat? *Lancet Infect Dis.* 2004;4(4):240−245.
41. McDonald MI, Towers RJ, Andrews RM, Benger N, Currie BJ, Carapetis JR. Low rates of streptococcal pharyngitis and high rates of pyoderma in Australian aboriginal communities where acute rheumatic fever is hyperendemic. *Clin Infect Dis.* 2006;43(6):683−689.
42. Bowen AC, Mahe A, Hay RJ, et al. The global epidemiology of impetigo: a systematic review of the population prevalence of impetigo and pyoderma. *PLoS One.* 2015; 10(8):e0136789.
43. Williamson DA, Smeesters PR, Steer AC, et al. M-protein analysis of *Streptococcus pyogenes* isolates associated with acute rheumatic fever in New Zealand. *J Clin Microbiol.* 2015;53(11):3618−3620.
44. Romani L, Steer AC, Whitfeld MJ, Kaldor JM. Prevalence of scabies and impetigo worldwide: a systematic review. *Lancet Infect Dis.* 2015;15(8):960−967.
45. Fischer K, Holt D, Currie B, Kemp D. Scabies: important clinical consequences explained by new molecular studies. *Adv Parasitol.* 2012;79:339−373.
46. Stollerman GH. *Rheumatic Fever and Streptococcal Infection.* Grune & Stratton; 1975.
47. Coburn A. Observations on the mechanism of rheumatic fever. *Lancet.* 1936;228(5905):1025−1030.
48. Oli K, Porteous J. Prevalence of rheumatic heart disease among school children in Addis Ababa. *East Afr Med J.* 1999;76(11):601−605.
49. Rizvi SF, Khan MA, Kundi A, Marsh DR, Samad A, Pasha O. Status of rheumatic heart disease in rural Pakistan. *Heart.* 2004;90(4):394−399.
50. Riaz BK, Selim S, Karim MN, Chowdhury KN, Chowdhury SH, Rahman MR. Risk factors of rheumatic heart disease in Bangladesh: a case-control study. *J Health Popul Nutr.* 2013;31(1):70−77.
51. Engel ME, Stander R, Vogel J, Adeyemo AA, Mayosi BM. Genetic susceptibility to acute rheumatic fever: a systematic review and meta-analysis of twin studies. *PLoS One.* 2011;6(9):e25326.
52. Gurney JK, Stanley J, Baker MG, Wilson NJ, Sarfati D. Estimating the risk of acute rheumatic fever in New Zealand by age, ethnicity and deprivation. *Epidemiol Infect.* 2016; 144(14):3058−3067.
53. Kurahara DK, Grandinetti A, Galario J, et al. Ethnic differences for developing rheumatic fever in a low-income group living in Hawaii. *Ethn Dis.* 2006;16(2):357−361.
54. Steer AC. Historical aspects of rheumatic fever. *J Paediatr Child Health.* 2015;51(1):21−27.
55. Martin WJ, Steer AC, Smeesters PR, et al. Post-infectious group A streptococcal autoimmune syndromes and the heart. *Autoimmun Rev.* 2015;14(8):710−725.
56. Berdeli A, Celik HA, Ozyurek R, Aydin HH. Involvement of immunoglobulin FcgammaRIIA and FcgammaRIIIB gene polymorphisms in susceptibility to rheumatic fever. *Clin Biochem.* 2004;37(10):925−929.
57. Chou HT, Tsai CH, Tsai FJ. Association between angiotensin I-converting enzyme gene insertion/deletion polymorphism and risk of rheumatic heart disease. *Jpn Heart J.* 2004;45(6):949−957.
58. Berdeli A, Celik HA, Ozyurek R, Dogrusoz B, Aydin HH. TLR-2 gene Arg753Gln polymorphism is strongly associated with acute rheumatic fever in children. *J Mol Med (Berl).* 2005;83(7):535−541.

59. Messias-Reason IJ, Schafranski MD, Kremsner PG, Kun JF. Ficolin 2 (FCN2) functional polymorphisms and the risk of rheumatic fever and rheumatic heart disease. *Clin Exp Immunol.* 2009;157(3):395−399.

60. Col-Araz N, Pehlivan S, Baspinar O, Oguzkan-Balci S, Sever T, Balat A. Role of cytokine gene (IFN-gamma, TNF-alpha, TGF-beta1, IL-6, and IL-10) polymorphisms in pathogenesis of acute rheumatic fever in Turkish children. *Eur J Pediatr.* 2012;171(7):1103−1108.

61. Nepom GT, Erlich H. MHC class-II molecules and autoimmunity. *Annu Rev Immunol.* 1991;9:493−525.

62. Parks T, Mirabel MM, Kado J, et al. Association between a common immunoglobulin heavy chain allele and rheumatic heart disease risk in Oceania. *Nat Commun.* 2017;8:14946.

63. Gray LA, D'Antoine HA, Tong SYC, et al. Genome-wide analysis of genetic risk factors for rheumatic heart disease in Aboriginal Australians provides support for pathogenic molecular mimicry. *J Infect Dis.* 2017;216(11):1460−1470. https://doi.org/10.1093/infdis/jix497.

64. Entine M. A survey of dental diseases as a diagnostic aid in rheumatic fever. *JADA.* 1949;38(3):303−308.

65. Burton JP, Drummond BK, Chilcott CN, et al. Influence of the probiotic Streptococcus salivarius strain M18 on indices of dental health in children: a randomized double-blind, placebo-controlled trial. *J Med Microbiol.* 2013;62(6):875−884.

66. Strom BL, Abrutyn E, Berlin JA, et al. Risk factors for infective endocarditis: oral hygiene and nondental exposures. *Circulation.* 2000;102(23):2842−2848.

67. He J, Li Y, Cao Y, Xue J, Zhou X. The oral microbiome diversity and its relation to human diseases. *Folia Microbiologica.* 2015;60(1):69−80.

68. Tam YC, Harvey RF, Chan EC. Chondroitin sulfatase–producing and hyaluronidase–producing oral bacteria associated with periodontal disease. *J Can Dent Assoc.* 1982;48(2):115−120.

69. Homer KA, Denbow L, Whiley RA, Beighton D. Chondroitin sulfate depolymerase and hyaluronidase activities of viridans streptococci determined by a sensitive spectrophotometric assay. *J Clin Microbiol.* 1993;31(6):1648−1651.

70. Hynes WL, Walton SL. Hyaluronidases of gram-positive bacteria. *FEMS Microbiol Lett.* 2000;183(2):201−207.

71. Thornley S, Sundborn G, Schmidt-Uili SM. Rheumatic fever in New Zealand: what are the teeth trying to tell us? *Pac Health Dialog.* 2014;20(1):7−10.

72. Thornley S, Marshall RJ, Bach K, et al. Sugar, dental caries and the incidence of acute rheumatic fever: a cohort study of Maori and Pacific children. *J Epidemiol Community Health.* 2016.

73. Chassy BM, Beall JR, Bielawski RM, Porter EV, Donkersloot JA. Occurrence and distribution of sucrose-metabolizing enzymes in oral streptococci. *Infect Immun.* 1976;14(2):408−415.

74. Shelburne 3rd SA, Keith D, Horstmann N, et al. A direct link between carbohydrate utilization and virulence in the major human pathogen group A Streptococcus. *Proc Natl Acad Sci USA.* 2008;105(5):1698−1703.

75. Longo-Mbenza B, Bayekula M, Ngiyulu R, et al. Survey of rheumatic heart disease in school children of Kinshasa town. *Int J Cardiol.* 1998;63(3):287−294.

76. Saxena A, Ramakrishnan S, Roy A, et al. Prevalence and outcome of subclinical rheumatic heart disease in India: the RHEUMATIC (rheumatic heart echo utilisation and monitoring actuarial trends in Indian children) study. *Heart.* 2011;97(24):2018−2022.

77. Zaman MM, Yoshiike N, Rouf MA, et al. Association of rheumatic fever with serum albumin concentration and body iron stores in Bangladeshi children: case-control study. *BMJ.* 1998;317(7168):1287−1288.

78. Zaman MM, Yoshiike N, Chowdhury AH, et al. Nutritional factors associated with rheumatic fever. *J Trop Pediatr.* 1998;44(3):142−147.

79. Steer AC, Kado J, Wilson N, et al. High prevalence of rheumatic heart disease by clinical and echocardiographic screening among children in Fiji. *J Heart Valve Dis.* 2009;18(3):327−335. discussion 36.

80. Hewison M. Vitamin D and immune function: an overview. *Proc Nutr Soc.* 2012;71(1):50−61.

81. Nseir W, Mograbi J, Abu-Rahmeh Z, Mahamid M, Abu-Elheja O, Shalata A. The association between vitamin D levels and recurrent group A streptococcal tonsillopharyngitis in adults. *Int J Infect Dis.* 2012;16(10):e735−e738.

82. Vlajinac H, Adanja B, Marinkovic J, Jarebinski M. Influence of socio-economic and other factors on rheumatic fever occurrence. *Eur J Epidemiol.* 1991;7(6):702−704.

83. Zaman MM, Yoshiike N, Chowdhury AH, et al. Socioeconomic deprivation associated with acute rheumatic fever. A hospital-based case-control study in Bangladesh. *Paediatr Perinat Epidemiol.* 1997;11(3):322−332.

84. Grave PE. Social and environmental factors in the aetiology of rheumatic fever. *Med J Aust.* 1957;44(18):602−608.

85. Ba-Saddik IA, Munibari AA, Al-Naqeeb MS, et al. Prevalence of rheumatic heart disease among school-children in Aden, Yemen. *Ann Trop Paediatr.* 2011;31(1):37−46.

86. Okello E, Kakande B, Sebatta E, et al. Socioeconomic and environmental risk factors among rheumatic heart disease patients in Uganda. *PLoS One.* 2012;7(8):e43917.

87. Vendsborg P, Hansen LF, Olesen KH. Decreasing incidence of a history of acute rheumatic fever in chronic rheumatic heart disease. *Cardiologia.* 1968;53(6):332−340.

88. Gordis L. The virtual disappearance of rheumatic fever in the United States: lessons in the rise and fall of disease. T. Duckett Jones memorial lecture. *Circulation.* 1985;72(6):1155−1162.

89. Carapetis JR, Steer AC, Mulholland EK, Weber M. The global burden of group A streptococcal diseases. *Lancet Infect Dis.* 2005;5(11):685−694.

90. Carapetis JR. Rheumatic heart disease in Asia. *Circulation.* 2008;118(25):2748−2753.

91. White H, Walsh W, Brown A, et al. Rheumatic heart disease in indigenous populations. *Heart Lung Circ.* 2010; 19(5–6):273–281.

92. Milne RJ, Lennon DR, Stewart JM, Vander Hoorn S, Scuffham PA. Incidence of acute rheumatic fever in New Zealand children and youth. *J Paediatr Child Health.* 2012;48(8):685–691.

93. Richardson M, Elliman D, Maguire H, Simpson J, Nicoll A. Evidence base of incubation periods, periods of infectiousness and exclusion policies for the control of communicable diseases in schools and preschools. *Pediatr Infect Dis J.* 2001;20(4):380–391.

94. Danchin MH, Rogers S, Kelpie L, et al. Burden of acute sore throat and group A streptococcal pharyngitis in school-aged children and their families in Australia. *Pediatrics.* 2007;120(5):950–957.

95. Zimmer C. *Evolution: The Triumph of an Idea.* New York: HarperCollins; 2001.

96. Stolleman GH. Factors determining the attack rate of rheumatic fever. *J Am Med Assoc.* 1961;177(12):823–828.

97. Schneider WF, Chapman S, Schulz VB, Krause RM, Lancefield RC. Prevention of streptococcal pharyngitis among military personnel and their civilian dependents by mass prophylaxis. *N Engl J Med.* 1964;270:1205–1212.

98. Gray GC, Callahan JD, Hawksworth AW, Fisher CA, Gaydos JC. Respiratory diseases among US military personnel: countering emerging threats. *Emerg Infect Dis.* 1999;5(3):379.

99. Spitzer J, Hennessy E, Neville L. High group A streptococcal carriage in the Orthodox Jewish community of north Hackney. *Br J Gen Pract.* 2001;51(463):101–105.

100. McDonald MI, Towers RJ, Andrews R, et al. The dynamic nature of group A streptococcal epidemiology in tropical communities with high rates of rheumatic heart disease. *Epidemiol Infect.* 2008;136(4):529–539.

101. Gordis L, Lilienfeld A, Rodriguez R. Studies in the epidemiology and preventability of rheumatic fever. II. Socioeconomic factors and the incidence of acute attacks. *J Chronic Dis.* 1969;21(9):655–666.

102. Jaine R, Baker M, Venugopal K. Acute rheumatic fever associated with household crowding in a developed country. *Pediatr Infect Dis J.* 2011;30(4):315–319.

103. McLaren MJ, Hawkins DM, Koornhof HJ, et al. Epidemiology of rheumatic heart disease in black shcoolchildren of Soweto, Johannesburg. *Br Med J.* 1975;3(5981): 474–478.

104. Mirabel M, Fauchier T, Bacquelin R, et al. Echocardiography screening to detect rheumatic heart disease: a cohort study of schoolchildren in French Pacific Islands. *Int J Cardiol.* 2015;188:89–95.

105. Adanja B, Vlajinac H, Jarebinski M. Socioeconomic factors in the etiology of rheumatic fever. *J Hyg Epidemiol Microbiol Immunol.* 1988;32(3):329–335.

106. Vlajinac H, Adanja B, Jarebinski M. Socio-economic factors and rheumatic fever occurrence. Differences between patients with and without frequent sore throat. *J Hyg Epidemiol Microbiol Immunol.* 1989;33(4): 471–476.

107. Coggon D, Barker DJ, Inskip H, Wield G. Housing in early life and later mortality. *J Epidemiol Community Health.* 1993;47(5):345–348.

108. Eriksson JG, Kajantie E, Phillips DI, Osmond C, Thornburg KL, Barker DJ. The developmental origins of chronic rheumatic heart disease. *Am J Hum Biol.* 2013; 25(5):655–658.

109. Kramer A, Schwebke I, Kampf G. How long do nosocomial pathogens persist on inanimate surfaces? A systematic review. *BMC Infectious Diseases.* 2006;6:130.

110. Bygdeman S, Jacobsson E, Myrback KE, Wallmark G. Hemolytic streptococci among infants in a maternity department. Report of an outbreak. *Scand J Infect Dis.* 1978; 10(1):45–49.

111. Luby SP, Agboatwalla M, Feikin DR, et al. Effect of handwashing on child health: a randomised controlled trial. *Lancet.* 2005;366(9481):225–233.

112. Carapetis JR, Johnston F, Nadjamerrek J, Kairupan J. Skin sores in aboriginal children. *J Paediatr Child Health.* 1995; 31(6):563.

113. Claesson BE, Claesson UL. An outbreak of endometritis in a maternity unit caused by spread of group A streptococci from a showerhead. *J Hosp Infect.* 1985;6(3):304–311.

114. Wagenvoort JH, Penders RJ, Davies BI, et al. Similar environmental survival patterns of Streptococcus pyogenes strains of different epidemiologic backgrounds and clinical severity. *Eur J Clin Microbiol Infect Dis.* 2005;24(1):65–67.

115. Tay L, Chay SO. A three-year streptococcal survey among Singapore school children. Part I – carriership of streptococci. *Ann Acad Med Singapore.* 1981;10(1):14–24.

116. Nandi S, Kumar R, Ray P, Vohra H, Ganguly NK. Group A streptococcal sore throat in a periurban population of northern India: a one-year prospective study. *Bull World Health Organ.* 2001;79(6):528–533.

117. Rushdy AA, Cooke RP, Iversen AM, Pickering BJ. Boarding school outbreak of group A streptococcal pharyngitis. *Commun Dis Rep – CDR Rev.* 1995;5(7):R106–R108.

118. Gordis L. Effectiveness of comprehensive-care programs in preventing rheumatic fever. *N Engl J Med.* 1973; 289(7):331–335.

119. Arguedas A, Mohs E. Prevention of rheumatic fever in Costa Rica. *J Pediatr.* 1992;121(4):569–572.

120. WHO. WHO programme for the prevention of rheumatic fever/rheumatic heart disease in developing countries: report from Phase I (1986–90). *Bull World Health Organ.* 1992;70(2):213–218.

121. Eltohami EA, Hajar HA, Folger Jr GM. Acute rheumatic fever in an Arabian Gulf country–effect of climate, advantageous socioeconomic conditions, and access to medical care. *Angiology.* 1997;48(6):481–489.

122. Bach JF, Chalons S, Forier E, et al. 10-year educational programme aimed at rheumatic fever in two French Caribbean islands. *Lancet.* 1996;347(9002):644–648.

123. Anderson P, King J, Moss M, et al. Nurse-led school-based clinics for rheumatic fever prevention and skin infection management: evaluation of Mana Kidz programme in Counties Manukau. *N Z Med J.* 2016;129(1428):37–46.

124. Jack SJ, Williamson DA, Galloway Y, et al. Primary prevention of rheumatic fever in the 21st century: evaluation of a national programme. *Int J Epidemiol*; 2018. https://doi.org/10.1093/ije/dyy150.

125. GBD Causes of Death Collaborators. Global, regional, and national age-sex specific mortality for 264 causes of death, 1980-2016: a systematic analysis for the Global Burden of Disease Study 2016. *Lancet*. 2017; 390(10100):1151−1210.

126. WHO. *Global Health Estimates 2016: Deaths by Cause, Age, Sex, by Country and by Region, 2000−2016*. Geneva: World Health Organization; 2018.

127. GBD 2016 Disease and Injury Incidence and Prevalence Collaborators. Global, regional, and national incidence, prevalence, and years lived with disability for 328 diseases and injuries for 195 countries, 1990−2016: a systematic analysis for the Global Burden of Disease Study 2016. *Lancet*. 2017;390(10100): 1211−1259.

128. Zuhlke L, Engel ME, Karthikeyan G, et al. Characteristics, complications, and gaps in evidence-based interventions in rheumatic heart disease: the Global Rheumatic Heart Disease Registry (the REMEDY study). *Eur Heart J*. 2015;36(18), 1115-22a.

129. IHME. *GBD Results Tool*; 2018. http://ghdx.healthdata.org/gbd-results-tool.

130. Scheel A, Ssinabulya I, Aliku T, et al. Community study to uncover the full spectrum of rheumatic heart disease in Uganda. *Heart*. 2019;105(1):60−66.

131. Terreri MT, Ferraz MB, Goldenberg J, Len C, Hilario MOE. Resource utilization and cost of rheumatic fever. *J Rheumatol*. 2001;28(6):1394−1397.

132. Seo HY, Yoon SJ, Kim EJ, Oh IH, Lee YH, Kim YA. The economic burden of rheumatic heart disease in South Korea. *Rheumatol Int*. 2013;33(6):1505−1510.

133. Cannon JW, Jack S, Wu Y, et al. An economic case for a vaccine to prevent group A streptococcus skin infections. *Vaccine*. 2018;36(46):6968−6978.

134. Sandhu AT, Karthikeyan G, Bolger A, Okello E, Kazi DS. Abstract 19839: clinical and economic burden of rheumatic heart disease in low-income nations: estimating the cost-of-illness in India and Uganda. *Circulation*. 2014;130. A19839-9.

135. Heenan RC, Parks T, Bärnighausen T, Kado J, Bloom DE, Steer AC. The cost-of-illness due to rheumatic heart disease: national estimates for Fiji. *Trans R Soc Trop Med Hyg*. 2019 [In press].

136. Watkins DA, Chang AY. *The Economic Impact of Rheumatic Heart Disease in Low- and Middle-Income Countries*. DCP3 working paper #19; 2017. http://dcp-3.org/sites/default/files/resources/19.%20RHD%20Watkins%20%26%20Chang.pdf.

137. Oyebamiji O. *The Household Economic Impact of Rheumatic Heart Disease (RHD) in South Africa*. Cape Town: University of Cape Town; 2018.

CHAPTER 2

Pathogenesis of Acute Rheumatic Fever

LUIZA GUILHERME • ANDREW C. STEER • MADELEINE CUNNINGHAM

INTRODUCTION

A complete and comprehensive understanding of the pathogenesis of acute rheumatic fever (ARF) has eluded scientists for decades. ARF is a multiorgan inflammatory disorder affecting the heart (carditis), joints (arthritis and arthralgia), brain (Sydneham's chorea), skin (erythema marginatum), and subcutaneous tissue (subcutaneous nodules). Rheumatic heart disease (RHD) is characterized by typical heart valve lesions, classified clinically as regurgitation and stenosis,[1] and histopathologically by the presence of pathognomonic granulomatous Aschoff bodies.

It is well established that ARF follows infection with group A *Streptococcus* (GAS), otherwise known as *Streptococcus pyogenes*, through an inflammatory process in susceptible individuals,[2,3] and that RHD occurs as a result of a severe initial or multiple episodes of ARF. Researchers have attempted to unravel the inflammatory basis of the pathogenesis of ARF, focusing on humoral and cellular immune responses with molecular mimicry as the central mediator of cross-reactivity with GAS.[4] Molecular mimicry is where a foreign antigen shares sequence or structural similarities with self-antigens.[5] Many questions remain, including whether skin infection can trigger ARF, whether groups C and G streptococci might also lead to the disease,[6–8] and whether there is a genetic basis to susceptibility to ARF.

In this chapter, we outline the current understanding of the pathogenesis of ARF. We begin with a broad overview and describe the mediators of autoimmune response, and then delve more deeply into molecular mimicry, pathogenesis of carditis and RHD, the role of T cells in RHD, pathogenesis of Sydenham's chorea, and finally genetic susceptibility.

OVERVIEW OF THE PATHOGENESIS OF ACUTE RHEUMATIC FEVER

Pharyngeal infection with GAS leads to activation of cells of the innate immune system. Neutrophils, macrophages, and dendritic cells phagocytose the bacteria, and then present antigens to T cells, in turn leading to activation of humoral and cellular immune responses. The immune response becomes cross-reactive with human tissues in susceptible individuals—this is the driving mechanism of ARF.[1] The B- and T-cell response leads to antibody production and CD4+ T-cell activation. These cross-reactive antibodies and T cells are generated through the process of molecular mimicry whereby antigenic epitopes are shared between host and bacteria.[4,5,9,10] This autoimmune process is believed to be the basis of all of the clinical manifestations of ARF: carditis is caused by both cross-reactive antibodies and T cells, arthritis by immune complex deposition, chorea by antibody binding to neuronal cells and the skin, and subcutaneous manifestations by a delayed hypersensitivity reaction (Fig. 2.1).[1,5]

MEDIATORS OF AUTOIMMUNE REACTIONS

Although immunity against GAS is intended to eliminate the bacterium from our bodies, in some instances, the immune response against GAS turns into an autoimmune response.[4,6,9,10] Autoimmune T and B lymphocyte responses target antigens both of GAS and the human heart, brain, skin, and articular joint tissues. Heart-tissue cross-reactive antibodies may bind to the valvular endothelial tissue generating inflammation and consequently upregulation of the vascular cell adhesion molecule-1 (VCAM-1).[11]

Cytokines and chemokines are involved initially in the response against GAS as well as throughout the entire inflammatory process of clearance of the streptococcus and development of sequelae in the heart of ARF and chronic RHD patients.[12] Chemokines are important mediators of cellular migration. In an in vitro assay, autoreactive T cells were shown to

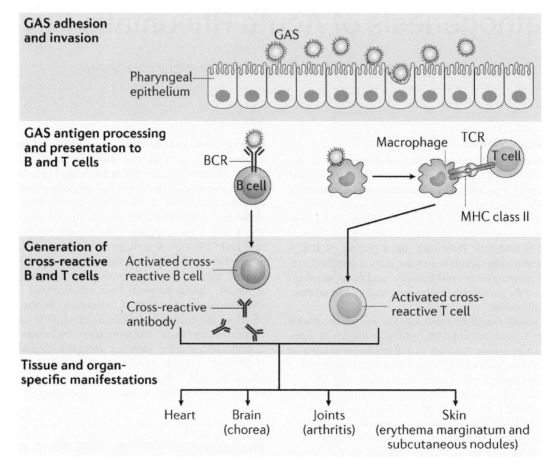

Nature Reviews | Disease Primers

FIG. 2.1 Generation of a cross-reactive immune response in acute rheumatic fever (ARF). Following GAS adhesion to and invasion of the pharyngeal epithelium, GAS antigens activate both B and T cells. Molecular mimicry between GAS group A carbohydrate and serotype-specific M protein and the host heart, brain, or joint tissues can lead to an autoimmune response, which causes the major manifestations of ARF. *BCR,* B-cell receptor; *TCR,* T-cell receptor. (Reproduced with permission from Carapetis JR et al.[1])

migrate into the inflamed heart tissue mainly toward a CXCL9/Mig gradient suggesting that these specific chemokines mediated both CD4[+] and CD8[+] T-cell recruitment into valvular heart tissue.[12] A cascade of soluble mediators consisting of cytokines such as IL-1, IL-2, IL-17, IFNγ, and TNF-α culminates in an inflammatory response that leads to tissue injury primarily in valves, leading to valvulitis with mild-to-severe functional consequences, and somewhat in the adjoining myocardium.[6,13−15]

MOLECULAR MIMICRY

Molecular mimicry is immune cross-recognition of conformational protein or carbohydrate structures and/or amino acid sequences with similarities between microbes and human tissues.[4,10,16] It is believed to be an important part of the pathogenesis of ARF including the development of autoimmunity and inflammation in the heart and brain.[4,10,17,18]

The development of autoimmune responses against the heart and the brain are thought to be primarily in response to the group A carbohydrate epitope N-acetyl-β-D-glucosamine (GlcNAc), the dominant epitope of the group A carbohydrate.[17] In one study, individuals with a diagnosis of RHD who made strong responses against the group A carbohydrate had a poor prognosis compared to those who did not have elevated anticarbohydrate antibodies.[19] Valvular carbohydrate epitopes are important in targeting an immune response against the valve.[20] Studies of human and mouse antistreptococcal/antimyosin monoclonal antibodies (mAbs) that reacted strongly with N-acetyl-glucosamine have demonstrated cytotoxicity for human cardiomyocytes or endothelium[17,21] and the antibodies also reacted with valvular endothelium in tissue sections of human valves.[17] Cytotoxic mAbs recognized α-helical laminin as part of the extracellular matrix in the basement membrane underlying the valvular endothelium. These data suggested that human antibody cross-reactivity with valve tissues is established through antimyosin/anti-N-acetyl-glucosamine/anti-laminin reactivity.[17,21]

CARDITIS AND RHEUMATIC HEART DISEASE

Rheumatic carditis is characterized by regurgitant lesions of the mitral and aortic valves (otherwise known as rheumatic valvulitis - see Chapter 3). Fig. 2.2 shows a diagram of the proposed pathogenesis of disease in the valve. Antibodies, potentially directed against the group A carbohydrate, react with valve endothelium to initiate inflammation at the valve surface and promote T-cell infiltration of the valve in RHD.[17,19,20,22,23] Cross-reactive T cells responsive to streptococcal M proteins and homologous α-helical protein antigens such as myosin, laminin, tropomyosin, or vimentin become activated and extravasate through activated endothelium into the valve where they differentiate into CD4+ TH1 cells producing γ IFN.[11,24−29]

Initial damage in RHD may originate at the chordae tendinae, where damage to the endothelium of these very delicate valve structures may begin the process of injury, edema, fibrosis, and scarring.[30] T cells infiltrate and congregate at the basement membrane of the valve[31] with upregulation of VCAM-1,[11] which allows

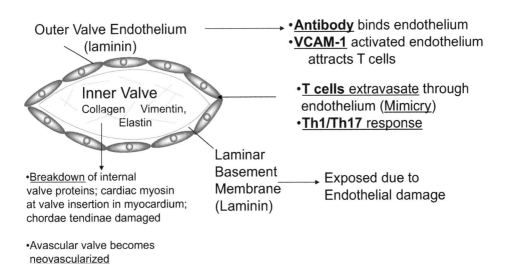

FIG. 2.2 Diagram of proposed pathogenesis of rheumatic heart disease as described in the text. Antistreptococcal antibodies directed against the group A streptococcus and the heart target the valve endothelium containing laminin.[17,21] The antiheart antibodies are proposed to lead to upregulation of VCAM-1 on the valve surface,[11] which then attracts T cells that enter the valve and lead to valve damage and continued heart disease with every streptococcal infection. T cells recognize the streptococcal M protein and α-helical proteins in the valve including laminin and vimentin. VCAM-1, vascular cell adhesion molecule-1. (Reproduced with permission from Cunningham MW[10])

the valve to be infiltrated by the T cells and leads to explosive valve injury with repeated streptococcal infections. Cross-reactive T cells penetrate the valve endothelium into an originally avascular valve.[11,24,26–29,32–39] T cells in peripheral blood of patients[40] and the valve[26,29,41,42] have been shown to be cross-reactive with M protein and cardiac proteins including cardiac myosin epitopes, and they are both CD4+ and CD8+ phenotypes, but the CD4+ phenotype and Th1 cells dominate. The development of scarring and fibrosis in the valve is part of the pathogenesis caused by γ-interferon (IFN)[6,13,42] production and IL-17A.[6,15] As the scarring promotes neovascularization and development of a blood supply into normally avascular valve tissue, T cells can subsequently enter the valve through blood vessels developed in the scar. In summary, cardiac valves with their thin avascular structure become inflamed and vascularized in acute rheumatic valvulitis. The healing process evolves after rheumatic valvulitis with a combination of neovascularization and tissue fibrosis.

Cardiac myosin is a major antigen in the myocardium that cross-reacts with antibodies and T cells produced in response to GAS infection. Using affinity-purified antimyosin antibodies from ARF patients, the cross-reactive streptococcal epitope has been further defined: a five-amino acid residue (Gln-Lys-Ser-Lys-Gln) of the N-terminal M5 and M6 proteins.[43] Later, several other cardiac myosin epitopes, identified as peptide sequences in light meromyosin (LMM), were also described as targets of both peripheral and heart-tissue infiltrating T-cell clones that demonstrated specific cross-reactivity between streptococcal M5 protein and cardiac myosin epitopes.[30,41] A high proportion (63.2%) of intralesional T-cell clones that recognized LMM peptides was observed, indicating that streptococcal-primed peripheral T-cell clones migrated to the heart and were maintained by their cross-reactivity with cardiac myosin in adjacent valve tissues or with other valve proteins such as vimentin and laminin.[41] Peptides in the S2 fragment of cardiac myosin are recognized by autoantibodies in rheumatic carditis.[40]

T-cell reactivity toward cardiac myosin epitopes in ARF and RHD patients may also trigger broader recognition of valvular proteins with structural or functional similarities, such as vimentin, laminin and others. RHD with more chronic disease displays more fibrosis, but the avascular valve becomes neovascularized to provide more blood vessels to the scar tissue in the valve, and with every streptococcal infection disease can explode in the valve leading to dysfunction and the need for valve replacement.

Increased but disorganized expression of vimentin, along with reduced expression of collagen VI, involved with repair and tissue integrity and a target for adhesion by GAS through collagen-binding proteins, was recently observed in ARF and RHD valvular tissue.[44–46] Noncross-reactive antibodies develop against collagen in RHD,[44,47] and may contribute to the pathogenesis of disease.[45] Once mimicry damages the valve, collagen is exposed to the immune system and antibodies develop against collagen.[47]

Cardiac myosin has an α-helical structure very similar to the streptococcal M protein.[43,48] Studies have shown that the structure of the M protein has regions of splayed helical amino acid sequence where the α-helix is disrupted due to irregularities in the amino acid periodicity required for the coiled-coil structure.[49] Antimyosin antibody only cross-reacts with the splayed regions of the α-helical coiled-coil streptococcal M protein structure, not if the splayed regions are closed and the structure is designed as a perfect helix.[49] Studies were undertaken to crystallize a portion of the streptococcal M1 protein to evaluate its virulence properties when portions of the amino acid sequence were mutated to eliminate the splayed α-helical regions, and also to investigate regions and structures responsible for eliciting or reacting with cross-reactive antibodies that participate in molecular mimicry.[49] The structural study revealed irregularities and instabilities in the coiled coil of the M1 fragment crystal. Similar structural instabilities and irregularities occur in myosin and tropomyosin that had previously been demonstrated to cross-react with the streptococcal M proteins.[43,50–52] Using mutation of specific amino acids, the study showed enhanced stability of the coiled-coil diminished the virulence properties of the M1 protein and reduced cross-reactivity of the M protein with cross-reactive autoantibodies that reacted with both cardiac myosin and GAS M proteins.[49] Thus, the stabilization of the α-helix to remove the splayed helical regions of the M protein led to a reduction of virulence and loss of cross-reactivity with heart reactive antibodies (Table 2.1).

T CELLS AND RHEUMATIC HEART DISEASE

T-cell clones isolated from mitral valves, papillary muscle, and the left atrium of patients with RHD have been shown to be responsive to several peptides of streptococcal M5 protein and proteins from heart tissue extracts.[26] In BALB/c mice immunized with human cardiac myosin, myosin-cross-reactive T-cell epitopes from the A, B repeat regions of the M5 protein were identified.[39] Thus, the regions of M protein that can induce heart cross-reactivity, cause disease in the heart, or be identified by T cells from lesions of rheumatic

TABLE 2.1
Major Events Leading to Autoimmune Reactions in Acute Rheumatic Fever and Rheumatic Heart Disease.

Several genes (bold) confer susceptibility to develop ARF/RHD, through alleles (parenthesis) that code for proteins that mediate both innate and adaptive immune response.
- Innate immunity: **TLR2** (−308A, −238G), **FCN2** (G/G/A), **MASP2** (371D, 377V, 439R), **MBL** (A, O) **MIF (-173CC)**, **FCγRIIa** (393A)
- Adaptive immune response: **HLA class II genes** (several HLA-DR and DQ alleles)
- Both innate and adaptive immune response: **ILRA** (A1/A1), **TNF-α** (−308A, −238G), **TGF-ß 1** (−509T,869T), **IL-10** (1082 G, A), **CTLA4** (49 GG), **IGHV** (4−61*02)

Throat and/or skin

- After GAS colonization, neutrophils, macrophages, and dendritic cells proceed to phagocytosis followed by antigen processing/presentation to T cells resulting in activation of both humoral and cellular immune response.

Peripheral blood

- Both B and T cells respond to the GAS infection. Antibodies (IgM and IgG) and T cells (mainly CD4$^+$) act as a natural defense against the bacteria.

In susceptible individuals, the immune response against the bacteria will trigger autoimmune reactions mediated by both antibodies and T cells, affecting diverse organs as follows:

Joints: Antigroup A carbohydrate and/or components of bacterial cell wall/membrane or M protein form immune complexes, activate complement cascade inducing transitory migratory arthritis.

Skin: Erythema marginatum and subcutaneous nodules

Brain: Basal ganglia: Antibodies from sera of Sydenham chorea patients bind to basal ganglia and neuronal cells. Gangliosides, tubulin, and dopamine receptors cross-react with N-acetyl ß-D-glucosamine, the dominant epitope of the group A carbohydrate and major cell wall streptococcal antigen.

Heart: Myocardium and valves
- Streptococcal antibodies activate adhesion molecules (VCAM/ICAM) on valve endothelium, facilitating infiltration of monocytes and T and B cells, leading to myocarditis/valvulitis. Antibodies anti-N-acetyl ß-D-glucosamine cross-react with cardiac myosin and laminin. Anticollagen antibodies may occur due to collagen exposure following valve damage.
- Heart-tissue infiltrating T cells recognize streptococcal M protein, cardiac myosin, vimentin, and other α-helical proteins by cross-reactivity. Cells producing inflammatory cytokines (IFNγ, TNFα, IL-17 and IL-23) are abundant.

ARF acute rheumatic fever; RHD rheumatic heart disease; GAS group A streptococcus; VCAM vascular cell adhesion molecule; ICAM intracellular adhesion molecule.

carditis and RHD have been investigated in rodents and humans. Six dominant myosin cross-reactive T-cell epitopes were recognized by T cells when reacted with the M5 molecule (Table 2.2)[39]. Listed in Table 2.2 include (1) the dominant Balb/c mouse T-cell epitopes or amino acid sequences of GAS M5 protein that react with T cells taken from BALB/c mice that have been immunized with the streptococcal M5 protein[39]; (2) the amino acid sequences of the GAS M5 protein that are recognized by T-cell clones from rheumatic heart valves[26]; and (3) amino acid sequences of the streptococcal M5 protein that have been previously reported to stimulate human T cells from ARF patients.[53,54] An important correlation/finding seen in Table 2.2 is that M5 peptides NT4/NT5 (GLKTENEGLKTENEGLKTE and KKEHEAENDKLKQQRDTL) and B1B2/B2 (VKDKIAKEQENKETIGTL and TIGTLKKILDETVKD-KIA), which were dominant cross-reactive T-cell epitopes in the M5 immunized BALB/c mouse, contain sequences similar to those M protein sequences

recognized by T cells from rheumatic valves.[26] Peptides NT4 and NT5 produced inflammatory infiltrates in the myocardium of rodents immunized with those peptides.[39] Amino acid sequences in the N-terminal portion of M5 protein that share homology with cardiac myosin may break immune tolerance and promote T cell-mediated inflammatory heart disease.[39] The correlation of similar or the same peptide sequences as observed in animal models as well as in T cells derived from human rheumatic heart valves suggests that these may be the peptides that lead to disease in humans. Certain HLA haplotypes may also predispose and enhance the recognition of these sequences and epitopes by T cells and increase susceptibility to RHD.

In humans with rheumatic carditis, T cells isolated and cloned from the peripheral blood or rheumatic mitral valves were shown to recognize streptococcal M5 peptides and LMM peptides.[29,30,41] The cross-reactive T cells taken from ARF and RHD heart valves mainly recognise three regions (residues 1-25, 81-103

TABLE 2.2
Myosin or Heart Cross-reactive T-Cell Epitopes of Streptococcal M5 Protein.

Peptide	Sequence	Origin of T-Cell Clone or Response
1–25	TVTRGTISDPQRAKEALDKYELENH[a]	ARF/Valve[26]
81–96	DKLKQQRDTLSTQKETLEREVQN[a]	ARF/Valve[26]
163–177	ETIGTLKKILDETVK[a]	ARF/Valve[26]
337–356	LRRDLDASREAKKQVEKAL	Normal/PBL[54]
347–366	AKKQVEKALEEANSKLAALE	Mice[53]/Normal PBL[54]
397–416	LKEQLAKQAEELAKLRAGKA	ARF/PBL[54]
NT4 40–58	GLKTENEGLKTENEGLKTE	BALB/c/Lymph node[34,b]
NT5 59–76	KKEHEAENDKLKQQRDTL	BALB/c/Lymph node[39,b]
B1B2 137–154	VKDKIAKEQENKETIGTL	BALB/c/Lymph node[39,b]
B2 150–167	TIGTLKKILDETVKDKIA	BALB/c/Lymph node[39,b]
C2A 254–271	EASRKGLRRDLDASREAK	BALB/c/Lymph node[39,b]
C3 293–308	KGLRRDLDASREAKKQ	BALB/c/Lymph node[39,b]

ARF, acute rheumatic fever, *PBL*, peripheral blood lymphocytes.
[a] Amino terminal TVTRGTIS sequence was taken from the M5 amino acid sequence published by Manjula et al.[103] and deviates from the M5 sequence published by Miller et al.[104] at positions 1 and 8. Other sequences (81–96) and (163–177) were taken from the PepM5 sequence as reported by Manjula.[103] These two sequences are found in the sequence as 67–89 and 174–188, respectively, as reported by Miller et al.[104] All other sequences shown earlier are from the M5 gene sequence reported by Miller et al.[104]
[b] BALB/c mice immunized with purified human cardiac myosin and the recovered lymph node lymphocytes were stimulated with each of the peptides in tritiated thymidine uptake assays.
Taken from Cunningham MW[25], with permission from ASM press.

and 163-177) of the amino-terminal region of the M protein and several valve proteins and peptides of human cardiac light meromyosin region, which is the smaller of the two subunits produced by tryptic digestion of human cardiac myosin.[26,29,30,41] To summarize, mimicry between M proteins and cardiac myosin stimulates cross-reactive T cells in the peripheral blood of the host during episodes of streptococcal infections and leads to heart disease.[24,28,30] The T cells then traffic to the valve once the endothelium of the valve becomes activated and inflamed.[11] This extravasation event at the valve endocardium allows the cross-reactive T cells to enter the valve where they recognize and proliferate to valvular proteins such as vimentin[23] and cardiac myosin from papillary muscle. T cells that remain in the valve survive if they continue to be stimulated by host α-helical proteins within the valve. The activated cross-reactive T cells when continually stimulated within the valve become pathogenic for the host and produce the Th1/Th17 mechanism of pathogenesis with scarring in the valve. Fig. 2.2 shows the events in rheumatic carditis that are a result of immune responses against the cross-reactive antigens of GAS.[4,10,11,17,25]

The granulomatous proinflammatory Th1 cell response and the presence of IFN gamma have been reported as dominant in rheumatic valves.[13] Studies of RHD have suggested that Th17 cells in peripheral blood are elevated with concomitant downregulation of the Treg phenotype.[15] In ARF and RHD, elevated numbers of Th17 cells, high IL-17A levels, and decreased T-regulatory cells were reported in peripheral blood.[15] Although less is known about Th17 cell responses in RHD, Th17 cells are important in GAS infections and have been identified in nasopharyngeal and tonsillar lymphoid tissues in animal models of streptococcal infection[55–57] or other streptococcal immunization animal models.[6] Different routes of bacterial infection may induce long-lived Th1 memory cells and short-lived Th17 cell responses in the mucosa.[56] IL-17A triggers effective immune responses against extracellular bacteria, such as promoting neutrophil responses.[58–61] However, the more chronic autoimmune IL17A response observed in chronic autoimmune disease may be important in RHD but this is not yet fully described. The Th17 cells found in human tonsils that are activated by GAS[62] may prove to be important in the premise put forth years ago by Wannamaker in his statement that GAS infections are the "chain that links the heart to the throat."[3] This could be the case if Th17 cells traffic during streptococcal infections in susceptible individuals from the tonsil to the valvular and myocardial tissues and if T-regulatory cells (or Tregs) become reduced during repetitive GAS infections, the Th17 cells may become chronically established in the heart. T-regulatory cells are known to protect the host against autoimmune disease.[61] It is also well known that Th1 and Th17 cells are plastic and may develop from each other, although the dominant T-cell program for each T helper cell type is established during development.[63−65]

SYDENHAM CHOREA

Human mAbs derived from patients with Sydenham chorea (SC) have been used to identify cross-reactive neuronal antibody targets in the brain. The mAbs as well as serum IgG from SC patients recognized mammalian lysoganglioside and GAS carbohydrate epitope N-acetyl-β-D-glucosamine (GlcNAc).[18] SC-derived mAbs and acute SC serum antibodies, as well as cerebrospinal fluid (CSF), reacted with lysoganglioside and targeted the surface of human neuronal cells leading to antibody-mediated neuronal cell signaling. Serum IgG antibodies that triggered the cell signaling in human neuronal cells were absorbed by anti-IgG beads.

The human chorea mAb 24.3.1 was constructed genetically to be a mouse IgG and in a model of SC in Tg mice expressing the antibody construct was shown to penetrate the brain.[66] Once the blood brain barrier was broken, 24.3.1 IgG penetrated into the substantia nigra or ventral tegmental area and penetrated dopaminergic neurons.[66] The chorea-derived antibody treatment of neuronal cells in culture led to production of excess tritiated dopamine. Mouse models directly receiving GAS immunization or passive transfer of anti-streptococcal antibodies have demonstrated behavioral alterations and antibody deposition in the brain.[67−70]

Studies collectively demonstrate that antineuronal IgG in SC patients targets a group of cross-reactive antigens in the brain,[18,71−74] including lysoganglioside, tubulin, and the dopamine receptors D1 and D2 (see Fig. 2.3). Therefore, SC may be characterized potentially as a dopamine receptor encephalitis where the autoantibodies signal the D2 receptor.[66] In Sydenham chorea, the anti-neuronal antibodies (IgG) are elevated in both serum and cerebrospinal fluid (CSF). In addition, serum and CSF (IgG) and SC-derived human mAbs signal human neuronal cells and activate calcium calmodulin dependent protein kinase II (CaMKII) in human

neuronal cells (SKNSH cell line).[18] Studies in SC patients have shown that the ratio of antidopamine D1 and D2 receptor antibodies correlated with symptoms[75] and suggest a dopamine receptor encephalitis in SC. Production and release of excess dopamine by neuronal cells in the basal ganglia may ultimately lead to an imbalance in central dopamine levels and lead to chorea and other movement and neuropsychiatric symptoms.

Studies in mice intranasally infected with GAS demonstrate the importance of infection and its role in opening the blood brain barrier, which must be broken to allow IgG to penetrate the brain. Intranasal streptococcal infection has been shown to lead to activated Th17 cells that then traverse the olfactory bulb and open the blood−brain barrier to proteins like IgG.[62,76] Upon opening the blood−brain barrier, IgG antineuronal autoantibodies can penetrate the brain and potentially lead to SC.

The studies suggest firstly that antistreptococcal antibodies against brain or caudate putamen in SC may be able to produce central nervous system dysfunction through a neuronal signal transduction and subsequent excess dopamine release mechanism and secondly that the neuronal targets of SC antibodies include lysoganglioside, tubulin, and the dopamine receptors.[18,66,71,72] The cross-reactive anti-GAS antibodies react with N-acetyl-β-D-glucosamine (GlcNAc) present on the rhamnose backbone of the group A carbohydrate.[18,72,77]

GENETIC SUSCEPTIBILITY TO ACUTE RHEUMATIC FEVER

Chapter 1 summarizes the epidemiological evidence for host genetic susceptibility to ARF/RHD. Several susceptibility genes in humans favor the development of ARF/RHD. Table 2.2 summarizes genes of the immune response that are involved with genetic susceptibility and some of the autoimmune mechanisms that lead to ARF and/or RHD. Some of the variant genes predisposing to ARF are involved in the first line of defense by recognition of GAS and activation of innate immunity such as toll-like receptor gene (TLR2), or by producing soluble mediators such as ficolin 2 gene (FCN2), mannan-binding lectin (MBL), and mannan-binding lectin serine protease (MASP2) genes that both activate the complement pathway to initially eliminate the bacteria after infection.[78−82] Other genes control the spread of the bacteria such as MIF (migratory inhibition factor) and CTLA4 gene (cytotoxic T lymphocyte-associated protein) that transmits an inhibitory signal to T cells, resulting in deficient or no immune response mediated by T cells.[83,84] Recently, a

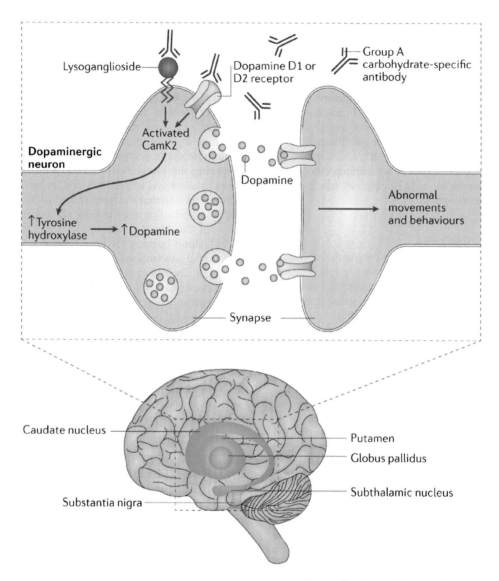

Nature Reviews | Disease Primers

FIG. 2.3 Proposed pathway for antineuronal autoantibodies against lysoganglioside and dopamine receptors D1 and D2 in Sydenham chorea.[1,5] The figure diagrams pre and postsynaptic neurons and the dopamine receptors and autoantibodies in Sydenham chorea. A cross-section of the basal ganglia reflects the regions that are targeted by the autoantibodies.[66] The evidence suggests that autoantibodies may target antigens in the basal ganglia including lysoganglioside, tubulin, and the dopamine receptors as well as antigens recognized by a human neuronal cell line and which are responsible for the calcium calmodulin dependent protein kinase II (CAMKII) signaling by the autoantibodies.[18] (Reproduced with permission from Carapetis JR et al.[1])

new polymorphism was described in the immunoglobulin gene by whole genome sequencing (GWAS), in which the allele IGHV4-61*02 was found in association with RHD in Oceania populations.[85] In Aboriginal

Australians, variation at HLA_DQA1-DQB1 appeared to be the major genetic risk factor for RHD.[86]

The adaptive immune response, which includes antibodies and T cells, is another type of immune defense against the streptococcus. This is activated by antigen presentation to T lymphocytes in the context of HLA class II antigens or alleles that are coded by the DRB1 gene that is located on the short arm of human chromosome 6. These have been described in association with streptococcal sequelae in several populations around the world. Briefly, the most frequent alleles associated with ARF and RHD are HLA-DRB1*07, -DRB1*04, -DRB1*09 that belong to the HLA-DR53 group and HLA-DRB1*01, DRB1*03, DRB*11, and DRB1*06 that belong to the HLA-DR52 group. It is of note that DRB1*04 and DRB1*0301 alleles were also described in association with impetigo as recently reviewed.[87−102] As stated in Chapter 1, the significance of candidate gene studies is unclear, and international, multicountry meta-analyses are needed to identify genetic determinants of ARF/RHD susceptibility.

ACKNOWLEDGMENTS

Research grants to MWC: (a) HL35280 and HL56267 from the National Heart Lung and Blood Institute and National Institute of Mental Health Bench to Bedside; (b) grants from the Oklahoma Center for the Advancement of Science and Technology and the American Heart Association. Declaration of financial interest: MWC is a chief scientific officer and consultant at Moleculera Labs, a company offering diagnostic testing for antineuronal autoantibodies in children with autoimmune movement and neuropsychiatric disorders.

Research grants to LG: FAPESP-2885-6 from "Fundaçao de Amparo a Pesquisa do Estado de Sao Paulo" and CNPQ-620418 from "Conselho Nacional de Desenvolvimento Científico e Tecnológico (CNPq)," Brazil.

REFERENCES

1. Carapetis JR, Beaton A, Cunningham MW, et al. Acute rheumatic fever and rheumatic heart disease. *Nature Reviews Disease Primers.* 2016;2:15084.
2. Bisno AL. Acute pharyngitis. *N Engl J Med.* 2001;344(3):205−211.
3. Wannamaker LW. The chain that links the throat to the heart. *Circulation.* 1973;48:9−18.
4. Cunningham MW. Rheumatic fever, autoimmunity, and molecular mimicry: the streptococcal connection. *Int Rev Immunol.* 2014;33(4):314−329.
5. Cunningham MW. *Molecular Mimicry, Autoimmunity and Infection: The Cross-Reactive Antigens of Group A Streptococci and Their Sequelae.* 2nd ed. American Society for Microbiology Press; 2018.
6. Sikder S, Williams NL, Sorenson AE, et al. Group G streptococcus induces an autoimmune IL-17A/IFN-gamma mediated carditis in the Lewis rat model of Rheumatic Heart Disease. *J Infect Dis.* 2017:324−335.
7. Collins CM, Kimura A, Bisno AL. Group G streptococcal M protein exhibits structural features analogous to those of class I M proteins of group A streptococci. *Infect Immun.* 1992;60:3689−3696.
8. Bisno A, Craven DE, McCabe WR. M proteins of group G streptococci isolated from bacteremic human infection. *Infect Immun.* 1987;55:753−757.
9. Guilherme L, Kalil J. Rheumatic fever and rheumatic heart disease: cellular mechanisms leading to autoimmune reactivity and disease. *J Clin Immunol.* 2010;30(1):17−23.
10. Cunningham MW. Streptococcus and rheumatic fever. *Curr Opin Rheumatol.* 2012;24(4):408−416.
11. Roberts S, Kosanke S, Dunn ST, Jankelow D, Duran CMG, Cunningham MW. Immune mechanisms in rheumatic carditis: focus on valvular endothelium. *J Infect Dis.* 2001;183:507−511.
12. Fae KC, Palacios SA, Nogueira LG, et al. CXCL9/Mig mediates T cells recruitment to valvular tissue lesions of chronic rheumatic heart disease patients. *Inflammation.* 2013;36(4):800−811.
13. Guilherme L, Cury P, Demarchi LM, et al. Rheumatic heart disease: proinflammatory cytokines play a role in the progression and maintenance of valvular lesions. *Am J Pathol.* 2004;165(5):1583−1591.
14. Guilherme L, Ramasawmy R, Kalil J. Rheumatic fever and rheumatic heart disease: genetics and pathogenesis. *Scand J Immunol.* 2007;66(2−3):199−207.
15. Bas HD, Baser K, Yavuz E, et al. A shift in the balance of regulatory T and T helper 17 cells in rheumatic heart disease. *J Investig Med.* 2014;62:78−83.
16. Shikhman AR, Greenspan NS, Cunningham MW. A subset of mouse monoclonal antibodies cross-reactive with cytoskeletal proteins and group A streptococcal M proteins recognizes N-acetyl-beta-D-glucosamine. *J Immunol.* 1993;151(7):3902−3913.
17. Galvin JE, Hemric ME, Ward K, Cunningham MW. Cytotoxic monoclonal antibody from rheumatic carditis reacts with human endothelium: implications in rheumatic heart disease. *J Clin Investig.* 2000;106:217−224.
18. Kirvan CA, Swedo SE, Heuser JS, Cunningham MW. Mimicry and autoantibody-mediated neuronal cell signaling in Sydenham chorea. *Nat Med.* 2003;9(7):914−920.
19. Dudding BA, Ayoub EM. Persistence of streptococcal group A antibody in patients with rheumatic valvular disease. *J Exp Med.* 1968;128:1081.
20. Goldstein I, Halpern B, Robert L. Immunological relationship between streptococcus A polysaccharide and the structural glycoproteins of heart valve. *Nature.* 1967;213:44−47.
21. Antone SM, Adderson EE, Mertens NMJ, Cunningham MW. Molecular analysis of V gene sequences encoding cytotoxic anti-streptococcal/anti-myosin monoclonal antibody 36.2.2 that recognizes

the heart cell surface protein laminin. *J Immunol.* 1997; 159:5422−5430.

22. Kaplan MH, Bolande R, Ratika L, Blair J. Presence of bound immunoglobulins and complement in the myocardium in acute rheumatic fever. *N Engl J Med.* 1964;271:637.

23. Gulizia JM, Cunningham MW, McManus BM. Immuno-reactivity of anti-streptococcal monoclonal antibodies to human heart valves. Evidence for multiple cross-reactive epitopes. *Am J Pathol.* 1991;138(2):285−301.

24. Cunningham MW. T cell Mimicry in inflammatory heart disease. *Mol Immunol.* 2004;40:1121−1127.

25. Cunningham MW. Autoimmunity and molecular mimicry in the pathogenesis of post-streptococcal heart disease. *Front Biosci.* 2003;8:s533−s543.

26. Guilherme L, Cunha-Neto E, Coelho V, et al. Human heart-filtrating T cell clones from rheumatic heart disease patients recognize both streptococcal and cardiac proteins. *Circulation.* 1995;92:415−420.

27. Guilherme L, Dulphy N, Douay C, et al. Molecular evidence for antigen-driven immune responses in cardiac lesions of rheumatic heart disease patients. *Int Immunol.* 2000;12(7):1063−1074.

28. Guilherme L, Oshiro SE, Fae KC, et al. T-cell reactivity against streptococcal antigens in the periphery mirrors reactivity of heart-infiltrating T lymphocytes in rheumatic heart disease patients. *Infect Immun.* 2001;69(9): 5345−5351.

29. Fae K, Kalil J, Toubert A, Guilherme L. Heart infiltrating T cell clones from a rheumatic heart disease patient display a common TCR usage and a degenerate antigen recognition pattern. *Mol Immunol.* 2004;40(14−15): 1129−1135.

30. Ellis NMJ, Li Y, Hildebrand W, Fischetti VA, Cunningham MW. T cell mimicry and epitope specificity of cross-reactive T cell clones from rheumatic heart disease. *J Immunol.* 2005;175:5448−5456.

31. Guilherme L, Kalil J. Rheumatic heart disease: molecules involved in valve tissue inflammation leading to the autoimmune process and anti-S. Pyogenes vaccine. *Front Immunol.* 2013;4:352.

32. Gibofsky A, Kerwar S, Zabriskie JB. *Rheumatic Fever: The Relationships between Host, Microbe and Genetics.* 1998.

33. Hutto JH, Ayoub EM. Cytotoxicity of lymphocytes from patients with rheumatic carditis to cardiac cells *in vitro.* In: Read SE, Zabriskie JB, eds. *Streptococcal Diseases and the Immune Response.* New York: Academic Press; 1980: 733−738.

34. Kemeny E, Grieve T, Marcus R, Sareli P, Zabriskie JB. Identification of mononuclear cells and T cell subsets in rheumatic valvulitis. *Clin Immunol Immunopathol.* 1989;52: 225−237.

35. Raizada V, Williams RC, Chopra P, et al. Tissue distribution of lymphocytes in rheumatic heart valves as defined by monoclonal anti-T cell antibodies. *Am J Med.* 1983;74: 90−96.

36. Read SE, Reid HF, Fischetti VA, et al. Serial studies on the cellular immune response to streptococcal antigens in acute and convalescent rheumatic fever patients in Trinidad. *J Clin Immunol.* 1986;6(6):433−441.

37. Bhatia R, Narula J, Reddy KS, et al. Lymphocyte subsets in acute rheumatic fever and rheumatic heart disease. *Clin Cardiol.* 1989;12(1):34−38.

38. Chopra P, Narula J, Kumar AS, Sachdeva S, Bhatia ML. Immunohistochemical characterisation of Aschoff nodules and endomyocardial inflammatory infiltrates in left atrial appendages from patients with chronic rheumatic heart disease. *Int J Cardiol.* 1988;20(1):99−105.

39. Cunningham MW, Antone SM, Smart M, Liu R, Kosanke S. Molecular analysis of human cardiac myosin-cross-reactive B- and T-cell epitopes of the group A streptococcal M5 protein. *Infect Immun.* 1997;65: 3913−3923.

40. Ellis NMJ, Kurahara D, Vohra H, et al. Priming the immune system for heart disease: a perspective on group A streptococci. *J Infect Dis.* 2010;202:1059.

41. Fae KC, da Silva DD, Oshiro SE, et al. Mimicry in recognition of cardiac myosin peptides by heart-intralesional T cell clones from rheumatic heart disease. *J Immunol.* 2006;176(9):5662−5670.

42. Guilherme L, Kalil J, Cunningham M. Molecular mimicry in the autoimmune pathogenesis of rheumatic heart disease. *Autoimmunity.* 2006;39(1):31−39.

43. Cunningham MW, McCormack JM, Fenderson PG, Ho MK, Beachey EH, Dale JB. Human and murine antibodies cross-reactive with streptococcal M protein and myosin recognize the sequence GLN-LYS-SER-LYS-GLN in M protein. *J Immunol.* 1989;143(8):2677−2683.

44. Dinkla K, Rohde M, Jansen WT, Kaplan EL, Chhatwal GS, Talay SR. Rheumatic fever-associated Streptococcus pyogenes isolates aggregate collagen. *J Clin Investig.* 2003; 111(12):1905−1912.

45. Tandon R, Sharma M, Chandrashekhar Y, Kotb M, Yacoub MH, Narula J. Revisiting the pathogenesis of rheumatic fever and carditis. *Nat Rev Cardiol.* 2013;10:171−177.

46. Martins CO, Demarchi L, Ferreira FM, et al. Rheumatic heart disease and myxomatous degeneration: differences and similarities of valve damage resulting from autoimmune reactions and matrix disorganization. *PLoS One.* 2017;12(1):e0170191.

47. Martins TB, Hoffman JL, Augustine NH, et al. Comprehensive analysis of antibody responses to streptococcal and tissue antigens in patients with acute rheumatic fever. *Int Immunol.* 2008;20(3):445−452.

48. Cunningham MW. Pathogenesis of group A streptococcal infections. *Clin Microbiol Rev.* 2000;13:470−511.

49. McNamara C, Zinkernagel AS, Macheboeuf P, Cunningham MW, Nizet V, Ghosh P. Coiled-coil irregularities and instabilities in group A streptococcus M1 are required for virulence. *Science.* 2008;319:1405−1408.

50. Dale JB, Beachey EH. Multiple, heart-cross-reactive epitopes of streptococcal M proteins. *J Exp Med.* 1985; 161(1):113−122.

51. Dale JB, Beachey EH. Epitopes of streptococcal M proteins shared with cardiac myosin. *J Exp Med.* 1985; 162(2):583−591.

52. Dale JB, Beachey EH. Sequence of myosin-cross-reactive epitopes of streptococcal M protein. *J Exp Med.* 1986; 164(5):1785–1790.

53. Pruksakorn S, Galbraith A, Houghten RA, Good MF. Conserved T and B cell epitopes on the M protein of group A streptococci. Induction of bactericidal antibodies. *J Immunol.* 1992;149:2729–2735.

54. Pruksakorn S, Currie B, Brandt E, et al. Identification of T cell autoepitopes that cross-react with the C-terminal segment of the M protein of group A streptococci. *Int Immunol.* 1994;6:1235–1244.

55. Dileepan T, Linehan JL, Moon JJ, Pepper M, Jenkins MK, Cleary PP. Robust antigen specific Th17 T cell response to group A Streptococcus is dependent on IL-6 and intra-nasal route of infection. *PLoS Pathogens.* 2011;7(9): e1002252.

56. Pepper M, Linehan JL, Pagan AJ, et al. Different routes of bacterial infection induce long-lived TH1 memory cells and short-lived TH17 cells. *Nat Immunol.* 2010;11(1): 83–89.

57. Wang B, Dileepan T, Briscoe S, et al. Induction of TGF-beta1 and TGF-beta1-dependent predominant Th17 differentiation by group A streptococcal infection. *Proc Natl Acad Sci USA.* 2010;107(13):5937–5942.

58. Weaver CT, Harrington LE, Mangan PR, Gavrieli M, Murphy KM. Th17: an effector CD4 T cell lineage with regulatory T cell ties. *Immunity.* 2006;24(6):677–688.

59. Weaver CT, Hatton RD, Mangan PR, Harrington LE. IL-17 family cytokines and the expanding diversity of effector T cell lineages. *Annu Rev Immunol.* 2007;25:821–852.

60. Peck A, Mellins ED. Precarious balance: Th17 cells in host defense. *Infect Immun.* 2010;78:32–38.

61. Cunningham MW. T regulatory cells: sentinels against autoimmune heart disease. *Circ Res.* 2006;99(10): 1024–1026.

62. Dileepan T, Smith ED, Knowland D, et al. Group A Streptococcus intranasal infection promotes CNS infiltration by streptococcal-specific Th17 cells. *J Clin Investig.* 2016; 126(1):303–317.

63. Bettelli E, Carrier Y, Gao W, et al. Reciprocal developmental pathways for the generation of pathogenic effector TH17 and regulatory T cells. *Nature.* 2006;441: 235–238.

64. Kuchroo VK, Das MP, Brown JA, et al. B7-1 and B7-2 costimulatory molecules activate differentially the Th1/Th2 developmental pathways: application to autoimmune disease therapy. *Cell.* 1995;80:707–718.

65. Mosman T, Coffman T. Th1 and Th2 cells: different patterns of lymphokine secretion lead to different functional properties. *Annu Rev Immunol.* 1989;7:145–173.

66. Cox CJ, Sharma M, Leckman JF, et al. Brain human monoclonal autoantibody from Sydenham chorea targets dopaminergic neurons in transgenic mice and signals dopamine d2 receptor: implications in human disease. *J Immunol.* 2013;191(11):5524–5541.

67. Brimberg L, Benhar I, Mascaro-Blanco A, et al. Behavioral, pharmacological, and immunological abnormalities after streptococcal exposure: a novel rat model of Sydenham chorea and related neuropsychiatric disorders. *Neuropsychopharmacology.* 2012;37(9): 2076–2087.

68. Lotan D, Benhar I, Alvarez K, et al. Behavioral and neural effects of intra-striatal infusion of anti-streptococcal antibodies in rats. *Brain Behav Immun.* 2014;38:249–262.

69. Hoffman KL, Hornig M, Yaddanapudi K, Jabado O, Lipkin WI. A murine model for neuropsychiatric disorders associated with group A beta-hemolytic streptococcal infection. *J Neurosci.* 2004;24(7):1780–1791.

70. Yaddanapudi K, Hornig M, Serge R, et al. Passive transfer of streptococcus-induced antibodies reproduces behavioral disturbances in a mouse model of pediatric autoimmune neuropsychiatric disorders associated with streptococcal infection. Mol Psychiatry; 15(7): 712-726.

71. Kirvan CA, Cox CJ, Swedo SE, Cunningham MW. Tubulin is a neuronal target of autoantibodies in Sydenham's chorea. *J Immunol.* 2007;178:7412–7421.

72. Kirvan CA, Swedo SE, Kurahara D, Cunningham MW. Streptococcal mimicry and antibody-mediated cell signaling in the pathogenesis of Sydenham's chorea. *Autoimmunity.* 2006;39(1):21–29.

73. Singer HS, Mascaro-Blanco A, Alvarez K, et al. Neuronal antibody biomarkers for Sydenham's chorea identify a new group of children with chronic recurrent episodic acute exacerbations of tic and obsessive compulsive symptoms following a streptococcal infection. *PLoS One.* 2015 (in press).

74. Kirvan CA, Galvin JE, Hilt S, Kosanke S, Cunningham MW. Identification of streptococcal m-protein cardiopathogenic epitopes in experimental autoimmune valvulitis. *J Cardiovasc Transl Res.* 2014;7(2):172–181.

75. Ben-Pazi H, Stoner JA, Cunningham MW. Dopamine receptor autoantibodies correlate with symptoms in sydenham's chorea. *PLoS One.* 2013;8(9):e73516.

76. Cutforth T, DeMille MM, Agalliu I, Agalliu D. CNS autoimmune disease after Streptococcus pyogenes infections: animal models, cellular mechanisms and genetic factors. *Future Neurol.* 2016;11(1):63–76.

77. McCarty M. Variation in the group specific carbohydrates of group A streptococci. II. Studies on the chemical basis for serological specificity of the carbohydrates. *J Exp Med.* 1956;104:629–643.

78. Messias Reason IJ, Schafranski MD, Jensenius JC, Steffensen R. The association between mannose-binding lectin gene polymorphism and rheumatic heart disease. *Hum Immunol.* 2006;67(12):991–998.

79. Ramasawmy R, Spina GS, Fae KC, et al. Association of mannose-binding lectin gene polymorphism but not of mannose-binding serine protease 2 with chronic severe aortic regurgitation of rheumatic etiology. *Clin Vaccine Immunol.* 2008;15(6):932–936.

80. Messias-Reason IJ, Schafranski MD, Kremsner PG, Kun JF. Ficolin 2 (FCN2) functional polymorphisms and the risk of rheumatic fever and rheumatic heart disease. *Clin Exp Immunol.* 2009;157(3):395–399.

81. Catarino SJ, Boldt AB, Beltrame MH, Nisihara RM, Schafranski MD, de Messias-Reason IJ. Association of

MASP2 polymorphisms and protein levels with rheumatic fever and rheumatic heart disease. *Hum Immunol.* 2014;75(12):1197–1202.

82. Guilherme L, Kohler KF, Postol E, Kalil J. Genes, autoimmunity, and pathogenesis of rheumatic heart disease. *Ann Pediatr Cardiol.* 2011;4:13–21.

83. Düzgün N, Duman T, Haydardedeoğlu FE, Tutkak H. Cytotoxic T lymphocyte-associated antigen-4 polymorphism in patients with rheumatic heart disease. *Tissue Antigens.* 2009;74(6):539–542.

84. Col-Araz N, Pehlivan S, Baspinar O, Sever T, Oguzkan-Balci S, Balat A. Association of macrophage migration inhibitory factor and mannose-binding lectin-2 gene polymorphisms in acute rheumatic fever. *Cardiol Young.* 2013;23(4):486–490.

85. Parks T, Mirabel M, Kado J, et al. Association between a common immunoglobulin heavy chain allele and rheumatic heart disease risk in Oceania. *Nat Commun.* 2017;8.

86. Gray LA, D'Antoine HA, Tong SYC, et al. Genome-wide analysis of genetic risk factors for rheumatic heart disease in aboriginal Australians provides support for pathogenic molecular mimicry. *J Infect Dis.* 2017;216(11):1460–1470.

87. Ayoub EM, Barrett DJ, Maclaren NK, Krischer JP. Association of class II human histocompatibility leukocyte antigens with rheumatic fever. *J Clin Investig.* 1986;77(6):2019–2026.

88. Maharaj B, Hammond MG, Appadoo B, Leary WP, Pudifin DJ. HLA-A, B, DR, and DQ antigens in black patients with severe chronic rheumatic heart disease. *Circulation.* 1987;76(2):259–261.

89. Monplaisir N, Valette I, Bach JF. HLA antigens in 88 cases of rheumatic fever observed in Martinique. *Tissue Antigens.* 1986;28(4):209–213.

90. Donadi EA, Smith AG, Louzada-Júnior P, Voltarelli JC, Nepom GT. HLA class I and class II profiles of patients presenting with Sydenham's chorea. *J Neurol.* 2000;247(2):122–128.

91. Hernández-Pacheco G, Aguilar-García J, Flores-Domínguez C, et al. MHC class II alleles in Mexican patients with rheumatic heart disease. *Int J Cardiol.* 2003;92(1):49–54.

92. Jhinghan B, Mehra NK, Reddy KS, Taneja V, Vaidya MC, Bhatia ML. HLA, blood groups and secretor status in patients with established rheumatic fever and rheumatic heart disease. *Tissue Antigens.* 1986;27(3):172–178.

93. Ozkan M, Carin M, Sönmez G, Senocak M, Ozdemir M, Yakut C. HLA antigens in Turkish race with rheumatic heart disease [see comment]. *Circulation.* 1993;87(6):1974–1978.

94. Anastasiou-Nana MI, Anderson JL, Carlquist JF, Nanas JN. HLA-DR typing and lymphocyte subset evaluation in rheumatic heart disease: a search for immune response factors. *Am Heart J.* 1986;112(5):992–997.

95. Rajapakse CN, Halim K, Al-Orainey I, Al-Nozha M, Al-Aska AK. A genetic marker for rheumatic heart disease. *Br Heart J.* 1987;58(6):659–662.

96. Olmez U, Turgay M, Ozenirler S, et al. Association of HLA class I and class II antigens with rheumatic fever in a Turkish population. *Scand J Rheumatol.* 1993;22(2):49–52.

97. Guédez Y, Kotby A, El-Demellawy M, et al. HLA class II associations with rheumatic heart disease are more evident and consistent among clinically homogeneous patients. *Circulation.* 1999;99(21):2784–2790.

98. Guilherme L, Weidebach W, Kiss MH, Snitcowsky R, Kalil J. Association of human leukocyte class II antigens with rheumatic fever or rheumatic heart disease in a Brazilian population. *Circulation.* 1991;83(6):1995–1998.

99. Visentainer JE, Pereira FC, Dalalio MM, Tsuneto LT, Donadio PR, Moliterno RA. Association of HLA-DR7 with rheumatic fever in the Brazilian population. *J Rheumatol.* 2000;27(6):1518–1520.

100. Haydardedeoğlu FE, Tutkak H, Köse K, Düzgün N. Genetic susceptibility to rheumatic heart disease and streptococcal pharyngitis: association with HLA-DR alleles. *Tissue Antigens.* 2006;68(4):293–296.

101. Stanevicha V, Eglite J, Sochnevs A, Gardovska D, Zavadska D, Shantere R. HLA class II associations with rheumatic heart disease among clinically homogeneous patients in children in Latvia. *Arthritis Res Ther.* 2003;5(6):R340–R346.

102. Koyanagi T, Koga Y, Nishi H, et al. DNA typing of HLA class II genes in Japanese patients with rheumatic heart disease. *J Mol Cell Cardiol.* 1996;28(6):1349–1353.

103. Manjula BN, Acharya AS, Mische SM, Fairwell T, Fischetti VA. The complete amino acid sequence of a biologically active 197-residue fragment of M protein isolated from type 5 group A streptococci. *J Biol Chem.* 1984;259(6):3686–3693.

104. Miller LC, Gray ED, Beachey EH, Kehoe MA. Antigenic variation among group A streptococcal M proteins: nucleotide sequence of the serotype 5 M protein gene and its' relationship with genes encoding types 6 and 24 M proteins. *J Biol Chem.* 1988;263:5668–5673.

CHAPTER 3

Clinical Evaluation and Diagnosis of Acute Rheumatic Fever

SCOTT DOUGHERTY • BRUNO NASCIMENTO • JONATHAN CARAPETIS

INTRODUCTION

The diagnosis of acute rheumatic fever (ARF) relies on a combination of clinical evaluation and laboratory studies. Diagnosis is usually made using the clinical criteria first formulated by T. Duckett Jones in 1944,[1] which have subsequently undergone multiple modifications, most recently in 2015.[2]

Acute fever and arthritis characterize the usual presentation of the disease, although in many patients it may not be acute, rheumatic, or febrile. Carditis and neurological manifestations may also be present or may emerge several months after the initial group A streptococcal (GAS) infection. Although the fleeting arthritis resolves without lasting damage, rheumatic carditis has a destructive effect on the heart valves, leading to the only chronic sequela of consequence in ARF: rheumatic heart disease (RHD). Severe RHD is associated with a number of important complications, including heart failure, stroke, atrial fibrillation, and infective endocarditis. The French physician Ernst-Charles Lasègue succinctly encapsulated the most important elements of ARF in 1884 when he said that "Pathologists have long known that rheumatic fever licks at the joints, but bites at the heart."

Although the Jones criteria have stood the test of time, the diagnostic process has not stood still. Marked shifts in ARF epidemiology, advances in echocardiography, and evidence that some clinical manifestations, such as joint involvement, are more variable than previously thought have all contributed to a significantly revised diagnostic landscape. In particular, the emergence of color-Doppler echocardiography in the 1990s led to a renaissance of new thinking in the subsequent 2 decades, highlighting the limitations of auscultation. National diagnostic guidelines from regions of the world where ARF remains endemic emerged,[3,4]

spearheading the development of new diagnostic standards that form the basis for how we think about ARF diagnosis in the 21st century. However, much work still lies ahead, particularly as we seek to bridge the gap between high RHD prevalence and low ARF incidence. New research is underway applying systems biology and genomics approaches to identify biological markers that could potentially allow for a precise and rapid diagnosis of ARF; either the holy grail is a single laboratory test for the diagnosis of ARF or at least an improvement to the Jones Criteria. Another advantage to these studies is that they will shine light on the immunological perturbations occurring in ARF, paving the way for clinical trials of immunotherapeutic agents that may ameliorate the cardiac valvular damage and prevent RHD.

This chapter will describe the detail of the clinical and laboratory manifestations of ARF. As alluded to above, there are many atypical scenarios and presentations. With this information, the reader can better understand the details of the diagnostic criteria and definitions in the second part of the chapter.

CLINICAL EVALUATION OF ACUTE RHEUMATIC FEVER

Careful diagnostic work-up is essential to make the diagnosis while excluding other etiologies. This may take some time. The importance of an accurate diagnosis of ARF is clear: overdiagnosis will expose the patient to the morbidity of lengthy treatment with 3-4 weekly penicillin injections, as well as potential harm from not being treated for their actual diagnosis; under diagnosis results in a missed opportunity for secondary prophylaxis, which in turn can lead to recurrent ARF and progressive RHD, with significant morbidity and early mortality.

Acute Rheumatic Fever and Rheumatic Heart Disease. https://doi.org/10.1016/B978-0-323-63982-8.00003-9

Risk Factors for Acute Rheumatic Fever

The clinical utility of any diagnostic criteria is dependent on the individual's pretest probability of having the disease and the background disease prevalence; careful consideration of any existing risk factors is therefore important when considering a diagnosis of ARF. The major established risk factors for ARF include frequency of exposure to GAS infection (throat and probably skin), age (the major period of vulnerability for ARF is between ages 4 and 20 years), host genetic factors (ARF is highly heritable but mechanisms are poorly understood), and poverty and social deprivation (leading to risk factors including poor quality housing and household crowding, malnutrition, and low utilization of and access to healthcare). These risk factors are discussed in detail in Chapter 1, and the clinical features of GAS infection are discussed in Chapter 10.

Without GAS there would be no ARF. In other words, exposure to GAS infection is essential for developing ARF. GAS pharyngitis has, until recently, been the only accepted cause of ARF, although contemporary epidemiological evidence suggests an association between GAS impetigo and ARF.[5] Many cases of GAS pharyngitis may be asymptomatic or cause only a mild sore throat. Older children and young adults are more likely to remember the pharyngitis (up to approximately 70% of patients) compared to young children (approximately 20% of patients), who therefore merit a higher index of suspicion when presenting with signs or symptoms consistent with ARF.[6]

CLINICAL FEATURES OF ACUTE RHEUMATIC FEVER

Following the initial GAS infection, there is usually a latency period during which the patient appears well before developing symptoms of ARF. This latency period, which is the same for initial as it is for recurrent attacks, averages 19 days in duration[7] with a range usually of 1–5 weeks,[8] although this may be significantly longer (up to 8 months) in those patients who develop isolated Sydenham chorea or indolent carditis.

The clinical profile of ARF is similar in all settings. The features that most often characterize ARF have been divided into major manifestations and minor manifestations. Clinical presentation may involve one or more of these manifestations, which can occur at various different points over the course of the illness: the mode of presentation can therefore be extremely variable (Box 3.1). Although classical descriptions

involve severe symptoms, particularly with joint pain and high fever, in some patients an episode may be asymptomatic or be so minor, resolving without intervention or with antiinflammatory medication, that affected individuals do not seek medical attention.

Major Manifestations

There are five major manifestations of ARF: joint symptoms (arthritis and arthralgia), carditis, chorea, and the skin manifestations erythema marginatum and subcutaneous nodules. These are termed "major" because they are relatively specific for ARF, although none is 100% specific.

Joint symptoms (arthritis and arthralgia)

Joint involvement is typically the presenting symptom of ARF. It is also the most common major manifestation, occurring in upwards of 75% of patients overall,[2,9,10] affecting almost all young adults, most teenagers (82%), and children (66%).[11] Joint involvement may qualify as a major manifestation or minor manifestation (see Diagnosis section).

Rheumatic joint involvement is notoriously variable, ranging from the classic migratory polyarthritis of large joints, to monoarthritis, polyarthralgia, and monoarthralgia. In the context of ARF, involvement of two or more joints is defined as polyarthritis. When joint symptoms are the sole major manifestation, the diagnosis of ARF may be problematic. Nevertheless, in

---

BOX 3.1
Modes of Presentation of Acute Rheumatic Fever

Acute presentations

Arthritis

Carditis

Subacute presentations

Sydenham chorea

Indolent carditis

Presentation with RHD

A large proportion of all ARF and RHD patients present with chronic RHD (40%–70% of cohort reports—see Chapters 5 and 6). Such patients have no known history or symptoms suggestive of ARF. This scenario is more common in poorer environments, where sequelae of RHD such as heart failure, stroke, infective endocarditis, and atrial fibrillation may be the first presentation of ARF or RHD.

RHD rheumatic heart disease; ARF acute rheumatic fever

patients from medium- to high-risk populations, ARF should always be included in the differential diagnosis of children and young adults presenting with arthritis and/or arthralgia.

The key to diagnosis is a detailed history and examination. It may take some time for the joint involvement to fully manifest (e.g., a monoarthritis on presentation may evolve into a polyarthritis several days later). Joint pain in ARF is usually asymmetrical, with a predilection for large joints including the knees, ankles, hips, elbows, and wrists (the leg joints are usually affected first). The small joints of the hands, feet, and spine are occasionally involved in ARF.

Rheumatic arthritis is usually extremely painful, often limiting movement and is often out of proportion to objective local signs of inflammation such as joint swelling, erythema, and increased temperature.[12] Any child who refuses to put any weight on the affected limb is however a "red flag" for serious illness, such as infection (e.g., septic arthritis) or malignancy (e.g., leukemia)—see Differential Diagnosis. A history of inability to walk due to hip pain is regarded by some guidelines[4] as arthritis, even if the signs of arthritis have resolved. The joint inflammation is characteristically transient, quickly disappearing from each joint often over a period of hours or just a few days and then appearing in another joint. Classically, multiple joints are often affected in quick succession, termed migratory arthritis. If subsequent joints are involved while preceding ones are still inflamed this can be termed "additive" polyarthritis, although this pattern is less specific to ARF than migratory polyarthritis. Joint involvement may number 6–16 in untreated patients.[11]

Polyarthralgia, although very common and highly nonspecific in low-risk populations, is considered a major manifestation in high-risk populations where it is more specific for ARF. The same applies to monoarthritis and monoarthralgia, which are both common manifestations of ARF in these populations. For example, aseptic monoarthritis was a major manifestation in 19% of high-risk children in Australia.[13] It is important however to first exclude septic arthritis in those who present with monoarthritis before diagnosing ARF. Close liaison with orthopedic colleagues may be necessary. The synovial fluid white cell count in joints affected by ARF contains 10,000–100,000 white blood cells/mm^3 (mostly neutrophils), while a count of >100,000 cells/mm^3 significantly increases the likelihood of the diagnosis of septic arthritis.[14] Other findings on synovial fluid analysis in rheumatic arthritis include a protein concentration of approximately 4 g/dL, normal glucose levels, and presence of a mucin clot.

Aspirin, naproxen, ibuprofen and other NSAIDs, and corticosteroids often produce a dramatic improvement in joint symptoms. The arthritis of ARF is so responsive to NSAIDs that rapid resolution is strongly supportive of the diagnosis of ARF. Conversely, if there is no improvement within 72 h of starting antiinflammatories, an alternative diagnosis should be considered. In patients who present with monoarthritis or monoarthralgia, it is important to withhold NSAIDs, instead using paracetamol or codeine for pain relief, to prevent masking any evolution of joint symptoms.[3,4] NSAIDs can be commenced once a second joint is involved, and the diagnosis is clear. Monoarthritis is now accepted as a major manifestation of ARF whether or not NSAIDs have been prescribed.[2–4] The indiscriminate use of NSAIDs in some low- and middle-income countries (LMICs) may in part be responsible for the apparent fall in incidence of ARF in these populations.

There is no evidence that temporarily withholding antiinflammatory therapy leads to worse outcomes. The only long-term sequela of rheumatic arthritis is Jaccoud arthropathy, although this is very rare. Originally thought to be associated only with ARF, Jaccoud arthropathy has since been shown to also occur with systemic lupus erythematosus (SLE), Sjögren syndrome, scleroderma, dermatomyositis, psoriatic arthritis, vasculitis, and ankylosing spondylitis.[15]

An episode of ARF lasts for approximately 3 months on average when unaltered by antiinflammatory medication. In most treated patients, the polyarthritis is severe for less than 1 week in two-thirds of cases and continues for another 1–2 weeks in the remainder before resolving completely. Symptoms persisting beyond 4 weeks should trigger a search for alternative pathologies, including juvenile idiopathic arthritis or SLE. Chronic ARF occurs in fewer than 5% of cases and is defined as the presence of active symptoms for more than 6 months.[11,16]

Carditis

Rheumatic carditis is the most important prognostic factor in ARF because carditis can evolve to chronic RHD. Depending on whether the diagnosis is made based on clinical assessment alone, or combined with echocardiography, the incidence of carditis during an initial attack of ARF ranges from 40% to 91%.[17–20] In the 1951 Bland and Duckett review of 1000 patients with ARF,[21] 65% were diagnosed with carditis and in the 1987 outbreak of ARF in Utah in the United States,[22] 91% had carditis when clinical examination was combined with echocardiographic evaluation. More recent studies that report both clinical and subclinical carditis show similar rates of carditis: for example, 85% of 66 children with definite or probable ARF had carditis.[23] In general, the younger the patient the higher the incidence of carditis during an episode of ARF.

Carditis can be found at presentation along with fever and arthritis although it often appears within 2–4 weeks of the acute illness, highlighting the importance of repeatedly examining the patient after initial presentation. The clinical findings of rheumatic carditis can be variable, ranging in severity from mild subclinical involvement (up to 53%)[24] to severe carditis (20%), leading to acute heart failure.[17] Death is also a rare but well-described complication of the acute illness. In most of those who present with ARF for the first time, however, carditis tends not to be severe: a New Zealand study of true first episodes of ARF found that severe carditis occurred in <10% of such patients.[25] In those with recurrent ARF, carditis almost invariably recurs if the initial episode involved the heart, and with each episode the cumulative heart valve damage can worsen. Internationally, acute carditis on chronic RHD may be as common as a true first episode of ARF. However, this chapter focuses on first episodes of ARF not chronic RHD.

Rheumatic carditis may involve all layers of the heart, including the pericardium (pericarditis), myocardium (myocarditis), and endocardium (endocarditis), hence some descriptions of rheumatic carditis use the term "pancarditis." It is worth emphasizing that the endocarditis part of rheumatic carditis is inflammatory and not infective in origin and is characterized by inflammation of the left-sided heart valves, leading to acute or subacute valvular regurgitation (valvulitis). Given that the term endocarditis is potentially confusing in this context, it should be avoided and valvulitis used instead.

Pericarditis and myocarditis rarely, if ever, occur without concomitant valvulitis.[2] Therefore, a diagnosis of rheumatic carditis should be reevaluated if clinical features of pericarditis or myocarditis occur in the absence of valvulitis.

Infrequently, carditis can also develop more subtly over several months after the GAS infection (known as indolent (insidious onset) carditis), and may be the only presenting feature of ARF. Indolent carditis is characterized by a subacute illness of several weeks or months with severe cardiac involvement and little or no joint symptoms. The presentation is with subacute heart failure in many cases. Younger children may have cardiac cachexia with weight loss.[4] In those patients with severe heart failure, heart valve surgery may be contraindicated due to severely impaired left ventricular function, with heart transplantation the only surgical option.[4]

Rheumatic Valvulitis. Valvulitis is the sine qua non of rheumatic carditis. It manifests as mitral regurgitation (MR) or aortic regurgitation (AR), or both, either clinically by detection of a corresponding murmur (Box 3.2) or subclinically by echocardiography (see next section). The mitral valve is almost always affected in rheumatic valvulitis, with the aortic valve also involved in up to one-third of cases. Isolated aortic valvulitis only occurs in 2% of patients and right-sided valvulitis only occurs in combination with the

---

BOX 3.2
Cardiac Examination in Rheumatic Valvulitis.

It is important to remember that clinical findings associated with acute valve regurgitation (e.g., in the setting of ARF) often differ significantly from those findings in chronic valve regurgitation (e.g., in setting of RHD)

Mitral Regurgitation. On palpation, the arterial pulse may be rapid and of low amplitude and the left ventricular impulse prominent with severe MR. On auscultation, acute MR may be detected as a blowing, pansystolic murmur that radiates to the back or axilla. It may also be short and soft, or may even be inaudible, owing to the rapid equilibration of left atrial and ventricular pressures. The murmur is best heard at the apex with the patient in the left lateral decubitus position using the diaphragm of the stethoscope. The murmur of rheumatic MR usually radiates to the axilla due to the posteriorly directed jet of MR secondary to AMVL prolapse. Less frequently, isolated PMVL prolapse occurs leading to an anteriorly directed jet of MR and this murmur is loudest at the lower left sternal edge. The most reliable auscultatory finding indicating a high regurgitant volume (severe MR) and left ventricular volume overload is a left-sided S3 gallop.

Carey Coombs Murmur. This middiastolic murmur is indicative of severe MR and is caused by increased blood flow across the mitral valve as a result of the high regurgitant volume. It is typically a short, middiastolic rumble and can be differentiated from the murmur of mitral stenosis by absence of an opening snap.

Aortic Regurgitation. On palpation, the typical signs of chronic aortic regurgitation, indicative of a hyperdynamic circulation, may be absent in acute aortic regurgitation. On auscultation, there is an early diastolic murmur best heart at the left sternal border that is low-pitched, quiet, and short (or sometimes inaudible in very severe regurgitation), due to rapid equilibration of aortic and left ventricular diastolic pressures. The murmur may be accentuated by asking the patient to sit up and lean forward while holding their breath after expiration. AR may also be difficult to define in the presence of tachycardia.

ARF acute rheumatic fever; RHD rheumatic heart disease; MR mitral regurgitation; AMVL anterior mitral valve leaflet; PMVL posterior mitral valve leaflet

left[26]: therefore, carditis cannot be diagnosed on the basis of right-sided regurgitation alone. It is also important to rule out volume and pressure overload from left-sided lesions before attributing even moderate tricuspid regurgitation to valvulitis.[4] Stenotic valvular lesions do not occur as part of the acute illness but occur after the transition from rheumatic carditis to the chronic valvular changes that define RHD, which evolve over months to years following one or more episodes of ARF.

In addition to acute/subacute valvular regurgitation, cardiomegaly and heart failure make up the three most common clinical manifestations of valvulitis.[3] Each of these features can be used to assess the severity of rheumatic carditis (Table 3.1), which helps guide appropriate medical and surgical management and determine the duration of secondary prophylaxis in the long term. In patients with both right- and left-sided lesions, diagnostic severity is determined by the left-sided lesion.[4]

Valvulitis may not always be evident at presentation. Those who do subsequently go on to develop valvulitis usually do so within 2 weeks[27] or, at the latest, within 4 weeks.[25] Therefore, if the initial echocardiogram is negative or equivocal, a second echocardiogram should be performed within 2–4 weeks of presentation to confidently exclude rheumatic valvulitis.

Subclinical carditis. Echocardiographic-based studies over the last 20 years have also revealed that a considerable number of patients with rheumatic valvulitis (up to 53%) do not have a murmur.[24] This has given rise to the term *subclinical carditis*, which refers exclusively to the circumstance where a patient is found to have pathological MR and/or AR on echocardiography but where classic auscultatory findings are not present or are not recognized by the examining clinician.[2]

The clinical course of subclinical carditis is similar to mild carditis detected by a murmur. A 2007 meta-analysis that included 23 studies from around the world showed that echocardiographic findings persisted or progressed in 44.7% of patients diagnosed with subclinical carditis.[28] Therefore, although a murmur remains an important manifestation of valvulitis, it is no longer the only means of diagnosing carditis: both clinical and subclinical carditis are now considered a major criterion of ARF by the American Heart Association[2] in both low- and moderate-to-high-risk settings (see Diagnosis of Acute Rheumatic Fever).

Pericarditis. Acute pericarditis often appears 7–10 days after the initial fever and arthritis and occurs in approximately 15% of patients.[29] Pericarditis should

TABLE 3.1
Grading the Severity of Rheumatic Carditis.

Severity	Clinical Features
Mild carditis	Mild mitral and/or aortic regurgitation clinically[a] and/or by echocardiography (see Table 3.6 for minimal echocardiographic criteria) No clinical evidence of heart failure and no cardiac chamber enlargement on echocardiography, CXR, or ECG
Moderate carditis	Any mitral or aortic valve lesion of moderate severity on clinical examination[a] **or** cardiac chamber enlargement seen on echocardiogram **or** any mitral or aortic valve lesion graded as moderate on echocardiogram • mitral regurgitation: Broad high-intensity proximal jet filling half the left atrium **or** a lesser volume high-intensity jet producing prominent blunting of pulmonary venous inflow • aortic regurgitation: The diameter of the regurgitant jet is 15%–30% of the diameter of the left ventricular outflow tract with flow reversal of the upper descending aorta
Severe carditis	Any impending or previous cardiac surgery **or** any valve lesion graded as severe on clinical examination[a] **or** any valve lesion associated with significant cardiomegaly or heart failure **or** any valve lesion graded as severe on echocardiogram • In children: Abnormal regurgitant color and Doppler flow pattern in pulmonary veins (mitral regurgitation) and Doppler reversal in the lower descending aorta (severe aortic regurgitation) • In adults: Doppler flow reversal in the pulmonary veins (severe MR) **or** abdominal aorta (for severe AR) are specific, if present, but can be more difficult to detect and their absence does not exclude severe regurgitation if not detected.

CXR chest X-ray; ECG electrocardiogram; MR mitral regurgitation; AR aortic regurgitation
[a] Clinical evaluation of the severity of valve lesions in discussed in detail in Chapter 5
Reproduced with permission from New Zealand[4] Heart Foundation

be suspected if the patient complains of chest pain or is found to have a friction rub or muffled heart sounds. The friction rub can mask cardiac murmurs. The early ECG changes that often characterize pericarditis (i.e., diffuse concave upward ST elevation with upright T waves and PR segment depression) are usually absent in rheumatic pericarditis.

The chest pain is usually precordial or retrosternal and may radiate to involve the trapezius ridge (bottom portion of the scapula), neck, left shoulder, or left arm. The chest pain is typically exacerbated on lying down or during inspiration and relieved by sitting up and bending forward. Rheumatic pericarditis may result in a pericardial effusion, which is usually small to moderate in size and only very rarely leads to cardiac tamponade (see Chapter 16). Constrictive pericarditis is also a very rare complication of ARF.[30]

Myocarditis. Rheumatic myocarditis is often asymptomatic. Different from many other forms of myocarditis, rheumatic myocarditis does not lead to impaired ventricular function in the absence of valvulitis[31] and does not produce elevated serum cardiac troponins.[32] Instead, the left ventricular enlargement and systolic dysfunction associated with severe carditis is secondary to volume overload from acute valve dysfunction. If troponins are elevated, this should raise suspicion of an alternative diagnosis such as viral myocarditis (see Differential Diagnosis (later) and Chapter 16).

Chorea

Rheumatic chorea, also known as Sydenham chorea or St Vitus' dance, is characterized by purposeless, involuntary movements of the trunk or extremities. Chorea is a neuropsychiatric disorder that occurs in 10%–30% of patients who have had ARF.[2] It is the most common form of acquired chorea in childhood (accounting for up to 96% of cases), most commonly occurring in those aged between 5 and 13 years and is rare after the age of 20 years.[33,34] Females are more frequently affected than males by a ratio of 2:1.[33]

Sydenham chorea has the longest latency period of all ARF manifestations, presenting 1–8 months after the initial GAS infection.[35] As a consequence, it only features as part of the acute illness in 5%–10% of patients, where it may be associated with other disease manifestations, although joint symptoms and chorea seldom occur simultaneously due to disparities in their respective latency periods. In other patients, it may be the only manifestation of ARF, developing several weeks to months after the acute illness when other features of the disease have typically disappeared. For this reason, chorea is considered a stand-alone criterion

for establishing the diagnosis of ARF, but only when other differential diagnoses have been excluded. Sydenham chorea is also commonly associated with carditis (28%–63% of cases),[36,37] regardless of the presence of cardiac murmurs. As with all patients suspected of having ARF, echocardiography should therefore be performed and the finding of subclinical carditis by echocardiography will support the diagnosis of chorea as a manifestation of ARF.

Sydenham chorea is characterized by chorea (involuntary, brief, jerky, uncoordinated movements of the limbs and face), hypotonia (which may be diffuse), emotional liability, and psychiatric manifestations. The caudate nucleus in the basal ganglia is involved and so there is no pyramidal tract or sensory involvement. Symptoms are often bilateral, although are frequently more marked on one side and are unilateral (hemichorea) in 20%–30% of cases.[33,38] Movements are accentuated by purposeful movement, excitement, and emotional stress, and disappear during sleep. Sometimes the movements are subtle and intermittent and might only be observed after a short period of observation. In severe cases, the chorea may impair the ability to eat and increase the risk of injury, requiring medication (see Chapter 4, Management of Acute Rheumatic Fever).

Speech can be explosive and dysarthric and the individual often has trouble counting rapidly. The tongue is sometimes said to resemble a "bag of worms" on inspection and some patients may demonstrate motor impersistence, involuntarily withdrawing the tongue when asked to protrude it for 30 s (known as a "darting tongue"). Facial involvement often leads to erratic movements that resemble grimaces, grins, and frowns. The handwriting can be clumsy and is a good objective means of monitoring the course of the disease. When examining the hands, there are three specific signs to look for:

1. *Milkmaid's grip:* when asked to grip the physician's fingers, the patient is unable to maintain grip, resulting in rhythmic squeezing and is another manifestation of motor impersistence
2. *Spooning sign:* flexion of the wrists and extension of the fingers when the hands are extended
3. *Pronator sign:* the arms and palms turn outwards (pronate) when the arm is held above the head

Psychiatric and cognitive disorders, such as attention deficit hyperactivity disorder and anxiety, are also commonly associated with Sydenham chorea and early recognition of these symptoms may aid in the management of the disorder.[39] Mental status however is usually normal and a confusional state suggests an alternative diagnosis, such as encephalitis.

Restlessness and abnormal behavior, such as easy crying and irritability and inappropriate laughing are also observed. In rare cases, patients may develop a transient psychosis, which can present many years after the initial onset of chorea symptoms. Not unsurprisingly, there is often a high burden of distress for the patient and their family, with missed school days and poor school performance, or self-isolation due to embarrassment, causing a significant reduction in functionality. However, no cases of permanent serious neurological deficits have been observed.

The manifestations of chorea may also wax and wane over its course, often during times of intercurrent illness and stress. It usually resolves gradually and the median duration of symptoms is 12—15 weeks,[7,40] although rarely symptoms may last 2—3 years.[36,41] Of all the ARF manifestations, chorea is one most likely to recur, doing so in 15%—30% of cases and usually within 2—3 years.[36,42] In most patients, recurrence is usually due to a repeat GAS infection. Some recurrences may occur despite faithful adherence to penicillin prophylaxis,[43,44] while other episodes may be seen with pregnancy (chorea gravidarum) or the oral contraceptive pill, suggesting a relation to hormonal factors.

Erythema Marginatum
Erythema marginatum is usually an evanescent, pink rash seen with pale centers and rounded or serpiginous margins.[2] This is a rare and difficult to detect manifestation, particularly in dark-skinned patients, hence careful inspection is required. Although estimates vary, it is usually observed in <6% of patients with ARF.[2] When present, it usually occurs early in the course of the illness but may also occur during recovery. It may also persist or recur after all other manifestations have resolved. It rarely occurs in isolation and is usually associated with carditis. Therefore, ARF should almost never be diagnosed on the basis of erythema marginatum alone[2] without the presence of other major criteria.

It is a distinctive rash and is neither painful nor pruritic. It appears as bright pink, slightly raised macules or papules that blanch under pressure. They are seen initially on the trunk and proximal ends of the extremities and never on the face. The lesions begin as a macule and expand centrifugally with central clearing (Fig. 3.1). Rapid migration (up to 2—10 mm in 12 h) is a characteristic feature of this rash and this movement can be documented with the use of ink markers on the skin (Fig. 3.2). The macules may be oval, ring, or crescentic shaped and the outer edge of the lesions is usually sharp whereas the inner edge is diffuse. The macules can fuse and coalesce to form a serpiginous pattern, and when circular, the rash

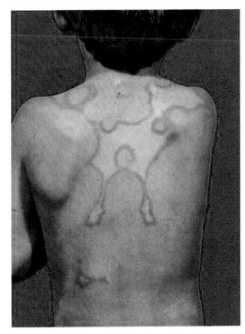

FIG. 3.1 Erythema marginatum in acute rheumatic fever demonstrating the characteristic pink rash with pale centres. Some of the margins are rounded while others are serpiginous. (Courtesy of Professor Mike South, Royal Children's Hospital, Melbourne; used with permission.)

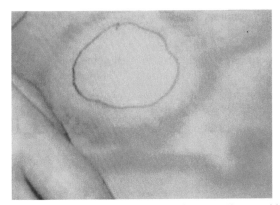

FIG. 3.2 Erythema marginatum demonstrating rapid migration: the pen mark shows the location of the rash around 60 min earlier. (Courtesy of Professor Mike South, Royal Children's Hospital, Melbourne; used with permission.)

is known as erythema annulare. It should not be confused with the circinate (circular) rash of Lyme disease, erythema chronicum migrans.

The rash may be characteristically evanescent, disappearing over a matter of hours and reappearing intermittently over the course of weeks, months, or even years; some lesions may appear and then disappear before the examiner's eyes, appearing like "smoke rings" beneath the skin. It may be more apparent or reappear after a warm shower or bath and it is not affected by antiinflammatory medication.

Subcutaneous Nodules

Similar to erythema marginatum, these are also rare, occurring in less than 2% of patients with ARF.[2] When present, they are highly specific for ARF but, similar to erythema marginatum, they rarely appear as a sole manifestation of the illness and should be accompanied by additional major criteria to establish a diagnosis of ARF. They are strongly associated with severe carditis and usually appear 1–2 weeks after the illness starts, lasting usually 1–2 weeks but rarely longer than a month.

The nodules are firm, round, painless, and freely mobile, usually 0.5–2.0 cm in diameter and are typically located over extensor surfaces (near bony prominences or tendons) of the elbows, wrists, knees, ankles, Achilles tendon, occiput, and the spinous processes of the thoracic and lumbar vertebrae (Fig. 3.3). The overlying skin is not inflamed. They are usually symmetrical and occur in crops of up to 12, but the average number is 3–4. The nodules of ARF may resemble those seen in rheumatoid arthritis, although the former are smaller and shorter lived. Although nodules most commonly occur on the elbow in both conditions, ARF nodules occur more commonly on the olecranon whereas rheumatoid nodules tend to be found 3–4 cm distally.[45]

Minor Manifestations

The four minor manifestations used in the diagnosis of ARF are as follows: fever, arthralgia, elevated acute phase

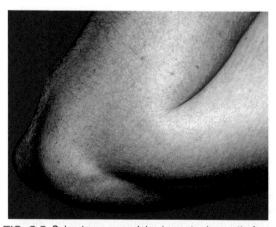

FIG. 3.3 Subcutaneous nodules in acute rheumatic fever located over the bony prominence of the extensor surface of the elbow. (Reproduced with permission from Beerman LB et al.[45a])

reactants (erythrocyte sedimentation rate, C-reactive protein, and white cell count), and first-degree heart block.

Fever

Most episodes of ARF are accompanied by fever (>90% of cases), unless the patient has taken antipyretics or presents with subacute or late-presenting manifestations, such as Sydenham chorea or indolent carditis. The fever may rise as high as 40°C, although there is no characteristic pattern and diurnal variations are common. Similar to arthritis and arthralgia, fever should respond rapidly to antiinflammatory treatment, usually decreasing within 1 week and rarely lasting more than 4 weeks. Documented fever before admission is also acceptable as a minor criterion, particularly if the patient has taken NSAIDs or paracetamol, which may suppress the fever.

Arthralgia

It is important to differentiate arthralgia from arthritis. In patients with ARF, several joints (polyarthralgia) are usually affected, although monoarthralgia may also be seen. Rheumatic polyarthralgia usually affects joints in the same pattern as rheumatic polyarthritis: that is, it is migratory, asymmetrical, and predominantly affects the large joints. If this pattern is not observed, alternative diagnoses should be considered. It is worth remembering that polyarthralgia and monoarthralgia are common in many other rheumatological and nonrheumatological disorders.

Elevated Acute Phase Reactants

Most guidelines, including the Jones criteria, recommend measuring the erythrocyte sedimentation rate (ESR) and/or the C-reactive protein (CRP) as part of the diagnostic work-up of ARF. The WHO diagnostic criteria differ slightly and recommend ESR and peripheral white blood cell (WBC) count.[46] The ESR and CRP are usually elevated in patients presenting with ARF (except in those with isolated Sydenham chorea), whereas Australian data showed that the WBC count is elevated ($>15 \times 10^9$/L) in only 25% of patients during an acute episode and is therefore much less sensitive for inflammation.[47]

The magnitude of the ESR is proportional to the degree of the inflammatory response. Most episodes of ARF produce an ESR >60 mm/h,[2] although antiinflammatories can reduce this figure. If there is concomitant heart failure, the ESR may also be decreased whereas the CRP may be elevated. The CRP is a direct measure of inflammation and typically rises and falls before the ESR (an indirect measure of inflammation) and thus may be a more precise reflection of the patient's rheumatic activity. The ESR might remain elevated for 3–6 months following recovery and chronic elevation (>6 months) is occasionally seen but poorly understood.[16]

First-Degree Heart Block

First-degree heart block is observed in 20%–60% of cases of ARF. In addition to valvulitis, it is a manifestation of carditis and is due to inflammation around the atrioventricular (AV) node as a consequence of myocarditis. First-degree heart block is due to delayed conduction from the atrium to the ventricle, defined as a prolonged age-adjusted PR interval (Table 3.2). It cannot be detected from history or examination alone and diagnosis is best confirmed using a 12-lead ECG, which should be performed on every patient suspected of having ARF.

First-degree heart block is almost universally benign and is occasionally a normal variant, often related to parasympathetic tone. Up to one-third of patients with uncomplicated GAS infections are also found to have first-degree heart block.[49] In the context of rheumatic carditis, any first-degree heart block should therefore be transient to distinguish from the normal variant. A prolonged PR interval on presentation that resolves over the following days to weeks may therefore be a useful clinical sign in patients whose symptoms were equivocal for ARF. If the PR interval has not normalized after 2 weeks, it is useful to repeat the ECG again after 1–2 months.[3,4]

Higher degrees of heart block and other arrhythmias are also occasionally observed in rheumatic carditis (Fig. 3.4). First-degree heart block may lead to an accelerated junctional rhythm, which has been detected in 9.4%–20% of ECGs from children with ARF[50,51] and may be a highly specific finding when present.[52] Second-degree heart block (2.6%) and rarely third-degree heart block (0.6%) may also complicate ARF.[50] Very rarely, patients with ARF may also present with syncope (1 of 508 pts[50]) or develop ventricular asystole, requiring temporary transvenous pacing. Interestingly, the echocardiograms of some of these patients revealed only minimal left-sided regurgitant lesions,[53] suggesting features of myocarditis with conduction system disease may dominate in rare circumstances.[53] Other conduction abnormalities reported in association with ARF include ventricular tachycardia, right and left bundle branch block, brady-tachyarrhythmia, and ventricular premature complexes. The larger case series reported that patients with advanced AV block or accelerated rhythm all reverted to sinus rhythm during convalescence.[50,53]

OTHER CLINICAL MANIFESTATIONS OF ACUTE RHEUMATIC FEVER

In the original 1944 Jones criteria,[1] epistaxis and abdominal pain were both considered minor criteria, although both were removed (due to lack of specificity) in the subsequent 1956 modification and have

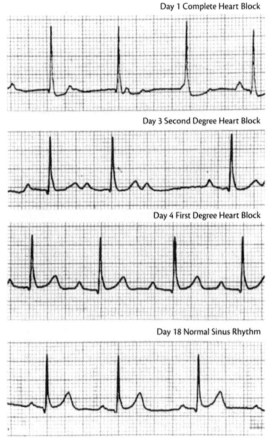

FIG. 3.4 Heart block in rheumatic carditis demonstrating complete heart block early in the disease, with improvement to secondary then first-degree heart block before return to sinus rhythm. (Reproduced from Bishop W et al.[53a])

TABLE 3.2	
Upper Limits of Normal of the PR Interval.	
Age (years)	**Duration (seconds)**
3–12	0.16
12–16	0.18
≥17	0.20

Adapted from Park MK.[48]

been absent since.[54] However, it is important to be aware that about 5% of patients with ARF will develop these features.[46] Particularly important is abdominal pain that can appear hours to days before the major manifestations and may mimic other acute abdominal conditions. The pain may be severe, is often epigastric or periumbilical, may be associated with guarding, and is sometimes indistinguishable from acute appendicitis.

Pulmonary manifestations ("rheumatic pneumonia") are also observed occasionally, usually in association with carditis and, like epistaxis and abdominal pain, were a minor criterion in the original Jones criteria. The clinical spectrum varies from mild (dyspnoea and nonproductive cough) to fulminant, with a variety of radiological patterns observed, including focal consolidation, diffuse bilateral infiltrates, pleural effusion, and confluent nodular lesions.[55,56] There are no specific diagnostic criteria for rheumatic pneumonia and it is likely that multiple etiologies contribute to this umbrella term, either as part of the rheumatic process (in which case steroids may help), or secondary to acute heart failure, uraemia, or intercurrent infection. Other less common clinical features include mild elevations of plasma transaminase levels and microscopic haematuria, pyuria, or proteinuria. Full blood count (FBC) may show a normochromic, normocytic anemia.

DIAGNOSTIC INVESTIGATIONS FOR ACUTE RHEUMATIC FEVER

The standard investigations used in the diagnostic work-up of ARF, when available, should include: select blood tests (FBC, ESR, CRP) and ECG (discussed earlier); and laboratory confirmation of a preceding GAS infection, Chest X-ray (CXR), and echocardiography (discussed here) (Table 3.3). Other nonroutine investigations may be required depending on the clinical picture and differential diagnoses being considered but typically include additional blood testing (e.g., rheumatology immunology, viral serology, ceruloplasmin levels), joint X-ray or ultrasound scan, and magnetic resonance imaging (MRI) of the brain and heart (Table 3.4).

Laboratory Evidence of a Preceding Group A Streptococcus Infection

Along with the major and minor manifestations, laboratory demonstration of a preceding GAS infection is a fundamental component of the diagnostic work-up of

patients suspected of ARF and is the keystone on which the Jones criteria rest (with exceptions, see later).

Laboratory confirmation of a preceding GAS infection can be achieved by three different means: throat culture, rapid antigen detection testing (RADT), or streptococcal serology.[2] It is important to note that because GAS can also exist in the throat in the carrier state, a positive throat culture or RADT result does not necessarily confirm active GAS infection. In contrast, serology testing, which measures the antibodies produced against GAS (antistreptococcal antibodies), tends to produce low antistreptococcal titers in the carrier state compared to GAS infection.

The usefulness of each test however is most dependent on the timing of the patient's presentation. Because it takes 2–3 weeks for the immune system to produce antistreptococcal antibodies, serology testing is often negative during the acute GAS infection and so culture and RADT are often more useful. However, because patients usually present with ARF several weeks after the infection that triggered it, detection of GAS is usually no longer possible whereas the antistreptococcal antibodies have often appeared by this time (throat cultures are only positive in approximately 25% of patients who present with ARF).[58,59] Streptococcal serology is therefore the most helpful test in the diagnosis of ARF.

Throat Culture

The gold standard for diagnosis of GAS pharyngitis is a positive throat culture. When performed correctly, it has a sensitivity of 90%–95% in detecting GAS.[60] Specimens should be obtained from the surface of both tonsils and the posterior pharyngeal wall. Other areas of the oropharynx are not acceptable.[6]

The sample should be cultured on a sheep-blood agar plate and incubated at 35–37°C for 18–24 h before reading. It is advisable to incubate for an additional 24 h if no growth is seen on the initial inspection before confirming a negative result. It is not possible to differentiate true GAS infection from the GAS carrier state based on the number of GAS colonies seen on the culture plate but generally patients with GAS pharyngitis are likely to have a more strongly positive culture. False-negative results may occur if the patient was treated with antibiotics shortly before the sample was collected.[6]

Rapid Antigen Detection Testing

RADT allows the identification of GAS pharyngitis directly from throat swabs and provides results within

TABLE 3.3
Investigations Used in the Diagnosis of Acute Rheumatic Fever.

RECOMMENDED FOR ALL CASES OF SUSPECTED ARF

Test	Result
ESR	≥30 mm/h (moderate- and high-risk populations) or ≥60 mm/h (low-risk populations) fulfills the minor criterion for elevated acute phase reactants.
CRP	≥3 mg/dL (≥28.57 nmol/L) fulfills the minor criterion for elevated acute phase reactants.
FBC	The white blood count is an insensitive marker of inflammation and only the WHO criteria[57] count it as a minor manifestation; FBC may show a normocytic normochromic anemia.
Blood culture	Should be requested if febrile and may prove useful if the patient has sepsis from an alternative diagnosis.
Throat culture/RADT	One of these tests should be performed in all patients to detect GAS in the throat. If a highly specific RADT is available a positive test can be considered confirmatory, but a negative test should be confirmed with throat culture, unless a validated molecular-based test is used..
Streptococcal serology	To seek evidence of antecedent GAS infection. Paired titers for ASO and ADB (12–28 days between acute titers and convalescent titers) are recommended. Single value acute titers above ULN can also be used, but local ULN values should ideally be available.
ECG	An age-adjusted (see main text) prolonged PR interval is a minor manifestation of carditis. Should be performed at initial assessment and, if the PR interval is prolonged, then repeated several weeks/months later to confirm resolution. Occasionally, higher degree of heart block or other arrhythmias are seen.
CXR	Important in patients with suspected carditis, looking for cardiomegaly and evidence of heart failure.
Echocardiogram	Important for **all patients**, even in the absence of a murmur. Allows for the detection of pathological mitral and/or aortic regurgitation and assessment of left ventricular size and function. Can also rule out other causes of cardiac murmur and exclude pericardial effusion.

ARF acute rheumatic fever; ESR erythrocyte sedimentation rate; CRP C-reactive protein; FBC full blood count; WHO World Health Organisation; RADT rapid antigen detection test; GAS group A streptococcus; ASO antistreptolysin O antibodies; ADB antideoxyribonuclease B antibodies; ULN upper limit of normal; ECG electrocardiogram; CXR chest X-ray

minutes. Rapid detection of GAS pharyngitis is advantageous because it allows prompt initiation of antibiotic therapy. Not only does this reduce the risk of poststreptococcal sequelae (ARF or poststreptococcal glomerulonephritis), it also provides relief of symptoms, reduces the risk of suppurative complications (such as peritonsillar abscess or cervical lymphadenitis), and reduces transmission rates.

There are several different testing kits, most of which use antibodies for the detection of group A carbohydrate antigen. More recent tests use molecular methods including nucleic acid amplification, and are reported to be highly sensitive and specific. Traditional RADT tests are highly specific, generally 95% or higher (when compared with standard throat culture), and false positive results are unusual.[61–63] The sensitivity however is lower at 70%–90%.[61,62] Therefore, if the RADT is positive, the patient can be treated for GAS pharyngitis without the need for throat culture but if the test is negative, a throat culture should be obtained, except if a validated molecular test is used.[6] Similar to throat cultures, RADT is often negative in patients who present with ARF.

Streptococcal Serology
The highest level of evidence of a recent streptococcal infection is by streptococcal serology as discussed eloquently in the 1992 AHA guidelines update.[58] Antistreptococcal antibodies are highly sensitive for previous GAS infection in the setting of ARF.[59] Antibodies are made in response to a whole host of streptococcal

TABLE 3.4
Tests for Differential Diagnoses of Acute Rheumatic Fever.

RECOMMENDED TESTS DEPEND ON CLINICAL FEATURES AND DIFFERENTIAL DIAGNOSIS	
Tests	**Result**
Autoimmune tests	These may include ANA (screen for connective tissue diseases), RF and anti-CCP (rheumatoid arthritis), and anti-dsDNA, anti-Sm, anti-Ro, and anti-La (SLE)
Microbiology tests	Tests for reactive arthritis: Cytomegalovirus, Epstein–Barr virus, mycoplasma, rubella (also postvaccination), hepatitis B virus, parvovirus, influenza, and Yersinia species and other gastrointestinal species, STI screen (namely chlamydia trachomatis)
Joint aspiration	Important investigation in any monoarthritis where there is diagnostic uncertainty. Send synovial fluid for urgent white cell count, gram stain and culture, polarized light microscopy (crystals).
Joint X-ray	To help exclude other causes of joint pain, such as slipped upper femoral epiphysis or other inflammatory arthritides (e.g., osteopenia and erosions in RA)
Joint ultrasound	Will help in determining if an effusion is present or not (differentiating between arthritis and arthralgia)
Choreiform tests	May include: Serum ceruloplasmin and 24-h urinary copper (any patient <40 years for Wilson's disease), brain MRI for focal or unilateral choreas (e.g., rule out structural lesion; there are no pathognomonic findings in Sydenham chorea and neuroimaging usually does not provide additional diagnostic information), genetic testing (e.g., Huntington disease), ANA (e.g., SLE), drug screen (e.g., cocaine, benzodiazepines)
Cardiac MRI[a]	In cases where the cause of heart failure is in doubt (e.g., viral myocarditis causing mechanical dysfunction)

ANA antinuclear antibodies; RF rheumatoid factor; anti-CCP anti-cyclic citrullinated peptide; anti-dsDNA anti-double-stranded deoxyribonucleic acid; SLE systemic lupus erythematosus; STI sexually transmitted infection; RA rheumatoid arthritis; MRI magnetic resonance imaging;
[a] Valvulitis, the major cardiac manifestation of ARF, is readily delineated by echocardiography, as is its impact on left ventricle size and function. Although the presence of valve inflammation may be apparent on late-enhancement cardiac MRI, there are few, if any, indications for cardiac MRI during ARF, except perhaps in the rare case presenting with severe left ventricular dysfunction in the absence of chronic valve involvement. In this situation, the finding of myocardial abnormalities such as fibrosis or edema on T2-weighted and late enhancement imaging suggests myocarditis or cardiomyopathy as an alternative or co-existing diagnosis.

antigens and many streptococcal antibody tests are available. However, only antistreptolysin O antibodies (ASO antibodies) and antideoxyribonuclease B antibodies (ADB antibodies) are routinely used in clinical practice.

Rising titers are preferred to single raised titers: a twofold or more increase in titer from acute to convalescence (usually 12−28 days apart) is considered the best evidence of an antecedent GAS infection.[2,64,65] However, given that ARF often manifests at the peak of the streptococcal antibody response (particularly ASO, which typically peaks during the first to third week of ARF), titers may already be at or near their peak at presentation

(therefore the twofold increase in titers may not be seen). Another issue, particularly in remote or resource-poor environments, is that it may be impractical to bring the patient back for the convalescent sample. Therefore, if only a single specimen is available, a single value above the upper limit of normal (ULN) at presentation is considered sufficient for a preceding GAS infection.[3] Published ULN criteria available with test kits may not be appropriate for the local population, so where possible locally derived ULNs should be used.

The ASO titer is the most widely used and best-understood test.[59] Age, geographic location, season, site of infection, and other factors all significantly influence the antibody level. Early antibiotic therapy can reduce the magnitude of the antibody response but will not abolish it. The ULN is defined as the highest ASO titer exceed by only 20% of the population.[66,67] Table 3.5 summarizes the normal values for children in tropical regions. Because of the high incidence of tonsilopharyngitis in elementary school children, ASO titers are often 200–300 Todd units/mL in healthy individuals while levels ≥500 Todd units/mL are good evidence of a recent GAS infection.[68] Furthermore, because 20% of individuals with ARF may have normal ASO titers,[69] additional ADB titers may be helpful. ASO levels start to fall after around 6–8 weeks after infection and ADB after 3 months.

Chest X-ray

CXR features are neither specific nor diagnostic of ARF but it remains an important investigation in all cases of ARF with suspected carditis, in particular looking for evidence of heart failure. Cardiomegaly (defined as a cardiothoracic ratio >50% on a posterior-anterior CXR view) may be seen due to left ventricular and left atrial enlargement. Isolated left atrial enlargement might also occur, particularly in the setting of MR. This can manifest as straightening of the left heart border or a double density on the right heart border on a frontal CXR. Occasionally, cardiomegaly may also be due to a pericardial effusion.

Echocardiography

The emergence of advanced echocardiography is arguably the single biggest advance in our diagnostic armamentarium since the initial conception of the Jones criteria and is currently the closest investigation to a diagnostic test for ARF in those who manifest carditis. It now plays a crucial role in the assessment of all patients with suspected ARF, having significantly improved both diagnostic sensitivity (e.g., through detection of subclinical carditis) and specificity (e.g., by ruling out carditis and other causes of heart disease).

Echocardiography also plays an important role in the assessment of disease severity in those with confirmed carditis. This includes assessing the degree of MR and AR, left ventricular size and function (Table 3.1), quantifying tricuspid regurgitation and pulmonary artery pressure, and confirming the presence and extent of a pericardial effusion and chronic valvular changes consistent with a diagnosis of RHD.

Diagnosis of Rheumatic Carditis by Echocardiography

The diagnosis of rheumatic carditis by echocardiography is predicated on the demonstration of pathological mitral and/or aortic regurgitation (i.e. rheumatic valvulitis-see Table 3.6). Note that some of these changes are based on color-Doppler. There may or may not be morphological features present (Table 3.7), especially if there is severe valvulitis or they may represent more long-standing chronic changes. Some echocardiography reports will then say there are acute and chronic changes. Note that echocardiography cannot date the duration of the changes. Once the inflammatory markers have settled, then from that time, any remaining valve changes should be termed chronic RHD.

The criteria in Table 3.6 provides a set of objective measures to distinguish physiological valvular regurgitation from pathological regurgitation, although it is important to realize these are not specific for rheumatic carditis and other disease states may also give rise to

---

TABLE 3.5
Upper Limit of Normal (80th Centile) Values for Serum Streptococcal Antibody Titers in Children and Adults in Tropical Settings Where GAS is Endemic.[70]

| Age Group (years) | UPPER LIMIT OF NORMAL (INTERNATIONAL UNITS/ML) | |
	ASO Titer	ADB Titer
1–4	170	366
5–14	276	499
15–24	238	473
25–34	177	390
≥35	127	265

ASO, Antistreptolysin O; *ADB*, Antideoxyribonuclease B; *GAS* group A streptococcus.

TABLE 3.6
Doppler Findings on Echocardiogram in Rheumatic Valvulitis.

Pathological Mitral Regurgitation (All Four Criteria Must be Met)	Pathological Aortic Regurgitation (All Four Criteria Must be Met)
Seen in at least two views	Seen in at least two views
Jet length ≥2 cm in at least one view	Jet length ≥1 cm in at least one view
Peak velocity >3 m/s	Peak velocity >3 m/s
Pan-systolic jet in at least one envelope	Pan-diastolic jet in at least one envelope

Reproduced with permission from Gewitz et al.[2]

TABLE 3.7
Morphological Findings on Echocardiogram in Rheumatic Valvulitis.

Acute Mitral Valve Changes	Aortic Valve Changes in Carditis or Chronic RHD
Annular dilatation	Irregular or focal leaflet thickening
Chordal elongation	Coaptation defect
Chordal rupture resulting in flail leaflet with severe mitral regurgitation	Restricted leaflet motion
Anterior (or less commonly posterior) leaflet tip prolapse	Leaflet prolapse
Beading/nodularity of leaflet tips	

Reproduced with permission from Gewitz et al.[2]

pathological regurgitation. The criteria in Table 3.6 are analogous to the World Heart Federation criteria used in the diagnosis of RHD,[71] meaning that the standard used to define pathological MR and AR associated with chronic RHD is the same as that for the MR and AR seen in ARF. Should there be any doubt regarding the etiology of MR or AR on echocardiography and in addition to the morphological changes discussed earlier, the following features support a diagnosis of acute carditis:

- Pathological regurgitation involving both the mitral and aortic valves
- A posteriorly directed mitral regurgitant jet, because the most common mechanism for MR in acute carditis is prolapse of the anterior mitral valve leaflet
- Evolution of valvulitis over weeks (increasing or decreasing in severity)

Pathological regurgitation should always be graded as either mild, moderate, or severe using continuous-wave and color-Doppler (Table 3.1), which allows stratification of the severity of carditis and helps guide management. Pressure and volume overload must be excluded before attributing tricuspid and pulmonary regurgitation to valvulitis. Assessment of the severity of valve lesions, LV size and function, the use of cardiac MRI when echocardiographic images are suboptimal, and the use of 3D echo are discussed in detail in Chapter 5.

The morphological changes listed in Table 3.7 are thought to underpin the mechanism of acute MR seen during ARF and are a direct result of inflammation of the entire valvular apparatus, namely annulitis (causing annular dilatation), chorditis (causing chordal elongation), and valvulitis (causing inflammation of the mitral valve leaflets), leading to prolapse of the anterior (or less commonly posterior) mitral valve leaflet[72] (see Chapter 4). The chronic mitral valve changes that characterize RHD evolve after ARF and represent a continuum of acute to chronic changes (see Chapter 5). The morphological changes seen in the aortic valve can be seen in ARF and similarly evolve to chronic RHD with time.

It is not uncommon for ARF to occur on a background of RHD, where acute carditis may coexist with chronic valvular insufficiency. Therefore, in the absence of pericarditis, involvement of a new valve, or worsening of a documented valvular lesion, it may be difficult to establish the diagnosis of acute carditis during an episode of ARF.

DIAGNOSIS OF ACUTE RHEUMATIC FEVER

Since its inception, the Jones criteria have widely been accepted as the clinical standard by which a diagnosis of ARF is made. The 2015 update of the Jones criteria is shown in Table 3.8. The initial diagnosis of ARF is made in the presence of two major manifestations or one major and two minor manifestations, with evidence of a preceding GAS infection. The diagnosis of recurrent ARF is made in the presence of two major manifestations, one major and two minor manifestations, or three minor manifestations, with evidence of a preceding GAS infection.[2] The exceptions are chorea and indolent carditis, which are still considered standalone criteria for establishing the diagnosis of ARF.

Before the 2015 revision, the criteria were last modified by the AHA in 1992[61] and reconfirmed in principle at an AHA-sponsored workshop in 2000.[73] The 1992 modified criteria were very helpful in describing joint manifestations, including that NSAIDs may abort the progression of arthritis, and details regarding the diagnosis of recent streptococcal pharyngitis (throat culture and streptococcal serology).[58,73] This update[61] clearly delineated the three circumstances in which ARF can be diagnosed without strictly adhering to the Jones criteria: (a) isolated chorea; (b) isolated indolent carditis; (c) presumptive ARF recurrence in the presence of only one major or several minor manifestations (if GAS infection was evident). However, no specific criteria for high-risk populations were included, nor echocardiography as a diagnostic tool, although its importance for ARF

TABLE 3.8
2015 AHA Revised Jones Criteria for the Diagnosis of Acute Rheumatic Fever.

A. FOR ALL PATIENT POPULATIONS WITH EVIDENCE OF PRECEDING GAS INFECTION

Diagnosis: Initial ARF	Two major manifestations or one major plus two minor manifestations
Diagnosis: Recurrent ARF	Two major or one major and two minor or three minor manifestations

B. MAJOR CRITERIA

Low-risk populations[a]	*Moderate- and high-risk populations*
Carditis[b]	Carditis[b]
• clinical and/or **subclinical**	• clinical and/or **subclinical**
Arthritis	Arthritis
• polyarthritis only	• **Monoarthritis** or polyarthritis
	• **Polyarthralgia**[c]
Chorea	Chorea
Erythema marginatum	Erythema marginatum
Subcutaneous nodules	Subcutaneous nodules

C. MINOR CRITERIA

Low-risk populations[a]	*Moderate- and high-risk populations*
Polyarthralgia	**Monoarthralgia**
Fever (≥38.5°C)	**Fever (≥38°C)**
ESR ≥60 mm in the first hour and/or CRP ≥3.0 mg/dL[d]	ESR **≥30 mm/h** and/or CRP ≥3.0 mg/dL[d]
Prolonged PR interval, after accounting for age variability (unless carditis is a major criterion)	Prolonged PR interval, after accounting for age variability (unless carditis is a major criterion)

Changes compared with the 1992 revision are highlighted in bold.
ARF indicates acute rheumatic fever; *CRP*, C-reactive protein; *ESR*, erythrocyte sedimentation rate; and *GAS*, group A streptococcal.
As in past versions of the criteria, erythema marginatum and subcutaneous nodules are rarely "stand-alone" major criteria. Additionally, joint manifestations can only be considered in either the major or minor categories but not both in the same patient.
[a] Low-risk populations are those with ARF incidence ≤2 per 100 000 school-aged children or all-age rheumatic heart disease prevalence of ≤1 per 1000 population per year.
[b] Subclinical carditis indicates echocardiographic valvulitis as defined in Table 3.6.
[c] Polyarthralgia should only be considered as a major manifestation in moderate-to-high-risk populations after exclusion of other causes. As in past versions of the criteria, erythema marginatum and subcutaneous nodules are rarely "stand-alone" major criteria. Additionally, joint manifestations can only be considered in either the major or minor categories but not both in the same patient.
[d] CRP value must be greater than upper limit of normal for laboratory. Furthermore, because ESR may evolve during the course of ARF, peak ESR values should be used.
Reproduced with permission from Gewitz et al.[2]

management and its use in the diagnosis of murmurs were discussed. The AHA had not accepted subclinical carditis as a major manifestation until 2015 when they correctly acknowledged 25 reports of countries using subclinical carditis in the diagnosis of ARF.[2]

RATIONALE FOR 2015 REVISION

The 2015 revision of the Jones criteria set out three important changes. First, it was recognized that one set of criteria was no longer adequate for all regions, given the marked disparities in the global distribution of ARF, with near eradication in High-income countries (HICs) over the last half century compared to very little change in most LMICs and poor populations within some HICs.[74–76] This shift in ARF epidemiology had important implications for the Jones criteria, where the clinical utility of the criteria is determined by the pretest probability of having ARF. Each of the Jones criteria revisions before 2015 responded to the declining incidence of ARF in the United States, increasing specificity because of the steadily reducing pretest probability. The aim was to avoid over diagnosis in low-risk populations, resulting in a progressive decrease in sensitivity. Inevitably, concerns began to emerge that the criteria were not sensitive enough in high-risk settings, particularly with evidence that strict adherence to the 1992 criteria resulted in missed diagnoses of ARF in some patients from endemic populations.[47]

In response to these observations, the Australian guidelines (2006, revised in 2012) were the first to use variable diagnostic criteria for low-risk (prioritizing specificity) and high-risk populations (prioritizing sensitivity). The 2015 AHA Jones criteria subsequently adopted the same approach. A key difference between the Australian guidelines and the Jones criteria is that the former provided a definition of high risk, whereas the latter provides a definition of low risk which, in practical terms, should be easier to define based on socioeconomic factors, helping to facilitate greater uniformity among healthcare providers when choosing a diagnostic pathway.[77] Low-risk populations are defined in the 2015 Jones revision as an ARF incidence of ≤2 per 100,000 school-aged children (usually 5–14 years old) per year, or an all-age RHD prevalence of ≤1 per 1000 population per year.[2]

In summary, the 2015 guidelines acknowledge the importance of including pretest probability in weighing sensitivity versus specificity: prioritizing specificity for low-risk populations and prioritizing sensitivity for moderate-to-high-risk populations.[77]

Second, in the 2015 Jones criteria, subclinical carditis was accepted as a major manifestation in all population groups, regardless of ARF risk. The role of echocardiography in ARF management was evaluated by several studies, and a substantial prevalence of subclinical carditis among patients with ARF was observed. A meta-analysis including 23 of these studies from five continents with different socioeconomic backgrounds found a pooled prevalence of subclinical carditis of 16.8%, with almost 45% of these patients demonstrating worsening of valvular involvement over time.[28] The addition of subclinical carditis as a major manifestation was therefore permitted by the 2006 and 2014 New Zealand guidelines (all populations), the 2006 and 2012 Australian guidelines (high-risk populations only), and the 2015 Jones criteria (all populations). It was also recommended that echocardiographic examination should be routine for all patients with confirmed or suspected ARF, with repeated studies for those negative on first evaluation for monitoring of

evolving cardiac disease.[2,77] In New Zealand, a country where ARF is frequently diagnosed and referred early to hospital, it was found that subclinical carditis could develop up to 4 weeks after presentation with joints symptoms.[25,27]

Finally, given the wide spectrum of rheumatic joint involvement observed in many high-risk patients with ARF, it was clear that if polyarthritis is considered the only major joint manifestation, a significant number of ARF diagnoses will be missed. Aseptic monoarthritis in particular is an important part of the clinical spectrum of ARF in high-risk populations, affecting up to 16%–18% of Australian Aboriginal children.[47] Accordingly, the Australian guidelines and Jones criteria have permitted greater diagnostic latitude beyond migratory polyarthritis in high-risk populations. The 2015 Jones criteria now includes aseptic monoarthritis and polyarthralgia as major manifestations and monoarthralgia as a minor manifestation in moderate-to-high-risk populations, while the diagnosis of joint involvement in low-risk populations remains unchanged.[2,77]

Modifications to the 2015 revision were also made to the minor manifestations in relation to fever and inflammation, also with the aim of improving sensitivity in moderate-to-high-risk populations. For these moderate-to-high-risk populations, the cut-off for fever was lowered to ≥38.0°C, based primarily on data from the endemic Australian Aboriginal population, and the ESR cut-off was lowered to ≥30 mm/h.[2,77] Cut-off values for temperature and ESR remained the same for low-risk populations and CRP cut-off values remain unchanged for all populations.

Possible Acute Rheumatic Fever

The 2015 update also provides for the option of "possible" ARF, where there is a strong clinical suspicion of ARF but the patient does not meet the diagnostic criteria. This may occur, for example, if all investigations are not available (e.g., laboratory data for acute phase inflammatory markers or echocardiography for subclinical carditis), there is incomplete or unclear documentation of clinical features, or the history is unreliable.[2] These issues are likely to be more relevant within resource-limited settings. In such circumstances, clinicians should use their clinical reasoning regarding diagnosis and treatment, following some recommendations: (a) Where there is genuine uncertainty, it is reasonable to consider offering 12 months of secondary prophylaxis followed by reevaluation with careful history and physical examination in addition to a repeat echocardiogram (*Class IIa; Level of Evidence C*); (b) In a patient with recurrent symptoms—especially joint manifestations—who has been adherent to prophylaxis recommendations but lacks serological evidence of streptococcal infection and echocardiographic evidence of valvulitis, it is reasonable to conclude that the recurrent symptoms are not likely related to ARF, and antibiotic prophylaxis may be discontinued *(Class IIa; Level of Evidence C)*.[2,77]

Rheumatic Fever Recurrences

All patients with an episode of ARF are at high risk of recurrent episodes of ARF.[58,59] The 1992 update emphasized that the complete set of Jones criteria may not be completely fulfilled.[58]

The 2015 Jones criteria define a recurrence of ARF as follows:

1. *With a reliable past history of ARF or established RHD, and in the face of GAS infection, two major or one major and two minor or three minor manifestations may be sufficient for a presumptive diagnosis(Class IIb; Level of Evidence C)*[2]
2. *When minor manifestations alone are present, the exclusion of other more likely causes of the clinical presentation is recommended before a diagnosis of ARF recurrence is made (Class I; Level of Evidence C)*[2]

The WHO recommendations[43] state that where there is established RHD, a recurrence of ARF can be diagnosed by the presence of two minor manifestations plus evidence of a preceding GAS infection. This can be useful if there is diagnostic difficulty, regardless of whether the degree of heart disease has changed.

INTERNATIONAL DIAGNOSTIC CRITERIA (AUSTRALIA, NEW ZEALAND, BRAZIL, INDIA)[3,4,78,79]

There is considerable heterogeneity between international ARF diagnostic guidelines regarding specific points of the Jones criteria. Table 3.9 compares the updated 2015 Jones criteria with the current version of four national guidelines from Australia, New Zealand, India, and Brazil.

DIFFERENTIAL DIAGNOSIS OF ACUTE RHEUMATIC FEVER

As discussed previously, none of the clinical manifestations of ARF are specific for the disease and no specific diagnostic test exists. Thus, the differential diagnosis in a patient suspected of having ARF may be extensive (Table 3.10).[2,77–79] A detailed evaluation must be performed, taking epidemiological factors, past medical history and clinical and laboratorial evidence of recent GAS infection into account. A classic case of ARF with migratory polyarthritis, minor criteria, and raised streptococcal antibody titers is relatively straight forward diagnostically. Similarly, in high prevalence regions a presentation with polyarthritis and carditis should be regarded as ARF until proved otherwise (even in regions without the availability of streptococcal serology). Many patients presenting with chronic RHD have no prior history of ARF. In some, the diagnosis of ARF was likely overlooked as a "missed opportunity." In others, it is likely the main feature was carditis that did not cause symptoms.

Because of the heterogenous manner in which ARF can manifest, a high index of suspicion is required to make the diagnosis while also considering the broad list of differential diagnoses for each clinical manifestation. In patients with nonmigratory or single joint involvement and no carditis, the diagnosis of ARF is particularly challenging and remains a diagnosis of exclusion: a selection of the tests mentioned in Table 3.4 may need to be performed.

Of note, poststreptococcal reactive arthritis (PSRA) is one of the most challenging differential diagnoses for ARF. In a retrospective study, clinical and laboratory features of both conditions were evaluated to determine whether the two diseases are separate clinical manifestations of the same disease or are in fact different diseases. One study found that ESR, C-reactive protein levels, duration of joint symptoms after initiation of antiinflammatory treatment, and relapse of joint symptoms after treatment cessation could be used to differentiate the two conditions, resulting in the correct diagnosis in >80% of the cases.[80] However, in high-risk populations, even a confident diagnosis of PSRA may represent a missed diagnosis of ARF, so clinicians may be best advised to either manage these cases as ARF or, as a minimum, to offer these patients 12 months of secondary prophylaxis with a repeat echocardiogram at that point: lack of evidence of rheumatic valvular changes could be sufficient evidence to cease prophylaxis.

ARF should be considered as a differential diagnosis in children with suspected septic arthritis and sterile joint fluid in endemic regions, especially considering that the rate of positive synovial fluid culture varies widely, with reports of as low as 16%.[81] Moreover, although monoarthritis is a major ARF criterion only in moderate-to-high-risk populations, this clinical finding has been previously described in ARF patients from industrialized countries, making the differentiation with septic arthritis even more challenging, and reinforcing the need for complimentary tests other than culture. In this setting, another important diagnosis to be considered is transient synovitis.

TABLE 3.9

Comparison Between International Acute Rheumatic Fever Diagnostic Guidelines and the 2015 Jones Criteria

Criteria:	Jones Criteria (2015)[2]	Australia (2012)[35]	New Zealand (2014)[30]	India (2008)[a,79]	Brazil (2009)[a,78]
Differentiation between high- and low-risk populations	Yes	Yes	No	No	No
Carditis	Clinical and/or **subclinical**[b]	High risk: Clinical and/or **subclinical**[b]; low risk: clinical.	Clinical and/or **subclinical**[b]	Clinical	Clinical
Joint manifestations	**Major:** Polyarthritis (all); monoarthritis/ polyarthritis/ polyarthralgia (moderate/high risk). **Minor:** Polyarthralgia (low risk); monoarthralgia (moderate/high risk).	**Major:** Polyarthritis (all); monoarthritis/ polyarthritis/ polyarthralgia (high risk). **Minor:** Polyarthralgia/ monoarthritis (low risk); monoarthralgia (high risk).	**Major:** Polyarthritis/ monoarthritis. **Minor:** Polyarthralgia	**Major:** Polyarthritis. **Minor:** Monoarthritis.	**Major:** Arthritis (any). **Minor:** Arthralgia (any).
Markers of inflammation	ESR ≥60 mm/h and/or CRP ≥3.0 mg/dL (low risk); ESR ≥30 mm/h and/or CRP ≥3.0 mg/dL (moderate/high risk).	ESR ≥30 mm/h and/or CRP ≥3.0 mg/dL (all groups).	ESR ≥50 mm/h and/or CRP ≥3.0 mg/dL.	Follow standard laboratory values.	Values not specified
Fever	≥38.5°C (low risk); ≥38.0°C (moderate/high risk).	≥38.0°C (all groups).	≥38.0°C.	Values not specified	Values not specified

[a] Both the Brazilian and Indian ARF diagnostic guidelines recognise subclinical carditis as a distinct entity but it is unclear if they count it as a major manifestation for diagnostic purposes

[b] Subclinical carditis: Seen only on echocardiography without auscultatory findings. *CRP*, C-reactive protein; *ESR*, erythrocyte sedimentation rate.

Other severe forms of cardiac disease, such as infective endocarditis, must also be considered, particularly in the presence of persistent fever of unknown origin (see Chapter 16). Sometimes the differential diagnosis of recurrent ARF can be difficult, especially in children with more severe clinical manifestations. Splenomegaly, vascular and immunologic phenomena, demonstration of vegetations on echocardiogram and positive blood cultures are indicative of infective endocarditis. Cardiac scintigraphy with Gallium can be used in selected cases.

SLE and other systemic autoimmune diseases frequently develop clinical manifestations that mimic ARF, such as arthralgia and transient arthritis. However, SLE affects multiple organs, including the kidneys, central nervous system, skin, and blood. Differentiation relies on clinical grounds and serologic studies may be informative.

TABLE 3.10
Differential Diagnoses of the Major Manifestations of Acute Rheumatic Fever[81–84].

Manifestations	Disease/Condition	Differentiating Signs/Symptoms	Differentiating Tests
Joint manifestations	Septic arthritis	Usually only one joint involved; not migratory; patient looks unwell.	Positive Gram stain from synovial fluid aspirate. Culture of an organism from joint aspirate. Elevated white cell count in blood and on microscopy (typically >100,000 cells/mm^3) of synovial fluid. May have positive blood culture.
	Juvenile idiopathic arthritis	Lasts longer than 6 weeks; may not have joint pain; uveitis may be present. Light pink rash in systemic form.	Positive connective tissue testing such as positive antinuclear antibody, anti-dsDNA.
	Viral arthropathy	History of viral illness.	Positive viral serology.
	Reactive arthritis	Usually develops 1–4 weeks following a gastrointestinal or urogenital infection. Most commonly occurs in young adults, affecting both men and women.	Evidence of a typical preceding extraarticular infection (e.g., Salmonella, Shigella, Yersinia, campylobacter, chlamydia trachomatis).
Joint manifestations, markers of inflammation	Gout and pseudogout	First metacarpophalangeal joint often affected; pain excruciating and often flaky red skin over affected joint.	Polarizing microscopy of synovial fluid or presence of gouty tophi.
Erythema, joint manifestations, fever and markers of inflammation	Lyme disease	Circular expanding rash with central clearing (erythema migrans); flu-like symptoms; acute neurological problems including Bell palsy; arthritis usually affects the knees.	Positive Borrelia burgdoferi serology.
Fever, markers of inflammation	Sickle cell anemia	Family history; signs and symptoms of anemia; not usually febrile unless infection has precipitated crisis.	Anemia and sickle cells on blood film.
	Leukemia	History may include lethargy, weight loss, night sweats, and bone pain.	Blast cells on film.
Carditis, fever, markers of inflammation	Infective endocarditis	Petechiae, Janeway lesions, Osler nodes, Roth spots, and splinter hemorrhages. Embolic complications (e.g., stroke, renal infarction)	Positive blood culture for organism causing endocarditis Echocardiogram; vegetations on valve
Carditis	Innocent murmur	Otherwise normal child; quiet murmur; never purely diastolic	Normal echocardiogram
	Mitral valve prolapse	Midsystolic click on cardiac auscultation.	Echocardiogram reveals characteristic billowing of one or both of the mitral valve leaflets into the left atrium during/toward the end of systole.
	Congenital heart disease	Undiagnosed heart murmurs	Echocardiography will reveal abnormalities
	Hypertrophic cardiomyopathy	Afebrile; may be asymptomatic.	

Continued

TABLE 3.10
Differential Diagnoses of the Major Manifestations of Acute Rheumatic Fever[81–84].—cont'd

Manifestations	Disease/Condition	Differentiating Signs/Symptoms	Differentiating Tests
			Echocardiography shows hypertrophy of left ventricle without dilatation of cavity
	Myocarditis	Usually follows a viral illness; chest pain and shortness of breath are common features.	Echocardiography shows impaired ventricular function and structurally normal heart valves +/- secondary MR Troponin and creatine kinase elevated. ECG may show low voltage QRS, saddle-shaped ST segments or T-wave changes. Cardiac MRI will demonstrate myocarditic inflammation. Cardiac muscle biopsy will demonstrate cardiac muscle inflammation (see Chapter 16).
	Pericarditis	Absence of the murmur of mitral regurgitation and/or aortic regurgitation	No other features of rheumatic carditis
Erythema marginatum	Systemic lupus erythematosus	Malar "butterfly" rash; joint pain typically affects hands and wrists; may have anemia.	Positive connective tissue testing such as positive antinuclear antibody, anti-dsDNA, and anti-Smith antibodies.
	Drug intoxication	History of recent ingestion; use of illicit drugs.	Drug screen, including phenytoin, amitriptyline, and metoclopramide.
Chorea/Neurological manifestations	Wilson disease	Hepatosplenomegaly and Kayser–Fleischer rings; may have a positive family history.	Decreased serum ceruloplasmin level; genetic testing. 24-h urinary copper excretion.
	Tic disorder	Can be motor or phonic tics; absence of fever or any other signs of acute rheumatic fever.	Psychiatric evaluation may reveal underlying cause.
	Encephalitis	Seizures, headache, fever, cognitive changes; sometimes photophobia and neck stiffness.	Electroencephalogram may show temporal lobe changes. MRI brain: Features depend on cause of encephalitis but may include temporal lobe hemorrhage or white matter lesions. Polymerase chain reaction of cerebrospinal fluid to detect viral DNA/RNA.
	Choreoathetoid cerebral palsy	Wide spectrum of symptoms depending on severity; features include difficulty maintaining posture, scissor walking, seizures, and learning difficulties.	Clinical diagnosis. CT may help to identify cerebral hemorrhage, and MRI can be useful to look for changes in

TABLE 3.10
Differential Diagnoses of the Major Manifestations of Acute Rheumatic Fever[81-84]—cont'd

Manifestations	Disease/Condition	Differentiating Signs/Symptoms	Differentiating Tests
			cerebral white matter in older children.
	Huntington chorea	May have associated symptoms of weight loss, depression, facial tics, impairment of rapid eye movement, and dementia. More likely if a parent is affected.	Genetic testing (autosomal dominant CAG trinucleotide repeat disorder).
	Intracranial tumor	May have headache, typically worse in the morning, with or without vomiting; may have papilledema; cranial nerve involvement possible.	CT/MRI of the brain.
	Hyperthyroidism	Tachycardia, tremor, weight loss. Goiter. Eye signs: Exophthalmos, lid lag and retraction, proptosis, complex ophthalmoplegias. Thyroid acropachy and pretibial myxoedema.	Thyroid function tests; typically elevated T4 and T3 with suppression of TSH in primary hyperthyroidism. Secondary hyperthyroidism will show elevated TSH levels.

ARF acute rheumatic fever; dsDNA double-stranded deoxyribonucleic acid; MR mitral regurgitation; ECG electrocardiogram; MRI magnetic resonance imaging; DNA deoxyribonucleic acid; RNA ribonucleic acid; CT computed tomography; TSH thyroid-stimulating hormone

As previously discussed, the diagnosis of Sydenham chorea may be reinforced by an echocardiogram demonstrating pathological regurgitation on the left-sided heart valves. It is important not to misinterpret other symptoms similar to chorea, such as tics and the phenothiazine-induced extrapyramidal syndrome. Table 3.10 provides a more detailed work-up of ARF differential diagnosis.

FUTURE RESEARCH DIRECTIONS

The regular revisions to the Jones Criteria, and emergence of ARF diagnostic criteria from other organizations and countries to respond to the needs of populations at highest risk of the disease, have all occurred because ARF diagnosis is imperfect. The application of any of these criteria still results in false-positive and false-negative diagnoses. ARF remains an imperfect clinical diagnosis, reliant on excluding many differential diagnoses, confirmation of recent GAS infection, clinical expertise in recognizing physical signs, various laboratory measures, ECG, and ideally echocardiography. In the era of "omic" sciences (genomics, proteomics, transcriptomics, metabolomics, etc.) that give previously unimaginable insights into human immunology, it is surprising that we are still relying

entirely on clinical criteria to diagnose ARF: an autoimmune disease that has a known precipitant (GAS).

Working toward Universal Diagnostic Criteria

As outlined earlier, the Australian diagnostic criteria issues in 2006 (updated in 2012) tried, for the first time, to respond to the needs for increased specificity in populations with decreasing disease incidence at the same time as increased sensitivity in populations with ongoing high incidence. It did so by asking the clinician to assess the prior risk of the patient, based on the level of ARF and RHD in their population. This approach was adopted and further refined in the most recent version of the Jones Criteria, thus reestablishing those criteria as the international standard, to be used in all countries and populations. However, as clinical criteria, they remain imperfect, so there is a need to continue to monitor their performance in different populations and refine them as needed. As new technologies emerge for clinical assessment, these may need to be added to the Jones Criteria if they can be shown to improve diagnostic accuracy, much as echocardiography has allowed the inclusion of subclinical carditis. Tools such as MRI may allow further refinement of the diagnosis of rheumatic carditis or arthritis in the near future.

The Search for a Molecular Signature in the Diagnosis of Acute Rheumatic Fever

Most studies to date have identified individual biomarkers that may have potential to improve accuracy of ARF diagnosis. The list of these is long, and covers a range of antibodies, adhesion molecules, complement components, T cell ratios, and other proteins (reviewed by de Dassel et al.[85]). There are promising signals, but none of these identified to date offer adequate promise as a single diagnostic test. However, next-generation sequencing (NGS) technologies should allow people with ARF, possible ARF and a range of other non-ARF conditions to be comprehensively profiled to identify a molecular signature (perhaps a range of biomarkers) that could be used together as a gold-standard diagnostic test (at best) or an additional feature to augment and improve the accuracy of the Jones Criteria (at worst). An important secondary benefit would be clearer definition of the immune perturbations that take place in ARF that could help identify potential treatments to reduce the development or progression of cardiac valvular damage. A recent small study took this approach to identify dysregulation in the interleukin-1β-granulocyte-macrophage colony-stimulating factor (GM-CSF) cytokine axis in ARF patients compared to controls, but also identified the potential for a widely used immunomodulatory agent, hydroxychloroquine, to suppress this dysregulation, thus opening the possibility of contributing not only to improved diagnosis, but also to treatment of ARF.[86]

More Appropriate Ways of Diagnosing Acute Rheumatic Fever in the 21st Century

The use of newer technologies such as NGS to improve the diagnosis of ARF will also require them to be affordable and practical in the settings where the disease is most common: low income countries. Although this poses challenges, it should not detract from pursuing this line of research. Indeed, recent experience suggests that adapting higher technology testing to resource-poor settings, including via point-of-care testing, may be more feasible than relying on more traditional laboratory testing.[87,88]

REFERENCES

1. Jones T. The diagnosis of acute rheumatic fever. *J Am Med Assoc.* 1944;126:481–484.
2. Gewitz MH, Baltimore RS, Tani LY, et al. Revision of the Jones Criteria for the diagnosis of acute rheumatic fever in the era of Doppler echocardiography: a scientific statement from the American Heart Association. *Circulation.* 2015;131(20):1806–1818.
3. RHD Australia (ARF/RHD writing group), National Heart Foundation of Australia, Cardiac Society of Australia and New Zealand. The Australian Guideline for Prevention, Diagnosis and Management of Acute Rheumatic Fever and Rheumatic Heart Disease (2nd ed.). Full guidelines2012:[1-136 pp.]. Available from: https://www.rhdaustralia.org.au/arf-rhd-guideline.
4. New Zealand Heart Foundation. *New Zealand Guidelines for Rheumatic Fever: Diagnosis, Management and Secondary Prevention of Acute Rheumatic Fever and Rheumatic Heart Disease: 2014 Update. Auckland.* 2014.
5. Parks T, Smeesters PR, Steer AC. Streptococcal skin infection and rheumatic heart disease. *Curr Opin Infect Dis.* 2012;25(2):145–153.
6. Shulman ST, Bisno AL, Clegg HW, et al. Clinical practice guideline for the diagnosis and management of group A streptococcal pharyngitis: 2012 update by the Infectious Diseases Society of America. *Clin Infect Dis.* 2012;55(10):1279–1282.
7. Lessof MH, Bywaters EG. The duration of chorea. *Br Med J.* 1956;1(4982):1520–1523.
8. Catanzaro FJ, Rammelkamp Jr CH, Chamovitz R. Prevention of rheumatic fever by treatment of streptococcal infections. II. Factors responsible for failures. *N Engl J Med.* 1958;259(2):53–57.
9. Steer AC, Kado J, Jenney AW, et al. Acute rheumatic fever and rheumatic heart disease in Fiji: prospective surveillance, 2005–2007. *Med J Aust.* 2009;190(3):133–135.
10. Feinstein AR, Spagnuolo M, Wood HF, Taranta A, Tursky E, Kleinberg E. Rheumatic fever in children and adolescents. A long-term epidemiologic study of subsequent prophylaxis, streptococcal infections, and clinical sequelae. VI. Clinical features of streptococcal infections and rheumatic recurrences. *Ann Intern Med.* 1964;60(Suppl 5):68–86.
11. Mody GM, Mayosi B. Acute rheumatic fever. In: Hochberg MC, Silman AJ, Smolen JS, Weinblatt ME, Weisman MH, eds. *Rheumatology.* 5th ed. Philadelphia, PA: Mosby; 2010:1093–1102.
12. Wallace MR, Garst PD, Papadimos TJ, Oldfield 3rd EC. The return of acute rheumatic fever in young adults. *J Am Med Assoc.* 1989;262(18):2557–2561.
13. Noonan S, Zurynski YA, Currie BJ, et al. A national prospective surveillance study of acute rheumatic fever in Australian children. *Pediatr Infect Dis J.* 2013;32(1):e26–32.
14. Margaretten ME, Kohlwes J, Moore D, Bent S. Does this adult patient have septic arthritis? *J Am Med Assoc.* 2007;297(13):1478–1488.
15. Santiago MB. Miscellaneous non-inflammatory musculoskeletal conditions. Jaccoud's arthropathy. *Best Pract Res Clin Rheumatol.* 2011;25(5):715–725.
16. Taranta A, Spagnuolo M, Feinstein AR. "Chronic" rheumatic fever. *Ann Intern Med.* 1962;56:367–388.
17. Veasy LG. Myocardial dysfunction in active rheumatic carditis. *J Am Coll Cardiol.* 1994;24(2):581–582.
18. Caldas AM, Terreri MT, Moises VA, et al. What is the true frequency of carditis in acute rheumatic fever? A prospective clinical and Doppler blind study of 56 children with up to 60 months of follow-up evaluation. *Pediatr Cardiol.* 2008;29(6):1048–1053.

19. Bhardwaj R, Sood A. Clinical profile of acute rheumatic fever patients in a tertiary care institute in present era. *J Assoc Phys India*. 2015;63(4):22−24.

20. Mayosi BM, Carapetis JR. Acute rheuamtic fever. In: Fuster V, O'Rourke R, Walsh R, Poole-Wilson P, eds. *Hurst's the Heart*. 12th ed. New York: McGraw Hill; 2007.

21. Bland EF, Duckett Jones T. Rheumatic fever and rheumatic heart disease; a twenty year report on 1000 patients followed since childhood. *Circulation*. 1951;4(6):836−843.

22. Veasy LG, Wiedmeier SE, Orsmond GS, et al. Resurgence of acute rheumatic fever in the intermountain area of the United States. *N Engl J Med*. 1987;316(8):421−427.

23. Wilson NJ, Voss L, Morreau J, Stewart J, Lennon D. New Zealand guidelines for the diagnosis of acute rheumatic fever: small increase in the incidence of definite cases compared to the American Heart Association Jones criteria. *N Z Med J*. 2013;126(1379):50−59.

24. Lanna CC, Tonelli E, Barros MV, Goulart EM, Mota CC. Subclinical rheumatic valvitis: a long-term follow-up. *Cardiol Young*. 2003;13(5):431−438.

25. Voss LM, Wilson NJ, Neutze JM, et al. Intravenous immunoglobulin in acute rheumatic fever: a randomized controlled trial. *Circulation*. 2001;103(3):401−406.

26. Remenyi B, ElGuindy A, Smith Jr SC, Yacoub M, Holmes Jr DR. Valvular aspects of rheumatic heart disease. *Lancet*. 2016;387(10025):1335−1346.

27. Abernethy M, Bass N, Sharpe N, et al. Doppler echocardiography and the early diagnosis of carditis in acute rheumatic fever. *Aust N Z J Med*. 1994;24(5):530−535.

28. Tubridy-Clark M, Carapetis JR. Subclinical carditis in rheumatic fever: a systematic review. *Int J Cardiol*. 2007;119(1):54−58.

29. reportWHO. Rheumatic Fever and Rheumatic Heart Disease. Technical Report Series No. 923. Geneva SWHO.

30. Lindinger ASA, Hoffmann W. Constrictive pericarditis due to acute rheumatic fever. *Eur Heart J*. 1987;8:241−244.

31. Gentles TL, Colan SD, Wilson NJ, Biosa R, Neutze JM. Left ventricular mechanics during and after acute rheumatic fever: contractile dysfunction is closely related to valve regurgitation. *J Am Coll Cardiol*. 2001;37(1):201−207.

32. Alehan D, Ayabakan C, Hallioglu O. Role of serum cardiac troponin T in the diagnosis of acute rheumatic fever and rheumatic carditis. *Heart*. 2004;90(6):689−690.

33. Zomorrodi A, Wald ER. Sydenham's chorea in western Pennsylvania. *Pediatrics*. 2006;117(4):e675−e679.

34. Demiroren K, Yavuz H, Cam L, Oran B, Karaaslan S, Demiroren S. Sydenham's chorea: a clinical follow-up of 65 patients. *J Child Neurol*. 2007;22(5):550−554.

35. Eshel G, Lahat E, Azizi E, Gross B, Aladjem M. Chorea as a manifestation of rheumatic fever–a 30-year survey (1960−1990). *Eur J Pediatr*. 1993;152(8):645−646.

36. Carapetis JR, Currie BJ. Rheumatic chorea in northern Australia: a clinical and epidemiological study. *Arch Dis Child*. 1999;80(4):353−358.

37. Elevli M, Celebi A, Tombul T, Gokalp AS. Cardiac involvement in Sydenham's chorea: clinical and Doppler echocardiographic findings. *Acta Paediatr*. 1999;88(10):1074−1077.

38. Kulkarni ML, Anees S. Sydenham's chorea. *Indian Pediatr*. 1996;33(2):112−115.

39. Punukollu M, Mushet N, Linney M, Hennessy C, Morton M. Neuropsychiatric manifestations of Sydenham's chorea: a systematic review. *Dev Med Child Neurol*. 2016;58(1):16−28.

40. Hitchens RA. Recurrent attacks of acute rheumatism in school-children. *Ann Rheum Dis*. 1958;17(3):293−302.

41. Cardoso F, Vargas AP, Oliveira LD, Guerra AA, Amaral SV. Persistent Sydenham's chorea. *Mov Disord*. 1999;14(5):805−807.

42. Gurkas E, Karalok ZS, Taskin BD, et al. Predictors of recurrence in Sydenham's chorea: clinical observation from a single center. *Brain Dev*. 2016;38(9):827−834.

43. Berrios X, Quesney F, Morales A, Blazquez J, Bisno AL. Are all recurrences of "pure" Sydenham chorea true recurrences of acute rheumatic fever? *J Pediatr*. 1985;107(6):867−872.

44. Terreri MT, Roja SC, Len CA, Faustino PC, Roberto AM, Hilario MO. Sydenham's chorea–clinical and evolutive characteristics. *Sao Paulo Med J*. 2002;120(1):16−19.

45. Baldwin JS, Kerr JM, Kuttner AG, Doyle EF. Observations on rheumatic nodules over a 30-year period. *J Pediatr*. 1960;56:465−470.

45a. Beerman LB, Kreutzer J, Allada V. Cardiology. In: Zitelli BJ, McIntire SC, Nowalk AJ, eds. *Atlas of Pediatric Physical Disorders*. 6th ed. Saunders: Philadelphia; 2012.

46. World Health Organisation. WHO expert consultation on rheumatic fever and rheumatic heart disease (2001: Geneva Switzerland). In: *Rheumatic Fever and Rheumatic Heart Disease: Report of a WHO Expert Consultation, Geneva, 29 October−1 November 2001. Geneva, Switzerland*. 2004.

47. Carapetis JR, Currie BJ. Rheumatic fever in a high incidence population: the importance of monoarthritis and low grade fever. *Arch Dis Child*. 2001;85(3):223−227.

48. Park MK. *Pcfp*. 2nd ed. Chicago: Year Book Medical; 1998.

49. Balli S, Oflaz MB, Kibar AE, Ece I. Rhythm and conduction analysis of patients with acute rheumatic fever. *Pediatr Cardiol*. 2013;34(2):383−389.

50. Clarke M, Keith JD. Atrioventricular conduction in acute rheumatic fever. *Br Heart J*. 1972;34(5):472−479.

51. Cristal N, Stern J, Gueron M. Atrioventricular dissociation in acute rheumatic fever. *Br Heart J*. 1971;33(1):12−15.

52. Ceviz N, Celik V, Olgun H, Karacan M. Accelerated junctional rhythm in children with acute rheumatic fever: is it specific to the disease? *Cardiol Young*. 2014;24(3):464−468.

53. Agnew R, Wilson N, Skinner J, Nicholson R. Beyond first degree heart block in acute rheumatic fever. *Cardiol Young*. 2019 (in press).

53a. Bishop W, Currie B, Carapetis J, Kilburn CA. subtle presentation of acute rheumatic fever in remote northern Australia. *Aust N Z J Med*. 1996;26(2):241−242.

54. JONES CRITERIA (modified) for guidance in the diagnosis of rheumatic fever. *Public Health Rep*. 1956;71(7):672−674.

55. Lustok MJ, Kuzma JF. Rheumatic fever pneumonitis: a clinical and pathologic study of 35 cases. *Ann Intern Med*. 1956;44(2):337−357.

56. Brown G, Goldring D, Behrer MR. Rheumatic pneumonia. *J Pediatr*. 1958;52(5):598−619.

57. World Health Organisation. *Rheumatic Fever and Rheumatic Heart Disease: Report of a WHO Expert Consultation*. Geneva, Switzerland: World Health Organization; 2004. Contract

No.: World Health Organisation Technical Report Series 923.

58. Guidelines for the diagnosis of rheumatic fever. Jones criteria, 1992 update. Special writing group of the committee on rheumatic fever, endocarditis, and Kawasaki disease of the council on cardiovascular disease in the young of the American heart association. *Jama*. 1992;268(15):2069–2073.

59. Steer AC, Smeesters PR, Curtis N. Streptococcal serology: secrets for the specialist. *Pediatr Infect Dis J*. 2015;34(11): 1250–1252.

60. Gerber MA. Diagnosis of pharyngitis: methodology of throat cultures. In: *Shulman ST ePmiaeodrfNYP*. 1984:61–72.

61. Gerber MA, Schulman S. Rapid diagnosis of pharyngitis caused by Group A Streptococci. *Clin Microbiol Rev*. 2004; 17(3):571–580.

62. Tanz RR, Gerber MA, Kabat W, Rippe J, Seshadri R, Shulman ST. Performance of a rapid antigen-detection test and throat culture in community pediatric offices: implications for management of pharyngitis. *Pediatrics*. 2009; 123(2):437–444.

63. Gerber MA. Comparison of throat cultures and rapid strep tests for diagnosis of streptococcal pharyngitis. *Pediatr Infect Dis J*. 1989;8(11):820–824.

64. Johnson DR, Kurlan R, Leckman J, Kaplan EL. The human immune response to streptococcal extracellular antigens: clinical, diagnostic, and potential pathogenetic implications. *Clin Infect Dis*. 2010;50(4):481–490.

65. Wannamaker LW, Ayoub EM. Antibody titers in acute rheumatic fever. *Circulation*. 1960;21:598–614.

66. Kaplan EL, Rothermel CD, Johnson DR. Antistreptolysin O and anti-deoxyribonuclease B titers: normal values for children ages 2 to 12 in the United States. *Pediatrics*. 1998;101(1 Pt 1):86–88.

67. Shet A, Kaplan EL. Clinical use and interpretation of group A streptococcal antibody tests: a practical approach for the pediatrician or primary care physician. *Pediatr Infect Dis J*. 2002;21(5):420–426. quiz 7-30.

68. Sethi S, Kaushik K, Mohandas K, Sengupta C, Singh S, Sharma M. Anti-streptolysin O titers in normal healthy children of 5–15 years. *Indian Pediatr*. 2003;40(11): 1068–1071.

69. Stollerman GH, Lewis AJ, Schultz I, Taranta A. Relationship of immune response to group A streptococci to the course of acute, chronic and recurrent rheumatic fever. *Am J Med*. 1956;20(2):163–169.

70. Steer AC, Vidmar S, Ritika R, et al. Normal ranges of streptococcal antibody titers are similar whether streptococci are endemic to the setting or not. *Clin Vaccine Immunol*. 2009;16(2):172–175.

71. Remenyi B, Wilson N, Steer A, et al. World Heart Federation criteria for echocardiographic diagnosis of rheumatic heart disease–an evidence-based guideline. *Nat Rev Cardiol*. 2012;9(5):297–309.

72. Marcus RH, Sareli P, Pocock WA, et al. Functional anatomy of severe mitral regurgitation in active rheumatic carditis. *Am J Cardiol*. 1989;63(9):577–584.

73. Ferrieri P, Jones Criteria Working G. Proceedings of the Jones criteria workshop. *Circulation*. 2002;106(19): 2521–2523.

74. Seckeler MD, Hoke TR. The worldwide epidemiology of acute rheumatic fever and rheumatic heart disease. *Clin Epidemiol*. 2011;3:67–84.

75. GBD 2013 Mortality and Causes of Death Collaborators. Global, regional, and national age-sex specific all-cause and cause-specific mortality for 240 cases of death, 1990–2013: a systemic analysis for the Global Burden of Disease Study 2013. *Lancet*. 2015;385:117–171.

76. Dougherty S, Beaton A, Nascimento BR, Zuhlke LJ, Khorsandi M, Wilson N. Prevention and control of rheumatic heart disease: overcoming core challenges in resource-poor environments. *Ann Pediatr Cardiol*. 2018; 11(1):68–78.

77. Beaton A, Carapetis J. The 2015 revision of the Jones criteria for the diagnosis of acute rheumatic fever: implications for practice in low-income and middle-income countries. *Heart Asia*. 2015;7(2):7–11.

78. Sociedade Brasileira de Cardiologia. Brazilian guidelines for the diagnosis, treatment and prevention of rheumatic fever. [Article in Portuguese]. *Arq Bras Cardiol*. 2009;93(3 Suppl 4):3–18.

79. Working Group on Pediatric Acute Rheumatic Fever and Cardiology Chapter of Indian Academy of Pediatrics, Saxena A, Krishna RK, et al. Consensus guidelines on pediatric acute rheumatic fever and rheumatic heart disease. *Indian Pediatr*. 2008;45:565–573.

80. Barash J, Mashiach E, Navon-Elkan P, et al. Differentiation of post-streptococcal reactive arthritis from acute rheumatic fever. *J Pediatr*. 2008;153(5):696–699.

81. Mataika R, Carapetis JR, Kado J, Steer AC. Acute rheumatic fever: an important differential diagnosis of septic arthritis. *J Trop Pediatr*. 2008;54(3):205–207.

82. Hallidie-Smith KA, Bywaters EG. The differential diagnosis of rheumatic fever. *Arch Dis Child*. 1958;33(170): 350–357.

83. Wallace MR, Lutwick LI, Ravishankar J. *Rheumatic Fever Differential Diagnoses*; April 2019. Medscape Online: Medscape Online. Available from: https://emedicine.medscape.com/article/236582-differential.

84. Steer A, Gibofsky A. *Acute Rheumatic Fever: Clinical Manifestations and Diagnosis*; April 2019. UpToDate: UpToDate. Available from: https://www.uptodate.com/contents/acute-rheumatic-fever-clinical-manifestations-and-diagnosis.

85. de Dassel JL, Ralph AP, Carapetis JR. Controlling acute rheumatic fever and rheumatic heart disease in developing countries: are we getting closer? *Curr Opin Pediatr*. 2015; 27(1):116–123.

86. Kim ML, Martin WJ, Minigo G, et al. Dysregulated IL-1beta-GM-CSF Axis in acute rheumatic fever that is limited by hydroxychloroquine. *Circulation*. 2018;138(23): 2648–2661.

87. Peeling RW, Mabey D. Point-of-care tests for diagnosing infections in the developing world. *Clin Microbiol Infect*. 2010;16(8):1062–1069.

88. Chin CD, Cheung YK, Laksanasopin T, et al. Mobile device for disease diagnosis and data tracking in resource-limited settings. *Clin Chem*. 2013;59(4):629–640.

CHAPTER 4

Management of Acute Rheumatic Fever

ANTOINETTE CILLIERS • MASOOD SADIQ

INTRODUCTION

Initial management of acute rheumatic fever (ARF) is based on establishing the diagnosis, eradication of the streptococcal organism, curtailment of normal physical activities, management of fever, joint manifestations, carditis and heart failure, and Sydenham chorea. Long-term care involves the commencement of prophylaxis against ARF and infective endocarditis, as well as patient/family/community education and public health measures (Table 4.1).[1]

Recommendations for the management of ARF have been sourced predominantly from the Indian Academy of Pediatrics (2008),[2] as well as the Australian (2012)[3] and New Zealand (2014)[4] consensus guidelines. These are based mainly on expert opinion, supported by various levels of evidence. There are few randomized controlled trials on the management of ARF and these do not cover all aspects of management. It is important to note that no treatment for ARF has been proven to slow the progression of valvular disease.

A medication summary (Table 4.2) with dosage regimens is provided based on these recommendations. In addition, patients should be monitored regularly for response to treatment and physicians should be mindful of contraindications to medications and drug allergies.

ESTABLISHING THE DIAGNOSIS

In most instances, admission to hospital is recommended as establishing the diagnosis takes time, requiring laboratory and echocardiographic evidence.[2–4] The consequences of under- and overdiagnosis cannot be overstated. The diagnosis and differential diagnosis of ARF are discussed in detail in Chapter 3.

Hospitalization also allows the opportunity for repeated education about ARF and the need for secondary prophylaxis.

ERADICATION OF THE GROUP A STREPTOCOCCUS

Penicillin is the most important medical treatment of ARF. Its introduction during the acute phase of ARF should eradicate the Group A Streptococcus (GAS) infection, which if persistent can induce chronic or relapsing autoimmune reactions.[5] Although penicillin is considered mandatory, this treatment has not been shown to alter the cardiac outcome after 1 year in controlled studies.[6]

Following hospital admission, oral penicillin V (Table 4.2) should be commenced in all cases whilst the diagnosis of ARF is being established[4]. Ordinarily, oral treatment should last for 10 days to reliably eradicate GAS[3,4]. However, once the diagnosis of ARF is established and providing that the patient is not in severe heart failure, the first dose of benzathine penicillin G (BPG) should also be started in hospital, at which point the oral penicillin is stopped[4]. BPG administration in these circumstances serves the dual purpose of eradication of GAS whilst also acting as the first dose of secondary prophylaxis. Education on the importance of secondary prophylaxis should also be provided at the same time[3,4]. Intravenous penicillin is not indicated.

There is emerging evidence that impetigo (skin sores) may play a role in the pathogenesis of ARF.[1] As such, bacterial cultures of impetigo should be taken and treatment of impetigo undertaken.

Rashes following previous antibiotic administration may lead to patients erroneously being labeled as allergic to penicillin (the vast majority are not). Penicillin allergy can be investigated by skin testing, preferably with input from an allergist. If this is unavailable and following careful investigation to ensure that it is safe to do so, an empiric course of penicillin should be given in hospital with close observation and treatment for anaphylaxis as required (see Chapter 11 for

TABLE 4.1
Management Protocol for Acute Rheumatic Fever.[1]

DIAGNOSIS

- Admission to hospital
- Investigations to confirm ARF and to exclude other pathologies (see Chapter 3)
  - Blood tests including acute phase reactants and serology for the streptococcal organism
  - Electrocardiogram
  - Echocardiographic evaluation

ERADICATION OF GAS

- Oral penicillin V[a] for 10 days OR single dose of intramuscular benzathine penicillin G
- Treatment of coexisting streptococcal impetigo

ARTHRITIS/ARTHRALGIA AND SYMPTOMATIC TREATMENT

- Paracetamol until the diagnosis has been confirmed
- NSAIDs (naproxen is preferably used)
  - Corticosteroids in cases where NSAIDs cannot be used

CARDITIS/HEART FAILURE

- Bed rest, fluid restriction, heart failure medications (furosemide, spironolactone, ACEI)
- Corticosteroids for severe heart failure if surgery is not indicated or unavailable
- Surgery for intractable heart failure associated with severe mitral or aortic regurgitation; preferable to defer surgery until acute rheumatic activity has resolved
  - See Chapter 16 for a full discussion on acute heart failure

CHOREA

- Penicillin V[a] orally or intramuscular benzathine penicillin G
- Haloperidol or carbamazepine can be considered if the abnormal movements interfere with daily activities
  - Valproic acid reserved for refractory cases
  - Multidisciplinary input as required for significant motor or neuropsychiatric manifestations

DISCHARGE PROCEDURE

- Discharge once there is clinical improvement and reduction in ESR or CRP
- Notification to health authorities
- Patient and family education
- Secondary prophylaxis (see Chapter 11)
- Outpatient follow-up

ACEI, angiotensin-converting enzyme inhibitor; *CRP*, C-reactive protein; *ESR*, erythrocyte sedimentation rate; *GAS*, group A streptococcal; *NSAIDs*, nonsteroidal antiinflammatory drugs.
[a] Also known as phenoxymethylpenicillin or penicillin V potassium (PVK)

further discussion on anaphylaxis and assessment of possible penicillin allergy). Erythromycin orally is the treatment of choice in those proven to have penicillin allergy (see Table 4.2).

GENERAL MEASURES AND SYMPTOMATIC RELIEF

Salicylates (aspirin) and nonsteroidal antiinflammatory drugs (NSAIDs) have been recommended for fever and joint pain but do not affect the prevalence or severity of clinical valve sequelae in the long term.[5]

Fever

Paracetamol can be prescribed in several circumstances: for fever and mild arthralgia; until the diagnosis of ARF is confirmed (see Arthritis and/or Arthralgia, below); until symptoms are relieved; or concomitantly when NSAIDs are started.[4]

Bed Rest and Diet

Most patients with suspected ARF should be admitted to hospital, which has benefits beyond establishing the diagnosis. If there is evidence of carditis, hospitalization also ensures that bed rest is adhered to (which

TABLE 4.2
Medication Table for Acute Rheumatic Fever.

	Australian Guidelines, 2012[3]	New Zealand Guidelines, 2014[4]	Other Recommendations
ANTIBIOTICS			
To treat the initial streptococcal infection			
Phenoxymethylpenicillin (Penicillin V), orally[a]	**Child**: 250 mg bd (for 10 days). **Adolescents and Adult**: 500 mg bd (for 10 days).	**Children <20 kg**: 250 mg 2–3 × daily (for 10 days). **Children and adults ≥20 kg**: 500 mg 2–3 × daily (for 10 days).	**Children:** 250 mg 2–3 × daily. **Adolescents or adults:** 250 mg 3–4 × daily, or 500 mg bd.[7]
Amoxicillin, orally[a]	–	**Once daily (for 10 days)**: 50 mg/kg (maximum dose 1000 mg daily). **OR:** Weight <30 kg: 750 mg once daily. Weight ≥30 kg: 1000 mg once daily. **Twice daily (for 10 days):** 25 mg/kg bd (maximum dose 1000 mg daily).	25–50 mg/kg/day tds. Total adult dose is 750–1500 mg/day × 10 days.[7]
Erythromycin ethyl succinate[b], orally. Used in those with penicillin allergy	**Child**: 20 mg/kg (maximum dose 800 mg) bd (for 10 days). **Adult**: 800 mg bd (for 10 days).	**Children and adults**: 40 mg/kg/day in 2–3 divided doses (for 10 days). Maximum dose 1600 mg daily.	–
Benzathine penicillin G by IM injection (Once the first dose is given, oral penicillin is stopped)	**<20 kg (single dose)**: 450 mg (600,000 units) **≥20 kg (single dose)**: 900 mg (1.2 million units)	**Children <30 kg (single dose)**: 450 mg (600,000 units). **Adults and children ≥30 kg (single dose):** 900 mg (1.2 million units).	1.2 million units IM, 600 000 units For children <27 kg.[7]
ANALGESICS			
Antiinflammatory drugs			
Paracetamol, orally. For fever and mild arthralgia or until diagnosis is confirmed. Duration: until symptoms are relieved or NSAIDs are started.	60 mg/kg/day given in 4–6 doses/day. Can increase to 90 mg/kg/day, if needed, under medical supervision. Maximum 4 grams daily.	60 mg/kg/day in 4–6 doses. Can increase to 90 mg/kg/day if required under medical supervision. Maximum 4 grams daily.	–
Naproxen, orally. For arthritis, or severe arthralgia (when ARF diagnosis is confirmed), until joint symptoms are relieved. Safer alternative to aspirin.	10–20 mg/kg/day (maximum 1250 mg/day), divided q12h.	10–20 mg/kg/day, divided q12h (maximum 1000 mg/day) until pain is relieved, then taper dose.	–
Ibuprofen, orally. Use as for naproxen. *No data to support its use in ARF*	30 mg/kg/day (maximum 1600 mg daily), divided tds.	5–10 mg/kg/dose 8 hourly until pain is relieved, then taper dose. Maximum 400 mg per dose.	–

Continued

TABLE 4.2
Medication Table for Acute Rheumatic Fever.—cont'd

	Australian Guidelines, 2012[3]	New Zealand Guidelines, 2014[4]	Other Recommendations
Aspirin, orally. Use as for naproxen.	Begin with 50–60 mg/kg/day, increasing if needed to 80–100 mg/kg/day (4–8 g/day in adults) given in 4–5 divided doses/day. If higher doses are required, reduce to 50–60 mg/kg/day when symptoms improve, and cease when symptom free for 1–2 weeks. Consider stopping in presence of acute viral illness, and it is recommended that children receiving aspirin during the influenza season (autumn/winter) also receive the influenza vaccine.	Not recommended due to concern about Reye's Syndrome.	–
HEART FAILURE DRUGS			
Diuretics			
Furosemide, orally or IV (can also be given IM). For heart failure signs and symptoms. Duration: until heart failure is controlled and carditis improved.	**Child:** 1–2 mg/kg stat, then 0.5–1 mg/kg/dose 6–24 hourly (maximum 6 mg/kg/day). **Adult:** 20–40 mg/dose, 6–24 hourly, up to 250–500 mg/day.	**Orally in children:** **1 month–12 years:** 0.5–2 mg/kg 2–3 times daily. Medium dose is 1 mg/kg bd. Maximum 6 mg/kg daily, not to exceed 80 mg/day. **12–18 years:** 20–40 mg daily (increase to 80–120 mg daily in resistant oedema). **Slow intravenous injection in children:** **1 month–12 years:** 0.5–1 mg/kg every 8 h as necessary. Maximum 2 mg/kg (40 mg) every 8 h. **12–18 years:** 20–40 mg every 8 h as necessary (resistant cases may require higher doses). **Adults:** 20–40 mg/dose 12–24 hourly up to a maximum dose of 250–500 mg/day.	–
Spironolactone, orally. Duration as for furosemide. Round dose to multiple of 6.25 mg (quarter of a 25 mg tablet) if liquid form not available	1–3 mg/kg/day (maximum 100 –200 mg/day) in 1–3 divided doses.	Orally in children: **1 month–12 years:** 1–3 mg/kg/day (maximum 100–200 mg/day) in 1–2 divided doses. **12-18 years:** 50–100 mg daily in 1–2 divided doses.	–

ACE inhibitors

Enalapril, orally. Duration as for furosemide.

Child: 0.1 mg/kg/day in 1–2 doses, increased gradually over 2 weeks.
Adult: Initially 2.5 mg daily. Maintenance 10–20 mg daily. Maximum 40 mg daily.

Children:
0.1 mg/kg/day in 1–2 doses increased gradually over 2 weeks.
Adults:
Initially 2.5 mg daily.
Maintenance 10–20 mg daily.
Maximum 40 mg daily.

–

Captopril, orally. Duration as for furosemide.

Child: Initial dose 0.1 mg/kg/dose. Beware of hypotension. Increase gradually over 2 weeks to 0.5–1 mg/kg/dose 8 hourly (maximum 2 mg/kg/dose 8 hourly).
Adult: Initial dose 2.5–5 mg. Maintenance dose 25–50 mg 8 hourly.

Children:
0.1–0.2 mg/kg/dose 8 hourly increasing in increments to 1–1.5 mg/kg/dose 8 hourly.
12–18 years:
12.5–25 mg 2–3 times a day increasing to a maximum of 150 mg daily in divided doses.
Adults:
Up to 50 mg 8 hourly.

–

Lisinopril, orally. Duration as for furosemide.

Child: 0.1–0.2 mg/kg once daily, up to 1 mg/kg/dose.
Adult: 2.5–20 mg once daily (maximum 40 mg/day).

Children:
Initially 70 mcg/kg (maximum 5 mg) once daily, increased in intervals of 1–2 weeks to a maximum of 600 mcg/kg (or 40 mg) once daily.
Adults:
2.5–20 mg once daily
Maximum of 40 mg daily.
Monitor blood pressure during initiation of therapy.

–

ADDITIONAL HEART FAILURE MEDICINES

Digoxin, orally or IV.
For heart failure/atrial fibrillation Seek advice from specialist regarding duration of use.
Intravenous use in children rarely indicated

Child: 15 mcg/kg initially, then 5 mcg/kg after 6 h, then 3–5 mcg/kg/ dose (maximum 125 mcg) 12 hourly.
Adult 125–250 mcg daily. *Check serum levels.*

Children:
15 mcg/kg oral stat and then 5 mcg/kg after 6 h, then 3–5 mcg/kg/dose 12 hourly. Maximum dose 125 mcg 12 hourly.
Adults:
62.5–500 mcg daily.
Check serum levels.

–

Prednisolone or **prednisone,** orally. For severe carditis, heart failure, or pericarditis with effusion (if acute heart surgery is not indicated) . Not evidence based and not shown to alter long-term outcome.
Usual duration: 1–3 weeks.

1–2 mg/kg/day (maximum 80 mg). If used >1 week, taper by 20% –25% per week.

1–2 mg/kg/day. If used >1 week, taper by 20%–25% per week.
Maximum dose: 60 mg daily.

Regime I[2]
Prednisolone: 2 mg/kg/day, maximum 80 mg/day till ESR normalizes—usually 2 weeks. Taper over 2–4 weeks, reduce dose by 2.5–5 mg every 3rd day.
Start aspirin: 50–75 mg/kg/day simultaneously, to complete total 12 weeks. (Level of evidence: class I)

Continued

TABLE 4.2
Medication Table for Acute Rheumatic Fever.—cont'd

	Australian Guidelines, 2012[3]	New Zealand Guidelines, 2014[4]	Other Recommendations
			Regime II[2] **Prednisolone:** same doses × 3–4 weeks. Taper slowly to cover total period of 10–12 weeks. (Level of evidence: class IIb)
Methylprednisolone sodium succinate ("Solu-Medrol"), IV *If no response to oral steroids.*	—	—	**Children 1–18 years:** 10–30 mg/kg/day, in 2 divided doses (maximum dose 1000 mg/day)[c] **Adults:** initial dose 10–40 mg over several minutes; for high-dose therapy, 30 mg/kg, may repeat every 4–6 hours[c]
SYDENHAM CHOREA			
Carbamazepine, orally. For severe chorea. Continue until chorea controlled for several weeks then trial off medication.	7–20 mg/kg/day (7–10 mg/kg/day usually sufficient) in divided doses, given 3 × daily.	7–20 mg/kg/day (7–10 mg/kg/day usually sufficient), given in divided doses tds.	–
Valproic acid, orally. For refractory chorea (hepatotoxic). Avoid in women of childbearing potential as teratogenic. Duration as for carbamazepine	15–20 mg/kg/day (can increase to 30 mg/kg/day) given In divided doses tds.	15–20 mg/kg/day (can increase to 30 mg/kg/day), given in divided doses tds.	–
Haloperidol	—	—	Start 0.025 mg/kg/day, increasing slowly monitoring effect to a maximum of 0.15 mg/kg/day.[41]
Prednisone	—	—	2 mg/kg/day for 4 weeks and then taper.[40]
Intravenous immunoglobulins (IVIG)	—	—	1 g/kg/day × 2 days.[44]

ARF, Acute Rheumatic Fever; *bd*, bis die (twice daily); *BPG* benzathine penicillin G; *ESR*, erythrocyte sedimentation rate; IM, intramuscular; *IV*, intravenously; *mcg*, micrograms; *NSAID*, nonsteroidal antiinflammatory drug; *po*, per oral; *stat*, statum (Latin word for immediately). *tds, ter die sumendum* (three times daily);

[a] Both Penicillin V and amoxicillin are equally effective in eradicating GAS. Oral penicillin V is best absorbed on an empty stomach whereas amoxicillin can be taken with food and is relatively palatable.

[b] There are other erythromycins available with different dosing regimens to erythromycin ethyl succinate. Check dosing with your local pharmacist.

[c] Administer by slow intravenous infusion over at least 30 min. Therapy should be continued only until the patient's condition has stabilised, usually not longer than 48–72 hours.

may not be feasible in a home environment, particularly in poorly-resourced countries). Resting allows reduction of workload on the heart and may prevent progression of the inflammatory process. Hospitalization also provides an ideal opportunity to educate patients and families about ARF. Further education by primary healthcare staff, using culturally appropriate educational materials, should be continued once the patient has returned home.

In the prepenicillin era there was evidence that bed rest was associated with a shorter duration of carditis and fewer relapses.[8] In the postpenicillin era, no randomized controlled trials have been undertaken to assess the effect of bed rest objectively. If mild, the mitral regurgitation in patients with carditis can diminish or disappear with bed rest. If the patient continues to exercise and the patient does not receive penicillin, rheumatic activity may persist and mitral regurgitation can worsen. The excessive workload on the heart of a patient with severe rheumatic mitral regurgitation produces a situation analogous to that of a child with active carditis and a mild valve lesion being forced to exercise continuously. Severe mitral regurgitation, with its associated hemodynamic overload, can aggravate rheumatic activity.[9] This concept is supported by the observation of rapid resolution of rheumatic activity postoperatively. The correction of the valve lesion results in removal of the excessive cardiac workload caused by the regurgitation.[9]

Although most patients with ARF need bed rest early in their illness, gradual mobilization is recommended once the initial symptoms have begun to resolve.[4,6] In those with heart failure or acute severe valve lesions, mobilisation should occur gradually over the first 4 weeks or until normalisation of the C-reactive protein (CRP) and the erythrocyte sedimentation rate (ESR) has normalised or dramatically reduced.[3]

In summary, in the absence of evidence, expert-based recommendation supports a role for bed rest initially, with the length of bed rest largely determined by the severity of carditis. In the absence of carditis, the patient can be mobilized once arthritis settles. No dietary restrictions are required except if the patient is in heart failure, then fluid and salt intake should be limited. Many patients with ARF are malnourished (pointing to rheumatic recurrence or an acute-on-chronic or indolent presentation) and their diet should be optimized with the help of a dietician and improvements should be monitored with weekly weight checks during their hospitalization.

MAJOR MANIFESTATIONS
Arthritis and/or Arthralgia

Early administration of NSAIDs may mask the development of migratory polyarthritis therefore it is recommended that joint pain and fever should be treated with paracetamol (and/or codeine) until the diagnosis of ARF is confirmed.[2-4,7] Although paracetamol may mask the fever, documented fever before admission can be used as a minor manifestation.[3,4] The arthritis of ARF is exquisitely responsive to treatment with NSAIDS. This response can be a useful diagnostic feature, as arthritis continuing unabated >3 days after starting NSAID therapy is unlikely to be due to ARF.[10]

Aspirin has traditionally been used to treat the fever, arthralgia, and arthritis of ARF. NSAIDs, particularly naproxen, have replaced aspirin in other childhood inflammatory diseases and because of its superior safety profile is being promoted as the first line antiinflammatory medication in patients with ARF and severe arthralgia or arthritis.[3,4,11] A small prospective, randomized trial comparing naproxen to aspirin in ARF showed that naproxen is as effective as and safer than aspirin. More patients in the aspirin group had adverse reactions such as elevation of hepatic enzymes, dyspepsia, vomiting, and adherence problems because of the higher number of doses per day.[12] Toxic effects also include tinnitus, headache, and tachypnoea, although these usually resolve within days after stopping the drug. Aspirin has also lost favor as the recommended choice for rheumatic arthritis because of the risk of developing Reye's syndrome in children with certain viral infections, particularly influenza.[3,4] The other advantage of naproxen is the twice-daily dosing regime and the fact that in some countries it is available as a suspension that is easier to administer to children.

Although naproxen is recommended as the treatment of choice, aspirin may still be used in resource constrained settings where it is easily available and cheaper, with close observation for any potential side effects. Ibuprofen is also often used but there is no published evidence of its effectiveness in ARF.[4] In those patients who are allergic to aspirin/NSAIDs or are unable to tolerate these drugs, low-dose oral steroids (prednisone or prednisolone) are a suitable alternative. Coadministration of a proton-pump inhibitor (e.g., omeprazole) should be considered if the patient develops gastrointestinal upset on aspirin or NSAIDs or is receiving steroid therapy.

The duration of therapy is arbitrarily based on the severity of illness and response to therapy, including improvement in inflammatory markers (ESR, CRP), and should be individualized. Most patients require treatment for only 1–2 weeks, but some cases may need 6–8 weeks. Fewer than 5% of patients require antiinflammatory treatment for 6 months or more. In cases where prolonged antiinflammatory therapy with aspirin is used (>2 weeks), drug levels should be monitored (if available) as the risk of salicylate toxicity is increased. If joint symptoms recur after reducing the dose or after stopping the drug (whether NSAIDs, aspirin or corticosteroids) it may be due to a "rebound phenomenon." This does not represent recurrence of ARF, and the patient should have an extension of their antiinflammatory treatment.

Carditis and Heart Failure
Carditis
Echocardiography should be performed in all patients with suspected ARF, regardless of the presence or absence of any murmurs, in order to confirm the presence and severity of carditis. The main manifestations of carditis are mitral regurgitation with or without aortic regurgitation and are discussed in detail in Chapters 3 and 16. Pericarditis (pericardial effusion) can also be present. First degree heart block is common. All degrees of carditis, including subclinical carditis,[13] require hospitalization. Patients with symptomatic moderate to severe valve regurgitation will benefit from diuretics, with or without ACE inhibitors (see section on Heart Failure and Chapters 6 and 16).[4] Steroids result in a more rapid resolution of the inflammation compared to aspirin,[14,15] and are often used in severe carditis with heart failure. However, there is little objective evidence to prove that they are beneficial over and above bed rest, fluid restriction, and heart failure medications.[1,9,16] Close observation is required as steroids may cause gastrointestinal bleeding and fluid retention, both of which can make the heart failure worse.

Advanced atrioventricular block
Advanced atrioventricular (AV) block with second-degree AV block, complete heart block and accelerated junctional rhythm should be monitored with cardiac monitoring and frequent ECGs.[17–21] Only rarely does a very slow rate occur with symptoms. In those with advanced AV block, rhythm monitoring will reveal return of AV synchrony for short periods initially, then permanently. Cardiac compromise is rarely seen. Anecdotally, pacing has been performed, usually because ARF was not recognized or the benign nature not understood. Thus, pacing should be avoided as return to sinus rhythm almost always

occurs spontaneously. If pacing is decided upon, a temporary pacing lead rather than permanent pacemaker implantation is recommended.[17] AV block is also present in ARF cases with accelerated junctional tachycardia[17,18] with the junctional rate faster than the sinus rate. Corticosteroids are often given for advanced AV block and seem intuitively logical, but this has not been tested in a randomized controlled trial. Both advanced AV block and junctional tachycardia have a high specificity for ARF.[17,19] In conclusion, the presence of advanced AV block in a patient with suspected ARF is useful diagnostically, requires cardiac monitoring, but is expected to resolve spontaneously.

Heart failure
General measures are summarized in Table 4.3. Patients with carditis and heart failure should be evaluated for associated anemia, intercurrent respiratory infections, infective endocarditis, and arrhythmias such as atrial fibrillation, all of which may worsen heart failure and should be treated accordingly. An urgent echocardiogram is essential to assess the severity of the heart valve lesions, assess ventricular size and function, and rule out a pericardial effusion. Infective endocarditis should be considered in all patients who are very ill or have a persistently high fever (see Chapter 16). Serial blood cultures should be taken and echocardiography will help to define the presence of intracardiac vegetations. An electrocardiogram will assist the confirmation of atrial fibrillation that may require treatment for rate

TABLE 4.3 Principles of Heart Failure Management in ARF.	
1	Bed rest
2	Monitor fluid balance and weight. Fluid and sodium restriction if congestive heart failure
3	Treat anemia, intercurrent respiratory infections, infective endocarditis
4	Treat malnutrition
5	Venous thrombo-prophylaxis in adults with prolonged bed rest
6	Cardiac medications: Diuretics first line management ACE inhibitor second line management
7	Arrhythmia management
8	Coronary care unit or intensive care unit if cardiogenic shock or respiratory failure (see Chapter 16)

and rhythm control and anticoagulation (see Chapters 6 and 16). Atrial fibrillation and infective endocarditis are usually associated with chronic valve disease.[2]

Heart-failure medications. The first line treatment for symptoms of heart failure and severe valve regurgitation in ARF is diuretics, such as furosemide or bumetanide. Many patients will respond to loop diuretics and bed rest. Thiazide diuretics or spironolactone may be added if the initial response to loop diuretics is inadequate. Oral diuretic and vasodilator therapy, including angiotensin converting enzyme inhibitors (ACEI) relieve symptoms by decreasing afterload and pulmonary venous pressure, but they do not alter the clinical evidence of rheumatic activity.[9] ACE inhibitors and beta blockers are usually reserved for those with impaired ventricular function once the patient is stable. Low-dose therapy should be started in stable patients with a progressive up-titration to the target dose.[22,23] Care must be taken with ACE inhibitors if there is hypotension. There is a risk of hyperkalemia with combined ACE inhibitor and spironolactone use.[4] Digoxin is usually reserved for patients with atrial fibrillation not controlled with beta blockers. Serum levels of digoxin should be monitored. The management of chronic heart failure is discussed in detail in Chapter 6.

If heart failure symptoms persist, intravenous diuretics and vasodilators (and inotropes if evidence of cardiogenic shock) may be required while awaiting cardiac surgery, although there is no evidence that any of these agents reduce mortality. Both dobutamine and dopamine have been shown to be effective inotropic agents in children with circulatory failure especially in low income countries where milrinone may not be available due to cost issues. Dobutamine and dopamine can induce tachycardias and tachyarrhythmias resulting in a mismatch between myocardial oxygen delivery and requirement; hence, they may be reserved only for patients with low cardiac output despite other therapies.[24,25] If available, milrinone is used to treat critically ill patients with heart failure where surgery is not immediately available.[2] The evaluation and management of acute heart failure, including cardiogenic shock, are discussed further in Chapter 16.

Antiinflammatory medications. Corticosteroids are not proven to be "lifesaving" treatment in patients who have severe active rheumatic carditis with heart failure. The cause of heart failure in rheumatic carditis is severe valvular regurgitation and not myocarditis; therefore, surgery is indicated in cases with intractable heart failure in the presence of severe mitral and/or aortic regurgitation. Depressed left ventricular function

may result from acute overload produced by severe valve regurgitation.[9,26]

A Cochrane review[16] of eight randomized control trials (most were published over 50 years ago) that involved 996 patients found that antiinflammatory treatment (namely aspirin, corticosteroids, and intravenous immunoglobulin) produced no significant difference in risk of cardiac disease at 1 year following ARF.[27] The type, dose, and duration of corticosteroids and other medications varied between the studies creating risk of bias due to the extensive heterogeneity between the trials. Severe outcomes such as death and the need for heart surgery were reported in only 3 of the 8 studies. There were a total of 8 deaths and 5 patients needing surgery, with 5/8 deaths and 4/5 surgical interventions occurring in the corticosteroid group. The data therefore refute a life-saving role for corticosteroid therapy in patients with carditis.[28] The extensive experience in South Africa supports the concept that the use of corticosteroids is ineffective for patients with significant carditis.[9] The same Cochrane meta-analysis[16] concluded that salicylates have no effect on the reduction of the incidence of residual rheumatic heart disease (RHD) and are therefore not recommended to treat carditis for the purposes of reducing severity of valve lesions.

In a small study of 24 patients, prednisone was shown to favorably affect clinical response (fall in heart rate and fall in clinical score) compared to aspirin. As expected, the erythrocyte sedimentation rate (ESR) fell more quickly with prednisone.[28] Another small randomized clinical trial of 18 patients comparing intravenous pulses of methylprednisolone to oral prednisone over 4 weeks in the management of acute severe rheumatic carditis with heart failure showed the oral prednisone group to have a greater response in reduction of heart rate, ESR, ejection fraction and left ventricular end-systolic diameter. There was one death in the methylprednisolone group.[29]

There has been a call to undertake a multicentre randomized controlled trial of corticosteroids versus placebo for ARF using echocardiographic end points for acute carditis (for example, at 6 weeks) and chronic RHD (at 6 months to 1 year).[1] Such a study would need to be powered to account for the natural improvement of carditis after the acute phase[27] but would provide an evidence-based approach to corticosteroid therapy for active rheumatic carditis. The research group could then study other immunomodulators, informed by an expanded understanding of ARF immunopathogenesis. There is no role for further small, underpowered studies of corticosteroid use in ARF.[1]

Corticosteroids seem empirically indicated in patients with significant symptoms or signs of pericarditis that is an occasional feature of ARF.

In conclusion, corticosteroid therapy is considered optional in patients with severe carditis (i.e. severe valvular regurgitation and/or pericarditis) and may be considered for those with heart failure in whom acute cardiac surgery is not indicated or not available.[4,26]

Heart valve surgery. Serial echocardiography to measure cardiac dimensions and function is invaluable in the assessment of valve disease[3,4] and the need for heart valve surgery. In many patients, the severity of the carditis stabilizes or improves over weeks to months, as the inflammatory phase resolves. Wherever possible, surgery is delayed until the active inflammation has settled,[4] as surgery during the acute inflammatory phase is associated with higher failure rates.[30,31]

If surgery is unavoidable in the presence of ARF, the rheumatic activity can resolve dramatically during the first few weeks postoperatively. The main reason for the postoperative resolution of rheumatic activity (as discussed before) is removal of the cardiac workload by correction of the valve lesion, and is similar to the effect of bed rest on reducing rheumatic activity.[9,30]

Mitral valve repair is achievable in most ARF cases; however, early surgery needs to be adjusted to allow for the remodeling process as the inflammation subsides, which may shrink the leaflets and shorten chordae.[30,32–34] Nevertheless repair may have to be considered in the very young patient with ARF and heart failure, if only to delay prosthetic valve implantation by a few years. The data on the outcome of these patients after repair however is contradictory and may vary according to institutional factors and surgical expertise. Surgical outcomes also depend on other aspects such as severity of disease, left ventricular function, nutritional status of the patient, adherence to secondary prophylaxis, and recurrences of ARF.

The very inflamed and oedematous tissue does make the repair challenging and the medium to long-term results suboptimal, resulting in frequent reoperation particularly if the carditis persists or recurs.[30,32–34] Excellent outcomes have been reported with repair surgery (90% survival and 75% freedom from reoperation at 10 years) when compared with valve replacement in patients under 20 years old.[35] Moreover, 50% of patients with an MV replacement were found to have a significant hemorrhagic or thromboembolic event within 11 years of operation.[35]

Despite the associated risks of prosthetic valve replacement (notably thromboembolism, need for anticoagulation, infection, hemolysis), valve replacement may have to be considered if surgical expertise does

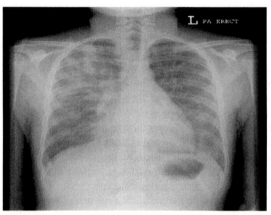

FIG. 4.1 Chest X-ray of a 10-year-old child showing acute pulmonary edema dominantly in the right upper zone, secondary to acute onset of severe mitral regurgitation associated with a flail posterior mitral valve leaflet. Note the relatively normal heart size.

not extend to mitral valve repair (indications for cardiac surgery are discussed in Chapter 6 and surgical details are discussed in Chapter 7).

Surgery can be lifesaving in patients where the principal cause of severe hemodynamic deterioration is ruptured chordae tendineae causing severe mitral regurgitation. In the acute setting, this results in the rapid rise of left atrial pressure due to a noncompliant left atrium. Pulmonary edema (Fig. 4.1) ensues, which can be unilateral.*,[2,4,36] Acute severe aortic regurgitation can also result in severe left ventricular failure not controlled by diuretics, inotropes, and corticosteroids. In this setting, cardiac valve surgery can also be lifesaving (see Chapter 16).[26,36]

Sydenham Chorea

Recommendations for optimal management remain inconsistent and are hampered by the side effects from pharmacotherapy.[37] Treatment is therefore mainly symptomatic, not evidence based, and is aimed at minimizing involuntary movements, incoordination and

---

*Most ARF patients with acute mitral regurgitation and pulmonary edema develop bilateral signs on chest X-ray. Occasionally, the pulmonary edema is unilateral (seen in approximately 2% of cases), most often affecting the right upper lobe and can be confused with pneumonia (particularly if the patient has concurrent fever). This is mostly seen in chordal rupture with a flail anterior mitral valve leaflet as a complication of rheumatic valvulitis. This radiological finding is secondary to a posteriorly-directed regurgitant jet that is directed towards the right superior pulmonary vein, causing a selective increase in hydrostatic pressure. The findings on chest X-ray often resolve rapidly after commencing diuretics, which helps clinch the diagnosis.

psychiatric symptoms, treatment of the immune and inflammatory response, and supportive measures.[37]

Sydenham chorea is strongly associated with carditis [38]; therefore, treatment with penicillin is indicated to eliminate the GAS. Patients who receive 10 days of penicillin, bed rest, and/or hospitalization have significantly better neurocognitive outcomes.[39]

Chorea is usually benign and self-limiting with resolution within about 6 months, but can have a relapsing course for up to 2−3 years.[39] Patients and the family need to be informed of the potential for chorea to continue for several months and to fluctuate during times of intercurrent illness and stress (see Chapter 3).

If, however, movements interfere with normal activities, or place the patient at risk of injury such as falling over, or are extremely distressing to the patient or their family, treatment can be considered. A multidisciplinary approach is ideal and may include pharmacotherapy, occupational therapy, physiotherapy, and support with schooling (missed school days and poor school performance can be a significant issue).

Several dopamine 2 (D2) receptor antagonists have been utilized in worldwide studies to treat chorea, the most common being the neuroleptics haloperidol and pimozide.[37] Sedatives such as phenobarbitone and diazepam are recommended in mild chorea.[2] In severe cases, carbamazepine and valproic acid are the preferred choices to haloperidol,[3,4] which has severe side effects such as drowsiness, dizziness, poor school performance, dystonia, and extrapyramidal signs and symptoms.[37] Carbamazepine has anticonvulsant and analgesic effects, and valproic acid is used as an anticonvulsant and mood stabilizer. It is recommended that carbamazepine be used as the first choice in cases of severe chorea[1] when movements become incapacitating for the patient to the point that they require assistance during activities of daily living.[1] Valproic acid should be kept for refractory cases because it has a possible liver toxic effect and is the most teratogenic of all anticonvulsants.[1]

Haloperidol may however be the first choice in many resource limited countries because it is more readily available and cost effective. The dose should be titrated to the maximum dose slowly.[37,40,41] There is the risk of inducing an acute movement disorder with D2 receptor antagonists, such as dystonia or akathisia. This can be treated with an anticholinergic such as diphenhydramine along with withdrawal or reduction in dosage of the offending drug.

A recent case report from South America describes successful use of levetiracetam, an anticonvulsant, for Sydenham's chorea.[42] This may warrant further investigation.

A response may not be seen for 1−2 weeks, and successful medication may only reduce but not eliminate symptoms. Medication should be continued for 2−4 weeks after chorea has subsided, and then withdrawn.[43] Recurrences are usually mild and can be managed conservatively, but in severe recurrences the medication can be restarted.[3]

Improvements in symptoms have also been reported using corticosteroids. Paz et al. showed in a randomized controlled trial comparing prednisone to placebo for 4 weeks that the intensity score and chorea remission time was significantly shorter in the prednisone group, but the recurrence rates were the same in the two groups.[40]

Immunomodulatory therapies such as plasma exchange to remove antineuronal antibodies and intravenous immunoglobulins (IVIG) to inactivate antineuronal antibodies have been compared with prednisone. The results were not statistically significant but clinical improvement was more apparent in the plasma exchange and IVIG groups.[35,44] Until more evidence is available, IVIG is not recommended, except for severe chorea refractory to all other treatments.[3]

The neuropsychiatric symptoms of Sydenham chorea, such as obsessive-compulsive disorder, attention-deficit hyperactive disorder, and affective disorders are also a significant concern and early recognition may aid in patient management. A multidisciplinary approach is best and should include referral to psychiatry, psychology, and neurology specialists.

DISCHARGE PROTOCOL
Each center managing ARF patients should consider a discharge planning protocol or check list.[4]

Discharge Criteria
The duration of treatment is dictated by the clinical response and improvement in inflammatory markers, such as the ESR and the C-reactive protein.[3,4,45]

Notification
Notification of ARF to public health authorities for infectious disease surveillance and for public health measures is mandatory in certain countries.[3,4]

Patient and Family Education
All patients should have a good understanding of the cause and symptoms of ARF and the need to have sore throats treated early for themselves as well as other family members.[3,4] Family members should be informed that they are at increased risk of ARF compared to the wider community.[4] Recent evidence supports offering echocardiographic screening for RHD for first-degree relatives of index cases.[46]

Prophylaxis

Secondary Prophylaxis: Patients and families should understand the reason for long-term secondary prophylaxis, and the consequences of not receiving all recommended treatments (see also Chapter 11).

The first dose of IM benzathine penicillin G is usually given in hospital. The patient and family should have a good understanding of where and by whom the benzathine penicillin G is being given: for example, community nursing services, local clinic, hospital clinic, or family doctor.

Anaphylaxis to benzathine penicillin G is rare. Anaphylaxis should be treated with epinephrine (adrenaline) 0.01 mg/kg (maximum dose of 0.5 mg) per single dose, injected intramuscularly into the mid-outer thigh. A fuller discussion of anaphylaxis is given in Chapter 11.

Infective endocarditis

Although the American Heart Association guidelines no longer list RHD as an indication for antibiotic prophylaxis, it is recommended that patients with established RHD or prosthetic valves receive antibiotic prophylaxis before procedures expected to produce bacteremia, especially for Streptococcus viridans (see Chapter 16).[1,4,47]

Refer to dental services at the time of diagnosis of ARF for evaluation and treatment, if indicated. The patient's family should also be educated on the importance of good dental hygiene.

Outpatient Follow-up

All patients should receive regular review and outpatient follow-up that should be arranged before discharge. Medical, cardiology, and psychiatry/psychology follow-up all may be required, the frequency of which will depend on the severity of the carditis and extent of continuing chorea.

REFERENCES

1. Carapetis JR, Beaton A, Cunningham MW, et al. Acute rheumatic fever and rheumatic heart disease. *Nat Rev Dis Primers*. 2016;2:15084.
2. Working Group on Pediatric Acute Rheumatic Fever and Cardiology Chapter of Indian Academy of Pediatrics, Saxena A, Krishna RK, et al. Consensus guidelines on pediatric acute rheumatic fever and rheumatic heart disease. *Indian Pediatr*. 2008;45:565−573.
3. RHD Australia (ARF/RHD writing group). *National heart Foundation of Australia, Cardiac Society of Australia and New Zealand. The Australian Guideline for Prevention, Diagnosis and Management of Acute Rheumatic Fever And Rheumatic Heart Disease*. Full guidelines. 2nd ed.; 2012, 1-136 pp. Available from: https://www.rhdaustralia.org.au/arf-rhd-guideline.
4. New Zealand Heart Foundation. New Zealand Guidelines for Rheumatic Fever: Diagnosis, Management and Secondary Prevention of Acute Rheumatic Fever and Rheumatic Heart Disease: 2014 Update. 2014. Auckland. https://www.heartfoundation.org.nz.
5. Marijon E, Mirabel M, Celermajer D, Jouven X. Rheumatic heart disease. *Lancet*. 2012;379:953−964.
6. Carapetis JR, McDonald M, Wilson NJ. Acute rheumatic fever. *Lancet*. 2005;366(9480):155−168.
7. World Health Organisation. *Rheumatic Fever and Rheumatic Heart Disease: Report of a WHO Expert Consultation*. Geneva, Switzerland: World Health Organization; 2004. Contract No: World Health Organisation Technical Report Series 923.
8. Markovitz M, Gordis L. *Rheumatic Fever*. 2nd ed. Philadelphia: WB Saunders; 1972.
9. Barlow JB, Marcus RH, Pocock WA, Barlow CW, Essop R, Sareli P. Mechanisms and management of heart failure in active rheumatic carditis. *S Afr Med J*. 1990;78(4):181−186.
10. Carapetis JR, Brown A, Wilson NJ, Edwards KN. Rheumatic Fever Guidelines Writing G. An Australian guideline for rheumatic fever and rheumatic heart disease: an abridged outline. *Med J Aust*. 2007;186(11):581−586.
11. Cetin II , Ekici F, Kocabas A, et al. The efficacy and safety of naproxen in acute rheumatic fever: the comparative results of 11-year experience with acetylsalicylic acid and naproxen. *Turk J Pediatr*. 2016;58(5):473−479.
12. Hashkes PJ, Tauber T, Somekh E, et al. Naproxen as an alternative to aspirin for the treatment of arthritis of rheumatic fever: a randomized trial. *J Pediatr*. 2003;143(3):399−401.
13. Beg A, Sadiq M. Subclinical valvulitis in children with acute rheumatic Fever. *Pediatr Cardiol*. 2008;29(3):619−623.
14. Kasliwal RR, Mehrotra R. Rheumatic fever: diagnosis and management. In: Kumar RR, ed. *ECAB Clinical Update: Cardiology-Rheumatic Heart Disease*. India: Elsevier; 2008:21−47.
15. Mishra TK, Das B, Routray S, Mishra H. Management of acute rheumatic fever: a re-appraisal. *JICC*. 2012;2(1):33−39.
16. Cilliers A, Manyemba J, Adler AJ, Saloojee H. Anti-inflammatory treatment for carditis in acute rheumatic fever. *Cochrane Database Syst Rev*. 2012;6:Cd003176.
17. Agnew J, Wilson N, Skinner J, Nicholson R. Beyond first-degree heart block in the diagnosis of acute rheumatic fever. *Cardiol Young*. 2019;29(6):744−748.
18. Balli S, Oflaz MB, Kibar AE, Ece I. Rhythm and conduction analysis of patients with acute rheumatic fever. *Pediatr Cardiol*. 2013;34(2):383−389.
19. Ceviz N, Celik V, Olgun H, Karacan M. Accelerated junctional rhythm in children with acute rheumatic fever: is it specific to the disease? *Cardiol Young*. 2014;24(3):464−468.
20. Karacan M, Isikay S, Olgun H, Ceviz N. Asymptomatic rhythm and conduction abnormalities in children with acute rheumatic fever: 24-hour electrocardiography study. *Cardiol Young*. 2010;20(6):620−630.
21. Zalzstein E, Maor R, Zucker N, Katz A. Advanced atrioventricular conduction block in acute rheumatic fever. *Cardiol Young*. 2003;13(6):506−508.

22. Hussey A, Weintraub RG. Drug treatment of heart failure in children: focus on recent recommendations from the ISHLT guidelines for the management of pediatric heart failure. *Pediatr Drugs.* 2016;18(2):89–99.

23. Alabed S, Sabouni A, Al Dakhoul S, Bdaiwi Y, Frobel-Mercier AK. Beta-blockers for congestive heart failure in children. *Cochrane Database Syst Rev.* 2016;1: CD007037.

24. Masarone D, Valente F, Rubino M, et al. Pediatric heart failure: a practical guide to diagnosis and management. *Pediatr Neonatol.* 2017;58(4):303–312.

25. Schweigmann U, Meierhofer C. Strategies for the treatment of acute heart failure in children. *Minerva Cardioangiol.* 2008;56(3):321–333.

26. Saxena A. Treatment of rheumatic carditis. *Indian J Pediatr.* 2002;69(6):513–516.

27. Voss LM, Wilson NJ, Neutze JM, et al. Intravenous immunoglobulin in acute rheumatic fever: a randomized controlled trial. *Circulation.* 2001;103(3):401–406.

28. Human DG, Hill ID, Fraser CB. Treatment choice in acute rheumatic carditis. *Arch Dis Child.* 1984;59(5):410–413.

29. Camara EJ, Braga JC, Alves-Silva LS, Camara GF, da Silva Lopes AA. Comparison of an intravenous pulse of methylprednisolone versus oral corticosteroid in severe acute rheumatic carditis: a randomized clinical trial. *Cardiol Young.* 2002;12(2):119–124.

30. Finucane K, Wilson N. Priorities in cardiac surgery for rheumatic heart disease. *Glob Heart.* 2013;8(3):213–220.

31. Webb RH, Grant C, Harnden A. Acute rheumatic fever. *BMJ.* 2015;351:h3443.

32. Antunes MJ. Challenges in rheumatic valvular disease: surgical strategies for mitral valve preservation. *Glob Cardiol Sci Pract.* 2015;2015:9.

33. Hillman ND, Tani LY, Veasy LG, et al. Current status of surgery for rheumatic carditis in children. *Ann Thorac Surg.* 2004;78(4):1403–1408.

34. Al Kasab S, Al Fagih M, Shahid M, Habbab M, Al Zaibag M. Valve surgery in acute rheumatic heart disease: one- to four- year follow-up. *Chest.* 1988;94(4):830–833.

35. Remenyi B, Webb R, Gentles T, et al. Improved long-term survival for rheumatic mitral valve repair compared to replacement in the young. *World J Pediatr Congenit Heart Surg.* 2013;4(2):155–164.

36. Anderson YWN, Nicholson R, Finucane K. Fulminant mitral regurgitation due to ruptured chordae tendinae in acute rheumatic fever. *J Paediatr Child Health.* 2007; 44(3):134–137.

37. Walker KG, Wilmshurst JM. An update on the treatment of Sydenham's chorea: the evidence for established and evolving interventions. *Therapeut Adv Neurol Disord.* 2010;3(5):301–309.

38. Demiroren K, Yavuz H, Cam L, Oran B, Karaaslan S, Demiroren S. Sydenham's chorea: a clinical follow-up of 65 patients. *J Child Neurol.* 2007;22(5):550–554.

39. Walker KG, Lawrenson J, Wilmshurst JM. Neuropsychiatric movement disorders following streptococcal infection. *Dev Med Child Neurol.* 2005;47(11):771–775.

40. Paz JA, Silva CA, Marques-Dias MJ. Randomized double-blind study with prednisone in Sydenham's chorea. *Pediatr Neurol.* 2006;34(4):264–269.

41. Shenker DM, Grossman HJ, Klawans HL. Treatment of Sydenham's chorea with haloperidol. *Dev Med Child Neurol.* 1973;15(1):19–24.

42. Sahin S, Cansu A. A New alternative drug with fewer adverse effects in the treatment of sydenham chorea: levetiracetam efficacy in a child. *Clin Neuropharmacol.* 2015; 38(4):144–146.

43. Aron AM, Freeman JM, Carter S. The natural history of sydenham's chorea. Review of the literature and long-term evaluation with emphasis on cardiac sequelae. *Am J Med.* 1965;38:83–95.

44. Garvey MA, Snider LA, Leitman SF, Werden R, Swedo SE. Treatment of Sydenham's chorea with intravenous immunoglobulin, plasma exchange, or prednisone. *J Child Neurol.* 2005;20(5):424–429.

45. Cilliers AM. Rheumatic fever and its management. *BMJ.* 2006;333(7579):1153–1156.

46. Aliku T, Sable C, Scheel A, et al. Targeted echocardiographic screening for latent rheumatic heart disease in Northern Uganda: evaluating familial risk following identification of an index case. *PLoS Neglected Tropical Diseases.* 2016;10(6):e0004727.

47. Nishimura RA, Carabello BA, Faxon DP, et al. ACC/AHA 2008 guideline update on valvular heart disease: focused update on infective endocarditis: a report of the American college of cardiology/American heart association task force on practice guidelines endorsed by the society of cardiovascular anesthesiologists, society for cardiovascular angiography and interventions, and society of thoracic surgeons. *J Am Coll Cardiol.* 2008;52(8):676–685.

CHAPTER 5

Clinical Evaluation and Diagnosis of Rheumatic Heart Disease

ARI HORTON • TOM GENTLES • BO REMENYI

INTRODUCTION

Until recently, the diagnosis and evaluation of rheumatic heart disease (RHD) was purely clinical in resource-poor settings where RHD has remained endemic. The advent of portable echocardiographic technology, however, now means that this valuable diagnostic tool is more widely available in resource-poor settings and in remote locations, thus transforming the diagnosis of both acute rheumatic fever (ARF) and RHD. In 2012, the first evidence-based echocardiographic guidelines were published to facilitate early diagnosis of mild RHD in individuals without a previous history of ARF.[1] This was followed by revision of the Jones criteria in 2015 to include echocardiographic findings in the diagnosis of ARF.[2] The most common manifestation of RHD in adults is multivalve and mixed valve disease. Current international guidelines focus on the evaluation of advanced single valve disease with either regurgitation or stenosis as the dominant pathology. A knowledge gap exists regarding the evaluation of multivalve and mixed valve diseases that characterize chronic RHD across the age spectrum.

A detailed review of the pathogenesis of ARF and RHD is presented in Chapter 2. RHD is the only significant long-term sequela of ARF and predominantly affects the left-sided cardiac valves.[3,4] Approximately 60% of patients who experience at least one episode of ARF will develop RHD.[5–9] Although acute rheumatic valvulitis is often reversible,[10–13] severe single or repeated episodes of ARF often lead to permanent scarring and chronic valvular dysfunction known as chronic

RHD.[14] Myocardial impairment and dilatation occur only in the setting of severe valve disease, and recovery can be expected if timely cardiosurgical correction of valvular dysfunction takes place.[15–17] The initial or recurrent episode of ARF may lead to a prolonged phase of inflammation and requires a long period of rest and recovery.[11,13] The pericardial effusion seen during the acute phase of ARF usually resolves with no long-term sequelae (see Chapter 3 for a more complete discussion of the clinical features of ARF).

EPIDEMIOLOGY OF RHEUMATIC HEART DISEASE

In 2015, an estimated 33.4 million people worldwide had RHD, resulting in 319,400 deaths and 10.5 million disability-adjusted life-years lost per annum.[18] Today, RHD predominantly affects those young people who live in marginalized communities or resource-poor settings.[18,19] Many affected populations live in rural and remote regions, some distance from diagnostic and specialist services.[20,21]

In childhood, by far the most common lesion in RHD is isolated mitral regurgitation (Fig. 5.1).[22] By adolescence and young adulthood, mixed multivalve disease involving both the aortic and mitral valves becomes the most common manifestation (Fig. 5.1).[22] Isolated aortic valve disease occurs in children but by adulthood it is rare, being more often associated with multivalve pathology (Fig. 5.1).[22] Pure mitral stenosis can occur as young as 10 years old but it is more

Acute Rheumatic Fever and Rheumatic Heart Disease. https://doi.org/10.1016/B978-0-323-63982-8.00005-2

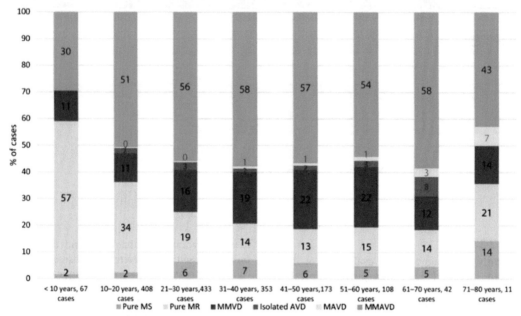

FIG. 5.1 The pattern of native rheumatic valve disease in 2475 children and adults with no percutaneous or surgical intervention. MS, mitral stenosis; MR, mitral regurgitation; MMVD, mixed mitral valve disease; AVD, aortic valve disease; MAVD, mixed aortic valve disease; MMAVD, mixed mitral and aortic valve disease. (Reproduced with permission from Zühlke et al.[22])

common during the third and fourth decades of life.[22] Chronic RHD is more common in women than men across all ages with unrecognized RHD affecting many women during their childbearing years leading to preventable morbidity and mortality for both mother and child (Fig. 5.2).[22,102,103,104]

DIAGNOSTIC CRITERIA FOR RHEUMATIC HEART DISEASE

The diagnosis of RHD often occurs late and usually because of complications of the illness, including heart failure (HF), infective endocarditis, arrhythmias, stroke, pregnancy-related complications, or sudden death.[22,23] A long latent phase of asymptomatic valvular heart disease, often without any preceding history or symptoms of ARF, is the most common scenario.[22] The Global Rheumatic Heart Disease Registry study (REMEDY) showed that the proportion of patients with RHD who had a previous history of ARF is 22.3% in low-income countries, 44.3% in lower-middle-income countries, and 59% of upper-middle-income countries.[22] Low public awareness of ARF and limited access to primary healthcare and diagnostic modalities are likely reasons for this

disparity.[2,24] Additionally, the current diagnostic guidelines may not be sufficiently sensitive to detect ARF in some high-risk populations.

The 2012 World Heart Federation (WHF) diagnostic criteria were developed by multinational collaboration to allow for standardized diagnosis of RHD with a focus on mild RHD in high-risk populations in individuals without a prior history of ARF (Table 5.1).[1] See Chapter 13 for discussions on RHD screening. The WHF definitions for pathologic aortic and mitral regurgitation have been adopted by the Jones criteria writing group to diagnose acute valvulitis in the setting of ARF.[2] The diagnosis of ARF is discussed in Chapter 3. Patients who present with ARF may have acute or "acute-on-chronic" RHD. This chapter explores the diagnosis of established chronic RHD.

Diagnosis of Chronic Rheumatic Heart Disease in Individuals with a History of Acute Rheumatic Fever

In individuals with a confirmed diagnosis of ARF, and once acute inflammation has subsided after weeks to months, as determined by normalization of inflammatory markers, the persistence of pathologic regurgitation of the mitral and/or aortic valves on echocardiography

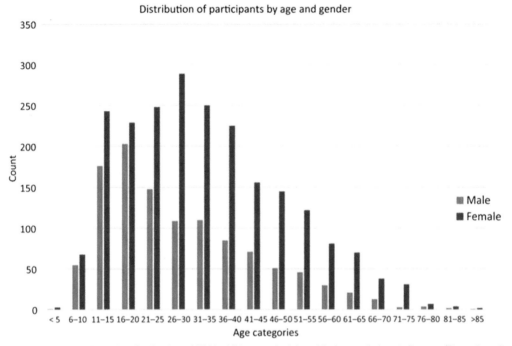

FIG. 5.2 Age and gender distribution of 3339 children and adults with rheumatic heart disease. (Reproduced with permission from Zühlke et al.[22])

(see Table 5.1) is pathognomonic for chronic RHD.[2] In circumstances where echocardiography is not available, one must rely on clinical acumen and the persistence of a mitral and/or aortic regurgitant murmur to confirm the diagnosis of chronic RHD.

Diagnosis of Rheumatic Heart Disease in Individuals Without a History of Acute Rheumatic Fever

Even after screening questions on history, practice shows that most patients in the world are diagnosed with RHD without any previous history of ARF.[22] Reasons for suspecting RHD and initiating a referral for clinical assessment and/or echocardiography may include the following: pathological murmur, exercise-induced chest pain, shortness of breath, HF, syncope, palpitations, atrial fibrillation, or stroke.

For the millions of young people in the world who already have established RHD, their best and most tangible hope for a longer and healthier life is to have their RHD detected at a stage when secondary prophylaxis has the greatest chance of modifying disease outcomes.[10–12,25] The 2012 WHF standardized echocardiographic criteria were developed with the aim of achieving rapid and consistent differentiation of mild RHD from normal echocardiographic findings in

individuals without a previous history of ARF.[1] The minimum diagnostic criteria in this setting are detailed above in Table 5.1.[1] Echocardiographic criteria for RHD are based on modalities that are available on basic portable machines: 2D, continuous-wave, and color-Doppler. The 2012 WHF guidelines clearly define what findings are consistent with definite and borderline RHD and also what are considered to be normal echocardiographic findings in children and adults.[1] The guidelines define the morphological features of RHD and also clearly state how to differentiate trivial or physiologic regurgitation from pathologic regurgitation. This differentiation is critically important in RHD where it can influence the decision to prescribe painful and long-term secondary antibiotic prophylaxis.

To diagnose definite RHD on echocardiography in individuals without a history of ARF, both morphologic features of RHD and functional aortic and/or mitral valvular regurgitation and/or stenosis must be present in the absence of congenital heart disease. The only exception to the rule is that in those aged ≤20 years, borderline RHD of both the aortic and mitral valves is classified as definite RHD.[1]

The borderline category only applies to those aged 20 years or younger, and it overlaps with normal findings in school-aged children.[26–28] The rationale

TABLE 5.1
2012 World Heart Federation Criteria for the Echocardiographic Diagnosis of Rheumatic Heart Disease.

Echocardiographic criteria for individuals aged ≤20 years

Definite RHD (either A, B, C, or D):

A) Pathological MR and at least two morphologic features of RHD of the MV
B) MS mean gradient ≥4 mmHg[a]
C) Pathological AR and at least two morphologic features of RHD of the AV[b]
D) Borderline disease of both the aortic and mitral valves[c]

Borderline RHD (either A, B, or C):

A) At least two morphological features of RHD of the MV without pathological MR or MS
B) Pathological MR
C) Pathological AR

Echocardiographic criteria for individuals aged >20 years

Definite RHD (either A, B, C, or D):

A) Pathological MR and at least two morphological features of RHD of the MV
B) MS mean gradient ≥4 mmHg[a]
C) Pathological AR and at least two morphological features of RHD of the AV, only in individuals aged <35 years[b]
D) Pathological AR and at least two morphological features of RHD of the MV

Echocardiographic criteria for pathological regurgitation (all four Doppler criteria must be met)

Pathological MR	Pathological AR
1. Seen in two views	1. Seen in two views
2. In at least one view, jet length ≥2 cm[d]	2. In at least one view, jet length ≥1 cm[d]
3. Velocity ≥3 m/s for one complete envelope	3. Peak velocity ≥3 m/s in early diastole
4. Pan-systolic jet in at least one envelope	4. Pan-diastolic jet in at least one envelope

Morphological features of RHD

Mitral Valve	Aortic Valve
1. AMVL thickening[e] ≥3mm (age-specific)[f]	1. Irregular or focal thickening[i]
2. Chordal thickening	2. Coaptation defect
3. Restricted leaflet motion[g]	3. Restricted leaflet motion
4. Excessive leaflet tip motion during systole[h]	4. Prolapse

RHD, rheumatic heart disease; MV, mitral valve; AV, aortic valve; MR, mitral regurgitation; MS, mitral stenosis; AR, aortic regurgitation; AMVL, anterior mitral valve leaflet.

[a] Congenital MV anomalies must be excluded. Furthermore, inflow obstruction due to nonrheumatic mitral annular calcification must be excluded in adults.

[b] Bicuspid AV, dilated aortic root, and hypertension must be excluded.

[c] Combined AR and MR in high prevalence regions and in the absence of congenital heart disease is regarded as rheumatic.

[d] A regurgitant jet length should be measured from the vena contracta to the last pixel of regurgitant color (blue or red).

[e] AMVL thickness should be measured during diastole at full excursion. Measurement should be taken at the thickest portion of the leaflet, including focal thickening, beading, and nodularity. Measurement should be performed on a frame with maximal separation of chordae from the leaflet tissue. Valve thickness can only be assessed if the images were acquired at optimal gain settings without harmonics and with a frequency of >2.0 MHz.

[f] Abnormal thickening of the AMVL is age-specific and defined as follows: ≥3 mm for individuals aged ≤20 years; ≥4 mm for individuals aged 21-40 years; and ≥5 mm for individuals aged >40 years. Valve thickness measurements obtained using harmonic imaging should be cautiously interpreted and a thickness up to 4 mm should be considered normal in those aged ≤20 years.

[g] Restricted leaflet motion of either the anterior or the posterior MV leaflet is usually the result of chordal shortening or fusion, commissural fusion, or leaflet thickening.

[h] Excessive leaflet tip motion is the result of elongation of the primary chords and is defined as displacement of the tip or edge of an involved leaflet towards the left atrium, resulting in abnormal coaptation and regurgitation. Excessive leaflet tip motion does not need to meet the standard echocardiographic definition of MV prolapse disease, as that refers to a different disease process. This feature applies to only those <35 years of age. In the presence of a flail MV leaflet in the young (<20 years of age), this single morphologic feature is sufficient to meet the morphologic criteria for RHD (that is, where the criteria state "at least two morphologic features of RHD of the MV" a flail leaflet in a person <20 years of age is sufficient).

[i] In the parasternal short-axis view, the right and noncoronary aortic cusp closure line often appears echogenic (thickened) in healthy individuals and this should be considered as normal.

Reproduced from Remenyi et al.[(1)]

for introducing a borderline category in this age group was to increase the sensitivity in those who live in endemic regions with a high pretest probability of disease.[1] The absolute clinical significance of borderline RHD is yet to be determined, though it is clear that those with borderline RHD are at an increased risk of both disease progression and morbidity.[29–31]

In those settings where echocardiography is not widely available, the diagnosis of RHD still relies on clinical auscultatory findings of valvular regurgitation or stenosis. Auscultatory findings do not address the etiology of disease and as such the pretest probability of RHD will determine diagnostic and management strategies.

CLINICAL ASSESSMENT AND FINDINGS

Mild-to-moderate RHD is almost always asymptomatic in children and young adults. In regions of the world where echocardiography is not widely available, diagnosis and referral to tertiary centers will be based on clinical assessments and findings. Each of the classical lesions is associated with a number of clinical features that help guide the assessment and give guidance regarding severity of disease. Clinical assessment needs to be supplemented with ECG, chest X-ray, and blood tests. Whenever available, echocardiography should be used to validate clinical findings and determine etiology and severity of valvular dysfunction.

Innocent Cardiac Murmurs

Innocent murmurs may complicate the clinical evaluation of high-risk children and adults when cardiac auscultation is used to diagnose RHD.[14] Figs. 5.3 and 5.4 demonstrate comparative phonographs and location of various innocent and pathologic murmurs. Cardiac auscultation is a fundamental process that requires active thought and listening, practice, and ongoing reinforcement of skills.

Innocent murmurs in the pediatric population

In the pediatric population, innocent murmurs occur in up to 25% of school age children on any given day and may confuse the clinical picture (Table 5.2).[32] Patients with innocent murmurs may have RHD, those without murmurs may have RHD, and those with murmurs and congenital heart disease may still have RHD.[32–34] An Australian study found that doctor identification of any murmur had 38.2% sensitivity, 75.1% specificity, and 5.1% positive predictive value and the corresponding values for pathological murmurs were 20.6%, 92.2%, and 8.3% in relation to RHD.[32]

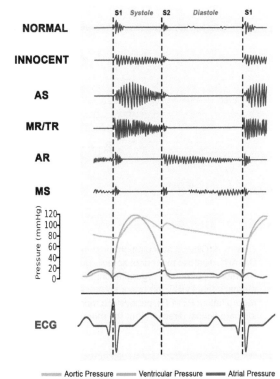

FIG. 5.3 Comparative phonograms for common valvular rheumatic heart disease lesions.
(Copyright: Dr Ari Horton.)

Still's murmur is the most common innocent murmur. It has a low-pitched musical or vibratory quality, best heard at the mid-to-lower sternal border and toward the apex and is not associated with any added sounds. Pulmonary flow murmurs are harsher and high-pitched, heard at the left upper sternal border, are often flow-dependent and vary with position, and disappear with Valsalva maneuver. Venous hum and carotid bruit are also common, but they are more easily distinguished from the pathologic murmurs of RHD. Venous hum is a continuous murmur that is heard below the clavicle and disappears when the patient is positioned supine, while the carotid bruit is localized to the carotid artery with or without any radiation. Innocent murmurs are associated with normal ECG and chest X-ray findings.

Pathological Murmurs in the Pediatric Population

The differentiation of innocent from pathological murmurs comes with critical thinking and

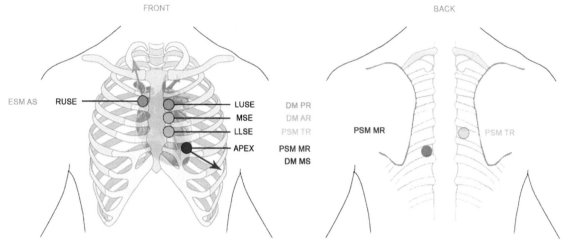

FIG. 5.4 Clinical auscultation for signs of rheumatic heart disease.
DM AR[a], diastolic murmur of aortic regurgitation; DM MS, diastolic murmur of mitral stenosis; DM PR, diastolic murmur of pulmonary regurgitation; ESM AS[a], ejection systolic murmur of aortic stenosis; LLSE, left lower sternal edge; LUSE, left upper sternal edge; MSE, midsternal edge; PSM MR[a], pansystolic murmur of mitral regurgitation; PSM TR, pansystolic murmur of tricuspid regurgitation; RUSE, right upper sternal edge. [a]Arrows indicate typical direction that the murmur radiates. (Copyright: Dr Ari Horton.)

TABLE 5.2
Key Differentiating Features on Examination Between Innocent and Pathological Murmurs.

Innocent	Pathological
Usually occur in systole	Can occur in systole, diastole, or both
Usually soft or vibratory	Harsh
Grade 1/6 or 2/6 only	Grade 1/6–6/6
Normal S1 and S2	Abnormal S2
Localized and do not radiate	Often radiate
No associated clicks or gallops	May be associated with added sounds (e.g., click)
Normal apex beat	May be associated with displaced apex beat
No parasternal heave or thrill	May be associated with a parasternal heave or thrill
Varies with respiration and position, often disappears on standing	Specific variation with respiration and position according to impact of maneuver on lesion
Not associated with other signs of heart disease	Associated with other signs of heart disease

assessment. The subtle differences lie in quality, pitch, location and radiation, added sounds and clicks, whilst dynamic maneuvers and positioning may assist (Table 5.2). In childhood, common congenital heart defects such as ventricular septal defects, atrial septal defects, pulmonary stenosis, and aortic stenosis (AS) are associated with pathological murmurs and require differentiation from RHD. Regurgitant lesions because of congenital mitral valve and aortic valve disease are less common, and echocardiography is usually required to differentiate congenital from rheumatic etiology.

Pathological Murmurs in the Adult Population

In the adult population, degenerative and acquired processes become the leading cause of pathological valvular disease. On clinical history and examination alone, it is often difficult to determine the etiology of valvular disease: consideration should be given to the age of the patient and to background prevalence of RHD, particularly when clinical decisions are made without the aid of echocardiography. Clinical findings in the diagnosis of RHD in regions without access to echocardiography remain critically important. The examination findings in severe RHD have been summarised in Table 5.3.

TABLE 5.3
Clinical Features Suggestive of severe Valvular Lesions on Clinical Examination.

	MITRAL		AORTIC	
	Regurgitation[a]	**Stenosis[a]**	**Regurgitation[a]**	**Stenosis[a]**
Apex	Thrusting ± thrill Inferolaterally displaced	Tapping Undisplaced	Thrusting Inferolaterally displaced	Heaving Minimally displaced
Pulse	Normal or jerky Commonly atrial fibrillation	Normal or low volume Often atrial fibrillation	Collapsing (or "water-hammer") See also box 5.1	Slow-rising
Heart sounds	Soft S1 Occasional S3	Loud S1 Short gap between S2 and the opening snap	Normal/soft S2 Occasional S3	Quiet or absent S2 Reversed split S2
Murmur	Does not correlate with severity	Long mid-diastolic murmur	Short early-diastolic murmur Austin Flint murmur	Does not correlate with severity
Other features	Evidence of left heart failure Carey Coombs murmur Signs of pulmonary hypertension[b]	Pulmonary congestion and right heart failure Signs of pulmonary hypertension[b]	Evidence of left heart failure Wide pulse pressure	Evidence of left heart failure

[a] In mixed valve disease, the dominant lesion can be determined by assessing the impact of any lesion on the above parameters. In mixed mitral valve disease, the most discriminating factors are the apex beat and auscultatory findings; in mixed aortic valve disease, it is the apex beat, pulse character, and blood pressure. In multivalve disease involving mitral and aortic regurgitation, the key discriminating features are the pulse and blood pressure: sinus rhythm in the presence of a high systolic BP and wide pulse pressure suggests that aortic regurgitation is the dominant lesion. In those with significant mitral stenosis, clinical signs of aortic valve disease may be less evident. On the other hand, if there is evidence of a severe aortic valve lesion in the context of mitral stenosis, this suggests that the mitral stenosis is not severe.
[b] Right ventricular parasternal heave, loud pulmonary component of S2 (P2), palpable (P2), murmur of tricuspid regurgitation, right heart failure.

Mitral Regurgitation
Clinical symptoms
Mitral regurgitation (MR) is the most common manifestation of RHD.[22] Symptoms develop as a result of increasing left atrial pressure, pulmonary venous hypertension and increased left ventricular (LV) end diastolic volumes and pressure. The acuity of the change in physiology often determines the severity of the symptoms and their recognition by patients and family members. Shortness of breath, especially during peak physical activity, may progress to shortness of breath at rest followed by clinical decompensation with HF and death. More rapid progression can occur in the setting of acute-on-chronic mitral valve disease or during significant intercurrent illnesses (see Chapter 16).

Clinical signs: mild-to-moderate mitral regurgitation
The hallmark of chronic MR is a harsh pansystolic murmur (Fig. 5.5) heard best at the apex with radiation to the axilla. The direction of the regurgitant jet is usually posterolateral (hence the radiation to the axilla) due to the typical retraction of the posterior mitral valve leaflet and prolapse of the anterior leaflet. It is often high-pitched, and the intensity does not increase with

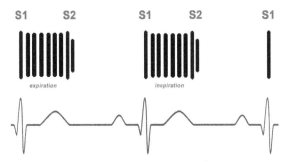

FIG. 5.5 Mitral regurgitation phonograms. (Copyright: Dr Ari Horton.)

inspiration, unlike the murmur of tricuspid regurgitation (TR). Less commonly, posterior mitral valve leaflet prolapse leads to an anteriorly-directed jet of MR with the pansystolic murmur heard medially at the lower left sternal edge. The LV apex will not be displaced in the setting of mild to moderate disease.

Clinical signs: moderate-to-severe mitral regurgitation
With progression of MR and ongoing ventricular dilatation, the apex beat becomes displaced laterally and

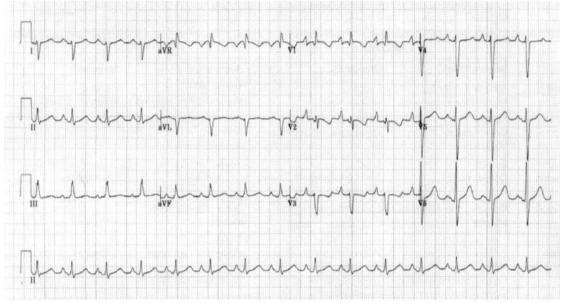

FIG. 5.6 ECG with classical findings of chronic RHD with severe mitral regurgitation. The ECG shows sinus rhythm with right axis deviation, biatrial dilatation, right ventricular hypertrophy, and right ventricular strain in the setting of severe pulmonary hypertension from left heart disease (see main text for further details).

inferiorly toward the axilla (Table 5.3). An associated middiastolic murmur related to increased transmitral flow may develop. This is often called as a Carey-Coombs murmur. It is heard best with the bell of the stethoscope, while the patient is in the left lateral position and the breath held in end-expiration. In the setting of significant left atrial dilatation, atrial fibrillation may develop leading to an irregularly irregular heartbeat.

Electrocardiogram

If there is acute valvulitis, the ECG may reveal first-degree heart block with a prolonged PR interval and or higher degrees of AV block (refer to age-specific normal ranges - see Chapter 3). In chronic RHD, the ECG is normal with mild-to-moderate mitral regurgitation. Moderate-to-severe disease often leads to classic ECG findings of left atrial enlargement with upright P waves in lead I, a bifid P wave in leads V1–V6 that gives the "M" pattern of P-mitrale. LV dilatation and hypertrophy leads to increased LV voltages (Fig. 5.6). Right axis deviation (negative QRS in lead I), positive QRS complexes (dominant R-waves) in V1-2 (suggesting right ventricular hypertrophy), ST depression and T wave inversion in V1-3 (suggesting right ventricular strain), and peaked P waves (P pulmonale, suggesting right atrial hypertrophy) may appear in the setting of severe pulmonary hypertension.

Chest X-ray

Chest X-ray (CXR) is normal in the setting of mild RHD, and it is helpful to exclude noncardiac pathologies that are common in resource-poor settings. As disease progresses, the CXR will demonstrate LV dilatation with cardiomegaly, left atrial enlargement with splaying of the carina, and pulmonary congestion with plethora if the MR is severe (Fig. 5.7).

Mitral Stenosis
Clinical symptoms

Pure mitral stenosis (MS) is rare in the first decade of life; however, it becomes more common during child-bearing years and has significant implications for pregnancy.[22,35,36] The symptoms of pregnancy and MS overlap (see Chapter 9).[36] Symptoms of MS develop as a result of progressive obstruction to LV inflow. The diastolic gradient between the left atrium and left ventricle is worsened with increased flow and heart rate, such as during illness, exercise or pregnancy, as well as in the presence of atrial fibrillation with a rapid ventricular rate. There is a clear correlation between the effective mitral valve orifice size and symptom onset and progression.[37,38] Initial symptoms of progressive exertional dyspnoea usually develop with a mitral valve area <2 cm^2, with the other symptoms of HF including orthopnoea and paroxysmal nocturnal dyspnoea manifesting as size decreases

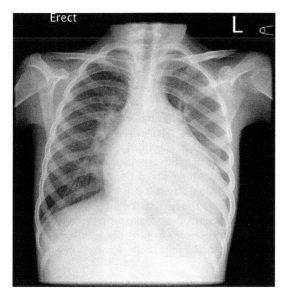

FIG. 5.7 Chest X-ray from a 14-year-old girl with severe mitral regurgitation, left ventricular dilatation, left ventricular dysfunction, pulmonary hypertension, and tricuspid regurgitation. Note the cardiomegaly, the dilated main pulmonary artery, and the splayed bronchi indicating left atrial enlargement. There is also evidence of pulmonary venous congestion and pulmonary vascular changes.

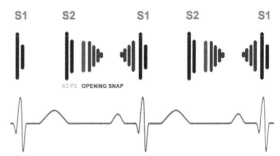

FIG. 5.8 Mitral stenosis phonograms. (Copyright: Dr Ari Horton.)

to <1.5 cm². [37,38] At advanced stages with massive left atrial enlargement, signs of cough, hemoptysis, chest pain, palpitations, and a hoarse voice (due to the left atrium mechanically compressing the left recurrent laryngeal nerve, known as Ortner's syndrome) begin to develop. Less commonly, patients present with symptoms related to arterial embolism from the left atrium, such as an ischemic stroke or peripheral arterial occlusion.

Clinical signs: mild to moderate
The clinical signs of MS include an opening snap followed immediately by a low-pitched, diastolic rumble or decrescendo murmur heard best at the apex with the patient in a left lateral position (Fig. 5.8). It is again accentuated by increasing heart rate with mild exercise. The duration of the murmur correlates with the severity of the MS. The opening snap is produced as the valve opens under the high left atrial pressures. The second phase of the murmur is in late diastole, as a result of atrial contraction, occurring immediately before the S1 sound creating a late diastolic, crescendo murmur.

In the presence of atrial fibrillation, the active LV filling phase does not take place and the latter part of the MS murmur disappears.

Clinical signs: moderate to severe
As MS worsens, left atrial pressure increases, forcing the mitral valve open earlier in diastole and the opening snap occurs earlier as does the initial decrescendo part of the murmur. Furthermore, as pulmonary hypertension increases, the pulse becomes small in volume and a right ventricular parasternal heave and loud or even palpable P2 become more prominent (Table 5.3). Less commonly patients may have signs of systemic embolism from the left atrium, especially if they have previously had episodes of atrial fibrillation, which further increases stroke risk in MS. [39]

Electrocardiogram
It is important to confirm the baseline rhythm, namely sinus rhythm or atrial fibrillation. Atrial fibrillation is rare under 20 years old even in the setting of severe MS. [39] Voltage criteria for left atrial enlargement, P-mitrale, and right ventricular hypertrophy are markers of severe disease.

Chest X-ray
Chest X-ray will demonstrate left atrial enlargement with a bulge sitting above the heart border in the left mediastinum with a splaying of the carina. Upper lobe diversion of blood flow and/or pulmonary congestion occurs in the setting of worsening HF. Calcification of the mitral valve apparatus may be seen on lateral CXR, especially in older patients. In the setting of established pulmonary hypertension, the main and hilar pulmonary arteries become prominent and there is also right ventricular hypertrophy on CXR.

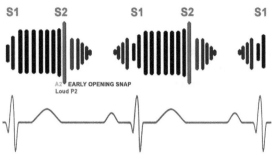

FIG. 5.9 Mixed mitral valve disease phonograms. (Copyright: Dr Ari Horton.)

Mixed Mitral Valve Disease
Clinical symptoms
With progression of RHD, severe mixed MS and MR often develops. The symptoms are insidious but are consistent with chronic progressive shortness of breath at rest, which is worse with any exertion. Exercise tolerance is often limited, and individuals will often self-limit activity. If pulmonary hypertension is present, then it may be associated with perioral cyanosis with activity.

Clinical signs: moderate to severe
There is both a short harsh pansystolic murmur at the apex and a short decrescendo diastolic murmur (Fig. 5.9). Signs of pulmonary hypertension are usually present. Particular attention to the apex beat and auscultatory findings can help to determine which lesion is dominant (Table 5.3).

Electrocardiogram
Voltage criteria for left atrial enlargement and right ventricular hypertrophy are markers of severe disease together with right ventricular strain.

Chest X-ray
Chest X-ray will demonstrate left atrial enlargement with a bulge sitting above the heart border in the left mediastinum with a splaying of the carina, upper lobe diversion of blood flow, and/or pulmonary congestion in the setting of worsening HF. In the setting of established pulmonary hypertension, the main and hilar pulmonary arteries become prominent on CXR.

Aortic Regurgitation
Clinical symptoms
Moderate to severe aortic regurgitation (AR) often remains stable for years until the left ventricle begins to fail after chronic volume overload. Late symptoms of chronic AR include dyspnea on exertion, sometimes accompanied by frank congestive failure with orthopnea, paroxysmal nocturnal dyspnea, and edema (see

Chapter 6). Severe AR carries a risk of decreased coronary perfusion pressure, which may manifest as angina despite normal coronary arteries. Initially, it may occur with exercise but eventually may develop at rest.

Clinical signs: mild-to-moderate aortic regurgitation
The clinical signs of mild-to-moderate AR include a soft, high-pitched blowing decrescendo early diastolic murmur best heard at the third intercostal space on the left sternal edge (Erb's point), at end-expiration with the patient sitting upright and leaning forward (Fig. 5.10). It is often also heard at the left lower sternal border and toward the apex, as the AR severity increases and jet lengthens, the flow is directed towards the apex of the heart. It decreases in intensity with inspiration. Generally, the length of the murmur correlates inversely with severity.

Clinical signs: moderate-to-severe aortic regurgitation
With progression to moderate-to-severe AR, the murmur at the left sternal edge shortens, and an added systolic ejection murmur develops at the right upper sternal edge reflecting increased stroke volume across the aortic valve. A characteristic Austin—Flint murmur may also be heard, which is a low-pitched middiastolic or presystolic murmur heard at the cardiac apex and radiating to the axilla, and this may be confused with the murmur of MS. This murmur is believed to be the result of the downward AR jet pressing on the anterior mitral valve leaflet, causing functional MS. The murmur is best heard in the left lateral decubitus position using the bell of the stethoscope at the apex.

In severe AR, abrupt distension and quick collapse of the pulses (known as the collapsing pulse or "water-hammer" pulse) may be visualized at the carotid artery (see box 5.1) or at the brachial, radial, ulnar, or femoral arteries. The collapsing pulse is defined as a pulse pressure that is greater than the diastolic pressure

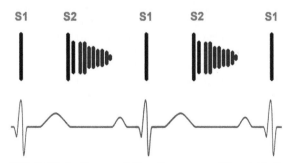

FIG. 5.10 Aortic regurgitation phonograms. (Copyright: Dr Ari Horton.)

BOX 5.1
Eponymous Signs in Chronic Severe Aortic Regurgitation[40, a]

- **Corrigan's sign**: visible carotid pulsation (common)
- **Traube's sign**: booming systolic and diastolic ("pistol shot") sounds heard whilst auscultating the femoral arteries (relatively uncommon)
- **de Musset's sign**: bobbing of the head with each heartbeat (uncommon)
- **Quincke's sign**: visible capillary pulsation in the nailbed (uncommon)
- **Durozier's sign**: systolic murmur heard over femoral artery when it is compressed proximally and a diastolic murmur when it is compressed distally (uncommon)
- **Müller's sign**: systolic pulsations of the uvula (uncommon)

---

[a]Note that these signs are usually not present in acute aortic regurgitation (see Chapter 16).

(i.e., the systolic pressure is double the diastolic pressure) and occurs as a result of the large stroke volume and aortic runoff from the aorta back to the left ventricle. The resulting wide pulse pressure is responsible for a variety of clinical signs associated with chronic severe AR (box 5.1).

The collapsing pulse may also be elicited by palpation. Holding the patient's arm at the wrist using the flat part of the fingers, the examiner lifts and straightens the arm vertically upwards. After a few seconds, the pulse should change in character from that of a prominent pulse to a tapping sensation. Lifting and straightening the arm accentuates the sign by emptying the arm more rapidly of blood due to gravity and straightens the natural kinks in the brachial artery and in the axillary/subclavian junction. These signs, however, are not specific for severe AR: anemia, thyrotoxicosis, arteriovenous malformations, and other high-flow states may also produce similar findings. Furthermore, it should be remembered that the pulse pressure narrows with the development of HF, attenuating the peripheral signs of AR.

In torrential AR (those at the most severe range of AR), the murmur is heard lying flat and the Korotkoff sounds may be heard almost down to the pressure of zero. Other clinical signs indicative of severe AR are summarised in Table 5.3.

Electrocardiogram
The electrocardiogram (ECG) often reveals a baseline tachycardia with or without increased LV voltages and nonspecific ST-T wave changes. Intermittent ischemia during exercise or periods of further vasodilatation may be seen infrequently.

Chest X-ray
In the setting of severe disease, the chest X-ray will demonstrate LV enlargement and may show a dilated ascending aorta.

Aortic Stenosis
Although isolated rheumatic AS is uncommon, it is important to understand the signs and symptoms of this uncommon manifestation of RHD. Clinical symptoms usually only result when there is a greater than 50% reduction in aortic valve area. Calcific AS in the elderly may occur in patients who had a history of ARF or RHD when younger. In this setting, the relative contribution of the calcific and the rheumatic processes may be uncertain. This concept and management of AS are discussed in more detail in Chapter 6.

Clinical symptoms
Mild to moderate AS is most often asymptomatic. Symptoms are gradual in onset, slowly progressive and are often initially associated with exercise only. Survival is excellent during the asymptomatic phase although with the development of symptoms, mortality exceeds 90% within a few years, with symptoms of HF or syncope associated with the worst prognosis followed by angina.

Clinical signs: mild to moderate
The classical murmur of AS is an ejection systolic murmur at the right upper sternal edge which may radiate toward the neck (Fig. 5.11). It is described as a high-pitched,

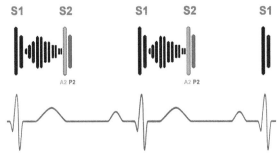

FIG. 5.11 Aortic stenosis phonograms. (Copyright: Dr Ari Horton.)

crescendo-decrescendo ejection systolic murmur with the peak in early systole. Intensity of the murmur is not a good marker of the severity of disease.

Clinical signs: moderate to severe

The murmur of AS will remain loudest at the right upper sternal border with radiation to the neck and to the apex. A loud, low-pitched, ejection systolic murmur is characteristically heard with a thrill over the aortic area and at the suprasternal notch. If the murmur radiates toward the apex (known as the Gallavardin phenomenon), it may be misinterpreted as mitral regurgitation, although the former tends to have a musical quality and does not radiate to the axilla. As the LV begins to fail, the ejection fraction declines resulting in a decreased intensity of the murmur with the peak intensity in later systole. The delay in closure of the aortic valve can also cause a paradoxically split S2. There are signs of a slowed and reduced carotid pulse upstroke (Table 5.3).

Electrocardiogram

ECG often demonstrates sinus rhythm with a baseline tachycardia and increased LV voltages meeting voltage criteria for LV hypertrophy. There may be secondary repolarization abnormalities, ST changes and T wave inversion in the lateral leads (leads I, aVL, and V5-6), consistent with LV strain.

Chest X-ray

Chest X-ray will often be normal in isolated AS unless there is associated mitral regurgitation. Calcification of the aortic valve may be visible on the lateral chest X-ray.

Tricuspid Regurgitation
Clinical symptoms

Tricuspid regurgitation is usually secondary to pulmonary hypertension due to MR or MS but may also be related (less commonly) to primary rheumatic disease of the tricuspid valve itself. Specific features of TR include abdominal discomfort and jaundice due to congestive hepatopathy, ascites due to increased porto-venous pressures, and weight loss due to indigestion and bowel wall edema, limiting appetite.

Clinical signs: mild to moderate

The early feature of TR is a low pitched pansystolic murmur at the left lower sternal edge (Fig. 5.12). It increases with inspiration. If secondary to pulmonary hypertension, it has a higher pitch and is associated with a loud pulmonary component of the second heart sound (P2).

Clinical signs: moderate to severe

The pathognomonic clinical sign of severe TR is a raised jugular venous pressure and if the pulsation is palpable

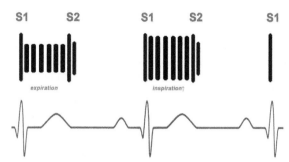

FIG. 5.12 Tricuspid regurgitation phonograms. (Copyright: Dr Ari Horton.)

and monomorphic, it is known as Lancisi's sign. Congestive hepatopathy is often associated with right-sided HF, jaundice, and tender hepatomegaly, which may be pulsatile. Occasionally, the systolic murmur of TR is transmitted to and heard over the liver. Peripheral edema, although nonspecific, is also often present. Anasarca (generalized swelling of the whole body) can occur in severe disease. Unilateral and bilateral pleural effusions are also seen frequently, particularly when the TR is secondary to left-sided valve disease.

Electrocardiogram

ECG may demonstrate right atrial enlargement and right ventricular hypertrophy with increased voltages. It may be associated with voltage criteria consistent with biventricular hypertrophy and potentially a right ventricular strain pattern (ST/T-wave changes present in the inferior leads II, III, aVF and V1-V4) in the setting of severe pulmonary hypertension.

Chest X-ray

Chest X-ray will generally reveal right ventricular dilatation and right atrial enlargement with an atrial bulge at the right mediastinal border. If the TR is secondary to severe MR or MS then cardiomegaly and pulmonary congestion may be present.

Pulmonary Regurgitation
Clinical symptoms

Pulmonary regurgitation (PR), the rarest of the valves directly involved in RHD, is mostly secondary to the raised mean diastolic pulmonary pressures that result from left-sided valve disease. It is asymptomatic until severe right ventricular dilatation leads to decreased exercise capacity.

Clinical signs: mild to moderate

PR is often difficult to differentiate from AR. It produces a soft, high-pitched, early diastolic decrescendo murmur at the left sternal edge (Fig. 5.13). Dynamic maneuvers can help to differentiate PR from AR. The

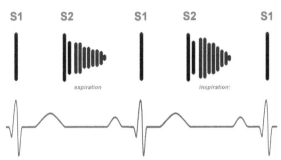

FIG. 5.13 Pulmonary regurgitation phonograms. (Copyright: Dr Ari Horton.)

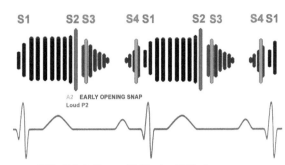

FIG. 5.14 Severe Multivalve RHD phonograms.

cardiac murmur of PR increases in intensity during inspiration, the opposite occurs in the setting of AR.

Clinical signs: moderate to severe
The diastolic murmur of PR will shorten as it becomes more severe. In the setting of RHD, clinical signs are usually of concomitant aortic, mitral, and tricuspid valve disease.

ECG
ECG changes usually represent concomitant severe mitral valve disease.

Chest X-ray
Chest X-ray will demonstrate right ventricular dilatation and enlarged pulmonary arteries with a prominent pulmonary knuckle.

Multivalve Rheumatic Heart Disease
The most common manifestation of RHD is multivalve disease, and the most common cause of multivalve disease is RHD.[22] Multivalve disease carries a high risk for ventricular dysfunction and symptomatic HF (see also Chapter 6).[16]

Clinical symptoms
In the setting of multivalve disease, clinical symptoms usually relate to the predominant valvular lesion and to heart failure, pulmonary hypertension and arrhythmias.

Clinical signs: severe multivalve disease
When multivalve disease is severe, the chest wall might be wasted with visible ribs and reduced subcutaneous fat or muscular tissue. There will be a visible hyperdynamic impulse with the apex beat wide and displaced to the anterior axillary line. There will be a visible and palpable pulmonic component with heavy closure of the pulmonic valve due to

pulmonary hypertension. The right ventricular heave may even lead to an asymmetric chest wall with the left side bulging in children. The heart sounds may be difficult to hear over the multiple murmurs, but there is often a loud P2 with the addition of a gallop rhythm (S3 and or S4). There will be loud, harsh systolic and diastolic murmurs heard throughout the chest that vary in intensity due to respiration and will radiate to the axilla and back (Fig. 5.14). Pedal edema, ascites, hepatomegaly with or without pulsatility, raised jugular venous pressure, and dilated neck veins with bounding pulses are all markers of severe disease (see Table 5.3).

ECG
The ECG will often demonstrate sinus tachycardia with both right and left atrial enlargement and right and LV hypertrophy. Atrial fibrillation may be present.

Chest X-ray
Chest X-ray will demonstrate significant cardiomegaly and pulmonary plethora with or without bilateral pleural effusions and ascites. There may be a widened mediastinum with enlarged pulmonary arteries.

ECHOCARDIOGRAPHY IN RHEUMATIC HEART DISEASE
Echocardiography is a noninvasive portable diagnostic tool that plays an essential role both in the diagnosis and management of valvular heart disease and in determining the etiology and severity of HF (Box 5.2). Left heart disease is also the most common cause of pulmonary hypertension in the modern era. Screening for pulmonary hypertension using echocardiography in patients with significant RHD is important because, untreated, morbidity and mortality levels are high and the diagnosis of pulmonary hypertension may be an indication for intervention (Box 5.3). Given that

---

BOX 5.2
Echocardiography is Vital in the Following Scenarios

- Determining the etiology and severity of heart disease and/or HF
- Diagnosis of RHD
- Grading the severity and delineating the mechanism of valvular dysfunction
- Serial assessments of LV size and function
- Determining the echocardiographic probability of the presence or absence of pulmonary hypertension
- Guiding the timing and nature of cardio-surgical intervention
- Confirming the duration of secondary prophylaxis, in accordance with guidelines (see Chapter 11)
- Screening for latent (clinical and subclinical) RHD (see Chapter 13)
- Screening for pericardial effusion in the setting of ARF.

---

echocardiography is much more sensitive and specific than clinical diagnosis and is more widely available than ever before (including point-of-care use and hand-held devices), it is now the primary means of diagnosing RHD in many regions of the world.[1,32,41,42] Resource-poor countries are evolving strategies such as task-shifting to make this vital tool available and affordable for the most remote and poorest populations.[43–45] Screening echocardiography with abbreviated protocols are being developed to facilitate task-shifting and rapid screening of large populations.

The following section will focus on the basic and advanced manifestations of RHD on echocardiography.

Grading the Severity of Valve Disease Using Echocardiography

As discussed above, limitations exist within the present echocardiographic grading systems to assess the severity of valvular dysfunction in the setting of RHD.[22,50,58,61,62] These limitations are related to the fact that RHD is often associated with the following:

- Multivalve disease states
- Mixed valvular disease states
- Eccentric and/or multiple regurgitant jets
- Cardiac arrhythmias
- Impaired ventricular function

Currently, there are no evidence-based echocardiographic grading systems that accommodate or compensate for the above variables that most commonly occur in the setting of RHD.[22,50,58,61,62] Despite this, the aim of echocardiographic assessment is to define the valve disease as mild, moderate, or severe. Tables 5.5–5.11 help guide severity of RHD in the setting of single valve

disease with a predominant hemodynamic lesion that is either regurgitant or stenotic and are discussed in the following sections. When reporting complex, mixed or multivalve rheumatic valve disease it is important to report the following parameters systematically:

1) overall grading of RHD
2) severity grading, Doppler parameters and morphological features of each valve including mechanism/pathology
3) left and right ventricular size, wall thickness and function
4) left and right atrial size
5) presence and degree or absence of pulmonary hypertension (See Box 5.3)
6) presence or absence of intracardiac thrombus
7) heart rate and cardiac rhythm
8) presence or absence of pericardial effusion.
9) any additional diagnostic features of importance for surgical planing
10) any other additional cardiac diagnoses

This facilitates better communication between treating teams and patients.

The differentiation of trivial from mild regurgitation is critical in the setting of RHD as the decision to prescribe long-term long-acting painful intramuscular penicillin injections could hinge on those findings. This differentiation from trivial to mild disease is also relevant in the diagnosis of definite ARF when considering rheumatic valvulitis/carditis. It is not relevant in many other cardiac conditions aside from suspected infective endocarditis as it does not change clinical management. For this reason, the 2012 WHF echocardiographic criteria were established with the aim of clearly defining how to differentiate normal echocardiographic findings from definite or borderline RHD (Table 5.1).

Mitral Valve Disease

The mitral valve is the most commonly affected valve in the setting of RHD.[22] Although the natural inclination is to classify mitral valve disease as purely regurgitant, mixed, or purely stenotic, the reality is that the hemodynamic effect is a continuum.[46]

Echocardiography of isolated mitral regurgitation

In children, isolated MR is the most common manifestation of RHD. Because RHD can affect the mitral valve annulus, leaflets, and chordae, echocardiographic interrogation needs to evaluate the entire mitral valve apparatus in order to understand the mechanism and nature of valvular dysfunction. Most classically, there is thickening of the mitral valve leaflets, with restrictive motion of the posterior mitral valve leaflet, subtle prolapse of the anterior mitral valve leaflet tip (as

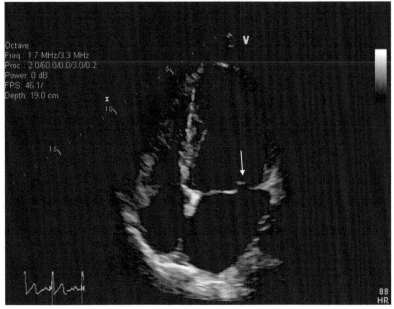

FIG. 5.15 Chronic rheumatic valve disease with restriction of the posterior leaflet of the mitral valve (white arrow).

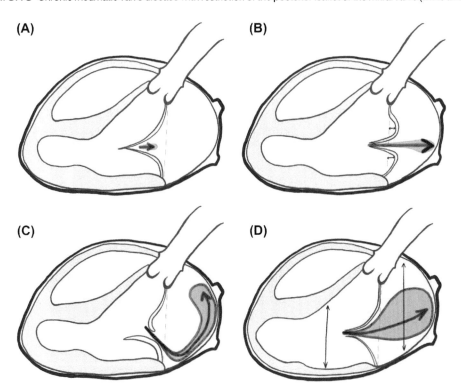

FIG. 5.16 Morphology and mechanisms of mitral regurgitation. (A) Normal heart with trivial central mitral regurgitation: physiological and normal finding; (B) mitral valve prolapsea with central, midsystolic regurgitant jet; (C) rheumatic heart disease with anterior mitral valve leaflet prolapse and severe, posteriorlydirected mitral regurgitation jet; (D) significantly dilated left heart with mitral annular dilatation and secondary, severe, and central mitral regurgitation: multiple possible etiologies, including chronic, severe primary mitral regurgitation with or without aortic regurgitation (common in rheumatic heart disease). A diagnosis of mitral valve prolapse requires prolapse of anterior mitral valve leaflet and/or posterior mitral valve leaflet 2 mm above the level of the mitral annulus. (Copyright: Dr Ari Horton.)

seen in Fig. 5.15), and a posteriorly-directed MR regurgitation jet. Fig. 5.16 is a diagrammatic representation of the different mitral valve morphologies and comparative mechanisms of mitral regurgitation commonly seen in normal, rheumatic, and non-rheumatic patients.

Physiological (trivial) MR can easily be distinguished from pathological MR related to RHD as detailed in Table 5.1. Milder degrees of regurgitation may be missed, unless all portions of the mitral valve leaflets are carefully assessed by performing a "sweeping" scan of the mitral valve in the parasternal and apical windows. Early in the disease process, especially in the setting of mild MR, the valve morphology may appear normal. During the acute stage of valvulitis, chordae elongate and the annulus dilates, leading to excessive leaflet motion of the anterior leaflet that then moves past the posterior leaflet resulting in malcoaptation, often leading to an eccentric, posteriorly-directed regurgitant jet. This stage is considered to be reversible, especially if the degree of regurgitation is only mild to moderate.[10-13]

If the chordae of the posterior leaflet are affected, then an anteriorly-directed regurgitant jet may occur. In more severe cases, chordal rupture can lead to a flail leaflet and acute severe MR, necessitating surgical correction. With time, particularly following repeated episodes of valvulitis, chronic scarring and fibrosis of the mitral valve apparatus ensues. In the chronic phase of RHD, leaflets subsequently thicken and retract and commissures and chordae eventually fuse, all of which result in restricted movement of the mitral valve leaflets. The classic deformed appearance of the anterior mitral valve leaflet is often described as a "dog-leg" or "hockey stick" deformity (Fig. 5.17). At this stage of the disease, the increased transmitral gradient may be flow-dependent as a result of moderate or severe MR, or secondary to the development of mixed mitral valve disease. Mitral valve planimetry is a useful way of differentiating the two processes because it is not based on haemodynamic variables.

Different segments of the mitral valve may evolve into restricted motion while others may have excessive motion or even become flail due to chordal rupture (Fig. 5.18). Assessment using the Carpentier classification is commonly used to optimize communication with surgical teams as this dictates surgical repair strategies for MR and mixed mitral valve disease (Table 5.4).[47] International standards require that all segments of the mitral valve are evaluated, which can be done using multiplanar 2D imaging together with real-time 3D echocardiography

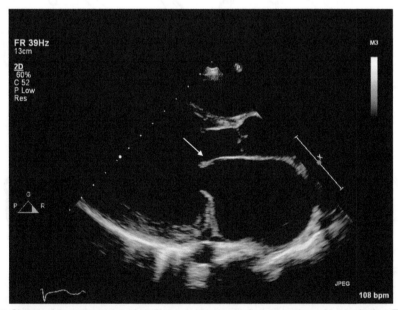

FIG. 5.17 Chronic rheumatic mitral valve disease with mixed mitral stenosis and regurgitation. The anterior mitral valve leaflet is thickened at the tip with the classic "dog-leg" or "hockey stick" deformity seen at full diastolic excursion (white arrow). The posterior leaflet is also thickened with restricted diastolic motion. The left atrium and left ventricle are severely dilated. There is also aortic valve disease with prolapse of the noncoronary cusp. The patient presented with endocarditis - there is a vegetation on the aortic valve that is apparent on the moving image.

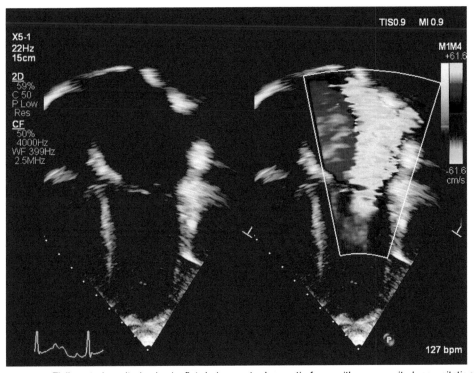

FIG. 5.18 Flail posterior mitral valve leaflet during acute rheumatic fever with severe mitral regurgitation.

TABLE 5.4
Carpentier's Functional Classification of Mitral Valve Insufficiency.

Type	Functional classification
I	Annular dilation with normal leaflet motion
II	Leaflet prolapse
IIa / IIIp	Prolapse of anterior mitral valve leaflet and restriction of posterior leaflet
III	Restricted leaflet motion

a, anterior; *p*, posterior.
Adapted from Chauvand et al.[47]

(RT3DE).[48] Fig. 5.19 shows the standard classification of the anatomy of the mitral valve both from the surgeon's view and the sonographer's view. There are a total of six segments or scallops: A1, A2, A3 of the anterior mitral valve leaflet and P1, P2, P3 of the posterior mitral valve leaflet. A1-P1 is the most lateral segment, and A3-P3 is the most medial segment.[48]

Grading of severity of MR on echocardiography is detailed in Table 5.5.[49,50] Many parameters, some

qualitative (the density of the continuous wave Doppler jet), some semiquantitative (pulmonary venous flow reversal, color jet area), and some quantitative (vena contracta width, effective regurgitant orifice area, regurgitant volume) are used to define the severity of MR. None of them can be relied on isolation, and there are limitations to each method of assessment.

The American Society of Echocardiography algorithm is a useful guide for categorising mild, moderate, and severe MR but does not specifically relate to rheumatic MR.[49]

An accurate measurement of LV end-systolic dimension (LVESD), left ventricular end-diastolic dimension (LVEDD), and systolic function by M-mode or 2D imaging must be obtained, as current guidelines for timing of surgery are partly based on these measurements.[51,52] The assessment of both cardiac size and cardiac function are more accurate using Simpson's and area—length methods to determine LV volumes. Generally, enlargement of the left ventricle or left atrium indicates at least moderate MR. In children, cardiac measurements should be indexed to body surface area and expressed as Z-scores (or standard deviations). Normal cardiac structures are between Z scores of −2.0 to +2.0. Z-score calculators can be found at http://parameterz.

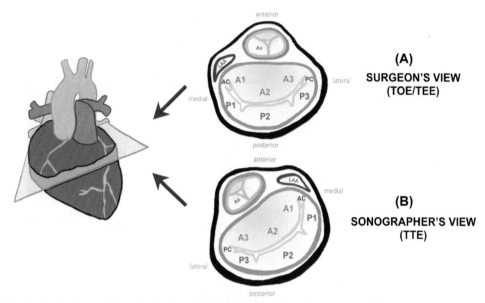

(A)
SURGEON'S VIEW
(TOE/TEE)

(B)
SONOGRAPHER'S VIEW
(TTE)

FIG. 5.19 Anatomy of the mitral valve. (A) Surgeon's view from above using RT3DE Trans-oesophageal echocardiography (TOE/TEE). (B) Sonographer's view from below using trans-thoracic echocardiography (TTE); Anterior leaflet of the MV has 3 segments with A1 anterior segment, A2 middle segment, A3 posterior segment. The posterior leaflet of the MV has 3 scallops with P1 anterolateral scallop, P2 middle scallop, P3 posteromedial scallop. AC anterior commissure and PC posterior commissure, LAA left atrial appendage, Ao Aortic Valve position relative to mitral valve. (Copyright: Dr Ari Horton.)

TABLE 5.5
Qualitative and Quantitative Parameters useful in Grading Mitral Valve Regurgitation Severity on Echocardiography.

Parameter	Mild	Moderate	Severe
Structural parameters			
LA size	Normal[a]	Normal or dilated	Usually dilated[b]
LV size	Normal[a]	Normal or dilated	Usually dilated[b]
Mitral leaflets or support apparatus	Normal or abnormal	Normal or abnormal	Abnormal including mechanism of prolapse/failure of coaptation/flail leaflet
Doppler parameters			
Color flow jet area[c]	Small, central jet (usually <4cm^2 or <20% of LA area)	Variable	Large central jet (usually >10 cm^2 or >40% of LA area) or variable size wall-impinging jet swirling in LA
Mitral inflow—PW	A-wave dominant[d]	Variable	E-wave dominant[a] (E usually ≥1.2 m/s)
Jet intensity—CW	Incomplete or faint	Dense	Dense
Jet contour CW	Parabolic	Usually parabolic	Early peaking—triangular
Pulmonary vein flow	Systolic dominance[e]	Systolic blunting[e]	Systolic flow reversal[f]

(continued)

TABLE 5.5
Qualitative and Quantitative Parameters useful in Grading Mitral Valve Regurgitation Severity on Echocardiography.—cont'd

Parameter	Mild	Moderate	Severe
Quantitative parameters[g]			
VC width (cm)	<0.3	0.3 − 0.69	≥0.7
R Vol (mL/beat)	<30	30 − 44; 45 − 59[h]	≥60
RF (%)	<30	30 − 39; 40 − 49[h]	≥50
EROA (cm²)	<0.20	0.2 − 0.29; 0.3 − 0.39[h]	≥0.40

Doppler; CW, continuous wave Doppler; LA, left atrium; LV, left ventricle.
[a]Unless there are other reasons for LA or LV dilation. Normal 2D measurements: LV minor axis ≤2.8cm/m², LV end-diastolic volume ≤82ml/m², maximal LA anteroposterior diameter ≤2cm/m², maximal LA volume ≤36 ml/m².[2,33,35]
[b]Exception: acute mitral regurgitation.
[c]At a Nyquist limit of 50-60 cm/s.
[d]Usually above 50 years of age or in conditions of impaired relaxation, in the absence of mitral stenosis or other causes of elevated LA pressure.
[e]Unless other reasons for systolic blunting (e.g., atrial fibrillation, elevated left atrial pressure).
[f]Pulmonary venous systolic flow reversal is specific but not sensitive for severe MR.
[g]Quantitative parameters can help subclassify the moderate regurgitation group into mild−moderate and moderate−severe.
[h]Grading of severity of MR subclassifies the moderate regurgitation group into "mild-to-moderate" (EROA of 0.20−0.29 cm², RF (%) of 30-39%, or a R Vol of 30−44 mL) and "moderate-to-severe" (EROA of 0.30−0.39 cm², RF (%) of 40-49%, or a R Vol of 45−59 mL).
Adapted and modified from the AHA/ACC/ASE[49] and ESC/EACVI[50] guidelines for evaluation and assessment of valvular regurgitation.

blogspot.com/2008/09/z-scoresof-cardiac-structures.html.

Echocardiographic findings in isolated mitral stenosis

With further commissural and chordal fusion, pure MS may ensue and may be associated with variable degrees of calcification, Fig. 5.20A and B.[53,54] In the setting of pure MS, leaflet motion is always restricted. In some regions of the world where ARF remains hyperendemic, progression to severe MS can be very rapid and affect children as young as 5−10 years old.[35,55] This has been called "juvenile mitral stenosis" or "malignant mitral stenosis".[35,55]

The severity of MS in adults is best characterized by the planimetered mitral valve area, measured directly in the short axis view, or calculated from the diastolic pressure half-time. In adults, severe MS is defined as a mitral valve area ≤1.0 cm² and usually corresponds to a transmitral mean gradient of >10 mmHg (Table 5.6)[56]. However, the mean pressure gradient

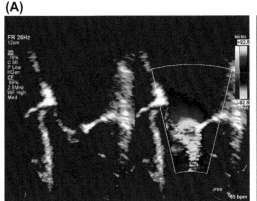
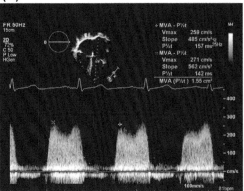

FIG. 5.20 Rheumatic mitral stenosis. **(A)** 2D and color Doppler from the apex in diastole. Note the restricted opening of both leafletsdespecially the posterior. **(B)** Continuous wave Doppler demonstrating the use of pressure half time to estimate mitral valve area. NOTE: a trace of the CW Doppler signal would provide an assessment of the mean mitral valve inflow gradient (in mmHg).

TABLE 5.6
Recommendations for Classification of Mitral Stenosis Severity in Adults.

	Mild	Moderate	Severe
Specific findings			
Valve area (cm^2)	1.5-2.5	1.0-1.5	<1.0
Supportive findings			
Mean gradient (mmHg)[a]	<5	5-10	>10
Pulmonary artery pressure (mmHg)	<30	30-50	>50

[a] At heart rates between 60 and 80 bpm and in sinus rhythm.
Adapted and modified from the AHA/ACC/ASE[56] and ESC/EACVI[61] guidelines for evaluation and assessment of valvular regurgitation.

TABLE 5.7
Grading of Mitral Valve Characteristics form the Echocardiographic Examination Using the Wilkins Score.

Grade	Mobility	Subvalvar thickening	Leaflet thickening	Calcification
1	Highly mobile valve with only leaflet tips restricted	Minimal thickening just below the mitral valve leaflets	Leaflets near normal in thickness (4-5 mm)	A single area of increased echo brightness
2	Leaflet mid and base portions have normal mobility	Thickening of chordal structures extending up to one-third of the chordal length	Mid-leaflets normal, considerable thickening of margins (5-8 mm)	Scattered areas of brightness confined to the leaflet margins
3	Valve continues to move forward in diastole, mainly from the base	Thickening extending to the distal third of the chords	Thickening extending through the entire leaflet (5-8 mm)	Brightness extending into the mid-portion of the leaflets
4	No or minimal forward movement of the leaflets in diastole	Extensive thickening and shortening of all chordal structures extending down to the papillary muscles	Considerable thickening of all leaflet tissue (>8-10 mm)	Extensive brightness throughout much of the leaflet tissue

Adopted from Wilkins G et al.[57] and Nishimura RA et al.[51]

across the mitral valve will rise with increased heart rate and with increased flow, such as concomitant MR. The mean pressure gradient should be measured using a Doppler trace of the inflow velocity using continuous-wave (CW) Doppler. Direct measurement of the mitral valve area using planimetry is not affected by flow dynamics. However, values derived from adult datasets cannot directly be applied to children with small body surface areas. In children, the mean transmitral gradient is the most commonly used method to assess severity with a mean gradient >15 mm Hg, or valve area of ≤1.0 cm^2/m^2 suggestive of severe disease.

Table 5.7 describes the grading of mitral valve echocardiographic morphologic features using the Wilkin's

score in the setting of MS to assess likelihood of a successful result following percutaneous mitral balloon commissurotomy (PMBC).[57] Four factors are evaluated in the Wilkin's score, each with a possible score of 0−4. A total score of 0 would therefore represent a completely normal valve, while higher scores (maximum 16) would represent severe anatomic disease with a lower chance of successful PMBC and durability. Pulmonary hypertension is common in MS and should be assessed as described in Box 5.3.

Echocardiography in mixed mitral valve disease
As disease progresses and further fusion of chordae and commissures develops, isolated MR may evolve into

---

BOX 5.3
Pulmonary Hypertension: Definition and Echocardiographic Features

- Pulmonary hypertension (pHT) is defined as a mean pulmonary artery pressure (mPAP) ≥20 mmHg at rest, as measured by right heart catherization[96,a]
  - For most adult patients in the modern era, including those with RHD, pHT secondary to left heart disease (WHO group 2) is the most common type
  - Echocardiographic features suggestive of left-heart disease causing pHT include[97]:
    - Greater than mild left-sided valvular heart disease (most relevant in RHD patients)
    - LV systolic dysfunction (dilated LV, reduced LVEF)[b]
    - LV diastolic dysfunction (E/e' >10, LA dilatation, LVH)[b]
- Although cardiac catheterization is required for formal diagnosis, echocardiography is the screening tool of choice for patients in whom there is clinical suspicion of pHT. Two useful echocardiographic correlates can be used to determine the probability of pHT:

1. **Peak tricuspid regurgitation velocity (TRmax)[c]**
   a. This measures the RV-RA pressure gradient[d] by continuous-wave Doppler and is the most common echocardiographic method for determining the probability of pHT[97,98]
   b. Measurements are best taken from the apical four chamber or parasternal axes, the maximal peak velocity measured using continuous wave doppler is classified as the TRmax

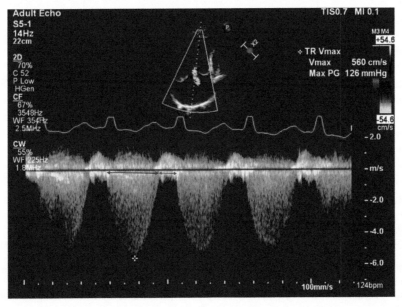

Measurement of the TRmax. This patient has severe pHT with systemic-level pulmonary pressure and prolonged systolic to diastolic duration ratio. The latter index[e] quantifies the time in systole (marked with red line) relative to the time in diastole (marked with blue line), and suggests severe impairment in global right ventricular function in this patient.
Figure reproduced with permission from Cordina et al.[99]

Continued

c. Once acquired, the TRmax can be used to report the echocardiographic probability of pHT in two main ways (although in general both are often used):

i) Using the TRmax with or without other echocardiographic features of pHT[98]:
- If the TRmax is >3.4 m/s, there is a high probability of pHT being present and evidence of other echocardiographic features of pHT are not required
- If the TRmax is ≤3.4, then the probability of pHT is assessed in combination with other echocardiographic features:

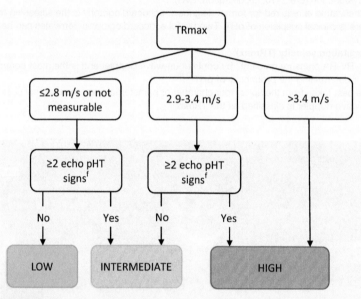

Flowchart to assess the probability of pHT using parameters identified from within ≥2 categories (ventricles, pulmonary artery, or the IVC/RA) in conjunction with peak TRmax

Reproduced with permission from Augustine et al.[97]

ii) Using the TRmax to estimate the pulmonary artery systolic pressure (PASP)[g]:
- This is useful in circumstances where the PASP is required to guide management of patients with pHT due to left heart disease
- In both the ESC[98] and AHA/ACC[100] valve guidelines, a PASP >50 mmHg in the presence of severe mitral valve disease is a IIa indication for cardiac surgery (see Chapter 6)
- The PASP is calculated by adding the estimated right atrial pressure[h] to the TRmax, using the modified Bernoulli equation:

$$PASP = 4(TRmax)^2 + RA\ pressure$$

2. **Pulmonary regurgitation peak velocity (PRpeak) or pulmonary regurgitation end diastolic velocity (PRend)**
   a. Pulmonary regurgitation provides a useful measure of pulmonary artery pressures, especially when tricuspid regurgitation is minimal or inaccurate[97,98]
   b. Measurements are taken in the parasternal short axis or parasternal RV outflow tract using continuous-wave Doppler:

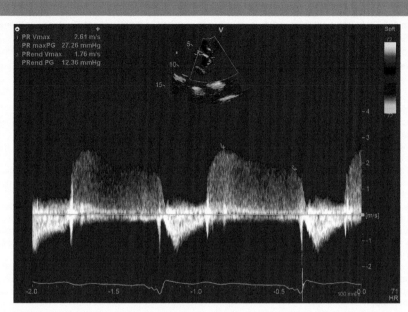

Measurement of the pulmonary regurgitation peak velocity (PRpeak) and pulmonary regurgitation end diastolic velocity (PRend). This Doppler signal was taken from a patient with RHD and significant left heart disease, with resultant pHT. This patient has severe pulmonary hypertension with a mean pulmonary artery pressure of 27mmHg (+RA pressure) and a pulmonary artery diastolic pressure of 12mmHg (+RA pressure).

c. The PRpeak, which measures the PA-RV pressure gradient, has been validated against cardiac catheterization for determining the mPAP[101]:

$$mPAP = 4(PRpeak)^2 + RA\ pressure$$

d. The pulmonary regurgitation end diastolic velocity (PRend) has also been validated against cardiac catherization for determining the PADP[101]:

$$PADP = 4(PRend)^2 + RA\ pressure$$

e. The mPAP can then be calculated from systolic (by the TRmax method) and diastolic (by the PRend method) pulmonary artery pressures:

$$mPAP = 2/3PADP + 1/3PASP\ \ where\ \ PASP = (4(TRmax)^2 + RAP$$

• In summary, a clinical diagnosis of pHT[i] is typically made in patients with RHD when there is significant left-sided valve disease to explain the degree of pHT (where the probability of pHT should be intermediate or high based on TRmax or the

Continued

PASP is >40 mmHg). Right heart catheterization is usually not required in these patients, unless another indication is present (e.g. PMBC for severe mitral stenosis)
- Management of pHT in RHD patients is directed at treating the left heart disease using medical, interventional, or surgical approaches — see Chapters 6-8

[a]The recent definition of pHT has been lowered from a mean of ≥25 mmHg to ≥20 mmHg[96]

[b]Chronic severe valve disease can also lead to systolic and/or diastolic dysfunction

[c]Absence of TR is insufficient to exclude pHT. Degree of TR does not correlate with peak TRmax. In the presence of severe TR, peak TRmax is significantly underestimated and should not be used alone to exclude pHT[97]

[d]The RV-RA pressure gradient (RVSP) will only be an accurate reflection of the pulmonary artery systolic pressure (PASP) if there is no right ventricular outflow tract obstruction or pulmonary stenosis

[e]Where a higher systolic to diastolic ratio is associated with impaired global right ventricular function, haemodynamics, functional capacity, and clinical outcomes. In children, a ratio of >1.4 is associated with an especially poor prognosis, although no specific cut-off points have been established in adults with pHT[99]

[f]Echocardiographic signs from at least two different categories (A/B/C) should be present to alter the echocardiographic probability of pHT when the peak TRmax is ≤3.4 m/s[3]. Category A (ventricles): RV/LV basal diameter ratio >1.0, flattening of the interventricular septum (LV eccentricity index >1.1 in systole and/or diastole); category B (pulmonary artery): RV outflow Doppler acceleration time <105 ms and/or middiastolic notching, early diastolic pulmonary regurgitation velocity >2.2 m/s; category C (IVC and RA): IVC diameter >2.1 cm with decreased respiratory collapse (<50% with sniff or <20% with quiet respiration), RA area (end-systole) >18 cm[2]

[g]pHT is suggested echocardiographically when the PASP is >40 mmHg in adults. However, the PASP may correlate poorly with values obtained at right heart catheterization, which may partly be due to variability in estimating the RA pressure. Recent ESC guidelines on pulmonary hypertenion[98] therefore propose that the TRmax together with other echocardiographic findings of pHT be used to report the echocardiographic probability of pHT and not PASP

[h]The RA pressure can be estimated using echocardiography based on the diameter and respiratory variation of the IVC. Normal pressure (0-5 mmHg): IVC diameter <2.1 cm + >50% collapse with sniff; intermediate (5-10 mmHg): when IVC diameter + collapse do not fit the definition of normal or high pressure; high pressure (10-20 mmHg): IVC diameter >2.1 cm + <50% collapse with sniff or <20% on quiet inspiration[98]. Note that this is not validated in the paediatric population

[i]It is worth emphasizing that the definition of PH is based on demonstrating *elevated mean pulmonary artery pressures* (mPAP) at right heart catherization, while the most common echocardiographic method uses the peak TRmax to estimate the *peak pulmonary artery systolic pressure* (PASP).

pHT, pulmonary hypertension; RHD, rheumatic heart disease; RV, right ventricular; RA, right atrial; RVSP, right-ventricular systolic pressure; PASP, pulmonary artery systolic pressure; TRmax, peak tricuspid regurgitation velocity; IVC, inferior vena cava; LV, left ventricle; LVEF, left ventricular ejection fraction; LVH, left ventricular hypertrophy; LA, left atrial dilatation; RV, right ventricle; PRpeak, pulmonary regurgitation peak velocity; PRend, pulmonary regurgitation end diastolic velocity; PADP, pulmonary artery diastolic pressure; mPAP, mean pulmonary artery pressure; PMBC, percutaneous mitral balloon commissurotomy

mixed mitral valve disease. The leaflets and chordae progressively thicken, retract and calcify. Grading of mixed stenotic and regurgitant lesions is challenging as there are no international guidelines. Pulmonary hypertension, LV and left atrial enlargement are all markers of moderate to severe disease. Impaired LV ejection fraction is always an ominous sign and should prompt urgent cardiosurgical referral.

Aortic Valve Disease

Mild AR is usually not associated with detectable structural or morphological valvular changes. Morphological changes may include leaflet tip prolapse (Fig. 5.21). In order of frequency, the left coronary cusp, then right coronary cusp and non-coronary cusp are most likely to prolapse. Central noncoaptation or eccentric regurgitation between retracted or rolled cusps are both common findings. With time, the leaflet tips thicken, retract, and roll, giving rise to the mixed effect of stenosis and regurgitation. One of the classical images in advanced aortic valve disease is a central triangular coaptation defect where all three leaflets are rolled and retracted. By this stage there is usually mixed stenosis and regurgitation (Fig. 5.22).[1] Isolated rheumatic AS is extremely uncommon in children and adolescents and usually takes decades to occur.[22]

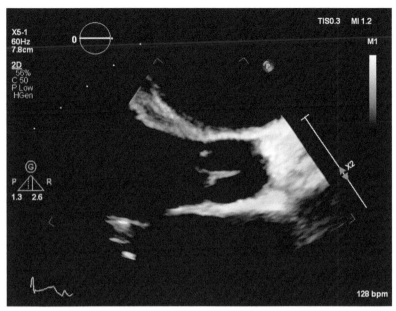

FIG. 5.21 A rheumatic aortic valve with prolapse of the anterior (right coronary) cusp.

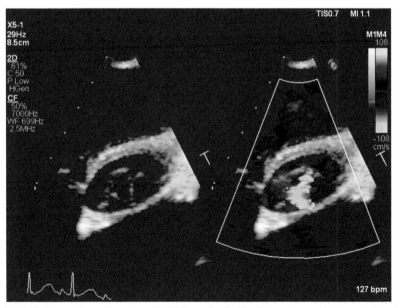

FIG. 5.22 A rheumatic aortic valve with thickened rolled leaflets and a central coaptation defect

Moderate or severe AR results in LV volume overload with progressive LV dilatation and hypertrophy. Initially, an increased end diastolic dimension helps maintain stroke volume, but eventually it leads to LV dysfunction and increased risk of mortality unless timely cardio-surgical intervention is performed (see Chapter 6).[58] Assessing the severity of aortic regurgitation by sampling for pandiastolic flow reversal in the descending thoracic

TABLE 5.8
Grading of Severity of Aortic Regurgitation.

Parameters	Mild	Moderate	Severe
Qualitative			
Aortic valve morphology	Normal/abnormal	Normal/abnormal	Abnormal including mechanism of flail leaflet/large coaptation defect
Colour flow AR jet width[a]	Small in central jets	Intermediate	Large in central jet, variable in eccentric jets
CW signal of AR jet	Incomplete/faint	Dense	Dense
Diastolic flow reversal in descending aorta	Brief, protodiastolic flow reversal	Intermediate	Holodiastolic flow reversal (end-diastolic velocity >20 cm/s)
Semiquantitative			
VC width (mm)	<3	Intermediate	>6
Pressure half-time (ms)[b]	>500	Intermediate	<200
Quantitative			
EROA (mm^2)	<10	10–19; 20–29[c]	≥30
R Vol (mL)	<30	30–44; 45–59[c]	≥60
LV size[d]	Normal	Usually normal	Usually dilated[e]

AR, aortic regurgitation; CW, continuous wave; LA, left atrium; EROA, effective regurgitant orifice area; LV, left ventricle; R Vol, regurgitant volume; VC, vena contracta.

[a] At a Nyquist limit of 50–60 cm/s.

[b] PHT is shortened with increasing LV diastolic pressure, vasodilator therapy, and in patients with a dilated compliant aorta or lengthened in chronic AR.

[c] Grading of the severity of AR classifies regurgitation as mild, moderate, or severe and subclassifies the moderate regurgitation group into "mild-to-moderate" (EROA of 10–19 mm^2 or an R Vol of 30–44 mL) and "moderate-to-severe" (EROA of 20–29 mm^2 or an R Vol of 45–59 mL).

[d] Unless for other reasons, the LV size is usually normal in patients with mild AR. In acute severe AR, the LV size is often normal. In chronic severe AR, the LV is classically dilated. Accepted cutoff values for nonsignificant LV enlargement: LV end-diastolic diameter <56 mm, LV end-diastolic volume <82 mL/m^2, LV end-systolic diameter <40 mm, LV end-systolic volume <30 mL/m^2.

[e] Exception in acute severe AR when chambers have not had a chance to dilate.

Adapted and modified from the AHA/ACC/ASE[49] and ESC/EACVI[58] guidelines for evaluation and assessment of valvular regurgitation

TABLE 5.9
Grading of Severity of Aortic Stenosis.

	Normal	Mild	Moderate	Severe
Peak velocity (m/s)	≤2.5 m/s	2.6–2.9	3.0–4.0	>4.0
AHA/ACC Mean gradient (mmHg)	–	<20	20–40	>40
ESC Mean gradient (mmHg)		<30	30–50	>50
AVA (cm^2)[a]	–	>1.5	1.0–1.5	<1.0
Indexed AVA (cm^2/m^2)	–	>0.85	0.60–0.85	<0.6
Velocity ratio	–	>0.50	0.25–0.50	<0.25

AVA, aortic valve area.

[a] AVA should be indexed for BSA if BSA <1.6 m^2 or >2 m^2.

Adapted and modified from Nishimura RA et al. [51] and Baumgartner H et al. [56,61,62].

aorta and abdominal aorta is critical, especially for the assessment of eccentric regurgitation, as the length and velocity of the reversed flow is proportional to the severity of aortic regurgitation. Useful methods for assessing the severity of AR and AS are detailed in Tables 5.8 and 5.9,[49,51,56,58] respectively.

Tricuspid Valve Disease

Most tricuspid valve disease in the setting of RHD is functional and the result of advanced left-sided pathology and pulmonary hypertension. Organic (primary) tricuspid valve disease as a direct result of RHD is less common but is well described and usually occurs in the setting of advanced multivalve RHD.[59] Rheumatic tricuspid valve disease rarely, if ever, occurs as an isolated lesion.[59] As the right ventricle fails in the setting of severe pulmonary hypertension, the right ventricular dilatation leads to annular dilatation and worsening of tricuspid regurgitation, with hepatic venous dilatation and bidirectional flow evident on Doppler. Useful methods for assessing the severity of tricuspid regurgitation are detailed in Table 5.10.[50] Similar to the pathology of mitral disease, tricuspid disease may progress to stenosis with leaflet thickening, chordal shortening, and commissural fusion.[59]

Pulmonary Valve Disease

Pulmonic valve involvement is exceedingly rare but has been described in the setting of multivalve disease and usually in the setting of secondary pulmonary hypertension.[60] The regurgitant jet can be useful as an adjunct for the determination of mean and peak pulmonary artery pressures and is a more direct measure than tricuspid

---

TABLE 5.10
Grading of Severity of Tricuspid Regurgitation.

Parameters	Mild	Moderate	Severe
Qualitative			
Tricuspid valve morphology	Normal/abnormal	Normal/abnormal	Abnormal/flail/large coaptation defect
Color flow TR jet[a]	Small, central	Intermediate	Very large central jet or eccentric wall impinging jet
CW signal of TR jet	Faint/parabolic	Dense/parabolic	Dense/triangular with early peaking (peak <2 m/s in massive TR)
Semiquantitative			
VC width (mm)[a]	Not defined	<7	≥7
PISA radius (mm)[b]	≤5	6−9	≥9
Hepatic vein flow[c]	Systolic dominance	Systolic blunting	Systolic flow reversal
Tricuspid inflow	Normal	Normal	E-wave dominant (≥1 cm/s)[d]
RA/IVC dimension[e]	Normal	Often dilated RA	Usually significantly dilated right atrium and dilated IVC
Quantitative			
EROA (mm^2)	Not defined	Not defined	≥40
R Vol (mL)	Not defined	Not defined	≥45

CW, continuous wave; EROA, effective regurgitant orifice area; RA, right atrium; RV, right ventricle; R Vol, regurgitant volume; TR, tricuspid regurgitation; VC, vena contracta.
[a] At a Nyquist limit of 50−60 cm/s.
[b] Baseline Nyquist limit shift of 28 cm/s.
[c] Unless other reasons of systolic blunting (atrial fibrillation, elevated RA pressure).
[d] In the absence of other causes of elevated RA pressure.
[e] Unless for other reasons, the RA and RV size and IVC are usually normal in patients with mild TR. An end-systolic RV eccentricity index >2 is in favor of severe TR. In acute severe TR, the RV size is often normal. In chronic severe TR, the RV is classically dilated. Accepted cutoff values for nonsignificant right-sided chambers enlargement (measurements obtained from the apical four-chamber view): Mid RV dimension ≤33 mm, RV end-diastolic area ≤28 cm^2, RV end-systolic area ≤16 cm^2, RV fractional area change >32%, maximal RA volume ≤33 mL/m^2. An IVC diameter <1.5 cm is considered normal.
Adapted and modified from Zohgbi WA et al.[49], Lancellotti P et al.[50] and Nishimura RA et al.[51]

TABLE 5.11
Grading the Severity of Pulmonary Regurgitation.

Parameters	Mild	Moderate	Severe
Qualitative			
Pulmonic valve morphology	Normal	Normal/abnormal	Abnormal
Color flow PR jet width[a]	Small, usually <10 mm in length with a narrow origin	Intermediate	Large, with a wide origin; may be brief in duration
CW signal of PR jet[b]	Faint/slow deceleration	Dense/variable	Dense/steep deceleration, early termination of diastolic flow
Pulmonic vs. aortic flow by PW	Normal or slightly increased	Intermediate	Greatly increased
Semiquantitative			
VC width (mm)	Not defined	Not defined	Not defined
Quantitative			
EROA (mm^2)	Not defined	Not defined	Not defined
R Vol (mL)	Not defined	Not defined	Not defined
RV size[c]	Normal	Normal	Can be dilated

PR, pulmonic regurgitation; CW, continuous wave; EROA, effective regurgitant orifice area; PW, pulse wave; RV, right ventricle; R Vol, regurgitant volume; VC, vena contracta.
Adapted and modified from Zohgbi et al [49] and Lancellotti et al [58]
[a] Nyquist limit of 50–60 cm/s.
[b] Steep deceleration is not specific for severe PR.
[c] Unless for other reasons, the RV size is usually normal in patients with mild PR. In acute severe PR, the RV size is often normal. Accepted cutoff values for nonsignificant RV enlargement (measurements obtained from the apical four-chamber view): Mid RV dimension ≤33 mm, RV end-diastolic area ≤28 cm^2, RV end-systolic area ≤16 cm^2, RV fractional area change >32%, maximal.

valve peak velocity. Useful methods for assessing the severity of pulmonary valve regurgitation are detailed in Table 5.11.[49,58]

Evaluation of Prosthetic Valves

Valve replacement is not a cure for RHD as patients simply exchange native valve disease for prosthetic valve disease (a fact that must be emphasised to patients before surgery). In addition, the remaining native cardiac valves remain at risk of damage by ARF recurrences, which may necessitate further cardiosurgical procedures. For this reason, the National Australian guidelines recommend 6-monthly cardiology reviews and echocardiograms after RHD surgical procedures (Table 5.12).[52] This regimen is much more aggressive than the recommendations by the American Heart Association for non-rheumatic valvular disease.[51] Such intense follow-up is justified especially in the young, as the long-term outcomes of both mechanical and bioprosthetic valve replacement in rheumatic patients remain very poor. A study in the Pacific Islands demonstrated that 10-year survival following mechanical valve replacement in young female adults was less than

50%.[63] Similarly, a study from New Zealand showed that event-free survival in children following mechanical valve replacement was equally poor with an actuarial survival of 52% at 10 years.[64] The small cohort of patients who underwent bioprosthetic valve replacement had very poor outcomes (see also Chapters 6 and 8).[64]

Bioprosthetic valves are prone to tissue degeneration especially in the young and may result in valvular regurgitation, stenosis, or mixed hemodynamic effects. Bioprosthetic valves are also at risk of valve dehiscence, infective endocarditis, and pannus formation. Clinical presentation is often insidious. Mechanical valves are at risk of the complications described earlier and also of acute valve thrombosis leading to abrupt impairment of leaflet function.

Transthoracic echocardiography provides accurate measurements of transvalvular velocities and pressure gradients as well as valvular and perivalvular regurgitation. Normal values vary from valve to valve. Therefore, it is important to perform a baseline assessment post replacement and then monitor for change over time. There might be changes in gradient related to

TABLE 5.12
Recommended clinical review for rheumatic heart disease.

Classification	Criteria[a]	Review and management plan	Frequency[b]
Priority 1 (severe)[c]	Severe valvular disease **or**	Doctor review	3–6 monthly
	moderate/severe valvular lesion with symptoms **or**	Cardiologist/physician/paediatrician review	3–6 monthly
	mechanical prosthetic valves, tissue prosthetic valves, and valve repairs, including balloon valvuloplasty	Echocardiography	3–6 monthly
Priority 2 (moderate)	Any moderate valve lesion in the absence of symptoms and with normal LV function	Doctor review	6-monthly
		ECG (optional)	Yearly
		Cardiologist/physician/paediatrician review	Yearly
		Echocardiography	Yearly
Priority 3 (mild)	ARF with no evidence of RHD **or**	Doctor review	Yearly
	trivial to mild valvular disease	Echocardiography	Children: 2 yearly[d] Adults: 2–3 yearly[d]
Priority 4 (inactive)	Patients with a history of ARF (no RHD) for whom secondary prophylaxis has been ceased	Medical review	Yearly
		Cardiologist/physician/paediatrician review	As referred with new symptoms

ARF, acute rheumatic fever; ECG, electrocardiogram; RHD, rheumatic heart disease.
[a] Serial echocardiographic assessments are required in the long-term management of RHD as an essential tool in determining the progress of cardiac damage and the optimal timing of surgery. Therefore, risk stratification should be based on clinical and echocardiographic findings (Grade D).
[b] Review frequency should be determined according to individual needs and local capacity. Most critically, the frequency of review should become more in the event of symptom onset, symptomatic deterioration, or a change in clinical findings.
[c] Any patient with severe valvular disease or moderate to severe valvular disease with symptoms should be referred for cardiological and surgical assessment as soon as possible.
[d] In patients with no evidence of valvular disease on echocardiography, who have no documented ARF recurrences, good adherence to secondary prophylaxis and no cardiac murmurs on examination at follow-up appointments, echocardiography may not be needed as frequently. Modified and updated from the 2012 RHD Australia Guidelines[52].

physiologic changes over time with somatic growth in children, increased weight, or in the setting of altered hyperdynamic states, such as fever or infection.

If there is a significant change in gradient across nonnative valves, then further evaluation is recommended. An X-ray image intensifier can be used to evaluate mechanical leaflet function. If available, it is recommended to evaluate non-native valvular dysfunction with transesophageal echocardiography, which may be able to better define the mechanism of dysfunction and

assess for thrombi, pannus formation, and identify any evidence for infective endocarditis. Acute prosthetic valve dysfunction and infective endocarditis are both discussed in detail in Chapter 16.

Monitoring Disease Progression and Resolution

Serial echocardiography is pivotal in monitoring disease progression or disease resolution, especially in the acute phase following an episode of ARF.

Progression to severe disease can occur without docu-mented episodes of ARF recurrences.[65] Improvements in echocardiographic findings most commonly occur in the setting of mild-to-moderate disease and with good adherence to secondary prophylaxis (see Chapter 11).[10–12,25,66] In the future, after results return from randomized control trials assessing the efficacy of sec-ondary prophylaxis in borderline and mild RHD, echo-cardiographic follow-up findings could influence management strategies by allowing for earlier cessation of secondary prophylaxis, necessitating updates to inter-national and national guidelines in the process.[52,67]

Serial assessments of the degree of valvular involve-ment, pulmonary hypertension, left atrial dimensions and area, LV size and volume using 2-D or newer 3-D modalities allow for optimization of medical and surgi-cal management strategies. Fractional shortening and/or ejection fraction as measured on echocardiography should be followed carefully, with any impairment of function an indication for referral to a cardiac center (see Chapters 6 and 8).

It is important to note that LV ejection fraction and fractional shortening are weak surrogates for cardiac contractility in the setting of significant combined aortic and mitral regurgitation. Altered loading conditions and dysrhythmias may underestimate the severity of impairment. Load-independent measures such as stress velocity index and strain measures may correlate more closely with true LV function under these circumstances.[15]

Recommendations for minimum timing intervals for follow-up have been suggested by multiple bodies including the Australian and New Zealand guide-lines.[52,68] All are conservative and determined by local availability of resources. More frequent follow-up may be appropriate for children and young adults who remain at the highest risk of ARF recurrence and hence progression of RHD. Table 5.12[52] makes best practice recommendations in relation to frequency of echocardi-ography and cardiology follow-up in a country with significant resources and high disease burden such as the Australian context.

Guide to Nature and Timing of Cardiosurgical Intervention

Echocardiographic parameters that guide timing of medical, catheter based, or surgical interventions are discussed in detail in Chapters 6. 2D and 3D echocardi-ography can accurately identify mechanisms of valvular dysfunction and evaluate suitability for percutaneous interventions and guide surgical mitral, aortic, and tricuspid valve repair strategies.[51]

3D Echocardiography and Rheumatic Valve Disease

Real-time 3D echocardiography (RT3DE) can contribute to pre- and perioperative decision-making by delineating the mechanism of regurgitation (Fig. 5.23A and B).[69] This is especially so in the case of mitral valve repair where RT3DE can demonstrate valve motion abnormalities, flail segments and perfora-tions which directly inform surgical strategy. This mo-dality has the advantage of providing images that are readily accessible to the surgical eye and are particularly

(A)

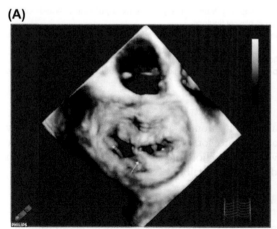

(B)

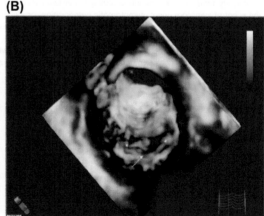

FIG. 5.23 3D transesophageal images of a rheumatic mitral valve viewed from **(A)** the left atrium and **(B)** the left ventricle. There is retraction of the posterior leaflet adjacent to both commissures (asterisks) and prolapse of its central portion (arrow).

useful in rheumatic mitral valve disease where there are often a number of abnormalities present in different areas of the coaptation zone. 2D transesophageal echocardiography and RT3DE also have a role in the immediate post-bypass echocardiogram as it can readily localize areas of regurgitation. The utility of 3D in assessment before aortic valve repair is less well established. Images of the aortic valve leaflets can be compromised by drop out, and very often the mechanism and site of regurgitation is readily demonstrable with 2D imaging.

Assessment of the severity of MS can be aided by 3D planimetry of the valve orifice, and multiplane imaging provides a more accurate measure of the mitral valve diastolic area than Doppler methods when compared to invasive measurement.[70,71] Assessment of the severity of regurgitation by measurement of the vena contracta with RT3DE may also be useful as it correlates well with Doppler measurement of the effective regurgitant orifice area.[72] Finally, there is little utility for RT3DE in the assessment of ARF except in the occasional case where valve surgery is necessary during the acute phase of the illness.

OTHER IMAGING AND DIAGNOSTIC MODALITIES

Cardiac Catheterization

The reader is referred to chapter 7 for a detailed discussion of the role of cardiac catheterization in RHD. Cardiac catheterization for hemodynamic assessment is rarely required to evaluate RHD in the young. Cardiac catheterization should be considered in adult patients when non-invasive tests are inconclusive, when cardiac MRI is not available or when there is a discrepancy between the findings on non-invasive testing and physical examination regarding severity of the valve lesion.[51] For adult patients who are at risk of coronary artery disease and are committed to valvular cardiac surgery, invasive coronary angiography is an appropriate choice of investigation when CT coronary angiogram is not available.[51] Percutaneous mitral balloon commissurotomy (PMBC) remains the procedure of choice in the setting of severe isolated MS with suitable valve morphology and in the absence of contraindications and is also discussed in Chapter 7.

Computed Tomography

Computed tomography (CT) scans have limited utility in the setting of RHD. Its primary role is to exclude significant coronary artery disease in the setting of significant valvular disease.[51]

Cardiac Magnetic Resonance Imaging

The role of cardiac magnetic resonance imaging (CMR) in the assessment and surveillance of RHD in childhood is limited. Myocardial fibrosis has been demonstrated with late gadolinium enhancement, but it remains unclear as to whether this finding is related to acute carditis or a consequence of volume-loading from chronic valve disease.[73,74] CMR provides gold-standard measures of LV size and function and as such has a role in patients with chronic rheumatic valve disease where echocardiographic image quality is poor or where measurements of LV size and function are borderline for intervention.[74,75] In addition, CMR can provide an accurate measure of regurgitant volume and is occasionally useful when the assessment of regurgitation with echocardiography is uncertain—particularly in the situation where apparently moderate mitral or AR is accompanied by significant dilatation of the left ventricle (Figs. 5.24 and 5.25).[75]

There may also be a role for CMR in the assessment of mixed valve disease, particularly of the aortic valve, where indications for intervention are not well defined and the combination of pressure and volume load

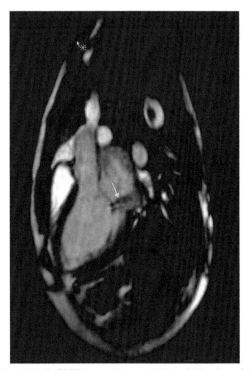

FIG. 5.24 A CMR image demonstrating thickening of the leaflet tips and regurgitation in a patient with rheumatic mitral valve disease.

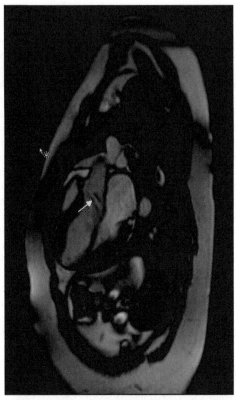

FIG. 5.25 A CMR image in a patient with rheumatic aortic valve disease demonstrating posteriorly-directed aortic regurgitation due to prolapse of the right coronary cusp of the aortic valve.

results in a varying degree of LV dilatation and hypertrophy.[75] In this situation, accurate serial measurement of LV mass and size, and assessment of myocardial fibrosis, may influence timing of surgery, although at the present time there are no data to support this approach. In the older patient with chronic mitral valve disease and atrial fibrillation, atrial wall fibrosis can be demonstrated with late enhancement CMR.[76] The degree of atrial fibrosis and remodeling on CMR may be predictive of outcome after atrial fibrillation intervention using ablation.[77]

Apart from these situations, there is little need for CMR in the assessment of RHD. CMR lacks the spatial and temporal resolution of echocardiography and as such its ability to assess the mechanism of regurgitation is limited. Moreover, criteria for surgical intervention that relate to LV chamber size and function have been derived from echocardiography and have not been validated in CMR. In addition, cost and availability are important factors that limit the utility of CMR in resource-poor settings.

EVALUATION OF HEART FAILURE

Heart failure is a clinical syndrome characterized by typical symptoms (dyspnoea, orthopnoea, ankle swelling, fatigue) and signs (pulmonary congestion, elevated jugular venous pressure). It develops when the heart is unable to pump sufficiently to maintain blood flow to meet the body's needs. The definition of HF is restricted only to patients in whom clinical symptoms are apparent (HF stages C and D) and excludes those with a background of risk factors for HF (HF stage A—such as a history of ARF) or asymptomatic structural or functional cardiac abnormalities (HF stage B—such as asymptomatic RHD). HF staging, as well as the natural history of valvular lesions, are discussed further in Chapter 6.

The etiologies of HF are wide-ranging but in the setting of RHD, HF occurs as a result of chronic, severe valvular dysfunction that in turn leads to ventricular dilatation and dysfunction, hypertrophy, pulmonary hypertension, and arrhythmias. This in turn impairs the ability of the ventricle to fill with or eject blood, resulting in reduced cardiac output and/or elevated intracardiac pressures.[78,79] If successful and timely cardio-surgical intervention takes place, particularly before LV decompensation occurs, the signs and symptoms of HF as a result of RHD are reversible.[15,16,80]

The most common symptom of HF is shortness of breath that is usually worse with exercise but as the disease progresses, shortness of breath will be present at rest or while lying down and may wake the person at night. HF classification is based on symptoms and degree of functional limitation, as defined by the New York Heart Association (Table 5.13).[81] As disease advances, it can lead to excessive tiredness, chest pain, peripheral edema, and ascites. Clinical findings may include abnormal blood pressure and heart rate, abnormal pulses, pulmonary edema, raised jugular venous pulse, hepatomegaly, ascites, and pedal edema.

Echocardiography is the most useful non–invasive tool to assess etiology and severity of HF. However, in rural and remote locations and resource-poor settings, this tool is often unavailable. In the setting of RHD, echocardiography allows determination of the nature and severity of valvular disease and associated ventricular dysfunction. Noting that, without other comorbidities, ventricular dysfunction in the setting of RHD

TABLE 5.13
New York Heart Association Functional Classification[81].

NYHA Class	Symptoms
I	No limitation of physical activity. Ordinary physical activity does not cause undue fatigue, palpitation, or dyspnea (shortness of breath).
II	Slight limitation of physical activity. Comfortable at rest. Ordinary physical activity results in fatigue, palpitation, or dyspnea (shortness of breath).
III	Marked limitation of physical activity. Comfortable at rest. Less than ordinary activity causes fatigue, palpitation, or dyspnea.
IV	Unable to carry on any physical activity without discomfort. Symptoms of HF at rest. If any physical activity is undertaken, discomfort increases.

only occurs when significant valvular dysfunction is present.[15,16,80] The medical management of chronic HF in those with RHD is discussed in Chapter 6. The etiology and precipitants of acute HF in the setting of ARF and RHD, along with the signs and symptoms, investigations, and management of these patients are discussed in detail in Chapter 16.

Clinical Investigations for Chronic Heart Failure

In many parts of the world, diagnosis of HF and RHD remains purely clinical. However, if available, blood tests with a combination of clinical history, examination and knowledge of the pretest probability of the etiology of HF can help refine the differential diagnosis and determine severity of disease. Blood cultures can be helpful to exclude concomitant bacterial infection and infective endocarditis. Serology and antibody testing can be useful to rule out differential diagnoses, for example, antinuclear and anticardiolipin antibody tests may be useful to exclude systemic lupus erythematosus. ECG, CXR, 6-min walk test, and exercise stress test can complement clinical assessment.

Full blood count

Full blood examination is useful for all patients at presentation. It is often normal in the setting of chronic RHD, but it is useful for looking at complications and comorbidities including anemia and infections, which can also precipitate HF in RHD. Transfusion triggers for anemia in the context of HF are discussed in Chapter 6.

Electrolytes and renal function testing

Acute and chronic kidney impairment can result from HF in the setting of RHD or as a complication of medical therapy. Regular monitoring of renal function and electrolytes is an essential component of medical therapy, in particular looking for creatinine and electrolyte disturbances (such as hyponatremia and hyperkalemia), which may complicate therapy with specific medications (see Chapters 6 and 16).

Troponin

Troponin might be slightly elevated in the setting of acute rheumatic carditis and is usually related to mild pericardial inflammation and is not usually associated with genuine myocarditis.[17] As such, it is generally not useful in the assessment of children with ARF or RHD.[17] However, in older patients it may help ascertain the etiology of chest pain when multiple potential etiologies of cardiac disease exists, for example, concomitant ischemic heart disease and valvular heart disease (see Table 16.7, Chapter 16).

Liver function testing and clotting profile

Liver function testing can reveal useful information regarding the impact of right HF on the liver (congestive hepatopathy), such as a mildly raised serum bilirubin levels (most common finding, occurring in up to 70% of patients) and mildly raised serum transaminases (occurs in about one-third of patients and typically no more than 2–3 times the upper limit of normal).[82] Hypoalbuminemia, which occurs in 30%–50% of patients and rarely falls to less than 2.5 g/dL, is most likely a consequence of malnutrition and protein-losing gastroenteropathy.[83] Mild elevations in the prothrombin time are seen in many patients, the cause of which is poorly understood. Extra caution should be exercised in those with evidence of congestive hepatopathy who also require anticoagulation (e.g., atrial fibrillation, mechanical heart valves) due to a potentially increased bleeding risk.

Inflammatory markers

C-reactive protein (CRP) and erythrocyte sedimentation rate (ESR) are useful markers of acute inflammation and may help to determine if the cardiac presentation is ARF, chronic RHD, or acute-on-chronic RHD.

Antibody testing

Anti-DNAse B and antistreptolysin O titer (ASOT) are primarily useful in determination of recent group A streptococcal infections in the setting of ARF. The absolute number does not reflect the severity of the ARF episode (see Chapter 3). It has limited to no utility in the setting of established RHD.

Biomarkers for heart failure

B-type natriuretic peptide (BNP) and pro B-type natriuretic peptide (NT-proBNP) are useful biomarkers of HF. The main clinical utility of either BNP or NT-proBNP is that a normal level helps to rule out chronic HF and thereby it can aid differentiation of respiratory versus cardiac cause of shortness of breath.[84] In specific circumstances like in the setting of MR, elevated BNP levels and a change in BNP are useful predictors of outcome.[85] Specifically, it helps to identify asymptomatic patients at higher risk of developing HF, LV dysfunction, or death.[86,87] See also Table 16.7, Chapter 16.

Exercise Stress Testing

Exercise testing is useful and recommended when there is a discrepancy between resting Doppler echocardiographic findings and clinical symptoms or signs. Exercise testing (e.g., treadmill testing) can confirm the absence of symptoms (patients with cardiac disease who complete 3 stages (9 minutes) of the Bruce protocol are usually considered asymptomatic), assess the hemodynamic response to exercise (changes in heart rate and blood pressure and pulmonary artery pressure) and determine prognosis.[51] In those with mitral valve disease, bicycle or treadmill stress testing can be combined with Doppler echocardiography (usually performed at rest after termination of exercise) to assess exercise pulmonary pressures (a pulmonary artery systolic pressure >60 mmHg with exercise would be a significant finding). Functional exercise capacity can also be assessed with a 6-minute walking test. The advantage of a 6-min walk test is that it is inexpensive and can be used in all environments including in low-resource settings. It can also be used to identify exertional desaturation, a sign of pulmonary hypertension. It is a simple, safe, and powerful method to assess the prognosis of patients with NYHA class II and III HF in the setting of nonvalvular heart disease.[51]

DISEASE PROGRESSION AND NATURAL HISTORY

The long-term outcomes in RHD, as well as disease progression and resolution, are related to three major factors: severity at diagnosis, recurrent episodes of ARF, and access to tertiary medical care.[11,23] As such, disease progression, morbidity and mortality due to RHD are greatest in endemic zones in low-middle income countries.[22,23]

Before the availability of penicillin and the introduction of secondary prophylaxis, 20-year mortality for ARF and RHD in the United States was as high as 30%–80%, with most individuals dying before the age of 30 years.[54,88] In resource-poor countries, untreated patients continue to suffer from poor outcomes with annual mortality in the range of 3.0%–12.5% and a mean age of death <25 years.[89–91] In the absence of secondary prophylaxis, 44%–80% of children with ARF or RHD will progress to severe cardiac disease.[54,88] On secondary prophylaxis, the long-term prognosis of mild-to-moderate carditis in the absence of a recurrent episode of ARF is very good, with the majority (65%–70%) of patients having no detectable disease after 10 years.[10–12,25] Those who experience ARF recurrence or develop severe RHD following the first episode have a much poorer prognosis.[11,14,66,92] The majority of patients with severe RHD will require cardiac surgery or succumb. An Australian study demonstrated that 50% of children with severe RHD will require cardiac surgery within a space of 2 years from diagnosis.[93]

Practical and financial limitations together have resulted in a generation of children in endemic countries unable to access both secondary prophylaxis and medical or surgical intervention.[94,95]

FUTURE DIRECTIONS

The future for the clinical evaluation and diagnosis of RHD around the world lies in the development of affordable, accessible echocardiography with task-shifting of screening and diagnosis. These need to be employed effectively in hyperendemic communities to empower them to care for their people and improve knowledge, experience, and outcomes for future generations. More research and advocacy is needed to better guide efforts for an end-game for RHD from primordial prevention to global cardiac surgical care.

REFERENCES

1. Remenyi B, Wilson N, Steer A, et al. World heart federation criteria for echocardiographic diagnosis of rheumatic heart disease—an evidence-based guideline. *Nat Rev Cardiol.* 2012;9:297–309.
2. Gewitz MH, Baltimore RS, Tani LY, et al. Revision of the Jones criteria for the diagnosis of acute rheumatic fever in the era of Doppler echocardiography: a scientific statement from the American heart association. *Circulation.* 2015;131:1806–1818.

3. Guilherme L, Kalil J, Cunningham M. Molecular mimicry in the autoimmune pathogenesis of rheumatic heart disease. *Autoimmunity*. 2006;39:31−39.

4. Denny FW, Wannamaker LW, Brink WR, Rammelkamp Jr CH, Custer EA. Prevention of rheumatic fever; treatment of the preceding streptococcic infection. *JAMA*. 1950;143:151−153.

5. Carapetis JR, Currie BJ, Mathews JD. Cumulative incidence of rheumatic fever in an endemic region: a guide to the susceptibility of the population? *Epidemiol Infect*. 2000;124:239−244.

6. Vasan RS, Shrivastava S, Vijayakumar M, Narang R, Lister BC, Narula J. Echocardiographic evaluation of patients with acute rheumatic fever and rheumatic carditis. *Circulation*. 1996;94:73−82.

7. Steer AC, Kado J, Jenney AW, et al. Acute rheumatic fever and rheumatic heart disease in Fiji: prospective surveillance, 2005−2007. *Med J Aust*. 2009;190:133−135.

8. Carapetis JR, Steer AC, Mulholland EK, Weber M. The global burden of group A streptococcal diseases. *Lancet Infect Dis*. 2005;5:685−694.

9. Lawrence JG, Carapetis JR, Griffiths K, Edwards K, Condon JR. Acute rheumatic Fever and rheumatic heart disease: incidence and progression in the northern territory of Australia, 1997 to 2010. *Circulation*. 2013;128: 492−501.

10. Tompkins DG, Boxerbaum B, Liebman J. Long-term prognosis of rheumatic fever patients receiving regular intramuscular benzathine penicillin. *Circulation*. 1972; 45:543−551.

11. Majeed HA, Batnager S, Yousof AM, Khuffash F, Yusuf AR. Acute rheumatic fever and the evolution of rheumatic heart disease: a prospective 12 year follow-up report. *J Clin Epidemiol*. 1992;45:871−875.

12. Kassem AS, El-Walili TM, Zaher SR, Ayman M. Reversibility of mitral regurgitation following rheumatic fever: clinical profile and echocardiographic evaluation. *Indian J Pediatr*. 1995;62:717−723.

13. Feinstein AR, Wood HF, Spagnuolo M, et al. Rheumatic fever in children and adolescents. A long-term epidemiologic study of subsequent prophylaxis, streptococcal infections, and clinical sequelae. Vii. Cardiac changes and sequelae. *Ann Intern Med*. 1964;60(Suppl 5):87−123.

14. Meira ZM, Goulart EM, Colosimo EA, Mota CC. Long term follow up of rheumatic fever and predictors of severe rheumatic valvar disease in Brazilian children and adolescents. *Heart*. 2005;91:1019−1022.

15. Gentles TL, Colan SD, Wilson NJ, Biosa R, Neutze JM. Left ventricular mechanics during and after acute rheumatic fever: contractile dysfunction is closely related to valve regurgitation. *J Am Coll Cardiol*. 2001;37: 201−207.

16. Gentles TL, Finucane AK, Remenyi B, Kerr AR, Wilson NJ. Ventricular function before and after surgery for isolated and combined regurgitation in the young. *Ann Thorac Surg*. 2015;100:1383−1389.

17. Kamblock J, Payot L, Iung B, et al. Does rheumatic myocarditis really exists? Systematic study with echocardiography and cardiac troponin I blood levels. *Eur Heart J*. 2003;24:855−862.

18. Watkins DA, Johnson CO, Colquhoun SM, et al. Global, regional, and national burden of rheumatic heart disease, 1990−2015. *N Engl J Med*. 2017;377:713−722.

19. Carapetis JR, Beaton A, Cunningham MW, et al. Acute rheumatic fever and rheumatic heart disease. *Nat Rev Dis Primers*. 2016;2:15084.

20. Roberts K, Maguire G, Brown A, et al. Rheumatic heart disease in Indigenous children in northern Australia: differences in prevalence and the challenges of screening. *Med J Aust*. 2015;203:219.

21. Okello E, Kakande B, Sebatta E, et al. Socioeconomic and environmental risk factors among rheumatic heart disease patients in Uganda. *PLoS One*. 2012;7:e43917.

22. Zuhlke L, Engel ME, Karthikeyan G, et al. Characteristics, complications, and gaps in evidence-based interventions in rheumatic heart disease: the global rheumatic heart disease registry (the REMEDY study). *Eur Heart J*. 2015; 36:1115−1122.

23. Zuhlke L, Karthikeyan G, Engel ME, et al. Clinical outcomes in 3343 children and adults with rheumatic heart disease from 14 low- and middle-income countries: two-year follow-up of the global rheumatic heart disease registry (the REMEDY study). *Circulation*. 2016;134: 1456−1466.

24. Dajani AS, Ayoub E, Bierman FZ, et al. Guidelines for the diagnosis of rheumatic fever: Jones criteria, 1992 update. 1992;268:2069−2073.

25. Feinstein AR, Spagnuolo M, Wood HF, Taranta A, Tursky E, Kleinberg E. Rheumatic fever in children and adolescents. A long-term epidemiologic study of subsequent prophylaxis, streptococcal infections, and clinical sequelae. Vi. Clinical features of streptococcal infections and rheumatic recurrences. *Ann Intern Med*. 1964; 60(Suppl 5):68−86.

26. Roberts K, Maguire G, Brown A, et al. Echocardiographic screening for rheumatic heart disease in high and low risk Australian children. *Circulation*. 2014;129: 1953−1961.

27. Webb RH, Gentles TL, Stirling JW, Lee M, O'Donnell C, Wilson NJ. Valvular regurgitation using portable echocardiography in a healthy student population: implications for rheumatic heart disease screening. *J Am Soc Echocardiogr*. 2015;28:981−988.

28. Clark BC, Krishnan A, McCarter R, Scheel J, Sable C, Beaton A. Using a low-risk population to estimate the specificity of the world heart federation criteria for the diagnosis of rheumatic heart disease. *J Am Soc Echocardiogr*. 2016;29(3):253−258.

29. Engelman D, Mataika RL, Ah Kee M, et al. Clinical outcomes for young people with screening-detected and clinically-diagnosed rheumatic heart disease in Fiji. *Int J Cardiol*. 2017;240:422−427.

30. Engelman D, Wheaton GR, Mataika RL, et al. Screening-detected rheumatic heart disease can progress to severe disease. *Heart Asia.* 2016;8:67–73.

31. Remond M, Atkinson D, White A, et al. Are minor echo-cardiographic changes associated with an increased risk of acute rheumatic fever or progression to rheumatic heart disease? *Int J Cardiol.* 2015;198:117–122.

32. Roberts KV, Brown AD, Maguire GP, Atkinson DN, Carapetis JR. Utility of auscultatory screening for detecting rheumatic heart disease in high-risk children in Australia's northern territory. *Med J Aust.* 2013;199: 196–199.

33. Marijon E, Celermajer DS, Tafflet M, et al. Rheumatic heart disease screening by echocardiography the inadequacy of world health organization criteria for optimizing the diagnosis of subclinical disease. *Circulation.* 2009;120:663–668.

34. Carapetis JR, Hardy M, Fakakovikaetau T, et al. Evaluation of a screening protocol using auscultation and portable echocardiography to detect asymptomatic rheumatic heart disease in Tongan school children. *Nat Clin Pract Cardiovasc Med.* 2008;5:411–417.

35. Tadele H, Mekonnen W, Tefera E. Rheumatic mitral stenosis in children: more accelerated course in sub-Saharan patients. *BMC Cardiovasc Disord.* 2013;13:95.

36. Beaton A, Okello E, Scheel A, et al. Impact of heart disease on maternal, fetal and neonatal outcomes in a low-resource setting. *Heart.* 2018;105(10):755–760.

37. Sagie A, Freitas N, Padial LR, et al. Doppler echocardiographic assessment of long-term progression of mitral stenosis in 103 patients: valve area and right heart disease. *J Am Coll Cardiol.* 1996;28:472–479.

38. Carabello BA. Modern management of mitral stenosis. *Circulation.* 2005;112:432–437.

39. Negi PC, Sondhi S, Rana V, et al. Prevalence, risk determinants and consequences of atrial fibrillation in rheumatic heart disease: 6 years hospital based-Himachal Pradesh- rheumatic fever/rheumatic heart disease (HP-RF/RHD) registry. *Indian Heart J.* 2018;70(Suppl 3): S68–S73.

40. Lindman BR, Otto CM. Aortic valve disease. In: Zipes DP, Libby P, Bonow RO, Mann DL, Tomaselli GF, eds. *Braunwald's Heart Disease, A Textbook of Cardiovascular Medicine.* Philadelphia: Elsevier; 2019:1389–1414.

41. Marijon E, Ou P, Celermajer DS, et al. Prevalence of rheumatic heart disease detected by echocardiographic screening. *N Engl J Med.* 2007;357:470–476.

42. Beaton A, Aliku T, Okello E, et al. The utility of handheld echocardiography for early diagnosis of rheumatic heart disease. *J Am Soc Echocardiogr.* 2014;27:42–49.

43. Engelman D, Kado JH, Remenyi B, et al. Focused cardiac ultrasound screening for rheumatic heart disease by briefly trained health workers: a study of diagnostic accuracy. *Lancet Glob Health.* 2016;4:e386–e394.

44. Nascimento BR, Sable C, Nunes MCP, et al. Comparison between different strategies of rheumatic heart disease echocardiographic screening in Brazil: data from the PROVAR (rheumatic valve disease screening program) study. *JAMA.* 2018;7.

45. Godown J, Lu JC, Beaton A, et al. Handheld echocardiography versus auscultation for detection of rheumatic heart disease. *Pediatrics.* 2015;135:e939–e944.

46. Marcus RH, Sareli P, Pocock WA, Barlow JB. The spectrum of severe rheumatic mitral valve disease in a developing country. Correlations among clinical presentation, surgical pathologic findings, and hemodynamic sequelae. *Ann Intern Med.* 1994;120:177–183.

47. Chauvaud S, Fuzellier J-F, Berrebi A, Deloche A, Fabiani J-N, Carpentier A. Long-term (29 Years) results of reconstructive surgery in rheumatic mitral valve insufficiency. *Circulation.* 2001;104. I-12–I-15.

48. Hahn RT, Abraham T, Adams MS, et al. Guidelines for performing a comprehensive transesophageal echocardiographic examination: recommendations from the American society of echocardiography and the society of cardiovascular anesthesiologists. *J Am Soc Echocardiogr.* 2013;26:921–964.

49. Zoghbi WA, Adams D, Bonow RO, et al. Recommendations for noninvasive evaluation of native valvular regurgitation: a report from the American society of echocardiography developed in collaboration with the society for cardiovascular magnetic resonance. *J Am Soc Echocardiogr.* 2017;30:303–371.

50. Lancellotti P, Moura L, Pierard LA, et al. European association of echocardiography recommendations for the assessment of valvular regurgitation. Part 2: mitral and tricuspid regurgitation (native valve disease). *Eur J Echocardiogr.* 2010;11:307–332.

51. Nishimura RA, Otto CM, Bonow RO, et al. 2014 AHA/ACC guideline for the management of patients with valvular heart disease: a report of the American college of cardiology/American heart association task force on practice guidelines. *J Am Coll Cardiol.* 2014;63: e57–185.

52. RHD Australia (ARF/RHD writing group). *National Heart Foundation of Australia and the Cardiac Society of Australia and New Zealand. Australian Guideline for Prevention, Diagnosis and Management of Acute Rheumatic Fever and Rheumatic Heart Disease.* 2nd ed. 2012.

53. Walsh BJ, Bland EF, Jones TD. Pure mitral stenosis in young persons. *Arch Intern Med.* 1940;65:321.

54. Bland E, Jones T. Rheumatic fever and rheumatic heart disease. A twenty-year report on 1,000 patients followed since childhood. *Circulation.* 1951;4:836–843.

55. Roy S, Bhatia M, Lazaro E, Ramalingaswami V. Juvenile mitral stenosis in India. *Lancet.* 1963;282:1193–1196.

56. Baumgartner H, Hung J, Bermejo J, et al. Echocardiographic assessment of valve stenosis: EAE/ASE recommendations for clinical practice. *Eur J Echocardiogr.* 2009;10: 1–25.

57. Wilkins G, Weyman AE, Abascal V, Block P, Palacios I. Percutaneous balloon dilatation of the mitral valve: an

analysis of echocardiographic variables related to outcome and the mechanism of dilatation. *Br Heart J.* 1988;60: 299−308.

58. Lancellotti P, Tribouilloy C, Hagendorff A, et al. European Association of Echocardiography recommendations for the assessment of valvular regurgitation. Part 1: aortic and pulmonary regurgitation (native valve disease). *Eur J Echocardiogr.* 2010;11:223−244.

59. Sultan F, Moustafa SE, Tajik J, et al. Rheumatic tricuspid valve disease: an evidence-based systematic overview. *J Heart Valve Dis.* 2010;19:374−382.

60. Vela JE, Contreras R, Sosa FR. Rheumatic pulmonary valve disease. *Am J Cardiol.* 1969;23:12−18.

61. Baumgartner H, Hung J, Bermejo J, et al. Echocardiographic assessment of valve stenosis: EAE/ASE recommendations for clinical practice. *J Am Soc Echocardiogr.* 2009;22:1−23. quiz 101-2.

62. Baumgartner H, Hung J, Bermejo J, et al. Recommendations on the echocardiographic assessment of aortic valve stenosis: a focused update from the European association of cardiovascular imaging and the American society of echocardiography. *J Am Soc Echocardiogr.* 2017;30: 372−392.

63. Thomson Mangnall L, Sibbritt D, Fry M, Gallagher R. Short- and long-term outcomes after valve replacement surgery for rheumatic heart disease in the South Pacific, conducted by a fly-in/fly-out humanitarian surgical team: a 20-year retrospective study for the years 1991 to 2011. *J Thorac Cardiovasc Surg.* 2014;148:1996−2003.

64. Remenyi B, Webb R, Gentles T, et al. Improved long-term survival for rheumatic mitral valve repair compared to replacement in the young. *World J Pediatr Congenit Heart Surg.* 2013;4:155−164.

65. de Dassel JL, de Klerk N, Carapetis JR, Ralph AP. How many doses make a difference? An analysis of secondary prevention of rheumatic fever and rheumatic heart disease. *Circulation.* 2018;7:e010223.

66. Cannon J, Roberts K, Milne C, Carapetis JR. Rheumatic heart disease severity, progression and outcomes: a multi-state model. *JAMA.* 2017;6.

67. *WHO Expert Consultation on Rheumatic Fever and Rheumatic Heart Disease (2001: Geneva Switzerland). Expert Rheumatic Fever and Rheumatic Heart Disease: Report of a WHO Consultation, Geneva, 29 October - 1 November 2001. WHO Technical Report Series; 923. Geneva: World Health Organization.* 2004.

68. Lennon DWN, Sharpe N, R L. *New Zealand Guidelines for Rheumatic Fever: Diagnosis, Management and Secondary Prevention of Acute Rheumatic Fever and Rheumatic Heart Disease: 2014.* 2017.

69. Grewal J, Mankad S, Freeman WK, et al. Real-time three-dimensional transesophageal echocardiography in the intraoperative assessment of mitral valve disease. *J Am Soc Echocardiogr.* 2009;22:34−41.

70. Schlosshan D, Aggarwal G, Mathur G, Allan R, Cranney G. Real-time 3D transesophageal echocardiography for the evaluation of rheumatic mitral stenosis. *JACC Cardiovasc Imaging.* 2011;4:580−588.

71. Zamorano J, Cordeiro P, Sugeng L, et al. Real-time three-dimensional echocardiography for rheumatic mitral valve stenosis evaluation: an accurate and novel approach. *J Am Coll Cardiol.* 2004;43:2091−2096.

72. Yosefy C, Hung J, Chua S, et al. Direct measurement of vena contracta area by real-time 3-dimensional echocardiography for assessing severity of mitral regurgitation. *Am J Cardiol.* 2009;104:978−983.

73. Choi EY, Yoon SJ, Lim SH, et al. Detection of myocardial involvement of rheumatic heart disease with contrast-enhanced magnetic resonance imaging. *Int J Cardiol.* 2006;113:e36−e38.

74. Mavrogeni S, Schwitter J, van Rossum A, et al. Cardiac magnetic resonance imaging in myocardial inflammation in autoimmune rheumatic diseases: an appraisal of the diagnostic strengths and limitations of the Lake Louise criteria. *Int J Cardiol.* 2018;252:216−219.

75. Doherty JU, Kort S, Mehran R, Schoenhagen P, Soman P. ACC/AATS/AHA/ASE/ASNC/HRS/SCAI/SCCT/SCMR/STS 2017 appropriate use criteria for multimodality imaging in valvular heart disease: a report of the American college of cardiology appropriate use criteria task force, American association for thoracic surgery, American heart association, American society of echocardiography, American society of nuclear cardiology, heart rhythm society, society for cardiovascular angiography and interventions, society of cardiovascular computed tomography, society for cardiovascular magnetic resonance, and society of thoracic surgeons. *J Am Coll Cardiol.* 2017;70:1647−1672.

76. Zhu D, Wu Z, van der Geest RJ, et al. Accuracy of late gadolinium enhancement − magnetic resonance imaging in the measurement of left atrial substrate remodeling in patients with rheumatic mitral valve disease and persistent atrial fibrillation. *Int Heart J.* 2015;56:505−510.

77. Kainuma S, Masai T, Yoshitatsu M, et al. Advanced left-atrial fibrosis is associated with unsuccessful maze operation for valvular atrial fibrillation. *Eur J Cardiothorac Surg.* 2011;40:61−69.

78. Ponikowski P, Voors AA, Anker SD, et al. 2016 ESC guidelines for the diagnosis and treatment of acute and chronic heart failure: the Task Force for the diagnosis and treatment of acute and chronic heart failure of the European society of cardiology (ESC) developed with the special contribution of the heart failure association (HFA) of the ESC. *Eur Heart J.* 2016;37: 2129−2200.

79. Yancy CW, Jessup M, Bozkurt B, et al. 2013 ACCF/AHA guideline for the management of heart failure: executive summary: a report of the American college of cardiology foundation/American heart association task force on practice guidelines. *Circulation.* 2013;128: 1810−1852.

80. Gentles TL, French JK, Zeng I, Milsom PF, Finucane AK, Wilson NJ. Normalized end-systolic volume and preload reserve predict ventricular dysfunction following surgery for aortic regurgitation independent of body size. *JACC Cardiovasc Imaging.* 2012;5:626−633.

81. Criteria Committee of the New York Heart Association. *Nomenclature and Criteria for Diagnosis of Diseases of the Heart and Great Vessels Te*. Boston: Little, Brown & Co.; 1994.
82. Dunn GD, Hayes P, Breen KJ, Schenker S. The liver in congestive heart failure: a review. *Am J Med Sci*. 1973; 265:174–189.
83. Richman SM, Delman AJ, Grob D. Alterations in indices of liver function in congestive heart failure with particular reference to serum enzymes. *Am J Med*. 1961;30:211–225.
84. Maisel AS, Krishnaswamy P, Nowak RM, et al. Rapid measurement of B-type natriuretic peptide in the emergency diagnosis of heart failure. *N Engl J Med*. 2002; 347:161–167.
85. Abdel Fattah EM, Girgis HY, El Khashab K, Ashour ZA, Ezzat GM. B-type natriuretic peptide as an index of symptoms and severity of chronic rheumatic mitral regurgitation. *Heart Views*. 2016;17:7–12.
86. Pizarro R, Bazzino OO, Oberti PF, et al. Prospective validation of the prognostic usefulness of brain natriuretic peptide in asymptomatic patients with chronic severe mitral regurgitation. *J Am Coll Cardiol*. 2009;54:1099–1106.
87. Klaar U, Gabriel H, Bergler-Klein J, et al. Prognostic value of serial B-type natriuretic peptide measurement in asymptomatic organic mitral regurgitation. *Eur J Heart Fail*. 2011;13:163–169.
88. Cohn AE, L C. The natural history of rheumatic cardiac disease: a statistical study: I. Onset and duration of disease. *JAMA*. 1943;121:1–8.
89. Jaiyesimi F, Antia AU. Childhood rheumatic heart disease in Nigeria. *Trop Geogr Med*. 1981;33:8–13.
90. Gunther G, Asmera J, Parry E. Death from rheumatic heart disease in rural Ethiopia. *Lancet*. 2006;367:391.
91. Kumar R, Raizada A, Aggarwal AK, Ganguly NK. A community-based rheumatic fever/rheumatic heart disease cohort: twelve-year experience. *Indian Heart J*. 2002; 54:54–58.
92. Kamblock J, N'Guyen L, Pagis B, et al. Acute severe mitral regurgitation during first attacks of rheumatic fever: clinical spectrum, mechanisms and prognostic factors. *J Heart Valve Dis*. 2005;14:440–446.
93. Danzl DF, Pozos RS, Auerbach PS, et al. Multicenter hypothermia survey. *Ann Emerg Med*. 1987;16:1042–1055.
94. Davis K, Remenyi B, Draper AD, et al. Rheumatic heart disease in Timor-Leste school students: an echocardiography-based prevalence study. *Med J Aust*. 2018;208:303–307.
95. Beaton A, Okello E, Lwabi P, Mondo C, McCarter R, Sable C. Echocardiography screening for rheumatic heart disease in Ugandan school children. *Circulation*. 2012; 125:3127–3132.
96. Simonneau G, Montani D, Celermajer DS, Denton CP, Gatzoulis MA, Krowka M, et al. Haemodynamic definitions and updated clinical classification of pulmonary hypertension. *Eur Respir J*. 2019;53(1).
97. Augustine DX, Coates-Bradshaw LD, Willis J, Harkness A, Ring L, Grapsa J, et al. Echocardiographic assessment of pulmonary hypertension: a guideline protocol from the British Society of Echocardiography. *Echo Res Pract*. 2018;5(3): G11-G24.
98. Galie N, Humbert M, Vachiery JL, Gibbs S, Lang I, Torbicki A, et al. ESC/ERS Guidelines for the diagnosis and treatment of pulmonary hypertension: The Joint Task Force for the Diagnosis and Treatment of Pulmonary Hypertension of the European Society of Cardiology (ESC) and the European Respiratory Society (ERS): Endorsed by: Association for European Paediatric and Congenital Cardiology (AEPC), International Society for Heart and Lung Transplantation (ISHLT). *Eur Heart J*. 2016;37(1):67–119.
99. Cordina RL, Playford D, Lang I, Celermajer DS. State-of-the-Art Review: Echocardiography in Pulmonary Hypertension. *Heart Lung Circ*. 2019;28(9):1351–1364.
100. Nishimura RA, Otto CM, Bonow RO, Carabello BA, Erwin JP, 3rd, Fleisher LA, et al. 2017 AHA/ACC Focused Update of the 2014 AHA/ACC Guideline for the Management of Patients With Valvular Heart Disease: A Report of the American College of Cardiology/American Heart Association Task Force on Clinical Practice Guidelines. *J Am Coll Cardiol*. 2017;70(2):252–289.
101. Parasuraman S, Walker S, Loudon BL, et al. Assessment of pulmonary artery pressure by echocardiography-A comprehensive review. Int J Cardiol Heart Vasc. 2016; 12:45e51. 2016 Jul 4;12:45-51.
102. van Hagen IM, et al. Pregnancy outcomes in women with rheumatic mitral valve disease: results from the registry of pregnancy and cardiac disease. *Circulation*. 2018;137(8): 806–816.
103. Van Hagen IM, et al. Risks of pregnancy in women with rheumatic mitral valve disease: data from ROPAC, an ESC registry. *Eur. Heart J*. 2016;37(s1):1240–1241.
104. Watkins DA et al. The burden of antenatal heart disease in South Africa: a systematic review. Bmc Cardiovasc Disord. 2012;12:23.

Medical Management of Rheumatic Heart Disease

EMMY OKELLO • IFY R. MORDI • CHIM C. LANG • CRAIG SABLE • SCOTT DOUGHERTY • NIGEL WILSON

INTRODUCTION

Chronic ambulatory heart failure (HF) is usually the most common clinical manifestation of advanced rheumatic heart disease (RHD)[1]. HF in RHD patients typically develops after a chronic, often asymptomatic, period of progressive valvular heart disease, typically manifesting clinically only when the valve disease is severe (or less than severe in mixed or multivalve disease). The pathophysiology of rheumatic valvular lesions and how this relates to the timing of cardiac surgery or catheter-based intervention, as well as the medical management of chronic HF and valvular lesions, are discussed in this chapter. Antithrombotic therapy, particularly in the context of mechanical heart valves and atrial fibrillation, also plays an important role in the medical management of RHD and is discussed in detail at the end of the chapter. Surgical (Chapter 8) and catheter-based management (Chapter 7), acute HF and other emergency presentations (Chapter 16), and the management of pregnant women with RHD (Chapter 9) are discussed in detail in their relevant chapters.

The recommendations promulgated in this chapter are based around three important groups of guidelines, each addressing different aspects of the medical management of RHD. The Australian[2] and New Zealand[3] guidelines define the **principles of management of RHD,** which apply to all patients. The American College of Cardiology, American Heart Association, and Heart Failure Society of America (ACC/AHA/HFSA),[4,5] and the European Society of Cardiology (ESC)[6] provide extensive guidance on the **medical management of chronic heart failure**, the main cause of death in RHD. Finally, the AHA and ACC (AHA/ACC),[7,8] and the ESC[9] provide guidance on the assessment of, and indications for, surgical or catheter-based treatment of

valve disease and are discussed in the section **medical management of individual valve lesions**.

Each of these guidelines is updated every few years by leading world experts in the respective fields and most use class of recommendation (COR) and level of evidence (LOE) for each recommendation. It should be emphasized that the guidelines on HF and valvular heart disease reflect evidence-based management for patients in high-income countries, usually without resource restriction for medicines and complex cardiac interventions. Although the guidelines on HF are relevant to most patients with RHD, the relevance of the valvular heart disease guidelines for specific RHD lesions varies. They are highly relevant for mitral stenosis (MS), relevant for mitral regurgitation (MR) and aortic regurgitation (AR), but may be of less relevance for aortic stenosis (AS), where the guidelines have evolved in recent years from advances in the management of calcific AS in the elderly.

An important theme of the AHA/ACC[7,8] and ESC[9] valve disease guidelines is the overall strong evidence-based support for surgical and catheter-based intervention for severe or symptomatic valvular heart disease. In contrast, the guidelines acknowledge the relative lack of evidence-based support for pharmacological management of severe valvular heart disease to alter outcomes. There is also little RHD-specific evidence on optimal drug therapy in HF. The recommendation for medical therapy in RHD patients with HF and left ventricular dysfunction is therefore largely based on evidence from patients with HF with reduced ejection fraction (HFrEF). Moreover, most evidence-based management of RHD and HF is based on adult data. Management principles for RHD in the young are often extrapolated from published guidelines for adult patients. The

Acute Rheumatic Fever and Rheumatic Heart Disease. https://doi.org/10.1016/B978-0-323-63982-8.00006-4

limited specific data that underpin the guidelines on the timing of intervention in children are included.

PRINCIPLES OF MANAGEMENT OF RHEUMATIC HEART DISEASE

Managing patients with RHD is complex, expensive, and requires strong national health systems. Adequate primary, secondary, and tertiary services with specialists including cardiology, cardiothoracic surgery, pediatrics, general medicine, general practice, dentistry, obstetrics, and infectious diseases are often required.[9] A practical approach to the long-term management of RHD is provided by best practice guidelines from Australia and New Zealand and include the following: periodic clinical evaluation by a specialist experienced in RHD management, serial echocardiography for assessment of left ventricular and valve function, timely referral for heart surgery or catheter intervention, monitoring of anticoagulation for patients with atrial fibrillation (AF) or prosthetic valves, access to oral healthcare, annual influenza vaccination, and last but not least secondary prevention with penicillin prophylaxis (Table 6.1).[2,11,12] These overall management principles for RHD will always be paramount to avoid the complications of recurrences of acute rheumatic fever (ARF), infective endocarditis, and thromboembolism, and facilitate optimal ongoing care. The principles of secondary prevention, anticoagulation for prosthetic valves and AF, and optimizing oral healthcare are discussed at the end of this chapter.

MEDICAL MANAGEMENT OF CHRONIC HEART FAILURE IN RHEUMATIC HEART DISEASE

Multivalve and mixed valve disease is the most common disease pattern seen in RHD in most age groups (see Chapter 5). This has important implications for the prognosis and management of RHD because multivalve and mixed valve disease carries a high risk for left ventricular dysfunction and symptomatic HF,[13] even if the individual lesions are not classified as severe. This contrasts with single valve disease, where in general only severe lesions lead to HF.

Overview of Heart Failure Treatment

HF is a pathophysiological state in which a structural or functional cardiac disorder impairs the ability of the ventricle to fill with or eject blood at a rate that meets the requirements of metabolizing tissues.[4] It is the final pathway for a multitude of diseases that affect the heart: for RHD, this refers to moderate to severe, usually chronic, valvular heart disease. Common symptoms of HF include dyspnea, fatigue, restricted exercise tolerance, and congestion (fluid accumulation in the lungs, abdomen, and lower extremities), all of which are discussed in Chapters 5 and 16.

All patients with HF should be classified and staged, which is important for diagnosis and management. HF classification is based on symptoms and degree of functional limitation, as defined by the New York Heart Association (NYHA—see Chapter 5). HF staging is based on the ACCF/AHA system,[4] which emphasizes the progressive nature of HF (different from the NYHA classification, where the patient can move up or down classes depending on how well their symptoms are controlled) and defines the appropriate therapeutic approach for each stage (Fig. 6.1)[4]. Staging HF in this manner should help promote an approach to RHD management that reflects some of the core themes of this book—that is, the importance of identifying and treating patients at risk for RHD (history of ARF), the importance of closely monitoring patients with established RHD for evidence of HF or left ventricular dysfunction, and the importance of timely treatment of symptomatic RHD (surgical, interventional, and/or medical management).

TABLE 6.1
Best Practice Rheumatic Heart Disease Management Principles.

1. Access to a specialist RHD physician (pediatrician, physician, cardiologist or specialized nurse/physician assistant experienced in RHD management) for regular follow-up visits

2. Secondary prevention with penicillin prophylaxis (see also Chapter 11)

3. Access to echocardiography

4. Access to cardiothoracic and interventional cardiology services, if required

5. Adequate monitoring of anticoagulation therapy in patients with atrial fibrillation and/or mechanical prosthetic valves

6. Optimise oral healthcare, including routine dentistry reviews

7. Annual influenza vaccination

8. Prevention of infective endocarditis

RHD, rheumatic heart disease.

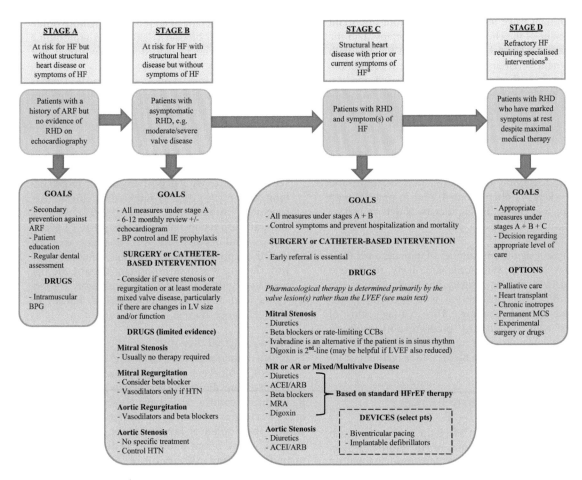

Adapted from Yancy et al.[3]

[a]Patients with HF have one or more symptoms of HF (e.g. dyspnoea, orthnopea, fatigue), which corresponds to HF stages C and D and excludes those with HF stages A and B. Patients with HF may or may not have a physical sign of heart failure (e.g. peripheral oedema, pulmonary crackles,elevated jugular venous pressure).

The clinical syndrome of HF may develop in patients with any LVEF - which is particularly relevant in patients with RHD. HF is typically categorized based on LVEF, which helps determine prognosis and management: HF with LVEF ≤40% (known as HFrEF; discussed in detail in the main text); HF with LVEF 41-49% (known as HFmrEF, which is managed similarly to HFrEF); and HF with LVEF ≥50% (causes include: significant valve disease (severe stenosis or regurgitation or at least moderate mixed regurgitation and stenosis), HFpEF,cardiomyopathy (hypertrophic or restrictive), pericardial disease (e.g. constrictive pericarditis), and right heart failure).

HF heart failure; ARF acute rheumatic fever; RHD rheumatic heart disease; HFrEF heart failure with reduced ejection fraction; MR mitral regurgitation; AR aortic regurgitation; HFmrEF heart failure with mid-range ejection fraction; HFpEF heart failure with preserved ejection fraction; BP blood pressure; HTN hypertension; IE infective endocarditis; LV left ventricular; ACEI angiotensin converting enzyme inhibitor; ARB angiotensin II receptor blocker; MRA mineralocorticoid receptor antagonist; ARNI angiotensin receptor-neprilysin inhibitor; HYD-ISN hydralazine and isosorbide dinitrate; MCS mechanical circulatory support

FIG. 6.1 Staging heart failure in the context of rheumatic heart disease. Adapted from Yancy et al.[4]

There are several different HF phenotypes, in part reflected by differences in left ventricular ejection fraction (LVEF). The LVEF is typically a key guide to medical therapy, most notably in HF patients with a LVEF ≤40% (known as heart failure with reduced ejection fraction (HFrEF)) due to the strong evidence base for disease-modifying therapies in this group. However, in patients with RHD presenting with HF symptoms, the dominant valve lesion is often a more important determinant of the choice of medical therapy than the LVEF (see also Fig. 6.1). For example, in patients with symptomatic severe mitral and/or aortic regurgitation, treatment is with standard guideline-based medical therapy for HFrEF, even if the LVEF is >40%. In symptomatic isolated mitral stenosis, the LVEF is usually normal and therapy is based on relieving symptoms of pulmonary congestion and controlling the heart rate. In severe symptomatic aortic stenosis, a combination of diuretics and ACEI are often used regardless of LVEF (started at low dose with gradual titration) and beta blockers are often avoided. And in patients with mixed or multivalve disease, therapy is determined by the dominant valve lesion, although is usually similar to that for HFrEF.

Because a significant number of patients with RHD who develop HF symptoms are likely to have a reduced LVEF and/or a significant regurgitant lesion (MR and/or AR), this section will focus on HFrEF guideline-directed therapy. The management of patients with isolated or predominantly stenotic lesions or asymptomatic regurgitant lesions is discussed later in the section Medical Management of Individual Valve Lesions.

Heart Failure Managment (HFrEF)
General management
The goals of management of HFrEF mainly focus on reducing morbidity (symptoms of HF, improving functional status and quality of life, decreasing hospitalization rates) and reducing mortality. Important general factors to consider include the following:

- **Lifestyle modification:** this should include cessation of smoking, avoidance of obesity, restriction or abstinence from alcohol, and daily weight monitoring to detect fluid accumulation. Recommendations regarding limiting salt intake vary: the ACCF/AHA HF guidelines suggest some degree of sodium restriction (e.g., <3 g/day),[4] whereas the 2016 ESC HF guidelines suggest avoiding excess sodium intake (<6 g/day).[6]
- **Hypertension:** consider antihypertensives if BP is ≥140/90 mmHg. In patients with HFrEF, hypertension should generally be managed with an angiotensin converting enzyme inhibitor (ACEI) (or an angiotensin II receptor blocker (ARB) or an angiotensin receptor-neprilysin inhibitor (ARNI)), a β-blocker, a diuretic, and/or a mineralocorticoid receptor antagonist (MRA), because these drugs are

also standard therapy in HFrEF.[15] A dihydropyridine calcium channel blocker (CCB), either amlodipine or felodipine, can be added if BP control is not achieved.
- **Anemia:** has an impact on prognosis in HF. There is no universally accepted hematocrit or hemoglobin level at which a blood transfusion should be given. The historically accepted trigger for transfusion has been a hemoglobin of <10 g/dL.[16] However, there is growing acceptance that transfusion triggers in general should be restrictive (hemoglobin trigger set at ≤7 g/dL, with a posttransfusion target hemoglobin of 9–10 g/dL) rather than liberal (hemoglobin trigger set at <10 g/dL, with a posttransfusion target hemoglobin of 10–12 g/dL), with several reports and meta-analyses showing that this approach leads to better outcomes.[17,18] Iron therapy is also an important therapeutic option and both oral and intravenous iron are recommended in the presence of iron deficiency or iron deficiency anemia.

Pharmacological therapy
Established therapies for HFrEF are loop diuretics, ACEI/ARB, β-blockers, MRAs, hydralazine combined with isosorbide dinitrate (HYD-ISDN), and digoxin. Randomized control trials have shown that each of these, with the exception of loop diuretics and digoxin, reduces the burden of hospitalization and improves survival.[4] More recent additions to the HFrEF armamentarium, valsartan/sacubitril, an ARNI, and the selective sinus node inhibitor (I_f-channel blocker), ivabradine, also reduce the risk of HF hospitalizations and mortality. It is important to remember that the evidence for these drugs focuses on non-RHD causes of HF and while they may help reduce HF-related morbidity and mortality in RHD, like they do in other causes of HF, there is no evidence that they alter the natural history of RHD or the need for interventional or surgical management. It is also important to remember that symptoms relieved by medications still mean that eligible patients should be considered for surgery.

ACC/AHA/HFSA recommendations[4,5,19] for initiating pharmacological therapy in a newly diagnosed patient with HFrEF (stage C heart failure) are summarized in Fig. 6.2 and the starting and target doses of recommended drugs are summarized in Table 6.2. ESC guidelines,[6] with few exceptions, make similar recommendations regarding the treatment of HFrEF. It is worth emphasizing that target doses of recommended medications should be aimed for, as far as possible, as these dosages are associated with the best evidence for improved outcomes.

Diuretics are usually started first in volume overloaded patients. Loop diuretics are recommended and furosemide is the most commonly used, although due to superior and more predictable absorption some patients respond better to bumetanide or torsemide. Thiazide-like diuretics (e.g., indapamide, metolazone) can be added to loop diuretics if there is a suboptimal

response. ACEI are typically added next, either during or after optimization of diuretic therapy, with β-blockers started once the patient is stable on ACEI therapy. Only evidence-based β-blockers should be used (see Table 6.2). In those patients who cannot tolerate ACEI (most often due to cough), an ARB should be offered instead.

In those patients that remain symptomatic (NYHA II–IV) after titration of an ACEI/ARB and a β-blocker, with an LVEF ≤35% and providing there are no contraindications, an MRA should be started. Inappropriate

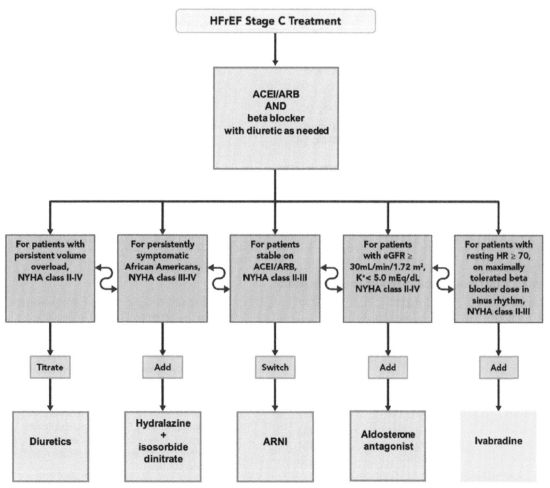

FIG. 6.2 Treatment algorithm for guideline-directed medical therapy of heart failure with reduced ejection fraction. Green squares indicate Class I guideline recommendations, while the yellow square indicates a Class II recommendation. ACEI angiotensin-converting enzyme inhibitor, ARB angiotensin receptor blocker, ARNI angiotensin receptor-neprilysin inhibitor, eGFR estimated glomerular filtration rate, HFrEF heart failure with reduced ejection fraction, HR heart rate, NYHA New York Heart Association. (Reproduced with permission from Yancy et al.[19])

TABLE 6.2
Starting and Target Doses of Disease-Modifying Drugs for Heart Failure with Reduced Ejection Fraction in Adults.

	Starting Dose	Target Dose	Comments
β-BLOCKERS			
Bisoprolol	1.25 mg OD	10 mg OD	Consider increasing dose every 2 weeks until maximum tolerated dose or target dose achieved
Carvedilol	3.125 mg OD	25–50 mg BID	
Metoprolol succinate	12.5–25 mg OD	200 mg OD	Monitor heart rate, blood pressure, and for signs of congestion after initiation and during titration
ANGIOTENSIN CONVERTING ENZYME INHIBITOR (ACEI)			
Captopril	6.25 mg TID	50 mg TID	Consider increasing dose every 2 weeks until maximum tolerated dose or target dose achieved
Enalapril	2.5 mg BID	10–20 mg BID	
Lisinopril	2.5–5 mg OD	20–40 mg OD	Monitor blood pressure, renal function, and potassium after initiation and during titration
Ramipril	1.25 mg OD	10 mg OD	
ANGIOTENSIN II RECEPTOR BLOCKER (ARB)			
Candesartan	4–8 mg OD	32 mg OD	Alternative in patients who cannot tolerate ACEI for reasons other than renal dysfunction or hyperkalemia (e.g., cough)
Losartan	25–50 mg OD	150 mg OD	
Valsartan	40 mg BID	160 mg BID	Monitoring as per ACEI
ANGIOTENSIN RECEPTOR-NEPRILYSIN INHIBITOR (ARNI)			
Sacubitril/valsartan	24/26 mg-49/51 mg BID	97/103 mg BID	Start 24/26 mg twice daily if taking equivalent of ≤10 mg daily of ramipril or equivalent of ≤160 mg daily of valsartan
			Start 49/51 mg twice daily if taking equivalent of >10 mg daily of ramipril or equivalent of >160 mg daily of valsartan
			Monitoring as per ACEI
MINERALOCORTICOID RECEPTOR ANTAGONISTS (MRA)			
Eplerenone	25 mg OD	50 mg OD	Consider increasing dose every 2 weeks until maximum tolerated dose or target dose achieved
Spironolactone	12.5–25 mg OD	25–50 mg OD	Monitor electrolytes and renal function 2–3 days after initiation and 7 days after titration. Afterward, check monthly for 3 months and 3 monthly thereafter
VASODILATORS			
Hydralazine	25 mg TID	75 mg TID	Consider increasing dose of ISDN and/or hydralazine every 2 weeks until maximum tolerated dose or target dose achieved
ISDN	20 mg TID	40 mg TID	
Fixed-dose combination ISDN/hydralazine	20/37.5 mg (one tab) TID	2 tabs TID	Monitor blood pressure after initiation and during titration
I$_F$-CHANNEL BLOCKER			
Ivabradine	2.5–5 mg BID	Titrate to heart rate 50–60 bpm Maximum dose 7.5 mg BID	If aged ≥75 years, start 2.5 mg twice daily; if aged <75 years, start 5 mg twice daily
			Monitor heart rate in at least 2–4 weeks: if <50 bpm, reduce dose by 2.5 mg twice daily; if 50–60 bpm maintain current dose; if >60 bpm increase dose by 2.5 mg twice daily

OD, omne in die (once daily); BID, bis in die (twice daily); TID, ter in die (three times daily); ISDN, isosorbide dinitrate; bpm, beats per minute.
Reproduced with permission from Yancy et al.[19]

use may be harmful and the potassium and creatinine must be checked within 1 week of commencing an MRA. For patients with ongoing HF symptoms (NYHA class II−III) and who have tolerated ACEI/ARB therapy, replacement by an ARNI is recommended to further reduce morbidity and mortality. If switching an ACEI to ARNI therapy, a 36-h washout is essential first to avoid angioedema (not required with ARBs).

For black patients who remain symptomatic (NYHA class III−IV) despite optimal treatment with diuretics, ACEI/ARB or ARNI, β-blocker, and an MRA, the addition of HYD-ISDN is recommended (isosorbide mononitrate is not recommended by the ACC/AHA/HFSA guideline). This strategy is particularly relevant in Africa, which has the largest burden of RHD, although data indicate that HYD-ISDN is rarely ever used for HF in these populations,[20] providing an opportunity for improved outcomes. HYD-ISDN can also be used in all patients who cannot tolerate an ACEI or ARB (or they are contraindicated) to reduce the risk of death. For those patients who are in sinus rhythm at a heart rate ≥70 bpm despite maximally tolerated β-blocker therapy (or in those for whom β-blockers are contraindicated or not tolerated), who remain symptomatic (NYHA class II or III) with an LVEF ≤35%, ivabradine is recommended.

Digoxin remains a therapeutic option in those patients in sinus rhythm who remain symptomatic despite an ACEI/ARB or ARNI, β-blocker, and an MRA. Although it has no effect on mortality, digoxin does reduce the risk of hospitalizations (both all-cause and HF hospitalizations). It is also indicated in patients with AF and a rapid ventricular rate (>110 bpm)[6], although for patients with HFrEF with AF requiring rate control, beta-blockers are preferred first line as they form part of the general treatment of HF. Should a second agent be required to achieve adequate rate control, digoxin can then be used. Digoxin is commonly used in patients with RHD (nearly 35% of patients in the REMEDY study)[2] particularly in those with MS, regardless of the presence of AF or HF. The main rationale for this is to reduce the heart rate and transmitral gradient, with the aim of improving symptoms. However REMEDY data at 2 years from enrollment suggests a possible association of digoxin use and increased mortality, particularly among those without AF or HF.[21]

Discussion of other types of HF, including refractory HF (stage D) and HF with LVEF ≥50% are beyond the scope of this book but are addressed in the ACC/AHA/HFSA and ESC HF guidelines.

MEDICAL MANAGEMENT OF INDIVIDUAL VALVE LESIONS

The clinical features and echocardiographic assessment of individual valve lesions are both discussed in detail in Chapter 5. Given that surgery is usually recommended for symptomatic severe valvular heart disease, it is worth emphasising here that decisions regarding surgery should be made in conjunction with cardiologists, cardiothoracic surgeons, and intensivists (as appropriate) in a multidisciplinary "heart team" approach. Risk assessment may be helped by the use of risk scores, such as those from the Society of Thoracic Surgeons[89] and European Association for Cardio-Thoracic Surgery (EuroSCORE II).[90] It is also worth emphasizing that patients who have undergone valve surgery should undergo 6-monthly cardiology review and echocardiogram[7] because the long-term outcomes of both mechanical and bioprosthetic valve replacement in RHD patients remain very poor. Finally, whilst the pathophysiology of valvular lesions is discussed here, the underlying valvular anatomic derangements are discussed in detail in chapter 8.

Chronic Mitral Regurgitation
Natural History and Pathophysiology of Mitral Regurgitation
Rheumatic MR results from thickening, retraction, and distortion of both the valve itself and the supporting structures. Annular dilatation and loss of the saddle shape of the mitral annulus,[22] elongation of the chordae tendinae (mostly the primary chords), and over the longer term, retraction of the thick intermediate chords, restricts the motion of both leaflets. Progression from mild-to-severe rheumatic MR can be halted or potentially reversed (when mild or moderate) by adherence to secondary penicillin prophylaxis.

The natural history of chronic MR has three distinct phases: compensated, transitional, and decompensated.[23−25] Progression between each phase can be insidious, emphasizing the importance of regular clinical and echocardiographic monitoring to identify early deleterious LV changes and proceeding to surgical correction before the establishment of irreversible LV damage. Over time, the natural history of untreated chronic severe MR is that of myocardial damage, HF, and eventual death.[8] The 2017 AHA/ACC update emphasize the concept that mitral regurgitation begets mitral regurgitation with a perpetual cycle of ever-increasing LV volumes and MR.[8]

Chronic MR imposes a volume load on the LV resulting in a series of myocardial adaptions, the most important of which is LV enlargement that maintains the total stroke volume and forward stroke volume. This represents the compensated phase, which often lasts several years, and most patients are asymptomatic. LV enlargement and eccentric hypertrophy develop, normalizing the systolic wall stress. Contractility and LVEF are both normal. When the echocardiographic LV end-diastolic dimension (LVEDD) is <60 mm and the LV end-systolic dimension (LVESD) is <40 mm, surgery is not indicated.

Eventually, compensatory mechanisms start to fail and structural and functional remodeling of the LV occurs. There is a decrease in LV contractile function and increase in wall stress (increased afterload). The onset of HF symptoms and/or development of LV systolic dysfunction (defined as LVEF <60%, often with LVESD ≥40 mm) heralds onset of the transitional phase and is an indication for surgery. Many patients, however, remain asymptomatic making this phase difficult to identify. If surgery is performed during this phase, a good clinical outcome is usually possible.

The decompensated phase is characterized by the onset of symptoms and progressive LV dilatation (LVEDD >70 mm, LVESD >45 mm) and a reduction in systolic function (LVEF <50%). Corrective surgery should be performed before the establishment of the decompensated phase because patients with chronic MR and LV dysfunction have higher postoperative mortality and persistent LV dysfunction.

In the current era, cardiac catheterization is not usually indicated as severity is apparent by clinical and echocardiographic assessment. It is pertinent, however, to understand the hemodynamics of symptomatic, decompensated, severe MR. A series of 219 patients with isolated severe MR, all NYHA class III-IV, underwent cardiac catheterization prior to cardiac surgery in the 1980s in South Africa. The mean left atrial (LA) pressure was 24 ± 9 mmHg, the LA V-wave was 46 ± 18 mmHg, and LV end-diastolic pressure was 16 ± 8 mmHg. Importantly, the right ventricular systolic pressure (RVSP), and pulmonary artery systolic pressure, was 50 ± 13 mmHg, as high as patients with pure MS.[26]

Mitral Regurgitation Medical Management

For patients with chronic asymptomatic MR, there is some evidence that β-blockers lead to possible benefit. A preliminary trial of 38 asymptomatic patients with moderate to severe isolated MR (cause of MR not specified) were randomized either to placebo or extended-release metoprolol for 2 years. LVEF and LV early diastolic filling time significantly improved with β-blocker therapy.[27] A retrospective study of 895 patients with severe MR (of multiple etiologies and normal LVEF) found that those who were treated with β-blockers had a significantly reduced risk of mortality, independent of whether the patients were managed medically or surgically.[28] In an Indian study looking specifically at RHD patients with chronic MR, therapy with metoprolol lowered NYHA class, left ventricular end-systolic and diastolic volumes, and brain natriuretic peptide over 3 months compared to controls. MR grade decreased from severe to moderate in 11% of those on metoprolol over 6 months of treatment (compared to none in the control group).[29] Symptomatic patients with moderate or severe MR and LVEF <60% (stage C HF) who are either awaiting valve surgery or surgery is not an option (usually either unfit for surgery or it is unavailable) should be managed with standard HFrEF therapy, as discussed earlier.

No published guidelines support the use of vasodilators in normotensive asymptomatic patients with chronic MR and normal LV systolic function.[7,9] However, there is some evidence that vasodilators may improve outcomes in symptomatic patients. A study on 47 patients with mildly symptomatic MR, 26 of whom had RHD, found that there was a significant reduction in left ventricular diameter and MR volume in those who received enalapril for 12 months, compared to placebo.[30] A Turkish study found that addition of an ACEI lowered left ventricular end diastolic volume and atrial natriuretic peptide levels after 20 days of treatment in a cohort of patients who were being treated with digoxin at baseline.[31,32] Finally, a study examined the impact of 6 months of treatment of enalapril and nicorandil, a balanced vasodilator, in 87 mildly symptomatic RHD patients with severe MR. Both drugs resulted in decreased left ventricular systolic volume and increased ejection fraction, and nicorandil was found to have a greater effect.[33]

Summary of the medical therapy of chronic MR:
- Mild MR is usually well tolerated and does not require any specific pharmacologic therapy
- Asymptomatic patients with moderate or severe MR and no evidence of LV dysfunction (stage B HF):
  - Limited evidence that β-blockers therapy leads to possible benefit
  - Vasodilators (e.g., ACEI or CCBs) are **not** indicated if the patient is normotensive
- Symptomatic patients with moderate or severe MR and LVEF <60% (stage C HF) that are both surgical and non-surgical candidates should be managed with standard HFrEF therapy

- All authorities and guidelines[2,3,7,8,34] recommend that the primary focus should be on surgical intervention. The AHA/ACC guidelines emphasize the natural history of untreated chronic severe MR, that of myocardial damage, HF, and eventual death.[8] Correction of the MR is indicated unless LV function is significantly impaired. The guidelines also emphasize that symptoms relieved by medications still mean that the patient should be considered for mitral valve surgery.
- Patients with hypertension without HF are treated with standard antihypertensive therapy, which may help reduce worsening of the MR.[7]

Indications for Cardiac Surgery for Mitral Regurgitation

As a general rule, repair, if possible, is preferred over valve replacement (see Chapter 8). Important reasons for this include avoiding the risk of complications associated with mechanical valves (thromboembolism, bleeding, nonadherence with oral anticoagulation (OAC), and OAC in women of childbearing age). Bioprosthetic valves in the mitral position have limited durability in children but have a key role in women of childbearing age wishing to have a pregnancy.

Key points regarding indications for referral for cardiac surgery for MR are summarized in the Australian Guideline for Prevention, Diagnosis and Management of Acute Rheumatic Fever and Rheumatic Heart Disease, second edition.[2] This is a useful checklist for health professionals such as specialist nurses, physicians, and noncardiologists regarding when to refer patients with severe MR to a cardiosurgical unit (Table 6.3).

Data for the LV end-systolic volume (LVESV) Z-score threshold is based on data from RHD patients in New Zealand, where the higher the preoperative LVESV Z-score the higher the risk of late postoperative LV dysfunction.[13,35,36]

More detailed descriptions of specific patient subsets and their indications for mitral valve surgery, as used by cardiologists assessing patients, and for decision-making at cardiosurgical units, are published in the extensively referenced AHA/ACC guidelines[7,8] and ESC guidelines,[9] using COR and LOE for each recommendation. It should be reemphasized that these guidelines are updated every few years and reflect evidence-based management for patients in high-income countries, usually without resource restrictions for complex cardiac interventions. Although there are no class 1A indications for mitral valve surgery, AHA/ACC class IB indications include the following:

- Mitral valve surgery is recommended for symptomatic patients with chronic severe primary MR and LVEF >30% *
- Mitral valve surgery is recommended for asymptomatic patients with chronic severe primary MR and LV dysfunction (LVEF 30%−60% and/or LVESD $\geq$40 mm)
- Mitral valve repair is recommended in preference to mitral valve replacement (MVR) when surgical treatment is indicated for patients with chronic severe primary MR limited to the posterior leaflet
- Mitral valve repair is recommended in preference to MVR when surgical treatment is indicated for patients with chronic severe primary MR involving the anterior leaflet or both leaflets when a successful and durable repair can be accomplished
- Concomitant mitral valve repair or MVR is indicated in patients with chronic severe primary MR undergoing cardiac surgery for other indications

Serial evaluation. Detecting any change in clinical status, as determined by history and physical examination, and any change in the severity of MR and LV function on echocardiography, are important goals of monitoring. See Table 5.10, Chapter 5 for further details on frequency of follow-up.

MITRAL STENOSIS
Natural History and Pathophysiology of Mitral Stenosis

Mitral stenosis is almost always rheumatic in origin; rare exceptions to this are seen in the elderly, where extensive calcification of the mitral valve apparatus can result in a similar syndrome. Commissural fusion is the pathognomonic lesion that underpins rheumatic MS. Females are more frequently affected, with 80% of those with MS in the REMEDY study being female.[1]

The normal mitral valve area is 4−6 cm^2 but obstructive symptoms only typically occur at $\leq$2 cm^2. The

---

*When assessing LV function preoperatively and considering the timing of surgery, it is important to remember that the true extent of intrinsic systolic dysfunction may not manifest fully until after surgery, which can lead to a "paradoxical" worsening of LVEF. This relates to preoperative LV mechanics, including end-systolic stress and afterload. For example, severe MR "unloads" the LV by providing a low-resistance pathway into the LA during systole. Therefore, in the presence of severe MR, a normally functioning LV should appear hyperdynamic. When LV function is depressed preoperatively, therefore, it may not recover and outcomes may be poor despite relief of symptoms due to the MR. Outcomes following cardiac surgery are discussed in more detail in Chapter 8.

TABLE 6.3
Indications for Referral for Cardiac Surgery due to Mitral Regurgitation in Adults and Children.[2,3]

ADULT PATIENTS WITH MODERATE OR SEVERE MR AND:

- NYHA class II-IV symptoms **or**
- Impaired LV systolic function (LVEF <60%) **or**
- LVESD ≥40 mm in adults or enlarged LVESD Z-score in children **or**
- Pulmonary hypertension (PASP >50 mmHg) **or**
- New onset atrial fibrillation

CHILDREN[a] WITH SEVERE MR[3] AND:

- Symptoms of breathlessness **or**
- Asymptomatic plus one of the following:
  - Impaired LV function (LVEF <60%)
  - LVESV z-score > +2.5
  - Pulmonary hypertension (PASP >50 mmHg)

MR, mitral regurgitation; NYHA, New York Heart Association; LV, left ventricular; LVEF, left ventricular ejection fraction; LVESD, left ventricular end-systolic dimension; LVESV, left ventricular end-systolic volume; PASP, pulmonary artery systolic pressure.
[a] Children defined as <16 years, or those with nonadult body habitus.

---

natural history of MS therefore begins with a typically prolonged asymptomatic period with little effect on mortality. This asymptomatic phase varies significantly between different populations. In some low- and middle-income countries, it may progress rapidly and lead to symptoms in teenagers or even children. For example, 20% of 275 patients with pure MS undergoing cardiac surgery in the 1980s in a South African series were under 20 years old.[26] On the other hand, the latency period can be as long as 5–40 years from ARF to symptoms in high-income countries.[7,37]

Patients with MS and NYHA class I or II have an excellent prognosis, with 10-year survival >80% at diagnosis. However, MS with NYHA classes III and IV symptoms are associated with a sharp decline in survival: without intervention this was estimated at 0%–15% over the ensuing 10 years in an earlier era.[38]

The hemodynamic hallmark of MS is an elevated transmitral pressure gradient resulting in elevated mean LA pressures and reduced LV filling. Pressure gradients are typically ≤5 mmHg at rest in mild MS and up to 25 mmHg in those with severe disease. The reduced mitral inflow usually "protects" the left ventricle from volume over load and its size will usually remain normal unless other conditions that cause overload coexist. These conditions may include hypertension, mixed mitral valve disease with MR, or multivalve disease with AR.

Because the transvalvular pressure gradient is a function of the square of the transvalvular flow rate (i.e. doubling the flow rate quadruples the pressure gradient), conditions which increase the heart rate

(such as exercise, atrial fibrillation, sepsis) and/or cardiac output (such as pregnancy or anemia) can precipitously increase the transmitral pressure gradient, leading to acute worsening of obstruction at the mitral valve in those with moderate or severe MS. These increased LA pressures are then reflected back into the pulmonary venous system, resulting in pulmonary congestion (or even frank pulmonary oedema) and, in some, hypotension (see also Chapter 16 for acute HF). Chronic elevation of LA pressures also leads to increased risk of thrombosis in situ, pulmonary hypertension, and eventually right HF. More than 60% of patients who die from MS do so from progressive right HF and/or pulmonary edema,[38,39] with the remaining deaths mostly secondary to systemic thromboembolism.[40] Important strategies in the medical management of rheumatic MS therefore may include rate and/or rhythm control, OAC in the setting of an enlarged LA or AF (see later), and treatment of pulmonary edema, pulmonary hypertension, and right HF.

Medical Management of Mitral Stenosis

The purpose of medical management of MS is broadly twofold: firstly, prevention and treatment of symptoms and complications and secondly, monitoring for timing of intervention.

Heart rate control can be an effective strategy in symptomatic MS, regardless of whether the patient is in sinus rhythm or AF.[41] Both selective and nonselective β-blockers achieve this well. β-Blockers are often used as first-line therapy, but nondihydropyridine CCBs with negative inotropic and chronotropic effects, such as diltiazem or verapamil, can also be used. The effect of these drugs on exercise tolerance however is uncertain.

Digoxin exerts a weakly positive inotropic and negative chronotropic effect on the heart, especially at rest. Because of its lack of effect on heart rate control during exercise and because many patients with MS have normal LV systolic function,[42,43] the role of digoxin in MS is limited. It may be more beneficial as a second line agent for rate control in patients with AF or in select patients with symptomatic left or right ventricular systolic dysfunction (see HFrEF, above).

More recently, ivabradine has been shown to have similar efficacy in hemodynamic improvement, exercise performance, and dyspnea when compared to metoprolol in patients with MS who are in sinus rhythm.[44] Therefore, ivabradine may be a useful adjunct to β-blockers for symptom management in MS or used as an alternative if β-blockers are contraindicated or not tolerated. The use of rate-limiting agents in truly asymptomatic patients with MS is more controversial. Although clinical practice varies, many patients, even with severe MS, do not require any specific treatment. Rate control in patients with MS who develop an acute tachyarrhythmia is discussed in Chapter 16.

Diuretics are useful when there is evidence of pulmonary congestion or right heat failure as they reduce preload. Loop diuretics are often used first-line but MRAs (spironolactone and eplerenone) and thiazide or thiazide-like diuretics (e.g., metolazone and chlorthalidone) can also be added.

Summary of the medical management of mitral stenosis:
1. Asymptomatic MS (any degree of severity)
   • Usually does not require any specific therapy
2. Symptomatic MS (usually moderate or severe)—see also Chapter 16
   • Heart rate control (β-blockers or non-dihydropyridine CCBs)
   • Consider digoxin second-line for heart rate control
   • Ivabradine is an alternative to β-blockers if the patient is in sinus rhythm
   • Diuretics for pulmonary vascular congestion or right heart failure
3. Diuretics, β-blockers, digoxin and CCBs may only transiently improve symptoms.
4. Symptoms are an indication to refer to a cardiosurgical unit.[1]
5. Anticoagulation with a target international normalized ratio (INR) between 2-3 is indicated in patients with evidence of AF, significant LA dilatation, or spontaneous LA contrast (see later)

Indications for Percutaneous Mitral Balloon Commissurotomy and Cardiac Surgery

In brief, any patient, child or adult, with severe symptomatic MS, a mitral valve area (MVA) of <1.5 cm², or pulmonary hypertension (RVSP 50 mmHg), meets the requirement for intervention (i.e., percutaneous mitral balloon commissurotomy (PMBC) or surgery) (Table 6.4).[2,3]

Whether the patient undergoes PMBC or not will depend on how favourable the valve is for PMBC and the presence or absence of contraindications (e.g., LA thrombus on transesophageal echocardiography (TEE))—see Chapter 7, and whether the patient is clinically favorable for surgery (see Chapter 8).[34] In many low- and middle-income countries (LMIC), availability and relative costs of PMBC and cardiac surgery may be the overriding factors for *which* intervention is undertaken.

In more detail, Class 1 recommendations for intervention for MS by the AHA/ACC are as follows[7]:
1. PMBC is indicated for severe MS (MVA <1.5 cm², stage D (see AHA/ACC guidelines for an explanation on the different stages of MS), and favorable valve morphology in the absence of contraindications) (LOE A)[45-49]
2. Mitral valve surgery for MS is indicated in severely symptomatic patients (NYHA class III/IV) with severe MS (MVA <1.5 cm², stage D), who are not high risk for surgery, and who are not candidates for or have failed previous PMBC (LOE B)[50-52]
3. Concomitant mitral valve surgery is indicated for patients with severe MS (MVA <1.5 cm², stage C or D) undergoing other cardiac surgery (LOE C)

Class 2 and other indications for PMBC or surgery are not based on high LOE and include the following: PMBC is reasonable for asymptomatic patients with

---

TABLE 6.4
Indications for Referral for Intervention in Patients With Mitral Stenosis (Child or Adult).[2,3]

Severe Mitral Stenosis With Either:

1. Symptoms **or**
2. Mitral valve area <1.5 cm² **or**
3. Pulmonary hypertension (PASP >50 mmHg)

PASP, pulmonary artery systolic pressure.

very severe MS (MVA ≤ 1 cm^2, stage C) and favorable valve morphology in the absence of contraindications.[7,8]

Serial evaluation

Monitoring helps optimize the timing of mitral valve intervention. Because many patients can have a long period of asymptomatic stable disease, it is important that intervention is not performed too early. If intervention is performed too late, however, the patient may develop HF, thromboembolism, pulmonary hypertension, or right heart failure.

An exercise test will help discriminate whether an apparently asymptomatic patient with moderate or severe MS is truly asymptomatic (see Chapter 5). In most LMICs, follow-up is recommended every 3 months with echocardiography performed every 6 months, as the first presentation is often late with advanced disease at first diagnosis (see Table 5.10, Chapter 5).

CHRONIC AORTIC REGURGITATION

Natural History and Pathophysiology of Aortic Regurgitation

Chronic severe AR imposes a volume load on the LV, resulting in an increased LV end-diastolic volume and elevated wall stress, ultimately resulting in eccentric LV hypertrophy. Forward stroke volume and cardiac output are initially maintained however, despite the regurgitant volume, because the eccentric hypertrophy and chamber dilatation increases the total stroke volume. Mild-to-moderate AR are both unlikely to lead to LV dilatation and remodeling in this way (and other causes should be sought if LV dilatation is observed), whereas almost all patients with chronic severe AR will at some point develop LV dilatation. The compensated phase, which is defined by an absence of symptoms, LVEF $\geq 55\%$, LVESD ≤ 45 mm, and LVEDD <60 mm,[53] generally evolves slowly over years to decades, before manifesting symptoms and/or LV dysfunction. In compensated patients, the risk of developing symptoms and/or LV dysfunction is $<6\%$ per year, and the risk of sudden death is very low at $<0.2\%$ per year. Moreover, patients with an LVESD <40 mm appear to have a benign prognosis, with no risk of developing any of these complications.[54] Because of these considerations, many of these patients are managed expectantly. An LVEF 51%–55%, LVESD 45–50 mm, or LVEDD 60–70 mm are considered to reflect the transitional phase.[53] As the heart enters the decompensated stage, the myocytes have reached maximum sarcomeric elongation such that further LV dilatation results in reduced contractility, culminating in a chronically decompensated state that is defined by an LVEF $\leq 50\%$, LVESD >55 mm, or LVEDD >75 mm.[53] Most patients with an LVEF $<50\%$ are likely to develop symptoms within 3 years ($>25\%$ per year) and once symptoms develop, mortality rates increase significantly. Severe AR with mild symptoms (NYHA II) is associated with a mortality rate of 6% per year, rising sharply to 25% per year for those with moderate to severe symptoms (NYHA III-IV).[57]

Accordingly, the timing of aortic valve surgery should ideally occur before development of the decompensated state: surgery is indicated in severe AR at the onset of symptoms, LV systolic dysfunction and/or severe LV dilatation. Current AHA/ACC[7,8] and ESC[9] recommendations reflect this approach. Patients are often unaware of any symptom deterioration before the advent of HF.[58,59]

Medical Management of Chronic Aortic Regurgitation

As yet, no medical therapy has been shown to slow down progression of AR and so treatment is predominantly targeted at symptom relief and treatment of underlying LV dysfunction and HF. For symptomatic patients with severe AR who are either awaiting surgery or surgery is not an option, medical therapy is similar to that for other causes of systolic HF, including diuretics, ACEI/ARB, β-blockers, MRAs, and HYD-ISDN (see HFrEF section above).

Treatment with ACEI/ARB and β-blockers have been shown to be beneficial in large population cohort studies in patients with AR and in particular those with LV dysfunction.[60–62] For asymptomatic patients with severe AR and LV dysfunction and for whom surgery is not an option, ACEI/ARB and β-blockers are reasonable options.[7] Recently, a small randomized controlled trial of 75 asymptomatic patients with moderate-to-severe AR comparing metoprolol versus placebo over 6 months found no effect on LV volumes or exercise capacity; however, this study was limited by sample size and the short duration of intervention.[63]

Because the regurgitant volume and the normal forward stroke volume are both ejected in chronic AR, systolic hypertension is both common and difficult to control. For these reasons, vasodilators, such as ACEI/ARB and dihydropyridine CCBs,[64,65] are favored[7,66] over β-blockers,[7] which may worsen the systolic hypertension because they can increase the stroke volume (by increasing the duration of diastole and thus the regurgitant volume).

Summary of the medical management of chronic AR:

1. Asymptomatic mild or moderate AR (stage B HF) is usually well tolerated with excellent survival rates and requires no specific therapy
   - If the patient has symptoms or LV dysfunction, another cause should be sought
2. Asymptomatic severe AR (stage B HF)
   a. Compensated disease (LVEF >50%, LVESD <45 mm, LVEDD <60 mm)
      i. No treatment necessary
   b. Transitional disease (LVEF >50%, LVESD 45–50 mm, LVEDD 60–70 mm)
      i. Exercise tolerance test should be considered[67]
      ii. If normal hemodynamic response: no treatment required
      iii. If abnormal hemodynamic response: vasodilators
   c. Decompensated AR (LVEF ≤50%, LVESD >50 mm, or LVEDD >70 mm)
      i. Awaiting surgery: vasodilators
      ii. Surgery contraindicated or not available: vasodilators and β-blockers[7]
3. Symptomatic severe AR (stage C HF)[7]
   a. Awaiting surgery: intense optimization with standard HFrEF therapy
   b. Surgery contraindicated or not available: standard HFrEF therapy
4. Chronic AR with hypertension
   a. Vasodilators
   b. β-Blockers may worsen systolic hypertension

Indications for Cardiac Surgery in Chronic Aortic Regurgitation

The indications for cardiac surgery in chronic AR for both adults and children are summarised in Table 6.5. All patients with symptomatic severe AR should be offered aortic valve replacement (AVR), regardless of LV systolic function (except in extreme cases).[7–9] Additionally, asymptomatic patients with severe AR and LV systolic dysfunction (LVEF <50%) should also be offered AVR. The presence of reduced LVEF has been identified as a strong marker of adverse prognosis post-AVR in patients with AR in several studies[59,68]; thus, intervention before the development of LV dysfunction is key. The final class I indication for AVR in patients with AR in both the AHA/ACC and ESC guidelines is for those with severe AR undergoing cardiac surgery for other indications. Often, determination of symptoms in patients is difficult due to the chronic nature of the disease but exercise testing can be useful in assessing symptomatic status and functional capacity (see Chapter 5).

TABLE 6.5
Indications for Cardiac Surgery for Aortic Regurgitation in Adults and Children.[3,4]
Adult with Moderate or Severe Aortic Regurgitation and:
A. Symptoms (NYHA II–IV)
B. Asymptomatic moderate or severe aortic regurgitation and: • LVEF <55% **or**   • LVESD ≥55 mm **or**   • LVEDD >70 mm **or**
Children with Severe Aortic Regurgitation and:
A. Symptoms of breathlessness
B. Asymptomatic plus one of the following: • LVESV z-score >4 **or**   • Impaired LV function (LVEF <50%)

NYHA, New York Heart Association; LVEF, left ventricular ejection fraction; LVESD, left ventricular end-systolic dimension; LVEDD, left ventricular end-diastolic dimension; LVESV, left ventricular end-systolic volume; LV, left ventricular.

AVR is reasonable (class IIa indication) in asymptomatic patients with severe AR, preserved systolic function (LVEF ≥50%), but with severe LV dilatation (left ventricular end-systolic diameter LVESD >50 mm).[7] The ESC guidelines also recommend considering surgery in this group of patients when LVEDD is greater than 70 mm.[9] In patients with a small body surface area, it may be appropriate to index LV diameters to body size (the ESC recommends an LVESD cut-off of 25 mm/m², which may also be associated with recovery of LV systolic function post-AVR).[9] The AHA/ACC guidelines differ from the ESC guidelines by suggesting that AVR is reasonable in patients with moderate AR undergoing other cardiac surgery (class IIa) and could be considered in asymptomatic patients with severe AR, preserved LV systolic function and progressive severe LV dilatation (LVEDD >65 mm) if surgical risk is low (class IIb) (Table 6.6).

Serial evaluation

Serial evaluation with transthoracic echocardiography (TTE) should also be performed to guide management and to optimize the timing of surgery. Both the AHA/ACC[7] and ESC[9] guidelines recommend that all patients with asymptomatic severe AR and preserved LV systolic function be assessed at least annually. Eliciting symptoms of HF, or less frequently angina, are important when staging AR. See Table 5.10, Chapter 5 for further details on frequency of follow-up.

TEE has a limited role in the evaluation of AR; however, it can provide accurate assessment of the proximal

TABLE 6.6
Indications for Surgery in Chronic Aortic Regurgitation based on AHA/ACC and ESC Guidelines.

	AMERICAN HEART ASSOCIATION/ AMERICAN COLLEGE OF CARDIOLOGY 2014/2017 GUIDELINES[8,9]		EUROPEAN SOCIETY OF CARDIOLOGY 2017 GUIDELINES[10]	
	Recommendation	Level of Evidence	Recommendation	Level of Evidence
SEVERE AORTIC REGURGITATION				
Symptomatic patients	I	B	I	B
Asymptomatic patients, LVEF <50%	I	B	I	C
Asymptomatic patients undergoing other cardiac surgery	I	C	I	C
Asymptomatic patients, LVESD >50 mm	IIa	B	IIa[a]	B
Asymptomatic patients, LVEDD >65 mm with low surgical risk	IIb	C	Not mentioned	
MODERATE AORTIC REGURGITATION				
Asymptomatic patients undergoing other cardiac surgery	IIb	C	Not mentioned	

LVEF—left ventricular ejection fraction; LVEDD—left ventricular end-diastolic dimension; LVESD—left ventricular end-systolic diameter; BSA—body surface area
[a] Also includes LVEDD >70 mm or LVESD >25 mm/m^2 BSA in patients with small body size.

ascending aorta and thus can be useful when there is concern regarding the need for and planning of aortic root surgery in addition to the aortic valve. In the future, it may become more useful when planning for transcatheter repair. Similarly, computed tomography (CT) can also be useful for accurate assessment of the aorta, as well as providing a noninvasive means of excluding significant coronary artery disease.

Use of cardiovascular magnetic resonance (CMR) for assessment of LV volumes, speckle-tracking echocardiography, or biomarkers such as natriuretic peptides may also provide additional information, particularly in identification of subclinical LV dysfunction before overt clinical deterioration, although their use in guiding timing of intervention remains purely adjunctive.[69–71] CMR can provide an accurate assessment of volumes and LVEF. The use of phase-contrast imaging can provide an assessment of the severity of AR.

AORTIC STENOSIS
Natural History and Pathophysiology of Aortic Stenosis
Rheumatic AS is one of three primary causes of valvular AS, the other two being congenital aortic valve disease

and calcific AS. Rheumatic AS is said to be uncommon and rarely occurs in isolation of other rheumatic valve pathology, where it is often accompanied by some degree of AR and/or mitral valve disease. However, 9% of those with RHD had AS in the contemporary REMEDY study,[1] with most (62%) found to have moderate-to-severe stenosis. The underlying pathogenesis of rheumatic AS involves commissural fusion. Calcification is not commonly seen in rheumatic AS, in contrast to congenital and calcific AS. Some elderly patients, in their sixth decade and beyond with calcific AS, may have had a history of ARF or RHD in childhood or early adulthood. In these patients, it may not be possible on echocardiographic grounds to definitively distinguish the etiology of the AS but it is unlikely to be primarily rheumatic.

In normal individuals, the aortic valve area (AVA) is approximately 3–4 cm^2. Only after this area is reduced to less than half of normal does a hemodynamically significant gradient develop, resulting in an increased impedance to LV ejection. Therefore, in a similar fashion to MS, there is often a prolonged asymptomatic period before the development of symptoms. Once AS is established, compensatory concentric left ventricular hypertrophy, necessary to maintain a normal wall stress, often sustains a large pressure gradient across the aortic valve for many years without decreasing cardiac output or increasing LV size. Survival is excellent during this phase.

Patients with AS and normal LV function generally do not develop symptoms until the stenosis is severe, which is defined at or beyond thresholds in four hemo-dynamic variables: peak Doppler aortic jet velocity ≥ 4 m/s, mean transaortic valve gradient (MG) of ≥ 40 mmHg, estimated aortic valve area ≤ 1 cm^2, or an indexed AVA ≤ 0.6 cm/m^2. In those with mixed aortic valve disease, patients may become symptomatic when the stenosis is less than severe. Symptom onset is a pivotal development in the natural history of AS, with mortality exceeding 90% within a few years. Those with HF symptoms have the worst prognosis, followed by syncope and then angina. Diastolic dysfunction can contribute to the development of symptoms and may persist after corrective surgery. Pulmonary hypertension is also a common complication of severe AS and is asso-ciated with a poorer prognosis.[72–75]

Echocardiographic assessment of the severity of AS predominantly relies on Doppler flow measurements through the aortic valve to derive flow gradients and AVA (via the continuity equation). Other measurements such as the Doppler velocity index and projected valve area at normal flow rate may also be used as adjunctive measures of stenosis severity. The reader is referred to Chapter 5.[34]

Medical Management of Aortic Stenosis

No medical therapy is proven to alter the pathophysio-logical processes in AS and improve prognosis. There is little role for long-term pharmacological management of AS of any etiology. Physical exertion should be limited to mild activity in those with severe symptom-atic AS, and competitive sports should be avoided.[76]

HF and hypertension should be treated as appro-priate. Hypertension, in addition to AS, imposes a dou-ble load on the LV and may lead to symptoms at an earlier stage of AS.[77] HF symptoms are often treated with ACEI and diuretics,[78] whereas β-blockers should be avoided in symptomatic AS with HF because they reduce contractility. Previously, it was thought that ACEI/ARB might be hazardous in patients with AS due to the reduction in afterload that theoretically might induce syncope; however, several studies have shown that these drugs are safe to use in this group of patients.[79–81] Although renin—angiotensin—aldosterone system blockade is safe in patients with AS, a recent small randomized trial only showed a trend in reducing LV mass and slowing progression of AS in patients given

ramipril versus placebo, so further work is required to determine whether ACEI/ARB provides any outcome benefit in AS.[82]

Indications for Surgery in Aortic Stenosis

The timing of AVR in patients with AS is typically driven by the echocardiographic AS severity (MG, peak Doppler jet velocity, and AVA) and the presence of symptoms. Indications for AVR in patients with severe AS are summarized in Table 6.7. AVR is recommended in patients with symptomatic severe AS (MG ≥ 40 mmHg or peak velocity ≥ 4 m/s), which is a class IB recommendation in both the AHA/ACC[7] and ESC guidelines,[9] irrespective of resting LVEF. The prog-nosis is so poor in symptomatic patients with severe AS that only those patients whose survival is estimated to be <1 year due to other comorbidities or those who are thought unlikely to survive any intervention should be considered unsuitable for AVR. The use of exercise testing to elucidate symptoms may also be useful (see Chapter 5), but is unnecessary and even contraindicated in symptomatic patients. It is noteworthy that these rec-ommendations are largely extrapolated from data from calcific aortic AS.

In addition, symptomatic patients with true low-flow (stroke volume ≤ 35 mL/m^2), low-gradient AS with reduced LVEF should have AVR if there is evidence of meeting the criteria for severe AS following an in-crease in flow using dobutamine stress echocardiogra-phy (DSE) (true severe AS). Those in whom the gradient remains <40 mmHg are described as having "pseudosevere AS" and should receive HF treatment in an attempt to increase LVEF and improve outcomes. Theoretically, those patients with true severe AS should have an improvement in LVEF following AVR.[83,84]

Given that the time to symptom onset can be very gradual and patients may have reduced their exertion over a long period of time and have adapted to this, a class I recommendation for AVR is given to those pa-tients with asymptomatic severe AS and LVEF $<50\%$ for which there is no other cause and in those undergo-ing other cardiac surgery in both sets of guidelines. AVR should also be considered in those patients with asymp-tomatic severe AS and an abnormal blood pressure response (decrease) during exercise. ESC guidelines give a class I recommendation for AVR in those patients who develop symptoms on exercise testing; however, AHA/ACC guidelines give this a class IIa recommendation.

A class IIa recommendation is also given to AVR in patients with moderate AS undergoing other cardiac surgery and a IIb recommendation is given to AVR

TABLE 6.7
Indications for Surgery in Aortic Stenosis based on AHA/ACC and ESC Guidelines.

	AMERICAN HEART ASSOCIATION/ AMERICAN COLLEGE OF CARDIOLOGY 2014/2017 GUIDELINES[8,9]		EUROPEAN SOCIETY OF CARDIOLOGY 2017 GUIDELINES[10]	
	Recommendation	Level of Evidence	Recommendation	Level of Evidence
SEVERE AS—SYMPTOMATIC				
Mean gradient ≥40 mmHg or peak velocity ≥4 m/s	I	B	I	B
Low-flow, low-gradient AS with reduced LVEF and evidence of contractile reserve during DSE	IIa	B	I	C
Asymptomatic patients undergoing other cardiac surgery	I	B	I	C
Low-flow, low-gradient AS with reduced LVEF without contractile reserve	Not mentioned		IIa[a]	C
Low-flow, low-gradient AS with preserved LVEF and AS thought to be the cause of symptoms	IIa	C	Not mentioned	
SEVERE AS—ASYMPTOMATIC [b]				
LVEF <50% due to AS	I	B	I	C

DSE—dobutamine stress echocardiography; AS—aortic stenosis; LVEF—left ventricular ejection fraction.
[a] ESC guidelines recommend adjunctive measures such as CT calcium scoring to help guide decision-making in this scenario.
[b] For class II indications—refer to the guidelines.

in patients with severe AS and rapid disease progression with low surgical risk in the AHA/ACC guidelines. The ESC guidelines give a class IIa recommendation for AVR in those patients with asymptomatic severe AS and extremely high peak velocity (>5.5 m/s), severe valve calcification and peak velocity progression of ≥0.3 m/s/year, markedly elevated natriuretic peptides and/or severe pulmonary hypertension (invasive pulmonary artery systolic pressure >60 mmHg at rest).

Transcatheter Aortic Valve Implantation

For patients with high-risk calcific AS too unwell for surgery, transcatheter aortic valve implantation (TAVI), first performed in 2002, is an established lifesaving option. Recent game-changing trials have also opened the door to TAVI as the default approach for most low-risk patients, demonstrating that TAVI is as safe and effective as surgery.[85,86] Conventional TAVI, however, relies on crushing the hydroxyapatite deposits to anchor the valves, and lack of such calcification is considered a relative contraindication.[9] Because rheumatic AS is usually noncalcific, this makes the use of TAVI potentially more hazardous and less successful in these patients, although it has been used successfully in a few instances.[87,88] The TAVI field is evolving rapidly, and new developments may in future make the procedure suited for rheumatic AS.

Serial evaluation

It is important to serially monitor patients with AS, both clinically for symptom status (asking specifically about HF symptoms, syncope, or evidence of angina) and echocardiographically for AS severity. Exercise testing is a useful adjunct to clarify the patient's symptom status. See also Table 5.10, Chapter 5.

TEE may have an additional role in assessment of AS and the aorta. Low-dose DSE is particularly useful in patients with AS and reduced LVEF, where often the AVA meets the criteria for severe AS but peak velocity and mean gradient do not.[91] There is very little proven role for other imaging modalities and biomarkers in rheumatic AS.

OTHER CHRONIC RHEUMATIC HEART DISEASE ENTITIES

Multivalve Disease and Mixed Valve Disease

Mixed valve and/or multivalve disease are the most common patterns of disease seen in RHD,[1] but there is less data for basing management decisions here than for the isolated valve disease already described.

Multivalve disease commonly manifests as mitral disease and aortic regurgitation, mitral disease and tricuspid disease, or three valve involvement with concomitant mitral, aortic, and tricuspid valve disease. Mixed valve disease (presence of both stenosis and regurgitation in the same valve) is particularly common in the mitral valve, and sometimes seen in the tricuspid valve.[1,92] Tricuspid and mitral regurgitation can also develop secondary to LV dilation.

Data on indications for intervention in multivalve and mixed valve disease are scarce, reflected as such in the AHA/ACC[7,8] and ESC guidelines.[9] Multivalve or mixed valve disease are a harbinger of poorer outcomes when compared to isolated lesions. In a series of untreated mixed mitral disease, only two-thirds were alive at 5 years and only one-third at 10 years.[93] Even in nonsevere disease, symptom onset and cardiac decompensation can occur in mixed mitral disease. Surgical intervention is often required, even if either lesion in isolation is not graded as severe, for example, mixed moderate MR and moderate MS.

The basic principle where one lesion is dominant over the other (e.g., severe MR plus mild AR) is that the pathophysiology, symptoms, and management all closely resemble the more severe lesion. In those patients where the severity of both lesions is balanced, the pathophysiological and clinical manifestations reflect the proximal lesion, which can often mask the manifestations of the distal lesion.[94] For example, significant AR may not be apparent in a patient with severe MS.

Concomitant MR and AR is a particularly deleterious combination, especially when both lesions are severe. Surgical treatment of both valves is necessary although postoperative outcomes, including persistence of symptoms, ventricular dysfunction and survival, are significantly worse compared to single valve disease.[13,95] Combined MR and AR confers a high risk for ventricular dysfunction in the young following surgery for ARF.[34] The implication is that the indication for intervention should be based on the LV size (dimensions and volumes) indications for MR rather than on the higher threshold of LV size for isolated AR.

If surgery is not an option in multivalve and mixed valve disease, treatment as per HFrEF recommendations (see above) may provide symptomatic improvement.

Tricuspid Valve Disease

Nearly one-third of patients in the REMEDY study had tricuspid regurgitation and significant pulmonary hypertension.[1] Treatment of pulmonary hypertension and right ventricular dysfunction is mostly directed at treating underlying left-sided valvular disease and left ventricular dysfunction. There are no data supporting use of pulmonary vasodilators before intervention. Loop diuretics may help in relief of systemic and hepatic congestion in both tricuspid stenosis and regurgitation but can exacerbate the low flow state that is present. In mixed tricuspid valve disease, surgery is often indicated in combination with surgery for one or both left sided valves. See Chapter 8.

Tricuspid valve stenosis can occur in combination with MS and other RHD valve lesions. A mean inflow gradient >5 mmHg is suggestive of severe disease. Tricuspid regurgitation may be secondary to a combination of direct rheumatic changes and pulmonary hypertension; it almost never occurs in isolation.[1] In rare cases of isolated tricuspid stenosis, balloon valvuloplasty may be indicated.

Prosthetic Valve Patients

The AHA/ACC valve guidelines and 2017 update provide detailed recommendations for assessment and management of prosthetic valves.[7,8] The first principle is that patients who have a valve replacement are not cured but still have serious heart disease. All too often RHD patients misunderstand that cardiac surgery is not curative. The surgical team needs to emphasize this and ensure linkage back to the medical (cardiology) team. Note that prosthetic valves include both mechanical and bioprosthetic valves.

Mechanical valves

Interestingly, after the initial TTE at 1−3 months following mechanical valve replacement, the AHA/ACC guidelines recommend yearly clinical follow up for mechanical valves but not yearly echocardiograms if the signs and symptoms indicate normal mechanical valve function. However, as alluded to previously, many patients with RHD continue to experience high morbidity and mortality following valve surgery and thus more aggressive follow-up is recommended (Table 5.10, Chapter 5). Furthermore, many patients require TTE for other reasons, such as LV systolic dysfunction, pulmonary hypertension, or other cardiac valve function. In the young, the development of patient prosthetic valve mismatch may occur with body growth.

For all these reasons 6-monthly clinical review, ideally with echocardiography, is recommended[1] for all RHD patients with prosthetic valves.

Bioprosthetic valves

The Australian guidelines recommend echocardiography 3-6 monthly[2] for bioprosthetic valves as deterioration can be subtle initially. Bioprosthetic valve dysfunction typically presents with the insidious onset of exertional dyspnea or with a louder systolic murmur (MR or AS) or a new diastolic murmur (AR or MS) on physical examination. More abrupt and severe symptoms may occur with bioprosthetic valve endocarditis or with degenerative rupture of a valve cusp. Management of acute prosthetic valve dysfunction is covered in Chapter 16.

GENERAL CARE PRINCIPALS FOR THE RHD PATIENT

Best practice RHD management principles are summarized in Table 6.1. Some of the principles not detailed earlier in the chapter warrant further discussion.

Secondary Prevention With Antibiotic Prophylaxis

Underpinning optimal long-term management of RHD is the secondary prevention of ARF recurrences that lead to progression of valve disease. It has long been shown that those with mild or moderate RHD are not at risk of progression to severe RHD and its complications as long as there is no recurrence of ARF. Resolution of RHD may also be seen.[11,96-98] For these patients, secondary antibiotic prophylaxis comprising regular 3-4 weekly long-acting intramuscular benzathine penicillin G injections is the single most important aspect of their medical management.

For patients with severe RHD, even in the absence of recurrences of ARF, disease progression occurs because of the irreversible damage to the cardiac valves, and impaired ventricular function due to longstanding ventricular overload. It is likely that prognosis for these patients is related more closely to the cardiac lesion than to recurrences of ARF.

The principles of secondary prevention for ARF and RHD are discussed in detail in Chapter 11. It is important that the duration of penicillin be reassessed in early adulthood based on the severity of disease at that time rather than making decisions for life based on the severity at first presentation with ARF or RHD.

Antithrombotic Therapy in Rheumatic Heart Disease

The unique social and epidemiological factors surrounding RHD influence the surgical decision-making of repair versus replacement.[99] The lack of access to surgery, especially reoperation, along with lack of surgical expertise in valve repair in many endemic countries mean that mechanical valves are performed more frequently than valve repairs (see Chapter 8). For RHD patients with prosthetic valves, OAC and INR monitoring become the most important aspects for quality survival. Successful INR monitoring for RHD patients receiving mechanical valves in LMICs can be achieved as reported from Rwanda.[100] Conversely, high rates of thromboembolism following prosthetic valve replacements have been found in other regions,[101] likely reflecting outcomes where there is suboptimal patient-health professional focus on optimal INR control. Constant vigilance to achieve good INR control is needed for all patients with prosthetic valves wherever they reside. Patient empowerment can be key to good outcomes.

Antithrombotics (OAC and/or anti-platelets) play a central role in the medical management of three broad groups of RHD patients: those with mechanical valve replacement, those with AF, and those in sinus rhythm with other specific risk factors for thromboembolism.

Antithrombotic Therapy for Prosthetic Valves

Vitamin K antagonists (VKA), namely warfarin, remain the mainstay of anticoagulation following mechanical valve replacement to prevent thromboembolic events and valve thrombosis. MVR is associated with higher rates of thromboembolic events compared to the aortic valve and this is reflected in the AHA/ACC and ESC guidelines, which both recommend higher INR targets for the former. There are a number of important differences between the AHA/ACC[7,8] and ESC[9] valvular guidelines on antithrombotic therapy following mechanical or bioprosthetic valve replacement (Tables 6.8 and 6.9). Nonvitamin K antagonist oral anticoagulants (NOACs), alternatively known as direct oral anticoagulants (DOACs), cannot be recommended for mechanical valve patients because they are associated with a significantly increased risk of thromboembolic complications.[9,102] Although both sets of guidelines recommend some form of antithrombotic therapy following bioprosthetic valve replacement, the evidence for this is limited. Acute valve thrombosis is discussed in Chapter 16.

TABLE 6.8
Long-Term Antithrombotic Management of Prosthetic Valves based on AHA/ACC and ESC Guidelines

	AMERICAN HEART ASSOCIATION/ AMERICAN COLLEGE OF CARDIOLOGY 2014/2017 GUIDELINES[7,8]	EUROPEAN SOCIETY OF CARDIOLOGY 2017 GUIDELINES[9]
MECHANICAL VALVES (ALL PATIENTS REQUIRE LIFELONG ANTITHROMBOTICS)		
Mechanical AVR	**VKA** plus **Aspirin 75–100 mg OD** No thromboembolic risk factors: *target INR 2.5 (2.0–3.0)* Thromboembolic risk factors[a]: *target INR 3.0 (2.5–3.5)*	**VKA only** See Table 6.9 for target INR
Mechanical MVR	**VKA** plus **Aspirin 75–100 mg OD** Target INR 3.0 (2.5–3.5)	**VKA only** See Table 6.9 for target INR
BIOPROSTHETIC VALVES		
Surgical bioprosthetic AVR	**VKA** (first 3–6 months only) plus **Aspirin 75-100 mg OD** (lifelong) Target INR 2.5 (2.0–3.0)	**Aspirin 75–100 mg OD** (first 3 months only)
Surgical bioprosthetic MVR	**VKA** (first 3–6 months only) plus **Aspirin 75-100 mg OD** (lifelong): Target INR 2.5 (2.0–3.0)	**VKA** (first 3 months only) Target INR 2.5 (2.0-3.0)
Transcatheter Aortic Valve Implantation (TAVI)	Consider **clopidogrel 75 mg OD** for the first 6 months in addition to lifelong **aspirin 75–100 mg OD**	Consider **DAPT** for the first 3 −6 months followed by lifelong **single antiplatelet therapy**

AVR aortic valve replacement, VKA vitaminK antagonist, MVR mitral valve replacement, DAPT dual antiplatelet therapy, OD omne in die (once daily).
[a] AHA/ACC thromboembolic risk factors: atrial fibrillation, previous thromboembolism, left ventricular dysfunction, hypercoagulable conditions.

TABLE 6.9
European Society of Cardiology Guidelines on Target International Normalized Ratio for Mechanical Prostheses.

Prosthesis Thrombogenicity	No Patient Risk Factors[a]	≥1 Risk Factor[a]
Low risk[b]	2.5 (2.0–3.0)	3.0 (2.5–3.5)
Medium risk[c]	3.0 (2.5–3.5)	3.5 (3.0–4.0)
High risk[d]	3.5 (3.0–4.0)	4.0 (3.5–4.5)

[a] Patient risk factors: mitral or tricuspid valve replacement, previous thromboembolism, atrial fibrillation, mitral stenosis of any grade, left ventricular ejection fraction <35%.
[b] Carbomedics, Medtronic Hall, ATS, Medtronic Open-Pivot, St-Jude Medical, Sorion Bicarbon, On-X*.
[c] Other bileaflet valves with insufficient data.
[d] Lillehei-Kaster, Omniscience, Starr-Edwards, Bjork-Shiley, and other tilting-disc valves. Reproduced with permission from Baumgartner et al.[9]
*The On-X aortic valve has a target INR of 1.8 (range 1.5–2.0).

Anticoagulation in Atrial Fibrillation

All patients with AF should be evaluated for the need of OAC. Stroke prevention is central to the management of AF and the latest recommendations by the ESC are presented in Fig. 6.3.[103] AF has traditionally been dichotomized into "valvular" and "nonvalvular" AF, although the terms are confusing. The definition of valvular AF varies slightly between major societies, but in recent guidelines only includes patients with mechanical heart valves or those with moderate or severe MS.[103–105] Therefore, patients who do not fulfill the definition of valvular AF, including those with other valvular pathologies such as MR, AR, and AS, should be considered to have nonvalvular AF.

Patients with valvular AF should receive OAC, unless contraindicated.[103] VKAs remain the anticoagulants of choice in these patients.[103] As stated earlier, NOACs are strictly contraindicated in patients with mechanical heart valves, whereas patients with significant MS were excluded from previous NOAC trials due to concerns that the MS might further augment the risk of thromboembolism brought by AF due to low flow in the left atrium, which does not apply to other forms of native valve disease. However, an international, multicentre, noninferiority trial comparing the NOAC rivaroxaban 20 mg once daily with VKAs for patients with rheumatic AF is currently ongoing

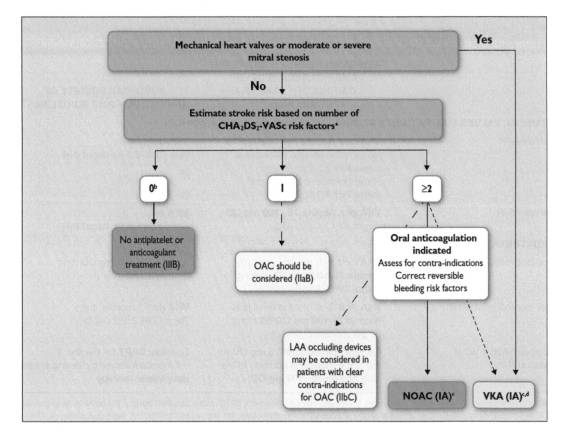

^a**C**ongestive heart failure, **H**ypertension, **A**ge ≥75 years (2 points), **D**iabetes, prior **S**troke/TIA/embolus (2 points), **V**ascular disease (prior myocardial infarction, peripheral arterial disease, or aortic plaque), **A**ge 65-74, female **S**ex
^bIncludes women without other stroke risk factors
^cIIaB for women with only one additional stroke risk factor
^dIB for patients with mechanical heart valves or mitral stenosis

AF atrial fibrillation, LAA left atrial appendage, non-vitamin K antagonist oral anticoagulant, OAC oral anticoagulation, VKA vitamin K antagonist

FIG. 6.3 European Society of Cardiology guidelines on stroke prevention in atrial fibrillation. Reproduced with permission from Kirchhof et al.[103]

(INVICTUS-VKA, NCT02832544). Inclusion criteria for increased risk of stroke are any one of the following: CHA$_2$DS$_2$-VASc score ≥2 (see later), moderate/severe MS, left atrial spontaneous echocardiographic contrast, or left atrial thrombus. As of 2019, the trial had recruited over 80% of the target sample size of 4500 patients, from over 150 centers in 24 RHD endemic countries in Asia, Africa, and Latin America. Results are expected in late 2021 (G Karthikeyan personal communication).

Conversely, the decision to anticoagulate patients with nonvalvular AF is based primarily on the 1-year risk of a thromboembolic event. In practice, OAC should be used in most patients with nonvalvular AF because the net clinical effect is almost universal, except in those at very low stroke risk.[103] The preferred tool for estimating thromboembolic risk is the CHA$_2$DS$_2$-VASc risk model[103,105] (see Fig. 6.3 for individual components of the risk model), which is widely used.[106] The CHA$_2$DS$_2$-VASc score represents a range of risk. A score of 0 is uncommon and is associated with an unadjusted (unadjusted for possible use of aspirin) ischemic stroke rate of 0.2% per year. This increases to 0.6% with a CHA_2DS_2-VASc score of 1 and 2.2% with a score of 2.[107] Actual stroke rates in RHD-endemic populations may however vary from these estimates. Depending on patient-specific characteristics, physician preference, drug availability, and affordability, the choice of OAC in these patients may be either a NOAC or VKA.[103]

Irrespective of the baseline risk, in patients with AF the use of VKAs reduces the risk of thromboembolic events (including stroke) by 64% and all-cause mortality by 26%, compared with control or placebo treatments.[108]

An important point is that the CHA_2DS_2-VASc score is gender-dependent. Female gender is considered an independent risk factor for stroke in those with AF. However, recent studies have suggested that in the absence of other stroke risk factors (CHA_2DS_2-VASc score of 0 in males and 1 in females), female gender carries a low stroke risk similar to males.[105] Conversely, females with ≥ 2 additional stroke risk factors (CHA_2DS_2-VASc score of ≥ 3 in females) appear to be at excess risk for stroke.[105] The latest ESC and American guidelines reflect these findings: for patients with nonvalvular AF and a CHA_2DS_2-VASc score of ≥ 2 in men or ≥ 3 in women, OAC is strongly recommended.[103,105] In men with a CHA_2DS_2-VASc score of 1, or 2 in women, OAC should be considered.[103,105] The rates of thromboembolism (including stroke) vary considerably in this group of patients due to differences in outcomes, populations, and anticoagulation status.[103] Clinical judgment and an individualized weighing of risk are important in determining which of these patients should be anticoagulated. Given that valvular heart disease probably has an additive effect on thromboembolic risk in those with AF,[103,109] most patients with RHD in this category are likely to benefit from OAC, providing adequate INR monitoring is available. Finally, in men with a CHA_2DS_2-VASc score of 0 or women with a CHA_2DS_2-VASc score of 1, OAC is not recommended (Fig. 6.3).[103,105]

An important caveat to the earlier recommendations is that those with AF who are being considered for cardioversion (either electrically or pharmacologically) will also require OAC, regardless of the CHA_2DS_2-VASc score.

Antiplatelet therapy as an alternative to OAC is not recommended by current ESC guidelines.[103] VKA therapy is better than single or dual antiplatelet therapy (aspirin and clopidogrel) at preventing stroke, systemic embolism, myocardial infarction, and vascular death. Additionally, bleeding rates with antiplatelets are similar to those on OAC.

Clinical risk scores for bleeding should also be considered before administering OAC. These include the HAS-BLED (hypertension, abnormal renal/liver function, stroke, bleeding history or predisposition, labile INR, elderly (>65 years), drugs/alcohol usage) and ABC (age, biomarkers, clinical history) bleeding scores. **A high bleeding risk score should not be used as an absolute cut-off to withhold or withdraw OAC.** Instead, these scores should be used as tools to identify and treat modifiable bleeding risk factors, such as hypertension, labile INR, excess alcohol (≥ 8 drinks/week), and medications that predispose to bleeding (e.g., antiplatelets, nonsteroidal antiinflammatories).[103]

Initiating warfarin therapy. Unfractionated heparin or low molecular weight heparin can be used to provide anticoagulation cover until the warfarin is therapeutic. Warfarin is prothrombic initially hence bridging with heparin for 48–72 h is required. The INR, full blood count, and renal function are checked at baseline as some patients may be coagulopathic and/or thrombocytopenic (e.g., due to liver disease). Warfarin can be started at a dose of 5 mg per day (or 2.5 mg per day in those with liver or kidney disease or heart failure, or in those who are frail, elderly, or malnourished) with a target INR range of 2–3. INR levels should be checked at least weekly during initiation of treatment and at least monthly when the INR is stable.[105] To maintain optimal INR control, the warfarin dose should not be increased by more than 10% at a time. Anticoagulation is usually lifelong.

Anticoagulation for patients in sinus rhythm and who have not had valve surgery
OAC is also indicated for patients in sinus rhythm with severe valve disease if (1) there is a previous history of thromboembolism, (2) presence of left atrial thrombus, (3) any grade of spontaneous echocardiographic contrast in the presence of MS (4) LA size: M-mode diameter >50 mm or LA volume >60 mL/m².[8]

Access to oral healthcare
RHD patients are at increased risk of developing infective endocarditis, a condition with significant morbidity and mortality. Oral bacteria have been identified as causative agents for infective endocarditis, underscoring the importance of meticulous dental and oral hygiene in those with RHD to reduce the risk of an oral source for bacteremia. Regular oral healthcare ideally includes the assessment and treatment of dental disease. Education about the prevention of dental disease should be part of the routine on-going management of RHD.

It is recommended that all patients with RHD (regardless of severity) undergo at least annual oral health review.[2,3] Dental recall intervals should be based on clinical risk.[52] Those with moderate/severe RHD, prosthetic cardiac valves, or higher dental risk factors (e.g., poor oral hygiene, chew betel nut, dry mouth, untreated dental caries, inflammatory periodontal disease) should be offered more frequent dental reviews.

Some dental procedures do have an increased risk of causing bacteremia. The effectiveness of additional antibiotic prophylaxis before dental procedures is controversial, however antibiotic prophylaxis is recommended for at-risk patients having at-risk dental procedures, for example those with prosthetic valves or those with previous history of infective endocarditis (see later).

Infective Endocarditis Prophylaxis

Many authorities no longer recommend that valvular heart disease patients require infective endocarditis prophylaxis as there is no published evidence to show that antibiotic prophylaxis prevents infective endocarditis. Cognisant of the high lifetime risk of infective endocarditis with its high risk of mortality or major morbidity, some guidelines[2,3] specifically do recommend antibiotic prophylaxis for RHD patients. Prophylaxis is recommended for people with chronic RHD of any severity, but is not recommended for those who have had previous ARF without carditis or for those who no longer have evidence of RHD.[2,3] RHD patients at very high risk of endocarditis are those with prosthetic heart valves (bioprosthetic or mechanical) and those with a history of previous endocarditis.

Persons with established RHD or prosthetic valves should receive antibiotic prophylaxis before procedures expected to produce bacteremia. Antibiotic prophylaxis should be considered in dental procedures involving manipulation of the gingival or the oral mucosa.[110,111]

Recommendations for dental procedures that do **not** require infective endocarditis prophylaxis include taking dental radiographs, placement or adjustment of orthodontic appliances and brackets, shedding of deciduous teeth, and bleeding from trauma to the lips or oral mucosa.[111]

Those already receiving penicillin for secondary prophylaxis should be offered a different antibiotic for prophylaxis of endocarditis.[3] Antibiotic prophylaxis against infective endocarditis in the context of RHD, including recommended antibiotics, is discussed further in Chapter 16. Appropriate antibiotics can also be found on the Heart Foundation of New Zealand website.[111]

REFERENCES

1. Zuhlke L, Engel ME, Karthikeyan G, et al. Characteristics, complications, and gaps in evidence-based interventions in rheumatic heart disease: the global rheumatic heart disease registry (the REMEDY study). *Eur Heart J.* 2015; 36(18), 1115-22a.
2. RHD Australia (ARF/RHD writing group), National Heart Foundation of Australia, Cardiac Society of Australia and New Zealand, *The Australian Guideline for Prevention, Diagnosis and Management of Acute Rheumatic Fever and Rheumatic Heart Disease.* 2nd ed., Full guidelines 2012: 1–136 pp. Available from: https://www.rhdaustralia.org.au/arf-rhd-guideline.
3. New Zealand Heart Foundation. *New Zealand Guidelines for Rheumatic Fever: Diagnosis, Management and Secondary Prevention of Acute Rheumatic Fever and Rheumatic Heart Disease: 2014 Update.* 2014. Auckland. https://www.heartfoundation.org.nz
4. Yancy CW, Jessup M, Bozkurt B, et al. 2013 ACCF/AHA guideline for the management of heart failure: executive summary: a report of the American college of cardiology foundation/american heart association task force on practice guidelines. *Circulation.* 2013;128(16): 1810–1852.
5. Yancy CW, Jessup M, Bozkurt B, et al. 2017 ACC/AHA/HFSA focused update of the 2013 ACCF/AHA guideline for the management of heart failure: a report of the American college of cardiology/American heart association task force on clinical practice guidelines and the heart failure society of America. *J Card Fail.* 2017;23(8): 628–651.
6. Ponikowski P, Voors AA, Anker SD, et al. 2016 ESC Guidelines for the diagnosis and treatment of acute and chronic heart failure: the task force for the diagnosis and treatment of acute and chronic heart failure of the European society of cardiology (ESC)Developed with the special contribution of the heart failure association (HFA) of the ESC. *Eur Heart J.* 2016;37(27): 2129–2200.
7. Nishimura RA, Otto CM, Bonow RO, et al. 2014 AHA/ACC guideline for the management of patients with valvular heart disease: a report of the American college of cardiology/American heart association task force on practice guidelines. *J Am Coll Cardiol.* 2014;63(22): e57–e185.
8. Nishimura RA, Otto CM, Bonow RO, et al. AHA/ACC focused update of the 2014 AHA/ACC guideline for the management of patients with valvular heart disease: a report of the American college of cardiology/American heart association task force on clinical practice guidelines. *J Am Coll Cardiol.* 2017;70(2):252–289.
9. Baumgartner H, Falk V, Bax JJ, et al. 2017 ESC/EACTS guidelines for the management of valvular heart disease. *Eur Heart J.* 2017;38(36):2739–2791.
10. Dougherty S, Beaton A, Nascimento BR, Zuhlke LJ, Khorsandi M, Wilson N. Prevention and control of rheumatic heart disease: overcoming core challenges in

resource-poor environments. *Ann Pediatr Cardiol.* 2018; 11(1):68–78.

11. Carapetis JR, Beaton A, Cunningham MW, et al. Acute rheumatic fever and rheumatic heart disease. *Nat Rev Dis Primers.* 2016;2:15084.

12. Oxman AD. Coordination of guidelines development. *CMAJ.* 1993;148(8):1285–1288.

13. Gentles TL, Finucane AK, Remenyi B, Kerr AR, Wilson NJ. Ventricular function before and after surgery for isolated and combined regurgitation in the young. *Ann Thorac Surg.* 2015;100(4):1383–1389.

14. Zhang W, Okello E, Nyakoojo W, Lwabi P, Mondo CK. Proportion of patients in the Uganda rheumatic heart disease registry with advanced disease requiring urgent surgical interventions. *Afr Health Sci.* 2015;15(4): 1182–1188.

15. Williams B, Mancia G, Spiering W, et al. 2018 ESC/ESH guidelines for the management of arterial hypertension: the task force for the management of arterial hypertension of the European society of cardiology and the European society of hypertension: the task force for the management of arterial hypertension of the European society of cardiology and the European society of hypertension. *J Hypertens.* 2018;36(10):1953–2041.

16. Hill SR, Carless PA, Henry DA, et al. Transfusion thresholds and other strategies for guiding allogeneic red blood cell transfusion. *Cochrane Database Syst Rev.* 2002;(2): CD002042.

17. Hebert PC, Wells G, Blajchman MA, et al. A multicenter, randomized, controlled clinical trial of transfusion requirements in critical care. Transfusion requirements in critical care investigators, canadian critical care trials group. *N Engl J Med.* 1999;340(6):409–417.

18. Hebert PC, Yetisir E, Martin C, et al. Is a low transfusion threshold safe in critically ill patients with cardiovascular diseases? *Crit Care Med.* 2001;29(2):227–234.

19. Yancy CW, Januzzi Jr JL, Allen LA, et al. 2017 ACC expert consensus decision pathway for optimization of heart failure treatment: answers to 10 pivotal issues about heart failure with reduced ejection fraction: a report of the American college of cardiology task force on expert consensus decision pathways. *J Am Coll Cardiol.* 2018; 71(2):201–230.

20. Damasceno A, Mayosi BM, Sani M, et al. The causes, treatment, and outcome of acute heart failure in 1006 Africans from 9 countries. *Arch Intern Med.* 2012;172(18): 1386–1394.

21. Karthikeyan G, Devasenapathy N, Zuhlke L, et al. Digoxin and clinical outcomes in the global rheumatic heart disease registry. *Heart.* 2018;105:350–352.

22. Yeong M, Silbery M, Finucane K, Wilson NJ, Gentles TL. Mitral valve geometry in paediatric rheumatic mitral regurgitation. *Pediatr Cardiol.* 2015;36(4):827–834.

23. Schuler G, Peterson KL, Johnson A, et al. Temporal response of left ventricular performance to mitral valve surgery. *Circulation.* 1979;59(6):1218–1231.

24. Borow KM, Green LH, Mann T, et al. End-systolic volume as a predictor of postoperative left ventricular

performance in volume overload from valvular regurgitation. *Am J Med.* 1980;68(5):655–663.

25. Crawford MH, Souchek J, Oprian CA, et al. Determinants of survival and left ventricular performance after mitral valve replacement. Department of veterans affairs cooperative study on valvular heart disease. *Circulation.* 1990;81(4):1173–1181.

26. Marcus RH, Sareli P, Pocock WA, Barlow JB. The spectrum of severe rheumatic mitral valve disease in a developing country. Correlations among clinical presentation, surgical pathologic findings, and hemodynamic sequelae. *Ann Intern Med.* 1994;120(3):177–183.

27. Ahmed MI, Aban I, Lloyd SG, et al. A randomized controlled phase IIb trial of beta(1)-receptor blockade for chronic degenerative mitral regurgitation. *J Am Coll Cardiol.* 2012;60(9):833–838.

28. Varadarajan P, Joshi N, Appel D, Duvvuri L, Pai RG. Effect of beta-blocker therapy on survival in patients with severe mitral regurgitation and normal left ventricular ejection fraction. *Am J Cardiol.* 2008;102(5):611–615.

29. Sahoo D, Kapoor A, Sinha A, et al. Targeting the sympatho-adrenergic link in chronic rheumatic mitral regurgitation: assessing the role of oral beta-blockers. *Cardiovasc Ther.* 2016;34(4):261–267.

30. Sampaio RO, Grinberg M, Leite JJ, et al. Effect of enalapril on left ventricular diameters and exercise capacity in asymptomatic or mildly symptomatic patients with regurgitation secondary to mitral valve prolapse or rheumatic heart disease. *Am J Cardiol.* 2005;96(1):117–121.

31. Kula S, Tunaoglu FS, Olgunturk R, Gokcora N. Atrial natriuretic peptide levels in rheumatic mitral regurgitation and response to angiotensin-converting enzyme inhibitors. *Can J Cardiol.* 2003;19(4):405–408.

32. Tunaoglu FS, Olgunturk R, Kula S, Oguz D. Effective regurgitant orifice area of rheumatic mitral insufficiency: response to angiotensin converting enzyme inhibitor treatment. *Anadolu Kardiyol Derg.* 2004;4(1):3–7.

33. Gupta DK, Kapoor A, Garg N, Tewari S, Sinha N. Beneficial effects of nicorandil versus enalapril in chronic rheumatic severe mitral regurgitation: six months follow up echocardiographic study. *J Heart Valve Dis.* 2001;10(2): 158–165.

34. Baumgartner H, Hung J, Bermejo J, et al. Recommendations on the echocardiographic assessment of aortic valve stenosis: a focused update from the European association of cardiovascular imaging and the American society of echocardiography. *J Am Soc Echocardiogr.* 2017;30(4): 372–392.

35. Remenyi B, Webb R, Gentles T, et al. Improve long-term survival for rheumatic mitral valve repair compare to replacement in the young. *World J Pediatr Congenit Heart Surg.* 2012;4(2):155–164.

36. Finucane K, Wilson N. Priorities in cardiac surgery for rheumatic heart disease. *Glob Heart.* 2013;8(3):213–220.

37. Horstkotte D, Niehues R, Strauer BE. Pathomorphological aspects, aetiology and natural history of acquired mitral valve stenosis. *Eur Heart J.* 1991;12(Suppl B): 55–60.

38. Rowe JC, Bland EF, Sprague HB, White PD. The course of mitral stenosis without surgery: ten- and twenty-year perspectives. *Ann Intern Med.* 1960;52:741−749.

39. Olesen KH. The natural history of 271 patients with mitral stenosis under medical treatment. *Br Heart J.* 1962;24:349−357.

40. Abernathy WS, Willis 3rd PW. Thromboembolic complications of rheumatic heart disease. *Cardiovasc Clin.* 1973;5(2):131−175.

41. Agrawal V, Kumar N, Lohiya B, et al. Metoprolol vs ivabradine in patients with mitral stenosis in sinus rhythm. *Int J Cardiol.* 2016;221:562−566.

42. Toutouzas P. Left ventricular function in mitral valve disease. *Herz.* 1984;9(5):297−305.

43. Gaasch WH, Folland ED. Left ventricular function in rheumatic mitral stenosis. *Eur Heart J.* 1991;12(Suppl B):66−69.

44. Saggu DK, Narain VS, Dwivedi SK, et al. Effect of ivabradine on heart rate and duration of exercise in patients with mild-to-moderate mitral stenosis: a randomized comparison with metoprolol. *J Cardiovasc Pharmacol.* 2015;65(6):552−554.

45. Arora R, Nair M, Kalra GS, Nigam M, Khalilullah M. Immediate and long-term results of balloon and surgical closed mitral valvotomy: a randomized comparative study. *Am Heart J.* 1993;125(4):1091−1094.

46. Cotrufo M, Renzulli A, Ismeno G, et al. Percutaneous mitral commissurotomy versus open mitral commissurotomy: a comparative study. *Eur J Cardiothorac Surg.* 1999;15(5):646−651. Discussion 51-2.

47. Patel JJ, Shama D, Mitha AS, et al. Balloon valvuloplasty versus closed commissurotomy for pliable mitral stenosis: a prospective hemodynamic study. *J Am Coll Cardiol.* 1991;18(5):1318−1322.

48. Ben Farhat M, Ayari M, Maatouk F, et al. Percutaneous balloon versus surgical closed and open mitral commissurotomy: seven-year follow-up results of a randomized trial. *Circulation.* 1998;97(3):245−250.

49. Ellis LB, Singh JB, Morales DD, Harken DE. Fifteen-to twenty-year study of one thousand patients undergoing closed mitral valvuloplasty. *Circulation.* 1973;48(2):357−364.

50. Iung B, Cormier B, Ducimetiere P, et al. Functional results 5 years after successful percutaneous mitral commissurotomy in a series of 528 patients and analysis of predictive factors. *J Am Coll Cardiol.* 1996;27(2):407−414.

51. John S, Bashi VV, Jairaj PS, et al. Closed mitral valvotomy: early results and long-term follow-up of 3724 consecutive patients. *Circulation.* 1983;68(5):891−896.

52. National Institute for Health and Care Excellence. *Dental Recall: Recall Interval between Routine Dental Examinations.* London: National Institute for Health and Care Excellence; 2004.

53. Bonow RO, Carabello BA, Chatterjee K, et al. 2008 focused update incorporated into the ACC/AHA 2006 guidelines for the management of patients with valvular heart disease: a report of the American college of cardiology/American heart association task force on practice guidelines (writing committee to revise the 1998 guidelines for the management of patients with valvular heart disease): endorsed by the society of cardiovascular anesthesiologists, society for cardiovascular angiography and interventions, and society of thoracic surgeons. *Circulation.* 2008;118(15):e523−e661.

54. Bonow RO, Lakatos E, Maron BJ, Epstein SE. Serial long-term assessment of the natural history of asymptomatic patients with chronic aortic regurgitation and normal left ventricular systolic function. *Circulation.* 1991;84(4):1625−1635.

55. Zoghbi WA, Adams D, Bonow RO, et al. Recommendations for noninvasive evaluation of native valvular regurgitation: a report from the American society of echocardiography developed in collaboration with the society for cardiovascular magnetic resonance. *J Am Soc Echocardiogr.* 2017;30(4):303−371.

56. Lancellotti P, Tribouilloy C, Hagendorff A, et al. Recommendations for the echocardiographic assessment of native valvular regurgitation: an executive summary from the European association of cardiovascular imaging. *Eur Heart J Cardiovasc Imaging.* 2013;14(7):611−644.

57. Dujardin KS, Enriquez-Sarano M, Schaff HV, Bailey KR, Seward JB, Tajik AJ. Mortality and morbidity of aortic regurgitation in clinical practice. A long-term follow-up study. *Circulation.* 1999;99(14):1851−1857.

58. Bhudia SK, McCarthy PM, Kumpati GS, et al. Improved outcomes after aortic valve surgery for chronic aortic regurgitation with severe left ventricular dysfunction. *J Am Coll Cardiol.* 2007;49(13):1465−1471.

59. Chaliki HP, Mohty D, Avierinos JF, et al. Outcomes after aortic valve replacement in patients with severe aortic regurgitation and markedly reduced left ventricular function. *Circulation.* 2002;106(21):2687−2693.

60. Elder DH, Wei L, Szwejkowski BR, et al. The impact of renin-angiotensin-aldosterone system blockade on heart failure outcomes and mortality in patients identified to have aortic regurgitation: a large population cohort study. *J Am Coll Cardiol.* 2011;58(20):2084−2091.

61. Sampat U, Varadarajan P, Turk R, Kamath A, Khandhar S, Pai RG. Effect of beta-blocker therapy on survival in patients with severe aortic regurgitation results from a cohort of 756 patients. *J Am Coll Cardiol.* 2009;54(5):452−457.

62. Zendaoui A, Lachance D, Roussel E, Couet J, Arsenault M. *Circ Heart Fail.* 2011;4(2):207−213.

63. Broch K, Urheim S, Lonnebakken MT, et al. Controlled release metoprolol for aortic regurgitation: a randomised clinical trial. *Heart.* 2016;102(3):191−197.

64. Scognamiglio R, Rahimtoola SH, Fasoli G, Nistri S, Dalla Volta S. Nifedipine in asymptomatic patients with severe aortic regurgitation and normal left ventricular function. *N Engl J Med.* 1994;331(11):689−694.

65. Evangelista A, Tornos P, Sambola A, Permanyer-Miralda G, Soler-Soler J. Long-term vasodilator therapy in patients with severe aortic regurgitation. *N Engl J Med.* 2005;353(13):1342−1349.

66. Vahanian A, Alfieri O, Andreotti F, et al. Guidelines on the management of valvular heart disease (version 2012): the joint task force on the management of valvular heart disease of the European society of cardiology (ESC) and the European association for cardio-thoracic surgery (EACTS). *Eur J Cardiothorac Surg.* 2012;42(4): S1–S44.

67. Shah RM, Singh M, Bhuriya R, Molnar J, Arora RR, Khosla S. Favorable effects of vasodilators on left ventricular remodeling in asymptomatic patients with chronic moderate-severe aortic regurgitation and normal ejection fraction: a meta-analysis of clinical trials. *Clin Cardiol.* 2012;35(10):619–625.

68. Tornos P, Sambola A, Permanyer-Miralda G, Evangelista A, Gomez Z, Soler-Soler J. Long-term outcome of surgically treated aortic regurgitation: influence of guideline adherence toward early surgery. *J Am Coll Cardiol.* 2006;47(5):1012–1017.

69. Pizarro R, Bazzino OO, Oberti PF, et al. Prospective validation of the prognostic usefulness of B-type natriuretic peptide in asymptomatic patients with chronic severe aortic regurgitation. *J Am Coll Cardiol.* 2011;58(16):1705–1714.

70. Lee JC, Branch KR, Hamilton-Craig C, Krieger EV. Evaluation of aortic regurgitation with cardiac magnetic resonance imaging: a systematic review. *Heart.* 2018;104(2): 103–110.

71. Olsen NT, Sogaard P, Larsson HB, et al. Speckle-tracking echocardiography for predicting outcome in chronic aortic regurgitation during conservative management and after surgery. *JACC Cardiovasc Imaging.* 2011;4(3): 223–230.

72. Chizner MA, Pearle DL, deLeon Jr AC. The natural history of aortic stenosis in adults. *Am Heart J.* 1980;99(4): 419–424.

73. Schwarz F, Baumann P, Manthey J, et al. The effect of aortic valve replacement on survival. *Circulation.* 1982; 66(5):1105–1110.

74. Kitai T, Honda S, Okada Y, et al. Clinical outcomes in non-surgically managed patients with very severe versus severe aortic stenosis. *Heart.* 2011;97(24):2029–2032.

75. Ben-Dor I, Pichard AD, Gonzalez MA, et al. Correlates and causes of death in patients with severe symptomatic aortic stenosis who are not eligible to participate in a clinical trial of transcatheter aortic valve implantation. *Circulation.* 2010;122(11 Suppl):S37–S42.

76. Bonow RO, Nishimura RA, Thompson PD, et al. Eligibility and disqualification recommendations for competitive athletes with cardiovascular abnormalities: task force 5: valvular heart disease: a scientific statement from the American heart association and American college of cardiology. *Circulation.* 2015;132(22): e292–e297.

77. Antonini-Canterin F, Huang G, Cervesato E, et al. Symptomatic aortic stenosis: does systemic hypertension play an additional role? *Hypertension.* 2003;41(6): 1268–1272.

78. Carabello BA, Paulus WJ. Aortic stenosis. *Lancet.* 2009; 373(9667):956–966.

79. O'Brien KD, Zhao XQ, Shavelle DM, et al. Hemodynamic effects of the angiotensin-converting enzyme inhibitor, ramipril, in patients with mild to moderate aortic stenosis and preserved left ventricular function. *J Investig Med.* 2004;52(3):185–191.

80. Chockalingam A, Venkatesan S, Subramaniam T, et al. Safety and efficacy of angiotensin-converting enzyme inhibitors in symptomatic severe aortic stenosis: symptomatic cardiac obstruction-pilot study of enalapril in aortic stenosis (SCOPE-AS). *Am Heart J.* 2004;147(4):E19.

81. Nadir MA, Wei L, Elder DH, et al. Impact of renin-angiotensin system blockade therapy on outcome in aortic stenosis. *J Am Coll Cardiol.* 2011;58(6):570–576.

82. Bull S, Loudon M, Francis JM, et al. A prospective, double-blind, randomized controlled trial of the angiotensin-converting enzyme inhibitor ramipril in aortic stenosis (RIAS trial). *Eur Heart J Cardiovasc Imaging.* 2015;16(8):834–841.

83. Tribouilloy C, Levy F, Rusinaru D, et al. Outcome after aortic valve replacement for low-flow/low-gradient aortic stenosis without contractile reserve on dobutamine stress echocardiography. *J Am Coll Cardiol.* 2009;53(20): 1865–1873.

84. Levy F, Laurent M, Monin JL, et al. Aortic valve replacement for low-flow/low-gradient aortic stenosis operative risk stratification and long-term outcome: a European multicenter study. *J Am Coll Cardiol.* 2008;51(15): 1466–1472.

85. Mack MJ, Leon MB, Thourani VH, et al. Transcatheter aortic-valve replacement with a balloon-expandable valve in low-risk patients. *N Engl J Med.* 2019;380(18): 1696–1705.

86. Popma JJ, Deeb GM, Yakubov SJ, et al. Transcatheter aortic-valve replacement with a self-expanding valve in low-risk patients. *N Engl J Med.* 2019;380(18): 1706–1715.

87. Bilge M, Saatci Yasar A, Alemdar R, Ali S. Transcatheter aortic valve implantation with the corevalve for the treatment of rheumatic aortic stenosis. *Anadolu Kardiyol Derg.* 2014;14(3):296–297.

88. Akujuo AC, Dellis SL, Britton LW, Bennett Jr EV. Transcatheter aortic and mitral valve implantation (TAMVI) in native rheumatic valves. *J Card Surg.* 2015;30(11): 813–816.

89. O'Brien SM, Shahian DM, Filardo G, et al. The society of thoracic surgeons 2008 cardiac surgery risk models: part 2–isolated valve surgery. *Ann Thorac Surg.* 2009;88(1 Suppl):S23–S42.

90. Nashef SA, Roques F, Sharples LD, et al. EuroSCORE II. *Eur J Cardiothorac Surg.* 2012;41(4):734–744. Discussion 44-5.

91. Picano E, Pibarot P, Lancellotti P, Monin JL, Bonow RO. The emerging role of exercise testing and stress echocardiography in valvular heart disease. *J Am Coll Cardiol.* 2009; 54(24):2251–2260.

92. Roberts WC, Sullivan MF. Clinical and necropsy observations early after simultaneous replacement of the mitral and aortic valves. *Am J Cardiol.* 1986;58(11):1067–1084.

93. McLean A, Waters M, Spencer E, Hadfield C. Experience with cardiac valve operations in cape York Peninsula and the torres strait islands, Australia. *Med J Aust.* 2007; 186(11):560–563.

94. Unger P, Clavel MA, Lindman BR, Mathieu P, Pibarot P. Pathophysiology and management of multivalvular disease. *Nat Rev Cardiol.* 2016;13(7):429–440.

95. Niles N, Borer JS, Kamen M, Hochreiter C, Devereux RB, Kligfield P. Preoperative left and right ventricular performance in combined aortic and mitral regurgitation and comparison with isolated aortic or mitral regurgitation. *Am J Cardiol.* 1990;65(20):1372–1378.

96. Carapetis JR, McDonald M, Wilson NJ. Acute rheumatic fever. *Lancet.* 2005;366(9480):155–168.

97. World Health Organisation, WHO Expert Consultation on Rheumatic Fever and Rheumatic Heart Disease (2001: Geneva Switzerland). *Rheumatic Fever and Rheumatic Heart Disease: Report of a WHO Expert Consultation, Geneva, 29 October–1 November 2001.* 2004. Geneva, Switzerland.

98. Tompkins D, Boxerbaum B, Liebman J. Long-term prognosis of rheumatic fever patients receiving regular intramuscular benzathine penicillin. *Circulation.* 1972;45: 543–551.

99. Okello E, Kakande B, Sebatta E, et al. Socioeconomic and environmental risk factors among rheumatic heart disease patients in Uganda. *PLoS One.* 2012;7(8):e43917.

100. Rusingiza EK, El-Khatib Z, Hedt-Gauthier B, et al. Outcomes for patients with rheumatic heart disease after cardiac surgery followed at rural district hospitals in Rwanda. *Heart.* 2018;104(20):1707–1713.

101. Thomson Mangnall L, Sibbritt D, Fry M, Gallagher R. Short- and long-term outcomes after valve replacement surgery for rheumatic heart disease in the South Pacific, conducted by a fly-in/fly-out humanitarian surgical team: a 20-year retrospective study for the years 1991 to 2011. *J Thorac Cardiovasc Surg.* 2014;148(5):1996–2003.

102. Eikelboom JW, Connolly SJ, Brueckmann M, et al. Dabigatran versus warfarin in patients with mechanical heart valves. *N Engl J Med.* 2013;369(13):1206–1214.

103. Kirchhof P, Benussi S, Kotecha D, et al. ESC Guidelines for the management of atrial fibrillation developed in collaboration with EACTS. *Eur Heart J.* 2016;37(38): 2893–2962.

104. Heidbuchel H, Verhamme P, Alings M, et al. Updated European heart rhythm association practical guide on the use of non-vitamin K antagonist anticoagulants in patients with non-valvular atrial fibrillation. *Europace.* 2015;17(10):1467–1507.

105. January CT, Wann LS, Calkins H, et al. 2019 AHA/ACC/HRS focused update of the 2014 AHA/ACC/HRS guideline for the management of patients with atrial fibrillation. *J AM Coll Cardiol.* 2019;74(1):104–132.

106. Kirchhof P, Curtis AB, Skanes AC, Gillis AM, Samuel Wann L, John Camm A. Atrial fibrillation guidelines across the atlantic: a comparison of the current recommendations of the European society of cardiology/European heart rhythm association/European association of cardiothoracic surgeons, the American college of cardiology foundation/American heart association/heart rhythm society, and the Canadian cardiovascular society. *Eur Heart J.* 2013;34(20):1471–1474.

107. Friberg L, Rosenqvist M, Lip GY. Evaluation of risk stratification schemes for ischaemic stroke and bleeding in 182 678 patients with atrial fibrillation: the Swedish atrial fibrillation cohort study. *Eur Heart J.* 2012;33(12): 1500–1510.

108. Hart RG, Pearce LA, Aguilar MI. Meta-analysis: antithrombotic therapy to prevent stroke in patients who have nonvalvular atrial fibrillation. *Ann Intern Med.* 2007;146(12):857–867.

109. Halperin JL, Hart RG. Atrial fibrillation and stroke: new ideas, persisting dilemmas. *Stroke.* 1988;19(8):937–941.

110. Habib G, Lancellotti P, Antunes MJ, et al. 2015 ESC guidelines for the management of infective endocarditis: the task force for the management of infective endocarditis of the European society of cardiology (ESC). Endorsed by: European association for cardio-thoracic surgery (EACTS), the European association of nuclear medicine (EANM). *Eur Heart J.* 2015;36(44):3075–3128.

111. New Zealand Heart Foundation. *New Zealand Guideline for Prevention of Infective Endocarditis Associated with Dental and Other Medical Interventions.* 2008. Auckland.

CHAPTER 7

Catheter-Based Evaluation and Treatment of Rheumatic Heart Disease

RAGHAV BANSAL • NAGENDRA BOOPATHY SENGUTTUVAN • GANESAN KARTHIKEYAN • MPIKO NTSEKHE

INTRODUCTION

Rheumatic heart disease (RHD) remains the most common cause of multivalvular heart disease worldwide, and a major cause of cardiac morbidity and mortality in low- and middle-income countries.[1]

The definitive management of patients with advanced rheumatic valvular disease includes replacement, repair, or mechanical opening of stenotic valves by either percutaneous (catheter-based) or surgical means. Appropriate management of sequelae such as atrial fibrillation and heart failure is also an essential component of the comprehensive care of such patients. Meticulous evaluation to establish an accurate pathological and hemodynamic diagnosis is needed to plan appropriate surgical or interventional therapy. As described in Chapter 5, the diagnosis of RHD is based on the combination of clinical history and examination, review of the electrocardiogram (ECG) and chest X-ray, and transthoracic echocardiography. Both transesophageal echocardiography and catheter-based invasive investigation may aid assessment of severity of RHD.

Before the advent of modern echocardiography, cardiac catheterization was considered an essential step before valve surgery.[2] Invasive evaluation was used: (1) to confirm the diagnosis and severity of valve disease; (2) to assess for the presence and severity of coexistent valve disease; (3) to document the presence and severity of pulmonary hypertension; (4) to estimate left ventricular function; and (5) for the evaluation of coexisting coronary artery disease (CAD).[2] Currently, the role of catheterization is much more restricted given the ability of echocardiography to provide many of the answers to these clinical questions.

There is limited published data about the availability of catheter laboratories in RHD endemic regions of the world, nor of volume, outcome, and impact of procedures performed where they do exist. However, it is reasonable to assume that the consequences of limited access to the sometimes lifesaving and life-prolonging catheter-based approaches to the diagnosis and treatment of RHD likely mirror those of the limited capacity for cardiac surgery in the same regions of the world.[3,4]

In this chapter, we provide an overview of the role of catheter-based investigation and treatment in patients with RHD. Specifically, we will review the indications for catheter-based evaluation, how to perform/technical aspects of the procedure, and discuss interpretation of the information obtained. We also discuss the indications for percutaneous mitral balloon commissurotomy (PMBC) and the role of aortic valvuloplasty and transcutaneous aortic valve implantation (TAVI) in patients with RHD.

INDICATIONS FOR CATHETER-BASED EVALUATION IN THE PATIENT WITH RHEUMATIC HEART DISEASE

Catheter-based measurements remain the gold standard for the evaluation of intracardiac chamber and vascular pressures, measuring pressure gradients across valves and between chambers, determining hemodynamic blood flow, stroke volume (SV), and cardiac output (CO), and providing direct accurate measures of oxygen content and saturation in all the chambers. Cardiac catheterization is therefore indicated: whenever there is a discrepancy between clinical information obtained from noninvasive evaluation (history, physical examination, ECG, chest X-ray and echocardiography); when there is doubt about the accuracy of the measured pulmonary artery pressure (PAP); when there is uncertainty regarding the severity of valve disease (common in cases of multivalvular involvement); and where echocardiography windows are poor and the quality of images do not allow for satisfactory analysis and interpretation.[5]

MEASUREMENTS IN THE CATHETERIZATION LABORATORY

Basics of Cardiac Catheterization and Pressure Measurement

Cardiac catheterization for full hemodynamic and valvular assessment in patients with RHD requires both arterial (for aortic and left ventricular pressure recording) and venous access (for right heart hemodynamics). Historically, femoral arterial and venous access were the most commonly used access routes. However, with growing evidence of improved safety and effectiveness of radial arterial access, it is likely that the use of radial/axillary vein or radial/femoral vein combinations will increase globally.[6]

Before the procedure, the fluid-filled pressure lines should be attached properly to a pressure transducer at one end and to the side port of a manifold attached to the cardiac catheter at the other, with the height of the transducer fixed to correspond with that of the patient's heart (approximately the midaxillary line, phlebostatic axis). The pressure lines should be clear of air bubbles and kinks and any radiographic contrast medium or blood should be flushed out from the tubing and the catheters to ensure proper pressure measurement and minimization of errors.

An end-hole catheter such as the Swan-Ganz catheter (a balloon floatation end-hole catheter) is the catheter of choice for right heart catheterization due to the advantage of easy positioning and accurate measurement of pulmonary capillary wedge pressure (PCWP).[7] Alternative catheters that are often used include stiffer end-hole catheters (e.g., Lehman, Cournand and Judkins right catheters). The use of end-hole catheters is particularly important when measurement of the PCWP is required (most right heart studies) as side-hole catheters such as NIH and Bermann catheters may introduce significant measurement error. Where severe tricuspid regurgitation is present, operators may experience difficulty with access to the right ventricle (RV) using balloon floatation catheters. Ventricle and stiffer nonballoon floatation catheters such as the

Judkins right coronary catheter or the use of an over a wire technique may help.

By convention, the right heart study measurements (see Table 7.1) are obtained before the left heart catheterization. Measurement of ventricular and aortic pressures and gradients are obtained using a pigtail catheter due to its atraumatic tip. However, if coronary angiography is to be undertaken, it is reasonable to start with coronary angiography before entering the left ventricle (LV) to reduce the risk of embolic complications.

Contour of Normal Pressure Waveforms and Common Artifacts

The atrial pressure waveform consists of three positive waves (a, c, and v waves) and two negative waves (x and y descent) (Fig. 7.1). Atrial contraction corresponds with the a wave and follows the P wave on the ECG. The a wave is followed by the x descent, which represents atrial relaxation and downward pulling of the tricuspid annulus as the RV contracts. The x descent is interrupted by a transient pressure increase, known as the c wave, which is caused by bulging of the closed tricuspid valve into the RA during right ventricular contraction. Both the a wave and x descent are absent in cases with atrial fibrillation. Passive atrial filling terminates the x descent which is followed by the v wave, which occurs near the end of (right) ventricular systole (the peak of atrial pressure). Opening of the tricuspid valve releases blood from the RA to the RV, resulting in a drop in atrial pressure and the final wave known as the y descent. The waveforms are similar for the left and the right atria, albeit that the mean pressures are slightly higher in the left atrium (LA), and the LA has a more prominent v wave.

The ventricular pressure waveform (Fig. 7.1) consists of a systolic and a diastolic phase. The systolic ejection phase begins with a steep rapid rise after the opening of the semilunar valve. The systolic ejection peak pressure occurs when the ventricular pressure equals the peak pressure of the connected great vessel. Both pressures

---

TABLE 7.1
Right Heart Catheterization Study.

The catheter procedure should aim to acquire:
1. PCWP and its contour
2. Pulmonary artery systolic, diastolic, and mean pressures
3. Pulmonary diastolic gradient (difference between diastolic pressure and wedge mean)
4. Right ventricular systolic and end-diastolic pressures and diastolic filling contour
5. Right atrial pressure and its contour
6. Cardiac output by the thermodilution method
7. Pulmonary vascular resistance (trans-pulmonary gradient/cardiac output)

PCWP pulmonary capillary wedge pressure

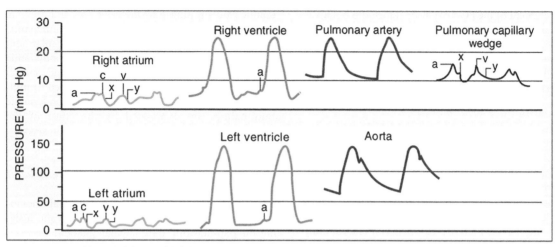

FIG. 7.1 Normal right- and left-heart pressures recorded from fluid-filled catheter systems in a human. Reproduced with permission from Pepine et al.[1]

then fall; the great vessel pressure falls to its nadir as diastole begins. The dicrotic notch is observed on the ventricular waveform that corresponds to the closure of the semilunar valves. The ventricular pressure then descends to close to zero, assuming no abnormalities of ventricular relaxation and compliance. Ventricular diastolic pressure typically consists of three independent phases: an energy-dependent early rapid filling phase; a period of passive ventricular filling called diastasis; and the final filling phase that corresponds to atrial systole and active emptying of the atria into the ventricle before AV valve closure.

An important aim of a well-performed hemodynamic study is to obtain and record all pressures within a short time span to avoid significant changes in hemodynamics that may occur over time. It is highly recommended to record simultaneous pressures for calculation of gradients across the mitral valve. Gradients across the tricuspid, pulmonary, and aortic valves are usually obtained as "pullback" measurements across the valve. Artifactual pressure waveform recordings can cause false readings. Common artifacts include damping artifacts when catheters have not been flushed correctly; errors in zeroing and calibration; and peripheral systolic pressure amplification due to summation of the reflected wave.

Blood samples should be taken from all appropriate cardiac chambers and blood vessels for oxygen saturation as they are required for the hemodynamic calculations. At a minimum, samples should include blood from the pulmonary artery (PA) (where venous blood from the superior vena cava, inferior vena cava, and coronary sinus are all mixed) and aorta. The samples should be collected in 2 mL heparinized syringes for

the purpose of measurement of CO by Fick's method and should be analyzed promptly to reduce error. Care should be taken to avoid any air bubbles in the sample. The spectrophotometric method may produce inaccurate results in the presence of abnormal hemoglobin. Reflectance oximetry is commonly used and is accurate if the oxygen saturation range is from 45% to 98%.[8] However, reliability decreases below 40% saturation, which is seen in mixed venous samples in low CO states and cyanotic congenital heart disease.

Estimation of Pulmonary Capillary Wedge Pressure

The PCWP, which is a surrogate of the left atrial pressure (LAP), is best measured with an end-hole catheter (often a Swan-Ganz catheter). This is placed in a distal branch of the PA with the inflated balloon completely occluding the antegrade flow, thus forming a continuum of blood between the distal PA, the pulmonary capillaries, and the pulmonary venous system draining into the LA. Although the PCWP waveform is similar to that from the atria (Fig. 7.1), it is delayed by as much as 50–150 ms due to the transmission through the pulmonary capillary bed and often appears more damped. These important differences need to be kept in mind when PCWP is used as a surrogate for LAP while valve gradient calculations are determined in mitral stenosis.

The ideal PCWP trace should have well defined a and v waves, a mean pressure that is equal to or less than the PA diastolic pressure, and an oxygen saturation of ≥95% (in the absence of pulmonary parenchymal diseases that distort normal gas exchange). Accurate measurement of the PCWP may be difficult to obtain as both over inflation and under inflation of the catheter balloon remain common source of errors. Over inflation leads to dampening of the pressure waveforms and underinflation leads to transmittance of the PAP and the overestimation of PCWP.

Estimation of Cardiac Output

The two most frequently used methods for estimating the CO are the Fick and thermodilution method. Using the Fick principle, the CO is calculated by dividing oxygen consumption (VO_2) by the arteriovenous oxygen difference, where the latter is assumed based on age, sex, and body surface area.[9] Although discrepancies may exist between the measured and estimated VO_2, direct measurement of VO_2 is rarely performed as it is technically demanding, time consuming, and expensive.[10] Blood samples from the aorta and the PA (mixed venous sample) are used to calculate the arteriovenous oxygen difference (Box 7.1). The Fick method looses accuracy in patients with significant mitral regurgitation or AR and should not be used in these conditions. It remains accurate however in low CO and tricuspid regurgitation.

The thermodilution technique uses specific catheters (such as the Swan-Ganz), which allow for the downstream placement of a thermistor in the PA to measure the temperature change (increase) of a fixed volume of cold saline injected into a proximal port. Automated complex calculations give the value of CO depending upon the temperature change noted at the distal thermistor. The major advantage of this technique is that it has significantly less measurement variability and better reliability compared to Fick's method. However, the thermodilution method becomes unreliable in the presence of intracardiac shunts, low flow states, in those with atrial fibrillation or severe tricuspid regurgitation.

HEMODYNAMIC ASSESSMENT OF VALVE FUNCTION

In patients with RHD, the catheter study allows determination of the nature and severity of the valve abnormality (stenosis, regurgitation, or both). The severity of stenotic valves is judged by the valve area and pressure gradients across the valves and the hemodynamic sequelae of the valve abnormality (ventricular and LAPs, etc.). The interpretation of any hemodynamic changes may include changes in the atrial and ventricular waveform exerted by the effect of isolated or multiple valvular lesions. As a rule, the hemodynamic abnormalities are dominated by the effect of the more proximal lesion and the lesion greater in severity.

Mitral Stenosis

The hemodynamic findings of mitral stenosis at cardiac catheterization

In patients with mitral stenosis (MS) the main hemodynamic abnormalities are an elevated LAP and a significant pan-diastolic transvalvular gradient between the LA and LV due to the pathological obstruction at the valve level. There is usually a close correlation between the magnitude of the mean diastolic gradient and the severity of mitral stenosis. Given that the LA empties into the LV in diastole, the diastolic filling time (DFT) is critical to the assessment of mitral valve gradient. If the DFT decreases, as it does during exercise, the reduced filling time results in an elevated transmitral gradient. Clinical variables such as anemia, thyrotoxicosis, and pregnancy that affect the CO may give apparent changes in the valve gradient and should be excluded when the CO is unexpectedly high. In patients with atrial fibrillation, the beat-to-beat variability of the RR interval makes single beat transmitral gradient an unreliable estimate of the severity of MS. In such patients, the average of multiple readings should be taken over a period of approximately 1 min to better estimate the mean gradient. The left ventricular end-diastolic pressure (LVEDP) remains normal or decreased throughout the disease course. The hemodynamic consequences of a chronically elevated LAP in MS include pulmonary venous hypertension, reactive pulmonary arterial hypertension, and a pressure-loaded RV.

The most accurate means of determining the mitral valve gradient is by direct measurement of the LA

BOX 7.1
Calculation of the Cardiac Output using the Fick Method.

$$\text{Fick Cardiac output (L/min)} = \frac{O_2 \text{ consumption (mL/min)}}{(A\text{-}VO_2) \times 1.36 \times Hb \times 10}$$

Where $A\text{-}VO_2$ is the arterial-venous oxygen saturation difference ($S_aO_2 - S_vO_2$), Hb is the haemoglobin concentration (mg/dL), and the constant 1.36 is the oxygen-carrying capacity of haemoglobin.

pressure (by the transseptal technique) with simultaneous measurement of the LV pressure over several cardiac cycles and integral quantification of the pressure difference in diastole (Fig. 7.2). However, the PCWP is typically used as a surrogate of the LAP due to its ease of measurement and because it avoids the transseptal puncture and its inherent risks. Simultaneous measurement of PCWP and left ventricular diastolic pressure allows for the determination of the gradient. There is a transmission delay in the PCWP waveform that needs to be accounted for by shifting the PCWP waveform to the left manually until the peak of the v wave just precedes or coincides with the downstroke of the left ventricular waveform.

Although the general consensus is that the PCWP is a satisfactory estimate of the LAP, use of the PCWP for measurement of the transvalvular gradient remains controversial with some experts. According to Lange et al., there is good correlation between phase-adjusted PCWP and LAP for calculation of the valve gradient and area.[11] However, phase adjustment may lead to overestimation according to others.[12] In practice, good correlation exists at lower wedge pressures (<25 mmHg) between PCWP and LAPs. The correlation is less reliable at higher wedge pressures.[13] Transseptal catheterization to obtain true transvalvular gradients should be considered when (1) PCWP >25 mmHg, (2) there is severe pulmonary arterial hypertension, (3) the quality of the PCWP waveforms is poor, (4) there are discrepant noninvasive gradients, and (5) prior prosthetic mitral valve implantation (due to altered LA mechanics).

The LAP waveform shows a prominent a wave due to the resistance to flow across the valve against atrial contraction (Fig. 7.2). In a dilated large and compliant LA, the increase in volume with the pulmonary venous return produces a smaller v wave. However, it is not

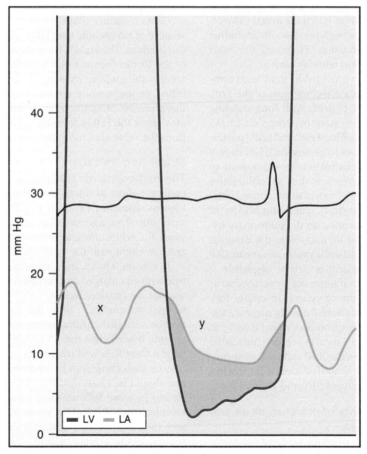

FIG. 7.2 Pressure gradient in a patient with mitral stenosis. The pressure in the left atrium (LA) exceeds the pressure in the left ventricle (LV) during diastole, producing a diastolic pressure gradient (green shaded area). (Reproduced with permission from Bashore.[54])

uncommon to find a prominent v wave in MS even in the absence of mitral regurgitation, due to a noncompliant, small LA. This prominent v wave can be differentiated from the v wave of mitral regurgitation by looking at the slope of the y descent, which is decreased in MS due to impaired left ventricular filling, while it remains steep in mitral regurgitation. It is important to note that diastasis (diastolic equalization of left atrial and left ventricular pressure) is never achieved in severe MS and there remains a persistent gradient even at end diastole (Fig. 7.2).

The contribution of atrial contraction to ventricular filling is less than 25% in normal individuals.[14] Intuitively, this should increase in MS due to incomplete LA emptying in the earlier part of diastole. However, the contribution of atrial contraction is paradoxically decreased in severe MS, despite the increased LAP and slower rate of deceleration of mitral flow.[15,16] The contribution of atrial contraction to LV filling decreases from 29% in mild MS to 9% in severe MS. This is reflected in the absence of a transmitted a wave in the LV diastolic tracing. A possible explanation is that the mitral valve offers increased resistance throughout diastole, including the period of atrial contraction. However, the exact reason for this phenomenon remains unclear.

Additional information provided by right heart catheterization in MS includes a direct measure of the PAP, which is often elevated in patients with long-standing symptomatic disease. Pulmonary hypertension in MS is usually the result of transmitted elevated LAP (postcapillary or pulmonary venous hypertension), but in very long standing disease it can include a component of pulmonary arterial hypertension due to obliterative changes in the pulmonary vasculature (mixed pre- and postcapillary hypertension). The contribution of pulmonary arterial hypertension to the pulmonary hypertension can be assessed by measuring the diastolic pulmonary gradient (PA diastolic pressure—mean LAP or wedge). Where the gradient is zero or negligible, it is safe to assume that the pulmonary hypertension is predominantly postcapillary or venous in origin. Pulmonary diastolic gradients above 7 mmHg suggest a significant precapillary contribution and worse long-term outcomes.[17] Values above 7 mmHg are also associated with a prominent a wave in the RAP and increased stiffness of the RV.[17] A cv wave should be looked for and implies the presence of significant tricuspid regurgitation.

Quantification of severity of mitral stenosis and calculation of valve area

Measurement of the mean diastolic gradient across the mitral valve gives an estimate of the severity of MS. Tracings should be measured on a scale of 0—50 mmHg at a fast speed (100 mm/s) to accurately record the gradient between LA and LV pressures. Modern laboratory automated computer algorithms can calculate the mean valve gradient. As previously described, the gradient and CO are affected by the hemodynamic status of the patient. Thus, calculation of mitral valve area (MVA) is important to provide an estimation of the severity of the stenosis that is independent of the hemodynamic status of the patient.

The Gorlin formula (Box 7.2), first derived by Dr. Richard Gorlin and his father using Torricelli's law, is applied for the calculation of valve areas.[18]

Accurate measurement of CO remains the Achilles' heel of Gorlin's formula. There may be a 10%—15% variation in the measurement of CO by assumed VO_2 even in the most stringent conditions. Other limitations of the formula include overestimation of the valve gradient and underestimation of the valve area in the presence of mitral regurgitation, and potential overestimation of the gradient severity due to atrial fibrillation.

Other formulae that have been used to measure the severity of MS include the Hakki formula (Box 7.2) and Cui method. The Hakkis formula is a simplified version of the Gorlin formula that is easier to remember, as it ignores the empiric constant, heart rate, and diastolic filling period/systolic ejection period.[20] However, in the presence of tachycardia or bradycardia, the valve area using the Hakki formula can vary by almost 20% from the valve area using the Gorlin formula.

Mitral Regurgitation
The hemodynamic findings in rheumatic mitral regurgitation at cardiac catheterization

Invasive assessment is rarely required for isolated rheumatic mitral regurgitation. However, it may be indicated when the echocardiographic severity of regurgitation is not consistent with the other clinical findings.

In chronic, severe, and compensated mitral regurgitation with an enlarged and compliant LA, PCWP and LAP tracings are characterized by an elevated mean LAP but normal waveforms.[21] With the onset of decompensation or with acute mitral regurgitation, the regurgitant volume overwhelms the LA compliance and leads to a large v wave followed by a steep y descent. This v wave may be high enough to be confused with a PAP tracing and should be carefully differentiated by looking at the timing (v wave follows the Twave on the ECG) and morphology. Although a prominent v wave may be seen in MS, a v wave 3 times the mean PCWP is highly specific for mitral regurgitation.[22] The a wave usually remains unaffected. Right heart catheterization may reveal elevated PAP. In acute mitral regurgitation, the pulmonary arterial trace may be characterized by a bifid

---

BOX 7.2
The Gorlin and Hakki Formulae.[a]

THE GORLIN FORMULAE

The original Gorlin formula was refined by Gorlin and Gorlin in 1951. However, in order to derive an accurate mitral valve area, cardiac output is corrected for the diastolic filling period (because mitral flow only occurs during diastole), producing the following equation:

$$MVA\left(cm^2\right) = \left[Cardiac\ output\left(\frac{mL}{min}\right) \div (DFR \times HR)\right] \div \left[37.7\sqrt{Mean\ gradient}\right]$$

The calculation is similar for the aortic valve: the cardiac output is divided by the actual systolic ejection period (because blood flow across the aortic valve only occurs during systole):

$$AVA\left(cm^2\right) = \left[Cardiac\ output\left(\frac{mL}{min}\right) \div (SEP \times HR)\right] \div \left[44.3\sqrt{Mean\ gradient}\right]$$

THE HAKKI FORMULAE

Hakki and colleagues proposed a simplified version of the above formulae. Because the diastolic filling period and systolic ejection period are relatively constant at normal heart rates, the Gorlin equations can be rewritten thus:

$$MVA\left(cm^2\right) = Cardiac\ output\left(\frac{L}{min}\right) \div \sqrt{Mean\ gradient}$$

Only the mean gradient was validated for the mitral valve area, whereas both the peak-to-peak and mean gradient can be used for the aortic valve area:

$$AVA\left(cm^2\right) = Cardiac\ output\left(\frac{L}{min}\right) \div \sqrt{Peak\text{-}to\text{-}peak\ or\ Mean\ gradient}$$

MVA, mitral valve area; AVA, aortic valve area; DFP, diastolic filling period (the period of opening to closure of the mitral valve); SEP, systolic ejection period (the period from opening to closure of the aortic valve); HR, heart rate (beats/min)

---

[a]Herrmann J. Cardiac Catherization. In: Zipes DP, Libby P, Bonow RO, Mann DL, Tomaselli GF, eds. Braunwald's Heart Disease A Textbook of Cardiovascular Medicine. 11th ed. Philadelphia: Elsevier; 2018:348–373.

---

appearance with a second peak in diastole that represents the reflected wave from the LA.

Chronic compensated mitral regurgitation is characterized by mild-to-moderate left ventricular dilatation with normal to elevated ejection fraction and normal filling pressures. With decompensation, the LV dilates further, LVEDP rises, and over time the LV ejection fraction falls (see also Chapter 6).

Left ventricular angiography with assessment of the density of contrast leaking to the LA is the most accurate invasive method of assessing the grade of mitral regurgitation. A relatively large injection should be used through a 6F catheter and care should be taken to avoid ectopy and entrapment of the mitral valve apparatus by the catheter. Mitral valve regurgitation severity can be graded as follows[23]:

1 + Contrast enters LA and clears with each beat
2 + Faint filling of entire LA but remains less dense as compared to LV

3 + Complete opacification of LA with density equal to that of LV
4 + Complete filling of LA on the first beat with greater density than that of LV; evidence of contrast in the pulmonary veins

Mixed Mitral Valve Disease

In the presence of combined chronic mitral regurgitation and stenosis, the hemodynamic findings are influenced by the compliance of the LA and LV and the degree of remodeling of the LV in response to the extra volume load from the mitral regurgitation.

The LAP in mixed mitral valve disease is usually significantly elevated with a prominent v wave followed by a slow long y descent reflecting the delayed emptying of blood into the ventricle caused by the stenotic component of the valve. The v wave is usually significantly greater than the a wave. As described earlier for MS, the contribution of atrial contraction to left ventricular filling is reduced and the *a* wave may not be reflected in the LVEDP tracing. The latter usually mirrors that encountered in isolated mitral regurgitation and depends on the stage of ventricular remodeling and compliance. Pulmonary venous hypertension is common, while the reactive obliterative pulmonary arteriopathy encountered in isolated longstanding MS is infrequent.[24]

Aortic Valve Disease

Echocardiography has almost entirely replaced cardiac catheterization in the diagnosis of aortic valve disease. The AHA/ACC guidelines recommend cardiac catheterization be reserved for patients with nondiagnostic echocardiography or when there is discordance between clinical findings and echocardiogram.[19]

Aortic Stenosis

At cardiac catheterization, assessment of the severity of aortic stenosis (AS) starts with identifying the density of calcification of the aortic valve, especially in degenerative aortic valve disease. AS severity is assessed by measuring the LV to aorta (LV-Ao) gradient. This could be done by having two arterial access points, with a pigtail catheter in the LV and another end-hole catheter in the aorta. Double-lumen catheters (Langston catheter, Vascular solutions, USA) can be used to measure the LV-Ao gradient simultaneously using single arterial access (Fig. 7.3). However, pull-back gradients using a single catheter are used in most cardiac catheterization labs. Care should be taken in the interpretation of pull-back gradients in the presence of atrial fibrillation because of the beat-to-beat variation in the SV and potential for over- or under-estimation of the gradient. Similarly, the use of the LV-femoral artery (LV-FA) pressure gradient as a surrogate for the LV-Ao gradient may be unreliable due to systolic peripheral arterial pressure amplification. The peak instantaneous echocardiographic gradient and the catheter mean gradient should be used for comparison/correlation of the two modalities.

Crossing the aortic valve from the aorta carries an increased risk of silent and clinically apparent strokes, particularly when the aortic valve is heavily calcified. Hence, it should be done only when necessary, for example, if echocardiographic assessment is judged unreliable.[41] There is no consensus on the optimal catheter and wire selection used to cross the aortic valve. Many operators favor the Amplatzer right 2 or Amplatzer left 1 with a straight tip guidewire (Terumo, Japan). In particularly difficult cases, an aortic root angiogram before crossing the valve may help to identify the location of the critical stenotic valve lumen, which also allows assessment of the degree of coexisting aortic regurgitation (AR).

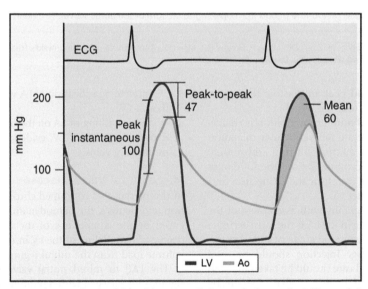

FIG. 7.3 There are various methods of describing an aortic transvalvular gradient. The peak-to-peak gradient (47 mmHg) is the difference between the maximal pressure in the LV and the maximal Ao pressure. The peak instantaneous gradient (100 mmHg) is the maximal pressure difference between the LV and Ao when the pressures are measured in the same moment (usually during early systole). The mean gradient (green shaded area) is the integral of the pressure difference between the LV and Ao during systole (60mmHg). (Reproduced with permission from Bashore.[54])

Once the gradients (peak-to-peak, mean and peak instantaneous gradients) have been measured (Fig. 7.3), the AV area (AVA) is traditionally calculated using the Gorlin formula and/or Hakki formula (Box 7.2). Some of the pitfalls associated with AV area calculation are the presence of AR, aorto-iliac stenosis, and peripheral amplification of systolic pressure. When the CO or SV index is low, the AVA may be falsely low as in low-flow, low-gradient AS (see Chapter 6). Hence, the LV-Ao gradient is commonly used to assess the severity of AS rather than AV area in the catheterization lab.

Characteristic findings of severe AS include a slow-rising and delayed upstroke on the aortic pressure trace (pulsus parvus et tardus), a large gradient between the LV and aorta, and elevated LV filling pressures with a rapid rise in the slope of diastolic filling tracing. Caraballo's sign, characterized by a rise in systolic aortic pressure by >5 mmHg compared to the LV pressure when the pigtail catheter is pulled back to the aorta, is a useful marker of severity when present.[42]

Aortic Regurgitation

The most frequently observed hemodynamic abnormality in patients with AR is low aortic diastolic pressure due to peripheral runoff, resulting in a wide pulse pressure. The pulse wave produced by LV ejection and the reflected wave, which are prominent in AR, summate in peripheral arteries. In some patients this may lead to a higher peripheral systolic pressure compared to the central aortic pressure, detected as a double peaked carotid waves (pulsus bisferiens—Fig. 7.4).

In severe AR, there may be a small apparent gradient or "aortic stenosis" created by high CO across a normal aortic valve area. The severity of AR is also assessed by a visual angiographic grading system proposed by Sellers[43] and by the regurgitant fraction method (Box 7.3).[44] Other less frequently used methods are a

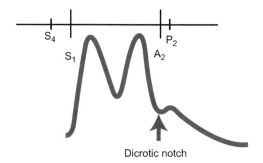

FIG. 7.4 Pulsus bisferiens in severe aortic regurgitation.

> **BOX 7.3**
> **The Sellers Grading System for Aortic Regurgitation[a].[43]**
>
> **Mild AR**: contrast cleared from the LV by next systole.
> **Moderate AR**: contrast does not cause complete opacification of the LV and it is cleared within three cardiac cycles.
> **Moderate-to-severe AR**: AR causes complete opacification of the LV with clearance within three cardiac cycles.
> **Severe AR**: opacification of the LV is greater than the aorta and it takes greater than three cardiac cycles to clear.

LV, left ventricle; AR, aortic regurgitation
[a]Based on visual estimation of the clearance of contrast from the LV with each beat and the degree of opacification of the LV

regurgitant fraction method that assesses the difference between the total SV and the forward SV.[44]

Tricuspid Valve Disease

Secondary functional tricuspid regurgitation (TR) is much more prevalent than primary rheumatic tricuspid disease. Right heart catheterization in patients with TR shows an attenuated x descent with a prominent cv wave (S wave) in the presence of severe tricuspid regurgitation.[49] If the TR is severe, it may lead to ventricularization of the right atrial waveform.

Isolated rheumatic tricuspid stenosis is extremely rare. It is almost always associated with rheumatic MS. The presence of tricuspid stenosis may mask the symptoms produced by MS. Right heart catheterization shows a prominent a wave with presence of an RA–RV gradient. Due to the presence of low chamber pressures with larger tricuspid valve sizes, the observed gradient in patients with tricuspid stenosis is mostly between 2 and 12 mmHg. Although a mean gradient >2 mmHg between the RA and RV is diagnostic of tricuspid stenosis, a mean gradient of ≥5 mmHg results in symptomatic obstruction, warranting intervention.[50] Similar to MS, Gorlin's formula could be used to calculate valve area. It is less validated for tricuspid stenosis compared to MS. In the presence of combined tricuspid and mitral stenosis, MS should be addressed first to avoid possible pulmonary edema due to unrestricted blood flow from the opened up tricuspid valve. An Inoue balloon is commonly used to cross the tricuspid valve. An algorithm has been proposed for RV entry from the RA using the Inoue balloon that may be used to complete tricuspid valvuloplasty after PMBC to complete the procedure safely.[51]

CATHETHER-BASED INTERVENTIONS IN RHEUMATIC HEART DISEASE

Mitral Stenosis

Percutaneous mitral balloon commissurotomy

The first surgical procedure for MS, a closed mitral commissurotomy, was first described in 1923 by Dr Elliot Cutler.[53] Open mitral commissurotomy replaced the initial technique in view of better outcomes in the early 1970s after the development of cardiopulmonary bypass (see Chapter 8). The concept of percutaneous balloon inflation of a stenosed mitral valve was first introduced by a cardiac surgeon, Kanji Inoue, in 1982.[26] The advent of percutaneous mitral balloon commissurotomy (PMBC), also called PTMC (percutaneous transvenous mitral commissurotomy) or PMBV (percutaneous mitral balloon valvuloplasty), has since revolutionized the management of rheumatic MS. Subsequently, use of a cylindrical balloon or double balloon was also introduced, but Inoue's single balloon method remains the most popular method in most parts of the world. PMBC shares a similar mechanism to the abandoned closed mitral commissurotomy.

Indications for Percutaneous Mitral Balloon Commissurotomy. Choosing the right patient remains the most important part of the procedure and involves good echocardiographic assessment of disease severity and valve morphology. The AHA/ACC guidelines recommend PMBC in any symptomatic patient with severe MS (MVA <1.5 cm^2) with suitable valve morphology in the absence of contraindications (Class I).[19] PMBC may also be attempted in patients who do not have suitable valve morphology but are considered high-risk surgical candidates (Class IIb). Asymptomatic patients with very severe MS (MVA $\leq$ 1 cm^2) with favorable valve morphology and in the absence of contraindications are also candidates for PMBC (Class IIa). Asymptomatic patients with PA hypertension or new onset atrial fibrillation may also be considered for PMBC (Class IIb).[19] See Chapter 6 for further details on the indications for PMBC and cardiac surgery in MS.

The Wilkins score is the most widely used grading of mitral valve echocardiographic morphologic features in the setting of MS to assess likelihood of a successful result following PMBC.[27] It assigns a score of 1–4 for each of the following: (1) valve calcification, (2) leaflet mobility, (3) leaflet thickening, and (4) subvalvular thickening (see Chapter 5, Table 5.5). A score of eight or less with less than moderate mitral regurgitation is considered suitable for performing PMBC. Other simpler scoring systems include the lung and Cormier score that integrate calcification as identified by fluoroscopy.[28] The success

of a PMBC procedure depends upon the pliability of the leaflets (especially the anterior mitral valve leaflet) and the severity of degeneration and calcification of the mitral valve and the subvalvular apparatus. It is important to rule out left atrial thrombus by transoesophageal echocardiography (TEE) as it remains an important contraindication for PMBC. If a clot is visualized, the patient should be adequately anticoagulated for a minimum of 6 weeks and reviewed again for left atrial thrombus before the procedure. Other contraindications to the procedure include (1) moderate or greater mitral regurgitation, (2) massive or bicommissural calcification, (3) severe aortic or tricuspid valve involvement requiring surgical intervention, and (4) severe concomitant CAD requiring surgery.

Percutaneous Mitral Balloon Commissurotomy Technique. Femoral access (5 French arterial access and 79 French venous access) is the standard site for performing PMBC. A simple formula is commonly used to calculate the balloon size based on the height of the patient (height [cm]/10 + 10), or sizing can be done directly by measuring the annular diameter in the apical 2-chamber view on the echocardiogram.[29] Alternatively, the commissural diameter of the mitral valve can be measured directly by echocardiography (maximal commissural diameter in the fully opened state in diastole on short axis view).[30] The Inoue balloon catheter (Toray, Tokyo, Japan) has special inflation characteristics that allow for optimal effect. The balloon has three components: the distal part inflates first followed by the proximal part, both by pressure inflation with a syringe. The middle waist part is the least compliant part and is last to inflate.

Before the PMBC, a right heart catheterization is often done first to allow for accurate hemodynamic assessment of the mitral valve gradient and area, as described earlier. Transseptal access is then gained with a Brockenbrough needle using fluoroscopic guidance in the AP (anteroposterior), RAO (right anterior oblique), and left lateral views, while a pigtail (via arterial access) remains in the noncoronary sinus to mark the location of the aortic root. TEE-guided transseptal access under conscious sedation is gaining in popularity as it allows for safe direct visualization of the puncture.[31] After femoral vein access, a Brockenbrough needle sheathed in Mullins sheath and dilator is placed in the superior vena cava and then pulled down slowly across the right atrium (RA) until the needle reaches the fossa ovalis in the AP view (here the tip is approximately one vertebral space below the location of the pigtail tip). The needle is then positioned with clockwise rotation in the lateral view until the tip faces posteriorly midway between the vertebral column and the tip of the pigtail catheter. The septal puncture is a critical step of the whole procedure. Accurate fossa ovalis puncture reduces the risk of perforation through the walls of either atria and the aorta and facilitates entry of the Inoue balloon into the LV. Once the optimal site is confirmed in multiple views, the Brockenbrough needle can be pushed across the septum into the LA. Entry into the LA can be confirmed by its characteristic pressure trace or by injecting a small amount of dye if there is doubt. The Mullins sheath and dilator are then advanced into the LA where the needle is safely removed and heparin is given to prevent thromboembolic complications.

Next, a coiled wire is inserted through the sheath into the LA and subcutaneous track in the groin and the atrial septum is then dilated using a septal dilator. The appropriately sized Inoue balloon catheter with its straight stylet is then introduced over the coil wire into the LA. The straight stylet is then removed and a loop is created in the balloon catheter in such a way that the tip faces toward the mitral valve. The coil wire is removed and a J-tipped stylet is introduced into the balloon catheter. The balloon is filled with $1-2$ mL of diluted contrast (1:4) so that the balloon faces toward the left ventricular inflow. The RAO view should be used for LV entry to ensure that the balloon catheter is well aligned with the LV axis. After LV entry, free movement of the balloon over the J stylet should be ensured using "the accordion maneuver" to prevent trapping of the balloon in the subvalvular apparatus. The distal balloon is then inflated and deformation of the balloon is carefully looked for. If there is any deformation suggestive of trapping in the subvalvular apparatus, the balloon inflation should be stopped, the balloon withdrawn back into the LA, and LV entry reattempted. If the distal balloon inflates well, the balloon catheter is pulled back into the valve until it gives a tug. Then, the inflation is completed with dilatation of the proximal and the middle part of the balloon resulting in mitral valve dilatation. The time period of dilatation should be kept as short as possible (dilatation followed by immediate deflation) due to the fall in CO while the balloon is in an inflated position. After balloon dilatation, the degree of success should be assessed by measuring the postcommissurotomy LAP and transvalvular gradient or planimetered estimation of the MVA. At this stage, one should carefully look at the LAP trace for mitral regurgitation, which is marked by a rise rather than a fall in the height of the v wave with or without a fall in the mean LAP.

Depending on the initial hemodynamic (gradient) and stenotic severity of MS, there are several measures of post-PMBC procedural success. These include, a postprocedure MVA >1.5 cm^2, a doubling of the preprocedure MVA, and a decrease in the preprocedure transvalvular gradient by $>50\%$. It may be useful to select the most severe measure of severity and apply the measure of success that best applies to it. For example, if the preprocedure MVA is 1.4 cm^2 and the gradient is 12 mmHg, reducing the gradient by $>50\%$ is a more valuable measure than get a postprocedure MVA to 1.6 cm^2, while the mean gradient remains well above 6 mmHg. If the dilatation is deemed unsuccessful, a second dilatation can be repeated if there is no mitral regurgitation. Echocardiographic assessment of valve area using the pressure half time method is unreliable immediately after PMBC due to rapidly changing left atrial compliance characteristics.[32]

Complications of Percutaneous Mitral Balloon Commissurotomy. The most common complication of the procedure is hemopericardium (0%−2% of cases), which may lead to cardiac tamponade.[33] This commonly occurs when the Brockenbrough needle accidently punctures the posterior wall of the RA, and rarely with manipulation of the coil wire or the balloon catheter in the left atrial appendage, a pulmonary vein, or left ventricular apex. Tamponade is managed with pericardiocentesis (pigtail drainage) and reversal of anticoagulation. The other common complication is mitral regurgitation, which in most cases is mild-to-moderate in severity and does not need any further intervention. Severe mitral regurgitation requiring intervention ranges from 1.4% to 9.4%.[34,35] Thromboembolic complications are best prevented by the early use of heparin. However, when they do occur their management should be dictated by the site of embolization and resources available.

Outcomes Following Percutaneous Mitral Balloon Commissurotomy. Significant improvement in functional status and quality of life has been reported after successful PMBC, with the best results reported in younger patients with favorable valvular anatomical characteristics. Survival without the need for reintervention and with good functional capacity is reported to be approximately 90% at 5−7 years after a successful PMBC procedure.[36,37] These results are similar to open mitral commissurotomy[38] and superior to closed mitral commissurotomy.[36] Event-free survival of up to 79% at 10 years and 43% at 15 years has been described in some cohorts[39,40] In the same series, freedom from restenosis was 85% at 5 years, 70% at 10 years, and 44% at 15 years. In the case of restenosis, a repeat PMBC is an option if the anatomy remains suitable. The factors favoring long-term prognosis include the presence of favorable anatomy initially, a successful procedure, a higher MVA achieved immediately after the procedure, and absence of significant mitral regurgitation.

Interventions in Rheumatic Aortic Valve Disease

Isolated AS due to RHD is relatively rare.[45] The preferred treatment of choice for patients with severe rheumatic AS, with or without other valve disease, is surgical aortic valve replacement. To date, there are no long-term catheter-based solutions for rheumatic aortic valve disease, in part due to the pliable nature of the aortic annulus.[46] Before the transcutaneous aortic valve implantation (TAVI) era (see Chapter 6), valvuloplasty for AS (widening of the stenotic AV using a balloon catheter inside the valve) was associated with high complication rates, with mortality up to 15% at 24 h and serious complications in up to 25% of patients, and was largely abandoned as a primary therapy for AS of all etiologies.[47] Aortic valvuloplasty for rheumatic AS is not recommended outside of clinical scenarios where patients are in hemodynamic trouble and the valvuloplasty is used as a bridge to aortic valve surgery.[48] Moreover, rheumatic AS is a relative contraindication to the procedure. Some elderly patients who present with "degenerative" AS may have a history of acute rheumatic fever and echocardiographic evidence for rheumatic AS (e.g., commissural fusion), in addition to marked calcific degeneration of the valve. The treatment algorithms in such patients would be as for degenerative disease.[46]

CONCLUSION

Diagnostic cardiac catheterization is rarely indicated in patients with rheumatic valvular heart disease in the modern era, but should still be regarded as the gold standard investigation where echocardiographic findings are discordant with the clinical picture. Diagnostic cardiac catheterization requires specific knowledge and skill as outlined in this chapter. The interventional cardiologist must also possess the skills to perform PMBC for the treatment of rheumatic MS. PMBC remains the procedure of choice for the management of severe rheumatic MS with suitable valvular anatomy. Isolated rheumatic tricuspid stenosis can also be successfully treated by balloon tricuspid valvuloplasty. The role of percutaneous interventions remains less well established for other rheumatic valvular lesions such as rheumatic mitral regurgitation and AS. There is a need to improve the availability of cardiac catheterization services, to address the unmet need in developing countries. An evaluation of the extent of the problem should be undertaken similar to cardiac surgical descriptions of the worldwide unmet need for cardiac surgery for RHD.[3,4]

REFERENCES

1. Pepine C, Hill JA, Lambert CR, eds. *Diagnostic and Therapeutic Cardiac Catheterization*. 3rd ed. Baltimore: Williams & Wilkins; 1998.
2. Rahimtoolah SH. The need for cardiac catheterization and angiography in valvular heart disease is *not* disproven. *Ann Intern Med*. 1982;97:433–439.
3. Reichert HA, Rath TE. Cardiac surgery in developing countries. *J Extra Corpor Technol*. 2017;49:98–106.
4. Zilla P, Bolman RM, Yacoub MH, et al. The Cape Town declaration on access to cardiac surgery in the developing world. *Cardiovasc J Afr*. 2018;29(4):256–259.
5. Kendrick AH, West J, Papouchado M, Rozkovec A. Direct Fick cardiac output: are assumed values of oxygen consumption acceptable? *Eur Heart J*. 1988;9:337.
6. DeRossa S, Torella D, Caiazzo G, et al. Left radial access for percutaneous coronary procedures: from neglected to performer? A meta-analysis of 14 studies including 7603 procedures. *Int J Cardiol*. 2014;171(1):66–72.
7. Callan P, Clark AL. Right heart catheterization: indications and interpretation. *Heart*. 2016;102:1–11.
8. Jensen LA, Onyskiw JE, Prasad NG. Meta-analysis of arterial oxygen saturation monitoring by pulse oximetry in adults. *Heart Lung*. 1998;27(6):387–408.
9. Fares WH, Blanchard SK, Stouffer GA, et al. Thermodilution and Fick cardiac outputs differ: impact on pulmonary hypertension evaluation. *Can Respir J*. 2012;19(4):261–266.
10. Thomassen B. Cardiac output in normal subjects under standard conditions: the repeatability of measurements by the Fick method. *Scand J Clin Lab Investig*. 1957;9:365.
11. Lange RA, Moore Jr DM, Cigarroa RG, Hillis LD. Use of pulmonary capillary wedge pressure to assess severity of mitral stenosis: is true left atrial pressure needed in this condition? *J Am Coll Cardiol*. 1989;13:825–831.
12. Nishimura RA, Rihal CS, Tajik AJ, Holmes Jr DR. Accurate measurement of transmitral gradient in patients with mitral stenosis : a simultaneous catheterization and Doppler echocardiography. *J Am Coll Cardiol*. 1994;24:152.
13. Walston A, Kendall ME. Comparison of pulmonary wedge and left atrial pressure in man. *Am Heart J*. 1973;86:159–164.
14. Prioli A, Marino P, Lanzoni L, et al. Increasing degrees of left ventricular filling impairment modulate left atrial function in humans. *Am J Cardiol*. 1998;82:756–761.
15. Meisner JS, Keren G, Pajaro OE, et al. Atrial contribution to ventricular filling in mitral stenosis. *Circulation*. 1991;84: 1469–1480.
16. Karthikeyan G. The value of rhythm control in mitral stenosis. *Heart*. 2006;92:1013–1016.
17. Naeije R, Vachiery JL, Yerly P, Vanderpool R. The transpulmonary pressure gradient for the diagnosis of pulmonary vascular disease. *Eur Respir J*. 2013;41:217–223.
18. Gorlin R, Gorlin SG. Hydraulic formula for calculation of the area of the stenotic mitral valve, other cardiac valves, and central circulatory shunts. *Am Heart J*. 1951;41:1–29.

19. Nishimura RA, Otto CM, Bonow RO, et al. AHA/ACC guideline for the management of patients with valvular heart disease. *J Am Coll Cardiol.* 2014;63(22):e57–e185.
20. Hakki AH, Iskandrian AS, Bemis CE, et al. A simplified formula for the calculation of stenotic cardiac valve areas. *Circulation.* 1981;63:1050–1055.
21. Braunwald E, Awe WV. The syndrome of severe mitral regurgitation with normal left atrial pressure. *Circulation.* 1963;27:31.
22. Feldman T, Grossman W. Valvular heart disease. In: Baim D, ed. *Grossman's Cardiac Catheterization, Angiography and Intervention.* 7th ed. Philadelphia, PA: Lipincott Williams and Wilkins; 2006:637–659.
23. Otto C. *Valvular Heart Disease.* Vol. 2. Saunders an Imprint of Elsevier; 2004:404–405.
24. *Hemodynamic Rounds. Interpretatoni of Cardiac Pathophysiology from Pressure Waveform Analysis:* Morton J Kern, MD.
25. Harken DE, Dexter L, Ellis LB, Farrand RE, Dickson III JF. The surgery of mitral stenosis: III: finger-fracture valvuloplasty. *Ann Surg.* 1951;134:722–742.
26. Inoue K, Owaki T, Nakamura T, Kitamura F, Miyamoto N. Clinical application of transvenous mitral commissurotomy by a new balloon catheter. *J Thorac Cardiovasc Surg.* 1984;87:394–402.
27. Wilkins GT, Weyman AE, Abascal VM, Block PC, Palacios IF. Percutaneous balloon dilatation of the mitral valve: an analysis of echocardiographic variables related to outcome and the mechanism of dilatation. *Br Heart J.* 1988;60:299–308.
28. Iung B, Cormier B, Ducimetiere P, et al. Immediate results of percutaneous mitral commissurotomy: a predictive model on a series of 1514 patients. *Circulation.* 1996;94: 2124–2130.
29. Lau KW, Hung JS. A simple balloon-sizing method in Inoue-balloon percutaneous transvenous mitral commissurotomy. *Cathet Cardiovasc Diagn.* 1994;33:120–129.
30. Sanati HR, Kiavar M, Salehi N, et al. Percutaneous mitral valvuloplasty—a new method for balloon sizing based on maximal commissural diameter to improve procedural results. *Am Heart Hosp J.* 2010;8(1):29–32.
31. Chiang CW, Huang HL, Ko YS. Echocardiography-guided balloon mitral valvotomy: transesophageal echocardiography versus intracardiac echocardiography. *J Heart Valve Dis.* 2007;16:596–601.
32. Thomas JD, Wilkins GT, Choong CY, et al. Inaccuracy of mitral pressure half-time immediately after percutaneous mitral valvotomy. Dependence on transmitral gradient and left atrial and ventricular compliance. *Circulation.* 1988;78:980–993.
33. Martinez-rios MA, Tovar S, Luna J, Eid-Lidt G. Percutaneous mitral commissurotomy. *Cardiol. Rev.* 1999;7: 108–116.
34. Chen CR, Cheng TO. Percutaneous balloon mitral valvuloplasty by the Inoue technique: a multicenter study of 4832 patients in China. *Am Heart J.* 1995;129:1197–1203.
35. Palacios IF, Sanchez PL, Harrell LC, Weyman AE, Block PC. Which patients benefit from percutaneous mitral balloon valvuloplasty? Prevalvuloplasty and postvalvuloplasty variables that predict long-term outcome. *Circulation.* 2002; 105:1465–1471.
36. Ben Farhat M, Ayari M, Maatouk F, et al. Percutaneous balloon versus surgical closed and open mitral commissurotomy: seven-year follow-up results of a randomized trial. *Circulation.* 1998;97:245–250.
37. Arora R, Kalra GS, Singh S, et al. Percutaneous transvenous mitral commissurotomy: immediate and long-term follow-up results. *Cathet Cardiovasc Interv.* 2002;55:450–456.
38. Reyes VP, Raju BS, Wynne J, et al. Percutaneous balloon valvuloplasty compared with open surgical commissurotomy for mitral stenosis. *N Engl J Med.* 1994;331: 961–967.
39. Fawzy ME, Shoukri M, Al Buraiki J, et al. Seventeen years' clinical and echocardiographic follow up of mitral balloon valvuloplasty in 520 patients, and predictors of long-term outcome. *J Heart Valve Dis.* 2007;16:454–460.
40. Fawzy ME, Shoukri M, Hassan W, Nambiar V, Stefadouros M, Canver CC. The impact of mitral valve morphology on the long-term outcome of mitral balloon valvuloplasty. *Cathet Cardiovasc Interv.* 2007;69:40–46.
41. Omran H, Schmidt H, Hackenbroch M, et al. Silent and apparent cerebral embolism after retrograde catheterisation of the aortic valve in valvular stenosis: a prospective, randomised study. *Lancet Lond Engl.* 2003;361(9365): 1241–1246.
42. Carabello BA, Barry WH, Grossman W. Changes in arterial pressure during left heart pullback in patients with aortic stenosis: a sign of severe aortic stenosis. *Am J Cardiol.* 1979;44(3):424–427.
43. Sellers RD, Levy MJ, Amplatz K, Lillehei CW. Left retrograde cardioangiography in acquired cardiac disease: technic, indications and interpretations in 700 cases. *Am J Cardiol.* 1964;14:437–447.
44. Baim DS. *Grossman's Cardiac Catheterization, Angiography, and Intervention.* Lippincott Williams & Wilkins; 2006, 846 pp.
45. Zühlke L, Karthikeyan G, Engel ME, et al. Clinical outcomes in 3343 children and adults with rheumatic heart disease from 14 low- and middle-income countries: two-year follow-up of the global rheumatic heart disease registry (the REMEDY study). *Circulation.* 2016;134(19): 1456–1466.
46. Ntsekhe M, Scherman J. TAVI for rheumatic aortic stenosis – the next frontier? *Int J Cardiol.* 2019;280:51–52.
47. NHLBI Balloon Valvuloplasty Registry Participants. Percutaneous balloon aortic valvuloplasty: acute and 30-day follow-up results in 674 patients from the NHLBI balloon valvuloplasty registry. *Circulation.* 1991;84(6): 2383–2397.
48. Baumgartner H, Falk V, Bax JJ, et al. ESC/EACTS guidelines for the management of valvular heart disease. *Eur Heart J.* 2017;38(36):2739–2791, 2017.
49. Senguttuvan NB, Karthikeyan G. Jugular venous C-V wave in severe tricuspid regurgitation. *N Engl J Med.* 2012 Jan 12; 366(2):e5.

50. Ewy GA. Tricuspid valve disease. In: Alpert J, Rahimtoola S, Dalen J, Valvular, eds. *Heart Disease*. 3rd ed. Lippincott Williams & Williams; 2000:377–392.

51. Bhargava B, Mathur A, Chandra S, Bahl VK. A simple algorithm: reply to the letter to the editor by Tejas Patel et al. *Cathet Cardiovasc Diagn*. 1997;40(3):334.

52. Herrmann J. Cardiac Catherization. In: Zipes DP, Libby P, Bonow RO, Mann DL, Tomaselli GF, eds. *Braunwald's Heart Disease A Textbook of Cardiovascular Medicine*. 11th edition. Philadelphia: Elsevier; 2018:348–373.

53. Cutler EC, Levine SA. Cardiotomy and valvulotomy for mitral stenosis: experimental observations and clinical notes concerning an operated case with recovery. *Bost Med Surg J*. 1923;188(26):1023–1027.

54. Bashore TM. *Invasive Cardiology: Principles and Techniques*. Philadelphia, BC Decker. 1990.

CHAPTER 8

Surgical Management of Rheumatic Valvular Heart Disease

MANUEL J. ANTUNES • KIRSTEN FINUCANE • A. SAMPATH KUMAR • GONÇALO F. COUTINHO

INTRODUCTION

New cases of acute rheumatic fever (ARF) have almost disappeared from most high-income countries (HICs), where rheumatic heart disease (RHD) is now a remnant of the past and usually only seen in the older population where it does not represent a problem significantly different from that of other etiologies of valve disease. By contrast, RHD remains an important health burden in low- and middle-income countries (LMICs), especially those in Asia, Oceania, Africa, and South America. A significant percentage of RHD patients eventually require surgery, mainly in young patients with a mean age of 20–25 years, although surgery is sometimes required in children less than 10 years old. Otherwise, patients may present in middle age or older with end-stage chronic rheumatic valvular heart disease, which is more characteristic of middle-high income countries.[1]

In the absence of recurrent ARF, the prognosis for those with mild and even moderate RHD is good.[2,3] However, continued medical management alone is insufficient for those with severe RHD. Those with severe functional valvular changes and dilated ventricles experience progressive cardiac deterioration over time (see Chapter 6). The major sequelae of chronic severe RHD includes infective endocarditis, atrial fibrillation, systolic and/or diastolic heart failure, thromboembolism, and secondary pulmonary hypertension. Timely and appropriately performed surgery and perioperative care will be required. This is frequently hindered because of delayed presentation or recognition, late referral, poor access to tertiary cardiac services, prohibitive cost, inadequate logistical or political support, and lack of long-term care and follow-up.

Cardiac surgery requires a complex infrastructure and the skills of a multidisciplinary team. In a significant number of LMICs, especially in Africa, these cardiac surgical facilities are either not available or are unable to cope with the very large demand.[4] The ratio of cardiac surgery centers per million inhabitants in subSaharan Africa (excluding South Africa) is 1:33, well below the ratio of 1:1 in Europe.[5] Even in better-developed countries, such as in India and other Southern Asian countries, the disease remains a significant health system burden. Outcomes for severe RHD are also reflected by the wealth of the country. In Ethiopia the mean age of death is 25 years,[6] in Fiji it is 37 years,[7] and in New Zealand 55 years.[8]

In sites with limited resources, there is frequently competition with congenital heart diseases, which may receive preferential case selection by the surgical teams. Surgery for congenital heart disease tends to be offered to children originating from wealthier population groups who have better access to healthcare, whereas rheumatic patients more often originate from poorer sectors of the population with poorer access and less advocacy for healthcare.

There may have been an improvement in these inequities in the 21st century. This has in part been driven by the efforts of humanitarian missions taking place in LMICs, some with a considerable degree of success leading to well-established local surgical facilities and teams. Nevertheless, there is still much to do, and unfortunately the economic development of LMICs is not sufficient to offset the shortcomings discussed earlier.

HISTORICAL BACKGROUND

In 1923, Dr. Elliott Cutler of the Peter Bent Brigham Hospital performed the world's first successful heart valve surgery—a closed mitral commissurotomy (CMC)—in a 12-year-old girl with rheumatic mitral stenosis (MS).[9] However, consistent clinical application was initiated only much later, in the 1940s and 1950s, initially by the "finger-fracture" technique via left thoracotomy and left atrial (LA) appendage, later advanced by Logan in 1959[10] with the development of the Tubbs mechanical dilator. Several modifications of the initial technique were since proposed, including right chest and transsternal approaches.

With the advent of open-heart surgery, CMC was progressively abandoned in favor of the open mitral commissurotomy (OMC) approach, initiated in the late 1950s and early 1960s. This method provides better visualization of the mitral valve apparatus and a more precisely directed commissurotomy, as well as improved techniques to repair the chordae tendinae and papillary muscles, when involved. However, CMC is still performed in many parts of the world today, particularly in LMICs and remote areas, as it remains a low-risk and inexpensive approach. It is also applicable to pregnant women and to patients with restenosis.

Finally, percutaneous mitral balloon commissurotomy (PMBC) was introduced by Inoue in 1984, and surgical mitral commissurotomy, both CMC and OMC, progressively has become a rarity in most technically advanced surgical centers, because the valves amenable to commissural split were treated by PMBC. Some surgeons rapidly lost the capability (and the will) to preserve more complex stenotic mitral valves.

A major development in the management of RHD was the introduction of valve replacement surgery. Aortic valve replacement with a mechanical valve prostheses was introduced by Albert Starr in 1961.[11] Dwight Harken pioneered mitral valve replacement in 1962,[12] which permitted treatment of valves with complex pathology not amenable to mitral commissurotomy or other type of repair. Stimulated by early beliefs of a simple and durable therapy for all kinds of mitral valve pathology, valve replacement became the most common procedure for the treatment of rheumatic mitral valve disease, even in developing countries. It is still generally thought to be less complicated surgically than repair and have a more predictable outcome.

Bioprostheses were introduced later, in the late 1960s, by Carpentier and others, ostensibly to avoid the thromboembolic complications of mechanical valves. However, it soon became clear that durability due to degeneration of the tissues was limited, especially in younger patients. It is now evident that mitral valve replacement with a mechanical or bioprosthetic valve has increased morbidity and mortality in the young compared to mitral valve repair. RHD patients often originate from endemic populations that are less educated, more disempowered, and largely nonadherent to care. In these settings, repeat surgery in those patients with previous mechanical or biological valves has a higher operative mortality because events tend to be more acute and catastrophic. Hence, the attention turned back to valve conservation procedures.

In the surgical treatment for aortic valve disease, the same considerations apply, although the incidence of prosthetic valve complications is lower. Perhaps, this can be attributed to the higher flow velocity in the left ventricular outflow tract, thus reducing the risk of thrombotic complications and requiring less intensive anticoagulation. Recently, percutaneous implantation of aortic and pulmonary heart valves has evolved. Percutaneous mitral valve implantation remains in the developmental stage,[13] and these techniques are generally unavailable in rheumatic-endemic regions due to lack of facilities and exceptionally high costs.

Lillehei initiated repair for mitral regurgitation (MR) in 1957, but it was the efforts of Carpentier, Duran, and others, in the late 1960s, that made it more scientific and broadened its applicability. However, repair for rheumatic mitral valve disease, beyond CMC or OMC, did not gain widespread acceptance in this era. The ongoing inflammatory process, which leads to scarring of the valve structures, was a limiting factor of long-term durability. The complex technical issues made repair unappealing in these patients, given the involvement of the entire mitral valve apparatus with fibrosis, thickening, shortening, and subsequent appearance of areas of calcification.

Nonetheless, Chauvaud et al., in 2001, claimed excellent results in an adult group of 951 patients, mostly rheumatic, who underwent mitral valve (MV) repair using Carpentier techniques (4% during the acute rheumatic phase) from 1970 to 1994. These included the following: annuloplasty (95%); chordal shortening (75%); chordal transfer (10%); chord resection (7%); pericardial leaflet extension (7.5%); or leaflet calcium stripping (5%).[14]

More recently, with the introduction of some technical modifications, better knowledge of the pathology and, above all, reports of excellent outcomes of mitral valve repair in comparison to replacement in other pathologies, especially degenerative mitral valve disease, led to renewed efforts by experienced surgeons to repair rheumatic pathology with a different eye. There are now widespread reports of excellent results of rheumatic mitral valve repair from multiple regions in the world.[15–28]

In summary, there has been considerable evolution of cardiac surgical techniques for valve surgery for severe RHD. Mitral valve repair is the hallmark of the competent rheumatic surgeon[29] but the unique features of rheumatic mitral valve disease mean that valve repair remains challenging. The remainder of the chapter describes in more detail specific rheumatic valve lesions and their surgical management.

ANATOMICAL FEATURES AND CLINICAL SPECTRUM OF SURGICAL RHEUMATIC HEART DISEASE

Mitral Valve Disease

The mitral valve is the commonest valve to require surgery in RHD. It is often the dominant lesion but in about 30% of cases there is also some aortic disease and in a further 15% of cases there is associated tricuspid valve disease.[30–32] Recurrent episodes of ARF result in cumulative damage to the mitral valve to a point where there is a significant impact on valve function. Disease pathologies vary by regions and age of presentation.[15,33] MR predominates in Oceania, and few children have advanced MS. Reports of MS are more common in children from India, Africa, and the Middle East due to later presentation after multiple rheumatic episodes and persistent inflammatory activity. Mixed MR and MS may be present.[34–36] By adulthood, MS becomes more prevalent throughout the world. The recent REMEDY study, which documented the pattern of native rheumatic valve disease in 2475 children and adults from across African and Asian countries, provides insight into contemporary patterns and presentation of RHD. Mixed aortic and mitral valve disease was the dominant lesion from the second decade onwards. Isolated MR was the most frequent lesion in those under 10 years old. Pure MS was seen more frequently from the third decade onwards, with the highest prevalence (14%) in the 71–80 year age group.[37]

The pathophysiology starts with annular dilatation and loss of the saddle shape of the mitral annulus.[38] Inflammatory softening of the chordae tendineae causes elongation of the chordal apparatus, particularly the longest chordae that are those leading to the anterior leaflet, although this elongation process can also involve the posterior leaflet chordae. These changes tend to predominantly affect the primary over the intermediate chords as they are thinner and more delicate, and eventually these chords can occasionally rupture. Chordal rupture leads to acute mitral regurgitation in patients with a first episode of ARF and, with a noncompliant LA, often leads to acute pulmonary edema (see Chapter 16).[39] Over the longer term, with recurrent episodes of ARF, there is retraction of the thick intermediate chords and this restricts the motion of both leaflets but seems to most commonly fix and retract the posterior leaflet, particularly at the P2 and P3 scallops.

Often, the restriction is more severe opposite the prolapsing anterior leaflet segment. The turbulent MR jet can cause fibrosis of the leaflet itself and the surrounding areas of the atrial wall. The edges of the leaflets that no longer coapt become thickened and rolled back. Loss of flexibility of the leaflet will impair the probability and durability of repair. In its most chronic state, these valves become grossly thickened with chordal apparatus that becomes matted together and so distorted that it is difficult to distinguish the apparatus from the leaflet itself.[16] The two leaflets fuse at the commissures, and fibrosis extends not just from the edges of the leaflet but all the way through the annulus. Eventually, a "fish-mouth" appearance of the valve occurs where there is very little free motion of either leaflet and just a fixed orifice that flaps in and out with systole and diastole but remains continuously open (Fig. 8.1). There is usually both severe MS and MR in this scenario that is no longer amenable to repair.

The patient with MR has an enlarged left ventricular end-diastolic dimension. The left ventricular end-systolic dimension (LVESD) is commonly well maintained with a normal left ventricular ejection fraction (LVEF). Over time, however, ventricular function starts to deteriorate with rising systolic dimensions and a falling LVEF. Ventricular dimensions should be normalized for body surface area in children.[17,40]

In the earlier stages, there can be severe regurgitation without symptoms. This is still a good stage at which to offer mitral valve repair if indicated by ventricular dimensions. Many such patients with severe asymptomatic MR are detected by echocardiographic screening programs.[41] The reader is also referred to Chapter 6 for a wider discussion on the indications for cardiac surgery for MR.

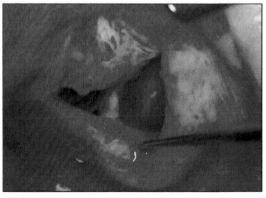

FIG. 8.1 Intraoperative view of a rheumatic mitral valve with a "fish-mouth" appearance resulting from severe generalized thickening of both leaflets and fusion of the commissures.

Aortic Valve Disease

Aortic valvular disease in the context of ARF can occur alone but is more commonly associated with at least mild mitral abnormalities.[31] The aortic leaflets soften and lose their elasticity during the acute inflammatory episode, and this causes the free edges of the leaflet to elongate. The longer the free edges get, the more prolapse can develop to the point where sometimes the free edges drop below the belly of the cusp. This often appears to affect one leaflet first that results in an asymmetric jet easily seen by echocardiography in the parasternal long axis view. At that point, repair is relatively straightforward as the other two leaflets can be almost normal in size and shape (Fig. 8.2).

In the longer term, however, the turbulent jet tends to create thickening at the leaflet edge and it then rolls back with loss of surface area of the leaflet. Additionally, the aortic regurgitation (AR) itself causes dilatation of the left ventricle and of the aortic annulus. As the annulus dilates, the surface of coaptation between the aortic leaflets deteriorates. Eventually, a triangular gap will appear in the center of the three leaflets that gradually enlarges. The typical chronic appearance of severe aortic rheumatic disease is a large triangular gap in the center of the aortic valve with all three leaflets appearing very shallow and retracted and with rolled edges.

As indicated earlier, the left ventricle gradually dilates with severe aortic regurgitation and both the diastolic and the systolic dimensions gradually increase with time. The LVEF usually remains normal but in a chronic state it deteriorates, particularly if there is combined aortic and mitral valve disease.[34,42] In those who present late with advanced disease, there is a risk that, even after combined surgery, left ventricular function will not return to normal and for that reason patients with combined aortic and mitral regurgitation should be treated more promptly than when there is single valve disease.[43]

However, during the acute phase of rheumatic carditis, mild and moderate AR can improve over time as the inflammatory markers settle. It is therefore reasonable to observe patients with combined disease carefully during the acute phase with the aim of avoiding acute aortic valve surgery.[31] Primary rheumatic aortic valve stenosis (AS) is rarely seen in RHD.

Tricuspid Valve Disease

Secondary tricuspid regurgitation (TR) is commonly seen in RHD patients and is usually secondary to severe mitral valve disease. Primary rheumatic tricuspid disease can occur as tricuspid stenosis, TR, or mixed valve disease. The pathological process of annular dilatation occurs primarily at the anterior and posterior portions of the annulus, corresponding to the right ventricular (RV) free wall.[44] The RV also dilates, which results in decreased leaflet apposition and further TR. TR is associated with, and allows assessment of, pulmonary hypertension. In the presence of severe TR, there is often significantly elevated right ventricular pressures and pulmonary hypertension.

Patients with more chronic and severe RHD have pathologic changes of the tricuspid valve that are similar to those which one finds on the mitral valve. Anterior and posterior leaflet chordae can be elongated significantly and septal leaflet chordae are retracted.[18] The leaflets themselves shrink, developing a thick rolled edge resulting in loss of leaflet area, and significant tricuspid valve stenosis occurs. Commonly, this involves the anterior leaflet that can be very difficult to correct if associated with a restricted septal leaflet that is held down against the right ventricular side of the basal ventricular septum.

Severe TR with pulmonary hypertension can result in the clinical scenario of a severely cachectic patient due to hepatic venous congestion leading to severe anorexia and vomiting. There is usually a severely dilated right atrium with associated atrial arrhythmias. The lungs may well be edematous in the context of left-sided valve disease, despite diuretics preoperatively. Patients with severe TR often have labile pulmonary artery pressures and pneumonias postoperatively.

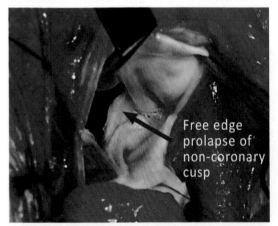

Free edge prolapse of non-coronary cusp

FIG. 8.2 Operative view of the aortic valve in a patient with severe aortic regurgitation, showing leaflet thickening, retraction, a central gap, and prolapse of the noncoronary cusp.

PREOPERATIVE DIAGNOSTIC WORK-UP

The roadmap to a precise diagnosis of RHD was developed in previous chapters of this book, in particular

Chapter 5. Here, we wish to stress particular aspects that are important to assist the surgical team in the design and conduction of the surgical treatment, as well as for the evaluation of the respective results.

Echocardiography—What Are Surgeons Looking for?

Serial ventricular dimensions, both diameter and volume measurements, in systole and diastole, normalized for body surface area to Z scores in children, are paramount in decision-making for threshold for cardiac surgery in chronic MR and AR. Fractional shortening and ejection fraction are reported with a comment on the patient's left and right ventricular function (see also Chapter 6). If there is impaired function, the estimated right ventricular pressure should also be reported to confirm or rule out the presence of pulmonary hypertension. The annuli are always measured and in children these are normalized by Z scores. A mean pressure gradient is measured through the mitral and/ or aortic valve if it is affected.

Over the last few decades, echocardiography has developed into an incredibly useful tool for the analysis of valve function with pictures now so accurate in real time detail that they enable surgeons to fine tune repairs with a shorter cross-clamp time.[45] Preoperative echocardiography has now become, in some aspects, better than direct visualization as the surgeon can now plan the specific steps for the repair.

The echocardiographer and surgeon need to work closely together in analyzing the mitral valve before attempting repair or deciding on replacement and for this reason it is crucial for there to be agreement on the terminology used. A commonly used terminology is to describe the anterior mitral leaflet with segments one, two and three (A1, A2, A3) lateral to medial and similarly to the posterior leaflet (P1, P2, P3). Degrees of prolapse of each segment are subjectively graded mild, moderate, or severe. The direction of the color jet and the degree of thickening of leaflets are described. Three-dimensional echocardiography allows visualization of the valve from the atria and ventricle (mitral disease) and from the ventricle and aorta (aortic disease) allowing "surgical views" of these valves.

Before surgery, the surgeon and cardiologist look at this data together to discuss the detail and review the images. If there was an aspect that was not clear, transesophageal echocardiographic (TEE) analysis is undertaken. This can also be performed "on the table" immediately before operation to lower cost and avoid a separate anesthetic for children.

Mitral valve analysis

Where a repair is being contemplated, there are a number of specific echocardiographic details that need to be analyzed by the surgeon. One needs to know the annulus and the Z score as this correlates with how much spare leaflet tissue is available.[38] Echocardiographic sweeps from back to front are necessary to analyze the relationship of the coapting edges of A1 to P1, A2 to P2, and A3 to P3. It is important to note the position of the leaflet tips in systole in relationship to the plane of the annulus as this allows an assessment of the degree of prolapse (mild, moderate, or severe) of any one of the specific segments.

The direction of the color jet in the left atrium also gives a clue as to which leaflet is prolapsing anterior or posterior. The most frequent scenario is a posteriorly directed jet of mitral regurgitation due to anterior leaflet prolapse. The short axis color flow imaging will reveal where the regurgitation is occurring at P1, P2, or P3 or a combination of any of the leaflets. This can influence how one adjusts gathering sutures during the annuloplasty. During systole and diastole, one should note how much movement there is in each of the leaflets. It is not uncommon for the posterior leaflet to be quite fixed and rigid.[19]

When analyzing prolapse of the anterior leaflet one should note whether it is the whole of the leaflet or actually just the outer rim of the leaflet prolapsing. This may occur when the primary chordae of the anterior leaflet are elongated and the intermediate chordae are at the correct length, this gives a "dog leg deformity" of the anterior leaflet (Fig. 8.3).

Less commonly, the posterior leaflet prolapses, and this results in an anteriorly directed jet of mitral regurgitation.

A mean mitral valve gradient over 6−8 mmHg indicates definite mitral stenosis with mean gradients below 4−5 mmHg attributable to severe regurgitation. If the left atrium is very large and out of proportion to the degree of regurgitation, that is cause to suspect significant mitral stenosis.

Aortic valve analysis

The size of the annulus at the sinuses and at the sinotubular junction is noted. The position of the bellies of each of the cusps should be observed. If one is hanging lower than the others in association with an eccentric jet, then this indicates a single leaflet prolapse. This is usually more easily repairable as two out of the three leaflets are relatively well preserved (Fig. 8.4). The direction of the regurgitant jet can be straight

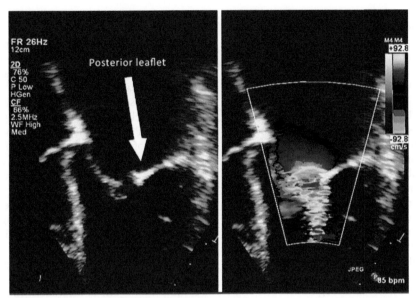

FIG. 8.3 Echocardiogram: Two-chamber view of mitral valve with severe regurgitation and stenosis. Note posterior leaflet thickening and restricted movement in diastole.

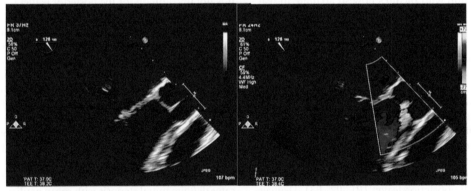

FIG. 8.4 Moderate aortic regurgitation due to single leaflet prolapse, repairable.

down the left ventricular outflow tract in the long axis view or it may be eccentric.

In a short-axis view, coaptation defects are noted where there appears to be a gap and where the color jet appears: is it a triangular jet in the middle indicating all three leaflets are retracted and failing to coapt or is it around one particular leaflet or at one particular commissure? The mobility and the thickness of the leaflets should also be observed. The position of the coronary origins should be noted as well, because occasionally there may be an unexpected coronary anomaly making homograft root replacement more complicated to perform.

Tricuspid valve analysis

Similar to the mitral valve, measuring the annulus size is important when analysing the tricuspid valve, although this may be a little bit more difficult to measure accurately than the mitral annulus. In other respects, the tricuspid valve can be analyzed on echocardiogram in a very similar way to the mitral valve including the mobility of the leaflets, any tethering effect on the chordae tendinae, the position of the tips, the direction of the color jet, and the presence of retraction or of prolapse of the leaflets. Preoperative transesophageal echocardiography (TTE) evaluation should also document the degree of RV dilatation and assess the severity of TR. However, there is no reliable method to judge how much of the TR is reversible when the left heart valve lesions are corrected[46]

Role of the preoperative three-dimensional and transesophageal echocardiogram. As a rule, all of this preoperative information can be obtained using two-dimensional and three-dimensional transthoracic echocardiography in younger children of normal weight.[47] Initially, TEE were performed on the operating table as the case began, but now some groups prefer to perform them as a separate procedure to enable more time to be spent analyzing the data, particularly 3-D echocardiography, to optimize the operating time.

Three-dimensional echocardiography has become extremely useful in giving surgeons greater detail of exactly where there is a problem with leaflet coaptation. There is a significant amount of skill and expertise required in developing good 3-D pictures, but this allows a surgical view like standing in the left atrium and watching the valve open and close in real time. Many surgeons attribute better repair results in recent years to 3-D echocardiography assessment. Following valve repair, TEE should be performed to assess the result.

Left and Right Catheterization—Coronary Angiography

In the era before echocardiography, angiography was useful in analyzing the size of the valve annuli, the motion of the leaflets, quantified valve stenosis and regurgitation, and evaluated left ventricular size and function. In the current era of echocardiography, these features are all assessed noninvasively. Cardiac catheterization is rarely required in the younger patient even if pulmonary hypertension is present as pulmonary hypertension resolves in the long term.

Nevertheless, there may be a role for left or right heart catheterization in an adult with significant ventricular dysfunction, to assess hemodynamics, and/or perform coronary angiography. Coronary angiography in particular is indicated before valve surgery in those with a history of cardiovascular disease or left ventricular dysfunction,[48] to name a few. Those with end-stage RHD following redo valve surgery in high-income countries require hemodynamic evaluation for consideration for transplantation. Catheter-based evaluation of the patient with RHD is discussed in detail in Chapter 7.

New Methods—CT Scan and Magnetic Resonance Imaging

Three-dimensional imaging such as computerized tomography (CT) scan and cardiac magnetic resonance imaging (MRI) have gone through major developments within the last decade and many of their functions have overtaken the original role of angiography. A CT scan is extremely useful in outlining coronary anatomy, and it can also demonstrate the calcification of a leaflet or of an aortic homograft in an adult or a redo situation. In redo aortic root surgery, it is helpful to know exactly the position of the cardiac structures behind the sternum that allows for safe reentry.

Cardiac MRI has the advantage of no radiation but has long acquisition times hence younger children require a general anesthetic. Cardiac MRI is highly accurate for left ventricular size and function and as the gold standard for right ventricular function is particularly useful for right ventricles not seen well on echocardiography. It can be used to measure regurgitant fractions of both the mitral and aortic valves where echocardiographic assessment is equivocal and it is particularly useful in very obese patients where echocardiographic views can be very limited.[29] Mechanical valve replacements can create artifacts that will affect measurements on MRI.

In summary, echocardiography remains the gold standard for the diagnostic work-up in rheumatic mitral, aortic, and tricuspid valvular disease. Close collaboration between surgeon and cardiologist to analyze valve abnormalities allows preoperative planning, the goal being a durable valve repair.

INDICATIONS FOR SURGERY AND SURGICAL TECHNIQUES
The Young Rheumatic Patient

Patients requiring surgery for rheumatic valvular heart disease cover a large spectrum from the asymptomatic schoolchild with chronic rheumatic regurgitation and a very repairable looking valve through to the severely symptomatic and cachectic teenager with poor social circumstances who has been hospitalized for some time with valves that do not look repairable.

Different from many of the lesions that cardiac surgeons operate on, rheumatic valve disease does not actually have a cure. Heart valves can usually be repaired but the repairs are not often perfect and nor are they always very durable. Over time, there is a significant chance that redo surgery will be required. Valve replacements may seem the best option, but mechanical valve insertions require lifelong anticoagulation (warfarin), which in this particular group of socially disadvantaged patients may actually carry greater risk than the original valve lesion.[17,49] On the other hand, bioprostheses still have very limited durability in children and teenagers, particularly in the mitral position, although they are a good option for woman of childbearing age. In the aortic position in children, homografts appear to allow for growth of the aortic annulus and last approximately 10 years.

Finally, there are also patients with very severely dilated left ventricles whose systolic function has become so impaired that surgery is not recommended. Sadly, there are certain circumstances where one elects for medical treatment only (see Chapter 6).

Data from our own patient cohort (KF) have suggested that repair of the mitral valve is more durable and left ventricle (LV) functions better postoperatively if it is performed before the left ventricle end-diastolic dimension Z scores are over four.[17]

The formal indications for surgery have already been covered in Chapter 6, but they include the dimensions of the left ventricle in systole and diastole, and these should be tabulated over a time span rather than just having one single set. Furthermore, they should be normalized to the patient's height and weight. Patients with ARF are treated conservatively unless the dimensions are steadily deteriorating and signs and symptoms of heart failure are not controlled by medical therapy.

The presence of pulmonary hypertension is a concern, as is the deterioration in systolic function of the left ventricle.[50] Very occasionally, the operation has to be undertaken acutely in the presence of pulmonary edema that does not resolve with intravenous diuretics or with a requirement for ventilation or inotropic support. In our experience, repairs during the acute phase of ARF are less reliable albeit lifesaving but postoperative survival is excellent.

It is important to know the local outcomes of surgical treatment for both valve repair and replacement in the context of rheumatic valve disease and not to assume that survival and postoperative complications are the same as for those with congenital heart disease or other degenerative heart diseases. Data from New Zealand and the Pacific island population have confirmed that survival in children is significantly better with repair and this is due to the complication rate associated with mechanical valve replacements.[17] Rates of sepsis, endocarditis, and warfarin-related complications are high in these socially disadvantaged patients, particularly in females.[36]

The evolution of the surgical approaches to the treatment of rheumatic valve disease was described in the introduction. The unique features of rheumatic mitral valve disease dictate the need for extensive valve repair techniques, especially valve leaflet debridement or stripping/peeling, resection, or pericardial patch extension, chordal shortening, anterior or posterior chordal transfer, expanded polytetrafluoroethylene (ePTFE) chordae substitutes, rigid or flexible annuloplasty, and biodegradable or homemade rings. Similar techniques may be used in aortic valve repair. In this section, some of the most important technical aspects are discussed.

Closed mitral commissurotomy for mitral stenosis

In this procedure, the traditional left anterolateral thoracotomy, through the submammary fifth intercostal space, is used. The pericardium is opened anterior and parallel to the phrenic nerve. The LA appendage is entered, unless clot is palpated, in which case the left atrium is entered via the left superior pulmonary vein. A Tubbs dilator is introduced via the apex of the left ventricle and guided to the mitral orifice by the operator's finger introduced in the left atrium (Fig. 8.5). In most cases, the Tubbs dilator is set at 3.6–3.8 cm for adult females, and 3.9–4.1 cm for adult males.[20]

Other approaches to the left atrium have also been described. De and Pezzella[51] from Vietnam described the finger fracture technique for redo CMC via the right chest (Fig. 8.5). Cooley et al.[52] in 1959, described a right thoracotomy and transsternal approach, and Cosio Pascal and Ibarra-Perez,[53] in 1974, suggested a median sternotomy approach. This had the advantage of easier conversion to OMC when CMC is not feasible as in the case of unstable hemodynamics, a friable or torn LA appendage, the presence of palpable LA clot, or a mitral valve area (MVA) < 0.6 cm, all making finger or dilator dilatation difficult or hazardous.

If only one commissure is opened, there should be no further attempts to dilate the other commissure, because of the risk of increasing regurgitation. Furthermore, if MR results from the initial dilatation, further dilatation attempts should be abandoned. Conversion of CMC to OMC or MV replacement during the left chest approach requires the use of cardiopulmonary bypass (CPB). This necessitates cannulation of the femoral artery or thoracic aorta, and femoral vein, pulmonary artery or right atrial appendage, if it can be reached.[20]

Intraoperative TEE may be used to better evaluate the anatomy, guide the operator's finger and Tubbs dilator during the commissurotomy, and assess the intraoperative result, that is, residual stenosis and/or new or increased regurgitation.[54,55]

The major criteria for CMC success are pure commissural fusion, pliable leaflets, thin and nonfused chordae, absence of calcification, and no mitral incompetence. The ideal patient has isolated mitral stenosis and is in sinus rhythm. These predictors of surgical success, not surprisingly, are similar to predictors of percutaneous balloon mitral valvuloplasty (see Chapter 7).

Mitral commissurotomy

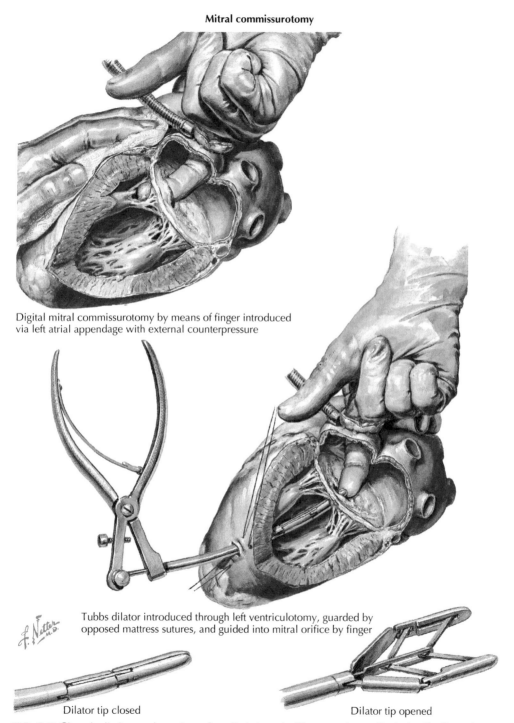

Digital mitral commissurotomy by means of finger introduced via left atrial appendage with external counterpressure

Tubbs dilator introduced through left ventriculotomy, guarded by opposed mattress sutures, and guided into mitral orifice by finger

Dilator tip closed

Dilator tip opened

FIG. 8.5 Closed mitral commissurotomy for mitral stenosis. The upper image illustrates the finger fracture technique, with the finger introduced via the left atrium (shown for historical interest as this is no longer currently performed). The lower image illustrates use of the Tubb's dilator, which is introduced via the apex of the left ventricle and guided to the mitral orifice via the operator's finger, which is introduced via the left atrium. (Reproduced with permission from The Netter Collection of Medical Illustrations.[53a])

Open mitral commissurotomy for mitral stenosis
This procedure is usually performed via a median sternotomy, under CPB and cardioplegic arrest. The left atrium is entered and any thrombus present removed. Retraction of both leaflets by nerve hooks may help to identify a furrow line in the commissures. A scalpel-blade incision is made commencing in the central valve orifice and progressively advanced to 3–4 mm from the annulus (Fig. 8.6). Fused chordae are separated with a knife or scissors and, when appropriate, the incision is carried down to the center of the papillary muscle.

Impaired valve pliability may be restored by peeling the fibrous layer covering the atrial surface of the leaflets. Calcifications are gently peeled or shaved off from the leaflets and the annular-leaflet junction. Some surgeons defend the routine use of a bilateral commissural plication as it shortens the posterior annulus and increases the coaptation length of the leaflets.

Competence of the mitral valve is assessed by injecting saline with a bulb syringe into the left ventricle through the mitral valve. If central mitral regurgitation persists, a complete posterior annuloplasty, from trigone to trigone, may be used, especially when the left atrium is very enlarged, to suspend the posterior annulus.[53,55]

At the end of the procedure, the atrial appendage may be closed from within the left atrium.

Repair for mitral valve regurgitation
The mitral valve anatomy and the classification of MR were well elucidated by Carpentier. Type I is characterized by normal leaflet length and motion but with either annular dilation or leaflet perforation, such as in endocarditis; type II MR is caused by leaflet prolapse, resulting from papillary muscle and chordal rupture or elongation; type III MR is caused by restricted leaflet motion (the Carpentier classification is summarised in Chapter 5).[21] Carpentier further stressed the importance of assessing MR, both with intraoperative TEE and surgical analysis. This includes the etiology, lesion or pathology, and dysfunction or pathophysiology.

The most prevalent mechanism of rheumatic MR is type IIIa restricted leaflet motion secondary to leaflet thickening and/or shortening or fusion of chordae. Type II, anterior leaflet prolapse secondary to chordal elongation, occurs in 30% of cases and type I, isolated annular dilatation, in 10%, usually in older patients where it can constitute one-third of the cases.

A variety of repair techniques for rheumatic MR have been reported.[14,20,22,56] These generally follow the principles and techniques initially proposed by Carpentier, which have a particular applicability in rheumatic MR, but have been recently enhanced by several modifications and new techniques.

Madesis et al.[22] have nicely summarized the surgical valve repair options available for rheumatic mitral valve disease, which include the following: commissurotomy with division of fused commissural chordae and/or papillary muscles; resection of secondary chordae; shortening or transposition of elongated chordae; artificial chordal replacement or reinforcement by ePTFE (Gore-Tex); leaflet thinning (removal of fibrous tissue);

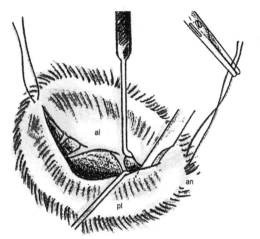
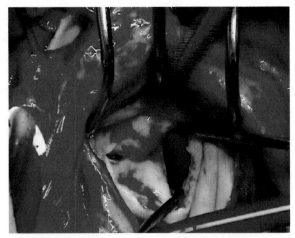

FIG. 8.6 Technique of open mitral commissurotomy. The illustration on the left is a diagrammatic representation of the procedure, whereas the image on the right is a surgeon's view. al, anterior leaflet; an, annulus; pl, posterior leaflet.

leaflet augmentation with autologous pericardium; partial replacement of the MV apparatus with a segment of an autologous tricuspid valve apparatus; ring or synthetic/autologous pericardial strip annuloplasty for annular disease; and posterior plication annuloplasty suture. Combinations of techniques are used, tailored to the valve pathology. This large array of armamentarium far exceeds that which is commonly used in degenerative disease, thus reflecting the greater complexity of rheumatic repair.

Treatment of elongated chordae, one of the most prevalent features in these cases, was originally done by one of several techniques of chordal shortening and/or transfer. Antunes et al.[23] used ePTFE (GoreTex CV-4) chordal substitution/reinforcement extensively with excellent results, and this is now the method preferred by many surgeons working in this field.

For leaflet extension, autologous pericardium soaked in glutaraldehyde for 5–10 min and then rinsed three separate times with saline is advisable.[25,57] For posterior leaflet extension, the annulus sutures should be placed before sewing in the pericardial patch to obviate tearing or dehiscence of the patch.

An annuloplasty ring is usually added at the end of the procedure for annular remodeling although some surgeons commence repair with the annuloplasty ring. We favor the rigid or semirigid device for rheumatic mitral etiology, given that the rheumatic annulus is fixed and deformed (Fig. 8.7). Flexible ring annuloplasty and biodegradable devices have also been used.[26]

Unfortunately, many of these current devices are not available or are too expensive for LMICs. Phan et al., from Vietnam, in a single center series of >2000 mitral valve repairs, utilizing the basic Carpentier techniques, favored the use of homemade rings to decrease cost: bands were used in patients <5 years old and rigid rings in patients >5 years old.[27]

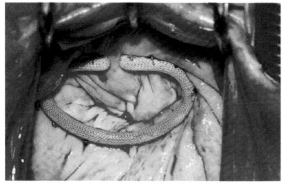

FIG. 8.7 Repaired mitral valve with a rigid annuloplasty ring (Carpentier-Edwards).

In conclusion, mitral repair for RHD entails a steep learning curve, a lesion-focused approach, a dedicated surgeon and team, the willingness to accept initial conversion to valve replacement, and early or long-term failure that may require subsequent reoperation, sometimes rerepair, usually valve replacement. It should be stressed that repair may require more operative time than valve replacement.

It is likely that a better appreciation of the disease process, application of newer surgical techniques, and better evaluation and surveillance with 2D and 3D echocardiography (both TTE and TEE) have increased the number of successful reports of valve repair for RHD, in both the mitral and aortic position.

Mitral valve replacement

It has long been accepted that a good mitral valve repair results in better long-term outcomes compared to valve replacement, with either a mechanical or bioprosthetic valve (Fig. 8.8).[28] Valve replacement, however, is recommended for patients who are judged too complex or unfavorable for valve repair, or fail PBMC, CMC, OMC, or repair.[58–60]

Selection of mechanical versus bioprosthetic valves is a major challenge in this group. This is related primarily to the problems with anticoagulation in the mechanical valve and the limited durability of the bioprostheses in patients <60 years old, together with the risks associated with redo surgery. Other important considerations include the noise of mechanical valves in thin patients and cost of bioprostheses, which are usually more expensive in LMICs.

Selection of valve prosthesis. The criteria for selection of a bioprostheses versus a mechanical valve (Fig. 8.9) have been outlined in both the European Society of Cardiology and American Heart Association/American College of Cardiology valvular heart disease guidelines.[48,61]

Reasons in favor of bioprosthetic valves include the following: informed patient choice (perhaps less important here); nonavailability or nonadherence with anticoagulation; lifestyle issues; bleeding disorders; reoperation for mechanical valve thrombosis despite good long-term anticoagulant control; young women contemplating pregnancy; and patients aged >65 years for prosthesis in aortic position or >70 years in mitral position.[48] Reasons in favor of mechanical prosthetic valves include the following: no contraindications to long-term anticoagulation; risk of accelerated structural valve deterioration; already on anticoagulation with a mechanical prosthesis in another valve position or

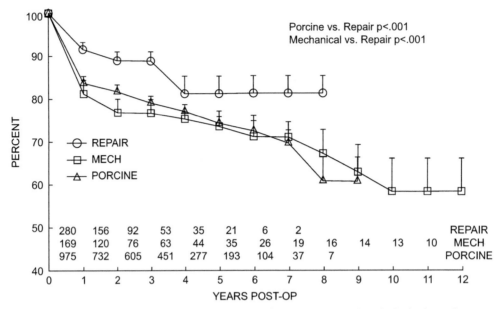

FIG. 8.8 Actuarial survival from all cardiac-related death after mitral valve repair and mitral valve replacement. (Reproduced with permission from Galloway et al.[28])

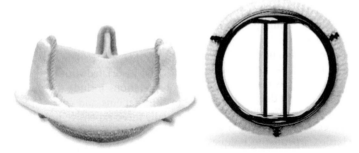

FIG. 8.9 The Edwards Magna (bioprosthetic) and St Jude Medical (mechanical) are the most commonly used prosthetic valves in current use.

due to high risk of thromboembolism; and age <60 years for prostheses in the aortic position and <65 years for prostheses in the mitral position.

In LMICs, bioprosthetic valve replacement may be performed in younger patients. In India, for example, life expectancy is, on average, 63–65 years. It therefore makes sense to consider implantation of tissue valves, thus avoiding anticoagulation, for patients over 40–45 years old.[62] However, in the much younger patients (<20–25 years old), bioprostheses degenerate exceedingly fast,[17] hence mechanical valves have to be used (Fig. 8.10). On the other hand, redo surgery in patients with previous mechanical valves may have a higher operative mortality than with bioprostheses, given that mechanical valve dysfunction tends to be more acute and

catastrophic compared to the more chronic clinical course with biological valves.[60]

Persistent efforts to improve the durability of tissue valves are continuously being made. The third generation valves have added antimineralization, along with surfactant and heat treatments. Stent designs have also improved.[63] However, the benefits of the third generation valves have not been evident so far.

Technique of valve replacement. The technical aspects of mitral valve replacement have been outlined by many surgeons.[56,64–66] An appreciation of the underlying pathology includes the following: adhesions from previous closed commissurotomy or other operations and the degree of any right and LA and left ventricular

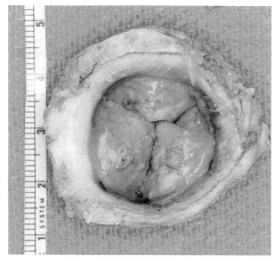

FIG. 8.10 Porcine bioprosthesis explanted from the mitral position due to severe stenosis after only 3 years of implantation in a 12-year old.

dilatation. Debridement and removal of all blood clots is important, although LA clots can be very adhesive. Obliteration or ligation of the LA appendage is now recommended in all adult cases. Concomitant LA reduction and/or Maze procedure may be performed.

The concept of preservation of the mitral valve apparatus was originally developed by Lillehei in 1964.[67] It offers the advantages of preserving LV geometry and function; reducing early and late mortality, and improving long-term survival and function; preventing left ventricular rupture; and preserving RV function.[68–72]

These advantages may accrue with preservation of both the anterior and posterior chordal apparatus. Some authors have been able to achieve preservation of the entire chordal apparatus in all of their patients undergoing mitral valve replacement (MVR).[72] Yet, this remains controversial in RHD given that in children, or those requiring double valve (aortic and mitral valve) replacement, or in rheumatic valves with advanced disease, total preservation may be difficult. Goretex sutures may be used to reestablish ventricular wall to annular continuity.

Surgery for aortic valve disease

Similar to what was discussed earlier for the mitral valve, the pathology and the demographics vary widely according to the two types of population. In general, patients from HICs are older (mean age 55 years) compared to those originating from LMICs, who are younger (mean age 25 years), poorer, uneducated,

and/or nonadherent to therapy. Hence, the same considerations about valve prostheses apply, although the rate of complications, especially thromboembolic, are lower in the aortic position. Mechanical valves may have greater applicability here, also because of better hemodynamic characteristics.

Frequently, aortic valve disease, of varying severity, accompanies severe mitral valve disease, the primary object of intervention. Hwang et al., from Seoul,[73] found that mild aortic valve disease in patients undergoing rheumatic mitral valve surgery could be left untreated, because a preventive aortic valve operation does not result in better clinical and echocardiographic outcomes. Even by 1988, Bernal and coworkers,[74] from Spain, described that long-term functional results of reparative procedures of nonsevere aortic valve disease in patients with predominant rheumatic mitral valve disease had been inadequate at 22 years of follow-up. According to these data, "conservative operations for rheumatic aortic valve disease do not seem appropriate."

Although the subject is still controversial, the Ross procedure, once thought to be a solution, does not appear to be suitable for young patients with RHD. Al-Halees et al.,[75] Kumar et al.,[76] and Alsoufi et al.[77] reported good short-term results but long-term durability came short of expectations in young rheumatic patients compared to the Ross procedure for congenital heart disease. However, it provides acceptable midterm results in carefully selected older (>30 years) patients with isolated rheumatic aortic valve disease. The advantages, especially in children or adolescents, include potential for growth, no need for anticoagulation and improved midterm durability. The disadvantages include technical complexity of implantation and requirement of a homograft for the right ventricular outflow construction.

Aortic valve repair. Aortic valve repair appears to be an alternative in some rheumatic cases. Talwar et al. reported on a small series of 61 patients, using several techniques: cusp thinning (95.2% of the cases); commissurotomy (73.8%); subcommissural annuloplasty (38.7%); commissural plication (19.4%); closure of perforation (3.3%); and decalcification of cusps (3.3%). Again, a complex procedure. They had a 95% survival and 87% freedom from significant AR after 10 years.[78]

Suri et al. point out that aortic cusp pliability, mobility, and calcification are less predictable with AV repair, thus affecting long-term durability. As the aortic cusps are retracted in most cases, cusp extension may provide adequate valve repair in a large proportion of children with rheumatic AR.[79]

Haluck et al.[80] reported that fresh autologous pericardium tended toward better durability than bovine pericardium. Other materials have also been experimented recently. Nosál et al.[81] found that the use of ePTFE leaflet extension is an effective technique for aortic valve reconstruction in congenital valvular disease. However, they alerted that long-term follow-up is necessary to assess the durability of this type of repair. Myers et al. reported a 75% freedom from reoperation 15 years after aortic cusp extension in a series of 78 patients, mean age 12 years at operation.[82] By contrast, d'Udekem and Sharma, in a reported debate, argued that cusp extension should be avoided in rheumatic cases because these patients are usually old enough to receive the same valve substitutes as adults, and lack of adherence with antibiotic prophylaxis will likely result in early reintervention.[83]

In conclusion, aortic valve repair in young rheumatics is feasible in a number of cases. Specific techniques are applicable to specific lesions. The procedure may be especially indicated in less than severe aortic lesions during MV repair. Generally, results are as durable as when compared to the mitral valve. Hence, it has the potential to be a good solution in younger adults, but application in older (>40 years) rheumatic patients is debatable. Perhaps, its use should be limited to simple, easy-to-correct lesions.

Aortic valve replacement. The technical aspects of routine aortic valve replacement have been well described before in the surgical literature and do not differ from those commonly used for other patients and pathologies. The aortotomy incision is either transverse or oblique onto the middle of the noncoronary sinus. After removal of the cusps, proper sizing of the annulus is important. Implantation of the valve is done with pledgeted or nonpledgeted mattress sutures, interrupted or continuous, and the prosthesis positioned in a supraannular, annular, or subannular fashion. Chart assessment of effective orifice area (EOA) should be utilized to avoid patient-prosthesis mismatch. Structures to be mindful of include the noncoronary to right commissure area where the AV node is located and the coronary orifices.

Tricuspid valve disease
Tricuspid regurgitation. The most common tricuspid valve (TV) problem is secondary TR due to left-sided mitral and/or aortic valve disease. It is a progressive disease that does not resolve with correction of the primary left-sided lesion alone. Hence, secondary TR is amenable to tricuspid annuloplasty. In secondary TR, a simple annuloplasty is usually sufficient. Currently, rings are used by most surgeons, although the choice between rigid and flexible is still a matter of debate.

However, there are reports attesting to excellent results of suture annuloplasty (DeVega or Kay or their modifications). Antunes et al.[46] prefer the DeVega repair for functional TR. This repair was modified with interposition of Teflon pledgets in each bite of the suture, to give it greater consistency. A Carpentier rigid ring repair was reserved primarily for organic disease, especially if stenosis was present.

Dreyfus et al.[44] developed the concept that annular dilatation can occur with or without TR. Hence, they recommended that repair be based on annular dilatation. Remodeling annuloplasty, albeit in nonrheumatic disease, was performed regardless of the degree of TR if the tricuspid diameter was >70 mm, as measured intraoperatively from the anteroseptal commissure to the anteroposterior commissure. At follow-up, there was a lower rate of progressive TR in those who had the annuloplasty.

Significant TR carries an increased perioperative risk. TR tends to persist or worsen even with a perfect mitral valve repair or replacement. In those with mild or moderate TR undergoing left-sided valve surgery, 25% are expected to progress postoperatively.[61] There is good evidence that residual TR has a significant impact on both the early postoperative course and on the long-term outcome,[31] including the need for reoperation for progressive TR.[61] Therefore, it is important to address moderate or severe TR at least with an annuloplasty at the time of mitral surgery.

The current consensus is that the tricuspid valve should be explored in all patients undergoing left-sided procedures, where functional or organic tricuspid disease is suspected or documented, be it at the initial operation or a subsequent reoperation. There is no reliable method to judge how much of the TR is reversible when the left heart valve lesions are corrected.[46]

Hence, the latest guidelines recommend that surgery of the tricuspid valve "should be considered in patients with mild or moderate secondary TR with dilated annulus ($\geq$40 mm or >21 mm/m^2) undergoing left-sided valve surgery" (Class IIa)—see Chapter 6.[48]

Tricuspid stenosis. Correction of organic disease with TV stenosis involves incising the anteroseptal commissure followed by the posteroseptal commissure. This creates a bicuspid valve. A ring annuloplasty usually follows.

TV replacement should be performed only as a last resort, in patients who have severe tricuspid stenosis, thickened and stiff leaflets, and diseased subvalvular structures that limit both anterior and posterior leaflet motion. However, patients with severe RV dysfunction should probably have valve replacement.

There is continued debate as to the choice of prosthesis, mechanical or biological. The same concepts discussed earlier for mitral valve replacement may apply to the tricuspid valve, but bioprostheses may be preferable here because of the possibility of percutaneous procedures when the prosthesis fails.

Alternatively, pericardial patch extension for organic tricuspid lesions with marked leaflet-edge rolling or contraction but good motion, with or without commissural fusion, is used by some.[84] This technique has also been recommended for patients with severe tethering of the leaflets in a very dilated ventricle. A ring must be always added to these procedures.

Multi valve surgery

Combined mitral and aortic valve regurgitation is a common scenario following ARF in the young. A small series from New Zealand warns of the risk for late ventricular dysfunction in this group, with the implication that indication for operation should be based on the lower LV dimensions pertaining to the MV rather than the aortic valve.[43] In the chronic RHD setting in adults, the valve with severe disease dominates the indications for cardiac surgery. When both valves have severe dysfunction, intervention on both is mandatory. On the other hand, there is little data or recommendation in the guidelines[48,61] relating to the decision to repair or replace a second valve with moderate disease, but, bearing in mind the evolutive nature of the rheumatic lesion, efforts should be made at eliminating or significantly decreasing the degree of regurgitation, especially if the valve can be repaired. Mild lesions need no intervention.

EARLY AND LONG-TERM OUTCOMES OF RHEUMATIC VALVE SURGERY

Immediate outcomes of heart valve surgery have improved significantly over the years due to refinement of surgical techniques, improvement of myocardial protection, and better postoperative care. Perioperative surgical results, including both morbidity and mortality, have generally not differed among different etiologies, particularly when comparing rheumatic with degenerative disease. Nevertheless, isolated valve surgery portends better results than multiple valve interventions, a common scenario in the rheumatic setting, or when combined with other procedures.

It is pertinent to reemphasize that RHD presents differently among the populations of HICs and those

of LMICs. To generalize, in the former, the disease appears in more advanced ages, the manifestations of valvular dysfunction developing in the latter decades. By contrast, in the latter, the disease emerges precociously, in the pediatric and adolescent years. Surgery may be required during the active phase of the disease. Besides the different clinical characteristics, RHD patients are often poor, with little or no education and have limited access to medical care. Therefore, the surgical results cannot be compared or generalized, but should be discussed in relation to each one of these different realities.

Accordingly, the best strategy for surgical treatment of the mitral valve (repair vs. replacement) in RHD is yet to be determined, in part due to the paucity of comparative long-term studies.[14,85–88] Socioeconomic factors mean medical follow-up is often incomplete.[17] The rationale for adopting MV repair techniques are partially related to the dire consequences of a prosthesis without close medical follow-up, namely thromboembolic or bleeding events, higher risk of endocarditis in mechanical valves, and early degeneration in the case of bioprostheses.[28,85] Moreover, there is evidence that long-term survival is also compromised with replacement and LV function may deteriorate throughout time.[89–92]

Perioperative Results

MVR is associated with worse perioperative outcomes than both mitral valve repair and aortic valve replacement (Table 8.1).[93]

TABLE 8.1 Operative Mortality After Surgery for Valvular Heart Disease.				
Surgery	EACTS	STS	UK	Germany
Aortic valve replacement, without combined CABG (%)	2.9	3.7	2.8	2.9
Mitral valve replacement, without combined CABG (%)	4.3	6.0	6.1	7.8
Mitral valve repair (%)	2.1	1.6	2.0	2.0

EACTS—European Association of Cardiothoracic Surgery; STS—Society of Thoracic Surgeons; UK—United Kingdom; CABG—Coronary Artery Bypass Grafting.
Reproduced with permission from Vahanian et al.[93]

In an analysis of the Society of Thoracic Surgeons database, over a 15-year period from 1993 to 2007, Vassileva et al. have shown that the operative mortality was almost double for multivalve surgery, which constituted 11% of the valve operations in the United States, in comparison with single valve procedures (10.7% vs. 5.7%, $P = .0001$).[94] In other series, multiple valve procedures constituted more than 25% of valve operations.[95]

There are several technical issues that might be responsible for the higher mortality in MVR: risk of AV block, especially when the posterior subvalvular apparatus is not preserved, or when debriding heavily calcified annuli; obstruction of the LV outflow tract (LVOT) and/or myocardial impingement by biological prosthetic struts; and obstruction of mechanical prosthetic discs by subvalvular constituents (leaflets, chordae tendinae and papillary muscle). Postoperative LV dysfunction is more an issue following mitral valve surgery than aortic valve surgery.

There are separate complications associated with MV repair: iatrogenic lesion of the circumflex artery by annuloplasty ring[96] and LVOT obstruction by systolic anterior movement of the mitral valve. The latter is rarer in rheumatic than in myxomatous valves.

In rheumatic valvular heart disease, contemporaneous surgical series have revealed operative mortality of 2%–4% for isolated aortic valve surgery or mitral valve replacement and 1%–2% for isolated mitral valve repair. However, there are still great discrepancies among different surgical centers. For instance, Wang and colleagues, from Taiwan, reported a hospital mortality of 3% for MV repair and 6.8% for replacement ($P = .65$), in a population with a mean age of 53.9 years, with no differences regarding other postoperative complications.[97] In a similar-aged population, Yau et al., from David Toronto's group, showed a hospital mortality of 0.7% for MV repair and 5.2%–5.6% for replacement ($P = .057$).[88] On the other hand, more recently, the Australia and New Zealand Society of Cardiac and Thoracic Surgeons reported the outcomes after mitral valve surgery for RHD, disclosing a similar 30-day mortality for MV repair and replacement (4.2% vs. 3.8%), in patients with a mean age around 60 years.[98] All these series are in developed countries in older patients.

The concept of heart valve centers of excellence in the treatment of valvular heart disease has emerged in recent years with the objective of delivering more consistent and better quality of care.[48,99] These centers should be equipped with "state-of-the-art" imaging devices (3D echocardiography, perioperative transesophageal echocardiography, cardiac CT, MRI), should have multidisciplinary teams with competence in valve repair/replacement, and should also report their outcomes (mortality, repair rates, durability of repair, reoperation rate) on a regular basis.

Perioperative results are significantly better in these centers, with mortality rates usually under 1% and repair rates greater than 95% in degenerative mitral disease. There are a lack of consensus statements and guidelines specifically pertaining to RHD surgery but we can suggest that one should aim at a mitral valve repair rate of 70%–80% and a mortality rate of 0.5% –2%. Most reports attest to lower mortality in centers with larger experiences.

We have recently analyzed our results (University Hospital of Coimbra, Portugal), during a 20-year period (1992–2012), in 1799 patients with rheumatic mitral valve disease (including associated procedures) and no previous MV surgery. Of these, 1470 had MV repair (81.7%) and 329 replacement, with a 30-day mortality of 1% and 1.8%, respectively ($P = .173$).

Long-Term Outcomes: Repair Versus Replacement
Mitral valve

As noted previously, rheumatic MV repair is not as straight-forward a procedure as degenerative etiology MV repairs. Rheumatic MV repair is associated with higher rates of reoperation. However, recent reports place rheumatic MV repair results at the same level of degenerative disease, when performed by dedicated surgeons in experienced centers. This is highly relevant for younger patient populations.

In a group of 329 patients below 18 years old, the surgeons from the National Heart Institute in Malaysia, documented a freedom from reoperation and valve failure rate of $92 \pm 5\%$ and $86 \pm 2\%$, and $87 \pm 4\%$ and $73 \pm 5\%$ ($P = .45$), respectively, at 5 and 10 years, comparable with that for degenerative valves ($92 \pm 2\%$ and $89 \pm 5\%$, and $92 \pm 5\%$ and $82 \pm 8\%$, respectively, $P = .79$). They concluded that the durability of MV repair for rheumatic disease in the current era had improved greatly and is comparable to that of degenerative disease.[57,100]

Talwar et al., from New Delhi, reported on 278 children (mean age $11.7 + 2.9$ years) who underwent mitral valve repair. Early mortality rate was 2.2%. After a mean follow-up of almost 6 years, actuarial, reoperation-free and event-free survivals were $95\% \pm 2\%$, $92\% \pm 2\%$, and $56\% \pm 4\%$, respectively. At 15 years, 86% of the patients remained free from reoperation.[101]

On the other hand, a group in São Paulo, Brazil, reported on 201 patients (mean age 26.9 ± 15.4 years) operated on from 1980 to 1997. After a mean follow-up of 10 years, the actuarial survival was 94% ± 2% and survival free from reoperation was 43% ± 14%. In their experience, patients less than 16 years old had lower survival rates, a finding that we had also seen before.[102]

Modifications of standard repair techniques, adherence to the importance of good leaflet coaptation, and strict quality control with stringent use of intraoperative TEE contributed to the improved long-term results.[57] In Coimbra, Portugal, we advocate the use of artificial chordae for correction of leaflet prolapse, rather than chordal shortening or chordal transfer, a lesson that has been learned from repairing anterior leaflet prolapse in degenerative disease.

Still, the few studies that have compared repair versus replacement in rheumatic patients seem to confer advantage in terms of survival and event-free survival with repair. Yau et al., in a population of 573 patients (mean age 54 ± 14 years), showed that MV repair was independently associated with a better survival than replacement ($P = .04$), despite higher rates of reoperation ($P = .005$). Freedom from thromboembolic complications, as expected, was also better in the repair group ($P < .001$).[88]

Cotrufo and associates ($n = 300$ patients, mean age 43 ± 12 years) revealed similar results with a nonsignificant better survival and freedom from embolic events, but a significantly worse reoperation rate after repair.[103] Wang et al. (92 patients, mean age 54 years) analyzed the midterm outcomes of rheumatic mitral repair versus replacement and found that MV repair was associated with lower surgical mortality and better survival, but higher repeat surgery rate.[97] More recently, however, Kim and colleagues, from South Korea (540 patients, mean age 49 ± 12 years) showed contradictory results, with no differences regarding adjusted survival, reoperation, and thromboembolic complications, although MVR patients had more anticoagulation therapy-related complications.[87]

Finally, Remenyi and colleagues, from New Zealand, analyzed the impact of MV repair versus replacement in a young population ($n = 82$) with RHD under 20 years old and demonstrated a greater overall survival and freedom from valve-related morbidity events, and long-term durability that equaled that of replacement.[17]

In a meta-analysis of 29 studies, where only three were of rheumatic etiology, Shuhaiber et al. failed to identify any overall survival difference between repair and replacement. However, these results should be interpreted with some caution, because of the retrospective nature of the studies, the small number of patients

enrolled, most patients were in the replacement group, and the heterogeneity of the populations studied.[91]

In summary, there appears to be a tendency to better results with repair; hence, there is an increasing acceptance of the need to repair by a larger number of surgeons and teams throughout the world. We have evaluated our own results (1491 patients with rheumatic MV disease, excluding associated procedures other than tricuspid valve surgery, mean age = 53 years) and demonstrated that MV replacement patients ($n = 290$) had reduced long-term survival in comparison with MV repair patients ($n = 1201$) (Fig. 8.11). This was also observed in the group of patients over 60 years old ($P = .001$).

Several factors were identified as independent risk factors of late mortality, MVR being one of the most significant in a multivariable analysis (Table 8.2). Older age, larger LVESD, larger LA, and higher pulmonary artery pressure were also all independent risk factors for decreased survival.

Aortic valve

There is scarce data comparing aortic valve (AV) repair and replacement in the rheumatic setting, as repair is seldom done and is performed only in specific cases, such as the pediatric population or when a prosthesis is judged to be contraindicated. The paucity of AV cusp tissue, especially with cusp restriction, thickening, or fenestrations, may preclude or render AV repair less predictable, thus affecting long-term durability.[79]

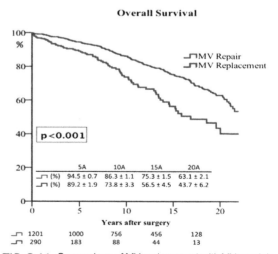

FIG. 8.11 Comparison of MV replacement with MV repair in patients with rheumatic mitral valve disease (Coimbra experience). MV, mitral valve.

TABLE 8.2
Cox Proportional Hazards Function to Determine the Independent Predictors of Late Mortality After Mitral Valve Surgery.

Variables	HR	CI 95%	P Value
Age	1.104	1.080–1.129	<0.0001
Renal disease	4.524	1.082–18.917	0.039
LVESD (mm)	1.052	1.025–1.080	<0.0001
LA (mm)	1.016	1.001–1.032	0.039
SPAP (mmHg)	1.013	1.003–1.023	0.012
MV replacement	1.541	1.021–2.326	0.039

HR—hazard ratio; CI—confidence interval; LA—left atrium; LV—left ventricle; SPAP—systolic pulmonary artery pressure; MV—mitral valve.

Duran and colleagues, from Saudi Arabia, described several surgical techniques in 50 young patients (mean age, 39.5 years) with rheumatic AR: (1) commissurotomy, (2) cusp free edge unfolding, (3) annuloplasty, and (4) supraaortic crest enlargement. Only four patients required reoperation for residual AR during a follow-up from 3 to 10 years.[104]

Talwar et al., from New Dehli,[78] described their experience with AV repair in 61 young patients (mean age 24 ± 9 years; 6–53 years). After a mean follow-up of 94 ± 46 months, 65% of patients had no/trivial or mild AR and four patients required reoperation for valve dysfunction, with no late deaths. Actuarial and reoperation-free survival at 160 months was 95% ± 3% and 85% ± 7%, respectively, and freedom from significant aortic stenosis (AS) or AR was 52% ± 17%.

How Far Can We Go With Repair?

As mentioned earlier, mitral valve repair techniques have evolved substantially in the last decades, and the excellent results obtained with degenerative disease have encouraged surgeons to go further in repairing rheumatic disease.[23] The use of rigid annuloplasty rings and of ePTFE chordae instead of the classical Carpenter's techniques, such as chordal transposition/transfer and shortening, constitute, in our opinion, the major advances. Leaflet peeling and extension by pericardial patch (glutaraldehyde-treated or fresh autologous pericardium, or bovine pericardium) have widened the range of repairable valves.[24,105]

There are instances when a strategy of MV repair should be pushed to the limit, such as in the case of patients from developing countries with poorer socioeconomic conditions, where mechanical prostheses could have catastrophic thromboembolic complications and

biological prostheses have very limited durability. We are firmly convinced that, in many of these cases, a suboptimal repair result may be more acceptable, because it delays the implantation of a prosthesis. By contrast, in older patients (>60–65 years) with good potential for adherence to the antithrombotic therapy required for a valve substitute, valve replacement should be considered if an optimal repair result cannot be expected.

From the analysis of 1799 patients with rheumatic MV disease, in our experience at Coimbra, several independent predictors or risk factors for failed repair were determined (Table 8.3).

These data were used in the development of a morphological rheumatic score to help in the decision to repair or replace the mitral valve.[106,107] The presence of calcification, anterior leaflet prolapse, degree of MR, and higher morphological scores were associated with lower probability of repair (Table 8.4).

Morphological scores >9 were associated with lower freedom from reoperation, suggesting that selected patients with those characteristics should have valve replacement (Fig. 8.12A). Furthermore, patients without an annuloplasty procedure also had poorer freedom from reoperation in comparison with those who had a ring (Fig. 8.12B). Patients with marked LA dilatation (>50 mm) also had poorer results.

THE ROLE OF NEW TECHNOLOGIES

Over the last decade, percutaneous valve intervention has rapidly emerged as an important innovation. Transcatheter aortic valve implantation (TAVI) for AS has substituted surgical replacement in many circumstances.[108] On the other hand, percutaneous mitral valve implantation has been slower in establishing itself and, for the moment, remains largely experimental. Many types of percutaneous prostheses are being developed for both aortic and mitral positions and further developments in this area are to be expected in the near future. Percutaneous repair of the mitral valve has also been actively implemented with devices designed to treat leaflet prolapse and annular dilatation.[108] With the exception of TAVI, the other procedures are, so far, used in extreme cases of impossible or very high-risk surgery, especially in elderly patients.

The application of these technologies in rheumatic patients in LMICs appears less probable in the foreseeable future for two reasons. First, the rheumatic pathology is less appropriate for current devices. Rheumatic AS is much rarer and typically lacks the extensive calcification characteristic of calcific AS, which affects the ability to safely anchor TAVI devices. AR is much more common in rheumatic cases and this lesion has, yet, precluded the use of percutaneous techniques. On the

TABLE 8.3
Multivariable Logistic Analysis to Determine the Independent Predictors of Failed Mitral Valve Repair.

Variables	OR	CI 95%	P Value
Gender (male)	0.54	0.34–0.84	0.007
Arterial hypertension	1.90	1.02–3.52	0.044
Diabetes	5.10	1.68–15.44	0.004
COPD	2.34	1.08–5.10	0.032
MV regurgitation (degree)	2.02	1.64–2.50	<0.0001
VALVE MORPHOLOGY:			
Annulus dilatation	0.30	0.14–0.65	0.003
Anterior leaflet prolapse	5.80	1.92–17.47	0.002
Annulus calcification	3.82	2.26–6.50	<0.0001
Commissure calcification	0.39	0.25–0.62	<0.0001
Morphological score	6.11	4.88–7.64	<0.0001

OR—odds ratio; CI—confidence interval; COPD—chronic obstructive pulmonary disease; MV—mitral valve.

TABLE 8.4
Intraoperative Morphological Score Based on the Analysis of 2344 Rheumatic Mitral Valves During Mitral Valve Surgery (Grading 4–12)[a].

Grade	Anterior Leaflet Pliability	Leaflet Thickening[b]	Subvalvular Thickening (Chordae)	Calcification (Site)
1	Pliable/minimal restriction	Minimal	Minimal	Absent/minimal
2	Mild–moderate restriction	Mild–moderate	Mild–moderate	Body of leaflet/commissures
3	Severe restriction (fixed)	Severe (all leaflet)	Severe (chordae shortening and/or fusion)	Free edge

ROC—receiver operating characteristic; AUC—area under the curve; CI—confidence interval.
[a] The higher the score the less favorable is the feasibility to repair. ROC analysis determined an AUC of 0.896 ($P < .001$, CI: 0.867–0.926) showing a very good predictive ability of the score. The estimated cut-off point for replacement was equal to or greater than 9.
[b] Minimal thickening implies a translucent leaflet, structurally almost normal. Severe thickening is considered when there is dense fibrous tissue with opaque or yellowish appearance. Mild–moderate leaflet/chordae thickening is in between those two grades.
Reproduced with permission from Coutinho et al.[106]

other hand, fibrosis of the mitral valve leaflets in rheumatic cases makes percutaneous intervention even more difficult. Second, the cost of these technologies is very high, in most cases more expensive than surgery, and is still prohibitive in LMICs.

A novel heart valve replacement offers hope for thousands with RHD has been announced a couple of years ago from Cape Town, South Africa.[109] The approach also entails task shifting, potentially utilizing general surgeons that are numerically more common than cardiac surgeons in LMICs. It is claimed that the technique does not require advanced cardiac surgical facilities or sophisticated cardiovascular imaging. An animal study has proven the concept, and clinical implantation is expected to commence soon. This device will be much less expensive than those currently in use because the prostheses is made of synthetic material, hence, easier to be mass produced.

CONCLUSIONS AND RECOMMENDATIONS

The burden of rheumatic valve disease still constitutes a major health problem in the developing countries of the

Freedom from reoperation

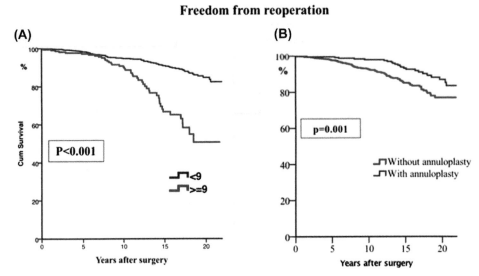

FIG. 8.12 **(A)** Freedom from reoperation between patients with a morphological score of 9 or above and under 9 (Coimbra experience). **(B)** Freedom from reoperation between patients who had an annuloplasty procedure with those who had not.

southern hemisphere and parts of Asia. All efforts to decrease the incidence of the disease and of its consequences are desirable. Better heart failure therapy and improved ARF prophylaxis have contributed to altering the course of the disease and to better long-term outcomes. Currently, however, there are literally millions of affected patients globally, and a significant proportion of these, especially children, adolescents, and young adults, who would benefit from valve surgery.[110] Zilla and colleagues have estimated the significant degree of under-delivery of lifesaving RHD surgery in LMICs.[111]

In these situations, valve replacement, especially of the mitral valve, constitutes a problem because these patients are often nonadherent to medical therapy, including anticoagulation.[49] Hence, whenever feasible, valve repair is recommended in children with rheumatic valvular heart disease, but it requires a considerable level of expertise that is associated with a significant caseload, which is not frequent under these circumstances.

In view of the young age of patients presenting with isolated mitral stenosis, PMBC is presently the first option, with surgical CMC as a subsequent procedure. This is especially important for young fertile females, as these two procedures can carry them through their maternal reproductive period without significant complications.

The evolution of the techniques of mitral valve repair, including use of ePTFE chordae versus shortening procedures and insertion of preshaped (rigid) rings, together with surgeons' increasing experience,

have improved the rate of repair and led to better surgical results for rheumatic MR.

Several works originating from rheumatic-endemic countries have confirmed better long-term survival and lower morbidity in patients subjected to mitral valve repair than replacement. Even freedom from reoperation, the main concern after repair, appears not to be inferior in high-volume surgical centers. Aortic valve repair is also possible in a number of cases but is less widely adopted among cardiac surgeons and the results are less predictable.

Surgeons must develop an attitude and interest in valve repair techniques that can easily be learned. Although patients who undergo valve repair at an early age are at risk of requiring additional surgery over time, mechanical valve replacement should be reserved for situations where more conservative approaches are not feasible. The percentage of valves requiring replacement decreases, as the experience of surgeons with mitral valve repair increases. Willingness to perform these challenging repairs is a fundamental challenge.

Acquiring the experience of valve repair is difficult in most low-volume centers. Referral to more experienced institutions or individual surgeons may be appropriate. The creation of regional reference centers, at national or supranational level, has been advocated by cardiologists and surgeons with significant experience in this environment. These would have the effect of creating the volume of cases necessary for acquiring expertise in more complex cases, essential in "training of the cardiovascular practitioners of the future," and become centers of research on endemic cardiovascular diseases (including RHD). This was expressed in the Addis Ababa Communiqué in 2016, which has since been endorsed by the African Union heads of state[112] and, more recently, by the Cape Town Declaration.[113]

In these young patients, even after a good repair, the inflammatory rheumatic process may continue its destructive scarring process and new bouts of the disease may occur, hence continued secondary prophylaxis is mandatory and realistic in the first 4 decades.[2] Some recommend lifelong prophylaxis (see Chapter 11).[54]

Finally, surgery for rheumatic valve disease in older adult patients (50–70 years) is a completely different question. In these cases, the rheumatic process is quiescent and valve repair follows the general lines adopted for other types of pathology. The main obstacle to repair is extensive fibrosis and calcification. Otherwise, the results are similar to those observed in nonrheumatic cases. Aortic valve repair may have some application in these cases, especially when the mitral valve is the primary indication for surgery.

As surgeons, we need to encourage the collection of more long-term data on outcomes and support projects to improve the medical follow-up and care of these patients. During their short surgical stay with us, we need to use that valuable time to educate them on how to look after their heart and valve. As we assess them for surgery and decide on repair or replacement, educational and social factors need to be considered. Cardiac surgery is only part of the continuum of care for chronic RHD.

REFERENCES

1. Carapetis JR, Steer AC, Mulholland EK, Weber M. The global burden of group A streptococcal diseases. *Lancet Infect Dis*. 2005;5(11):685–694.
2. Carapetis JR, Beaton A, Cunningham MW, et al. Acute rheumatic fever and rheumatic heart disease. *Nat Rev Dis Primers*. 2016;2:15084.
3. Tompkins DG, Boxerbaum B, Liebman J. Long-term prognosis of rheumatic fever patients receiving regular intramuscular benzathine penicillin. *Circulation*. 1972; 45(3):543–551.
4. Mirabel M, Grimaldi A, Freers J, Jouven X, Marijon E. Access to cardiac surgery in sub-Saharan Africa. *Lancet*. 2015;385(9968):606.
5. Yankah C, Fynn-Thompson F, Antunes M, et al. Cardiac surgery capacity in sub-Saharan Africa: quo vadis? *Thorac Cardiovasc Surg*. 2014;62(5):393–401.
6. Oli K, Asmera J. Rheumatic heart disease in Ethiopia: could it be more malignant? *Ethiop Med J*. 2004;42(1):1–8.
7. Parks T, Kado J, Miller AE, et al. Rheumatic heart disease-attributable mortality at ages 5-69 years in Fiji: a five-year, national, population-based record-linkage cohort study. *PLoS Negl Trop Dis*. 2015;9(9):e0004033.
8. Milne RJ, Lennon D, Stewart JM, Vander Hoorn S, Scuffham PA. Mortality and hospitalisation costs of rheumatic fever and rheumatic heart disease in New Zealand. *J Paediatr Child Health*. 2012;48(8):692–697.
9. Cutler EC, Levine SA. Cardiotomy and valvulotomy for mitral stenosis: experimental observations and clinical notes concerning an operated case with recovery. *Bost Med Surg J*. 1923;188(26):1023–1027.
10. Logan A, Turner R. Surgical treatment of mitral stenosis with particular reference to the transventricular approach with a mechanical dilator. *Lancet*. 1959;21(7108): 874–880.
11. Starr A, Edwards ML. Mitral replacement: clinical experience with a ball-valve prosthesis. *Ann Surg*. 1961;154: 726–740.
12. Harken DE, Taylor WJ, Lefemine AA, et al. Aortic valve replacement with a caged ball valve. *Am J Cardiol*. 1962; 9:292–299.
13. Lutter G, Quaden R, Iino K, et al. Mitral valved stent implantation. *Eur J Cardiothorac Surg*. 2010;38(3): 350–355.
14. Chauvaud S, Fuzellier J-F, Berrebi A, et al. Long-term (29 Years) results of reconstructive surgery in rheumatic mitral valve insufficiency. *Circulation*. 2001;104(suppl 1). I-12-I-5.
15. Mvondo CM, Pugliese M, Giamberti A, et al. Surgery for rheumatic mitral valve disease in sub-saharan African countries: why valve repair is still the best surgical option. *Pan Afr Med J*. 2016;24:307.
16. Kalangos A. The rheumatic mitral valve and repair techniques in children. *Semin Thorac Cardiovasc Surg Pediatr Card Surg Annu*. 2012;15(1):80–87.
17. Remenyi B, Webb R, Gentles T, et al. Improved long-term survival for rheumatic mitral valve repair compared to replacement in the young. *World J Pediatr Congenit Heart Surg*. 2013;4(2):155–164.
18. Bernal JM, Ponton A, Diaz B, et al. Combined mitral and tricuspid valve repair in rheumatic valve disease: fewer reoperations with prosthetic ring annuloplasty. *Circulation*. 2010;121(17):1934–1940.
19. Cardoso B, Loureiro P, Gomes I, et al. Mitral valve surgery for rheumatic lesions in young patients. *World J Pediatr Congenit Heart Surg*. 2016;7(3):321–328.
20. Antunes MJ. *Mitral Valve Repair*. Germany: Verlag R.S. Schulz; 1989.
21. Carpentier A, Adams D, Filsoufi F. *Carpentier's Reconstructive Valve Surgery*. Maryland Heights, Missouri: Saunders/Elsevier; 2010.
22. Madesis A, Tsakiridis K, Zarogoulidis P, et al. Review of mitral valve insufficiency: repair or replacement. *J Thorac Dis*. 2014;6(Suppl 1):S39–S51.
23. Antunes MJ. Repair of rheumatic mitral valve regurgitation: how far can we go? *Eur J Cardiothorac Surg*. 2013; 44(4):689–691.

24. Dillon J, Yakub MA, Nordin MN, Pau KK, Krishna Moorthy PS. Leaflet extension in rheumatic mitral valve reconstruction. *Eur J Cardiothorac Surg*. 2013;44(4): 682–689.

25. Mihos CG, Pineda AM, Capoulade R, Santana O. A systematic review of mitral valve repair with autologous pericardial leaflet augmentation for rheumatic mitral regurgitation. *Ann Thorac Surg*. 2016;102(4): 1400–1405.

26. Kalangos A, Christenson JT, Beghetti M, et al. Mitral valve repair for rheumatic valve disease in children: midterm results and impact of the use of a biodegradable mitral ring. *Ann Thorac Surg*. 2008;86(1):161–168. Discussion 8–9.

27. Van Phan N, Phuong PK, Vinh PN, et al. Mitral valvuloplasty with Carpentier's techniques. *Asian Cardiovasc Thorac Ann*. 1998;6(3):158–161.

28. Galloway AC, Colvin SB, Baumann FG, et al. A comparison of mitral valve reconstruction with mitral valve replacement: intermediate-term results. *Ann Thorac Surg*. 1989;47(5):655–662.

29. Myerson SG. Heart valve disease: investigation by cardiovascular magnetic resonance. *J Cardiovasc Magn Reson*. 2012;14:7.

30. Gilbert O, Wilson N, Finucane K. Early cardiac morbidity of rheumatic fever in children in New Zealand. *N Z Med J*. 2011;124(1343):57–64.

31. Namboodiri N, Remash K, Tharakan JA, et al. Natural history of aortic valve disease following intervention for rheumatic mitral valve disease. *J Heart Valve Dis*. 2009; 18(1):61–67.

32. Rusingiza EK, El-Khatib Z, Hedt-Gauthier B, et al. Outcomes for patients with rheumatic heart disease after cardiac surgery followed at rural district hospitals in Rwanda. *Heart*. 2018;104(20):1701–1713.

33. Zuhlke L, Karthikeyan G, Engel ME, et al. Clinical outcomes in 3343 children and adults with rheumatic heart disease from 14 low- and middle-income countries: two-year follow-up of the global rheumatic heart disease registry (the REMEDY study). *Circulation*. 2016;134(19): 1456–1466.

34. Marcus RH, Sareli P, Pocock WA, Barlow JB. The spectrum of severe rheumatic mitral valve disease in a developing country. Correlations among clinical presentation, surgical pathologic findings, and hemodynamic sequelae. *Ann Intern Med*. 1994;120(3):177–183.

35. Sani MU, Karaye KM, Borodo MM. Prevalence and pattern of rheumatic heart disease in the Nigerian savannah: an echocardiographic study. *Cardiovasc J Afr*. 2007;18(5):295–299.

36. Sriharibabu M, Himabindu Y, Kabir Z. Rheumatic heart disease in rural south India: a clinico-observational study. *J Cardiovasc Dis Res*. 2013;4(1):25–29.

37. Zuhlke L, Engel ME, Karthikeyan G, et al. Characteristics, complications, and gaps in evidence-based interventions in rheumatic heart disease: the global rheumatic heart disease registry (the REMEDY study). *Eur Heart J*. 2015; 36(18):1115–1122a.

38. Yeong M, Silbery M, Finucane K, Wilson NJ, Gentles TL. Mitral valve geometry in paediatric rheumatic mitral regurgitation. *Pediatr Cardiol*. 2015;36(4):827–834.

39. Anderson Y, W N, Nicholson R, Finucane K. Fulminant mitral regurgitation due to ruptured chordae tendinae in acute rheumatic fever. *J Paediatr Child Health*. 2007; 44(3):134–137.

40. Gentles TL, French JK, Zeng I, et al. Normalized end-systolic volume and pre-load reserve predict ventricular dysfunction following surgery for aortic regurgitation independent of body size. *JACC Cardiovasc Imaging*. 2012;5(6):626–633.

41. Wilson N. Rheumatic heart disease in indigenous populations–New Zealand experience. *Heart Lung Circ*. 2010;19(5–6):282–288.

42. Gentles TL, Colan SD, Wilson NJ, Biosa R, Neutze JM. Left ventricular mechanics during and after acute rheumatic fever: contractile dysfunction is closely related to valve regurgitation. *J Am Coll Cardiol*. 2001;37(1):201–207.

43. Gentles TL, Finucane AK, Remenyi B, Kerr AR, Wilson NJ. Ventricular function before and after surgery for isolated and combined regurgitation in the young. *Ann Thorac Surg*. 2015;100(4):1383–1389.

44. Dreyfus GD, Corbi PJ, Chan KM, Bahrami T. Secondary tricuspid regurgitation or dilatation: which should be the criteria for surgical repair? *Ann Thorac Surg*. 2005; 79(1):127–132.

45. Drake DH, Zimmerman KG, Hepner AM, Nichols CD. Echo-guided mitral repair. *Circ Cardiovasc Imaging*. 2014;7(1):132–141.

46. Antunes MJ, Barlow JB. Management of tricuspid valve regurgitation. *Heart*. 2007;93(2):271–276.

47. Saxena A. Echocardiographic diagnosis of chronic rheumatic valvular lesions. *Glob Heart*. 2013;8(3):203–212.

48. Baumgartner H, Falk V, Bax JJ, et al. 2017 ESC/EACTS Guidelines for the management of valvular heart disease. *Eur Heart J*. 2017;38(36):2739–2791.

49. Thomson Mangnall L, Sibbritt D, Fry M, Gallagher R. Short- and long-term outcomes after valve replacement surgery for rheumatic heart disease in the South Pacific, conducted by a fly-in/fly-out humanitarian surgical team: a 20-year retrospective study for the years 1991 to 2011. *J Thorac Cardiovasc Surg*. 2014;148(5):1996–2003.

50. Finucane K, Wilson N. Priorities in cardiac surgery for rheumatic heart disease. *Glob Heart*. 2013;8(3):213–220.

51. De DH, Pezzella AT. Closed mitral commissurotomy utilizing right thoracotomy approach. *Asian Cardiovasc Thorac Ann*. 2000;8(2):192–194.

52. Cooley DA, Stoneburner JM. Transventricular mitral valvotomy. *Surgery*. 1959;46(2):414–420.

53. Cosio-Pascal M, Ibarra-Perez C. Closed mitral commissurotomy through a midline sternotomy. A useful and potentially advantageous alternative to the left thoracotomy approach. *Am J Surg*. 1974;127(6):721–724.

53a. Netter, FH, The Netter Collection of Medical Illustrations - Heart. *Acquired Diseases of the Heart*. 191. https://www.netterimages.com/book-frank-h-netter-md-collection-of-medical-illustrations-heart-volume-5-9780914168850.html.

54. Akinci E, Degertekin M, Guler M, et al. Less invasive approaches for closed mitral commissurotomy. *Eur J Cardiothorac Surg.* 1998;14(3):274–278.

55. Victor S, Nayak VM. Closed mitral valvotomy: TEE probe or tactile control. *Ann Thorac Surg.* 1995;59(6):1622–1623.

56. Kumar AS. *Techniques in Valvular Heart Surgery.* 2nd ed. New Delhi, India: CBS Publishers; 2010.

57. Yakub MA, Dillon J, Krishna Moorthy PS, Pau KK, Nordin MN. Is rheumatic aetiology a predictor of poor outcome in the current era of mitral valve repair? Contemporary long-term results of mitral valve repair in rheumatic heart disease. *Eur J Cardiothorac Surg.* 2013;44(4):673–681.

58. Antunes MJ, Wessels A, Sadowski RG, et al. Medtronic Hall valve replacement in a third-world population group. A review of the performance of 1000 prostheses. *J Thorac Cardiovasc Surg.* 1988;95(6):980–993.

59. Jamieson WR, Gudas VM, Burr LH, et al. Mitral valve disease: if the mitral valve is not reparable/failed repair, is bioprosthesis suitable for replacement? *Eur J Cardiothorac Surg.* 2009;35(1):104–110.

60. Matsuyama K, Matsumoto M, Sugita T, et al. Long-term results of reoperative mitral valve surgery in patients with rheumatic disease. *Ann Thorac Surg.* 2003;76(6):1939–1943. Discussion 43.

61. Nishimura RA, Otto CM, Bonow RO, et al. 2014 AHA/ACC guideline for the management of patients with valvular heart disease: a report of the American college of cardiology/American heart association task force on practice guidelines. *J Am Coll Cardiol.* 2014;63(22):e57–185.

62. Talwar S, Sharma AK, Kumar AS. Tissue heart valve implantation in India; Indications, results and impact on quality of life. *Indian J Thorac Cardiovasc Surg.* 2008;24(1):10–14.

63. Chikwe J, Filsoufi F. Durability of tissue valves. *Semin Thorac Cardiovasc Surg.* 2011;23(1):18–23.

64. Doty DB, Doty RD. Mitral valve replacement. In: Doty DB, Doty RD, eds. *Cardiac Surgery: Operative Technique.* 2nd ed. Philadelphia, PA: Elsevier/Saunders; 2012:364–373.

65. Gudbjartsson T, Absi T, Aranki S. Mitral valve replacement. In: Cohn LH, ed. *Cardiac Surgery in the Adult.* New York, New York: McGraw Hill; 2008:1031–1068.

66. Khonsari S, Sintec CF. *Cardiac Surgery- Safeguards and Pitfalls in Operative Technique.* Philadelphia, PA: Lippincott Williams & and Wilkins; 2003.

67. Lillehei CW. New ideas and their acceptance. As it has related to preservation of chordae tendinea and certain other discoveries. *J Heart Valve Dis.* 1995;4(Suppl 2):S106–S114.

68. David TE. Mitral valve replacement with preservation of chordae tendinae: rationale and technical considerations. *Ann Thorac Surg.* 1986;41(6):680–682.

69. David TE, Burns RJ, Bacchus CM, Druck MN. Mitral valve replacement for mitral regurgitation with and without preservation of chordae tendineae. *J Thorac Cardiovasc Surg.* 1984;88(5 Pt 1):718–725.

70. Hetzer R, Bougioukas G, Franz M, Borst HG. Mitral valve replacement with preservation of papillary muscles and chordae tendineae – revival of a seemingly forgotten concept. I. Preliminary clinical report. *Thorac Cardiovasc Surg.* 1983;31(5):291–296.

71. Miller Jr DW, Johnson DD, Ivey TD. Does preservation of the posterior chordae tendineae enhance survival during mitral valve replacement? *Ann Thorac Surg.* 1979;28(1):22–27.

72. Turgeman Y, Atar S, Rosenfeld T. The subvalvular apparatus in rheumatic mitral stenosis: methods of assessment and therapeutic implications. *Chest.* 2003;124(5):1929–1936.

73. Hwang HY, Kim KH, Ahn H. Attitude after a mild aortic valve lesion during rheumatic mitral valve surgery. *J Thorac Cardiovasc Surg.* 2014;147(5):1540–1546.

74. Bernal JM, Fernandez-Vals M, Rabasa JM, et al. Repair of nonsevere rheumatic aortic valve disease during other valvular procedures: is it safe? *J Thorac Cardiovasc Surg.* 1998;115(5):1130–1135.

75. al-Halees Z, Kumar N, Gallo R, Gometza B, Duran CM. Pulmonary autograft for aortic valve replacement in rheumatic disease: a caveat. *Ann Thorac Surg.* 1995;60(2 Suppl):S172–S175. Discussion S6.

76. Sampath Kumar A, Talwar S, Saxena A, Singh R. Ross procedure in rheumatic aortic valve disease. *Eur J Cardiothorac Surg.* 2006;29(2):156–161.

77. Alsoufi B, Manlhiot C, Fadel B, et al. Is the ross procedure a suitable choice for aortic valve replacement in children with rheumatic aortic valve disease? *World J Pediatr Congenit Heart Surg.* 2012;3(1):8–15.

78. Talwar S, Saikrishna C, Saxena A, Kumar AS. Aortic valve repair for rheumatic aortic valve disease. *Ann Thorac Surg.* 2005;79(6):1921–1925.

79. Suri RM, Schaff HV. Aortic valve repair: defining the patient population and timing of the intervention. *J Thorac Cardiovasc Surg.* 2014;148(6):2477–2478.

80. Haluck RS, Richenbacher WE, Myers JL, et al. Pericardium as a thoracic aortic patch: glutaraldehyde-fixed and fresh autologous pericardium. *J Surg Res.* 1990;48(6):611–614.

81. Nosal M, Poruban R, Valentik P, et al. Initial experience with polytetrafluoroethylene leaflet extensions for aortic valve repair. *Eur J Cardiothorac Surg.* 2012;41(6):1255–1257. Discussion 8.

82. Myers PO, Tissot C, Christenson JT, et al. Aortic valve repair by cusp extension for rheumatic aortic insufficiency in children: long-term results and impact of extension material. *J Thorac Cardiovasc Surg.* 2010;140(4):836–844.

83. d'Udekem Y, Sharma V. Repair options in rheumatic aortic valve disease in young patients: potential problems with pericardial cusp extension. *World J Pediatr Congenit Heart Surg.* 2013;4(4):392–396.

84. Tang H, Xu Z, Zou L, et al. Valve repair with autologous pericardium for organic lesions in rheumatic tricuspid valve disease. *Ann Thorac Surg.* 2009;87(3):726–730.

85. Antunes MJ. Mitral valvuloplasty, a better alternative. Comparative study between valve reconstruction and

replacement for rheumatic mitral valve disease. *Eur J Cardiothorac Surg.* 1990;4(5):257–262. Discussion 63-4.

86. Choudhary SK, Dhareshwar J, Govil A, Airan B, Kumar AS. Open mitral commissurotomy in the current era: indications, technique, and results. *Ann Thorac Surg.* 2003;75(1):41–46.

87. Kim JB, Kim HJ, Moon DH, et al. Long-term outcomes after surgery for rheumatic mitral valve disease: valve repair versus mechanical valve replacement. *Eur J Cardiothorac Surg.* 2010;37(5):1039–1046.

88. Yau TM, El-Ghoneimi YA, Armstrong S, Ivanov J, David TE. Mitral valve repair and replacement for rheumatic disease. *J Thorac Cardiovasc Surg.* 2000;119(1):53–60.

89. Goldman ME, Mora F, Guarino T, Fuster V, Mindich BP. Mitral valvuloplasty is superior to valve replacement for preservation of left ventricular function: an intraoperative two-dimensional echocardiographic study. *J Am Coll Cardiol.* 1987;10(3):568–575.

90. Oliveira JM, Antunes MJ. Mitral valve repair: better than replacement. *Heart.* 2006;92(2):275–281.

91. Shuhaiber J, Anderson RJ. Meta-analysis of clinical outcomes following surgical mitral valve repair or replacement. *Eur J Cardiothorac Surg.* 2007;31(2):267–275.

92. Suri RM, Schaff HV, Dearani JA, et al. Survival advantage and improved durability of mitral repair for leaflet prolapse subsets in the current era. *Ann Thorac Surg.* 2006; 82(3):819–826.

93. Vahanian A, Alfieri O, Andreotti F, et al. Guidelines on the management of valvular heart disease (version 2012). *Eur Heart J.* 2012;33(19):2451–2496.

94. Vassileva CM, Li S, Thourani VH, et al. Outcome characteristics of multiple-valve surgery: comparison with single-valve procedures. *Innovations.* 2014;9(1):27–32.

95. John S, Ravikumar E, John CN, Bashi VV. 25-year experience with 456 combined mitral and aortic valve replacement for rheumatic heart disease. *Ann Thorac Surg.* 2000; 69(4):1167–1172.

96. Coutinho GF, Leite F, Antunes MJ. Circumflex artery injury during mitral valve repair: not well known, perhaps not so infrequent-lessons learned from a 6-case experience. *J Thorac Cardiovasc Surg.* 2017;154(5):1613–1620.

97. Wang YC, Tsai FC, Chu JJ, Lin PJ. Midterm outcomes of rheumatic mitral repair versus replacement. *Int Heart J.* 2008;49(5):565–576.

98. Russell EA, Walsh WF, Reid CM, et al. Outcomes after mitral valve surgery for rheumatic heart disease. *Heart Asia.* 2017;9(2):e010916.

99. Chambers JB, Prendergast B, Iung B, et al. Standards defining a 'heart valve centre': ESC working group on valvular heart disease European association for cardiothoracic surgery viewpoint. *Eur Heart J.* 2017;38(28): 2177–2183.

100. Dillon J, Yakub MA, Kong PK, et al. Comparative long-term results of mitral valve repair in adults with chronic rheumatic disease and degenerative disease: is repair for "burnt-out" rheumatic disease still inferior to repair for degenerative disease in the current era? *J Thorac Cardiovasc Surg.* 2015;149(3):771–777. Discussion 7-9.

101. Talwar S, Rajesh MR, Subramanian A, Saxena A, Kumar AS. Mitral valve repair in children with rheumatic heart disease. *J Thorac Cardiovasc Surg.* 2005;129(4):875–879.

102. Pomerantzeff PM, Brandao CM, Faber CM, et al. Mitral valve repair in rheumatic patients. *Heart Surg Forum.* 2000;3(4):273–276.

103. Cotrufo M, Renzulli A, Vitale N, et al. Long-term follow-up of open commissurotomy versus bileaflet valve replacement for rheumatic mitral stenosis. *Eur J Cardiothorac Surg.* 1997;12(3):335–339. Discussion 9-40.

104. Duran CG. Reconstructive techniques for rheumatic aortic valve disease. *J Card Surg.* 1988;3(1):23–28.

105. Zegdi R, Ould-Isselmou K, Fabiani JN, Deloche A. Pericardial patch anterior leaflet extension in rheumatic mitral insufficiency. *Eur J Cardiothorac Surg.* 2011;39(6): 1061–1063.

106. Coutinho GF, Bihun V, Correia PE, Antunes PE, Antunes MJ. Preservation of the subvalvular apparatus during mitral valve replacement of rheumatic valves does not affect long-term survival. *Eur J Cardiothorac Surg.* 2015;48(6):861–867. Discussion 7.

107. Coutinho GF, Branco CF, Jorge E, Correia PM, Antunes MJ. Mitral valve surgery after percutaneous mitral commissurotomy: is repair still feasible? *Eur J Cardiothorac Surg.* 2015;47(1):e1–6.

108. Saccocci M, Taramasso M, Maisano F. Mitral valve interventions in structural heart disease. *Curr Cardiol Rep.* 2018;20(6):49.

109. ESC Press Office. Novel heart valve replacement offers hope for thousands with rheumatic heart disease. In: *Technique Does Not Require Advanced Cardiac Surgical Facilities or Sophisticated Cardiovascular Imaging.* Cape Town, South Africa: European Society of Cardiology; 2016 [Press Release].

110. Petronio AS, Capranzano P, Barbato E, et al. Current status of transcatheter valve therapy in Europe: results from an EAPCI survey. *EuroIntervention.* 2016;12(7):890–895.

111. Zilla P, Yacoub M, Zuhlke L, et al. Global unmet needs in cardiac surgery. *Glob Heart.* 2018;13(4):293–303.

112. Watkins D, Zuhlke L, Engel M, et al. Seven key actions to eradicate rheumatic heart disease in Africa: the Addis Ababa communique. *Cardiovasc J Afr.* 2016;27(3):184–187.

113. Zilla P, Bolman RM, Yacoub MH, et al. The Cape Town declaration on access to cardiac surgery in the developing world. *S Afr Med J.* 2018;108(9):702–704.

CHAPTER 9

Rheumatic Heart Disease in Pregnancy

ANA MOCUMBI • ANDREA BEATON • PRIYA SOMA-PILLAY • SCOTT DOUGHERTY • KAREN SLIWA

INTRODUCTION

Heart disease is the highest indirect (nonobstetric) cause of mortality for pregnant women in both high-income countries (HICs) and low- and middle-income countries (LMICs).[1,2] Valvular heart disease is an important contributor to the burden of maternal disease, accounting for 15% of pregnancy-related complications in HICs, although this figure is significantly higher in LMICs owing to the much higher prevalence of rheumatic heart disease (RHD). In these resource-limited populations, RHD accounts for 50%–90% of maternal cardiac complications,[3] with rheumatic mitral stenosis (MS) being the single most common cause of cardiac maternal mortality.[4,5]

Damage to the cardiac valves, which is the hallmark of RHD, often leads to significant valvular heart disease and left ventricular dysfunction. These changes, coupled with the marked physiological adaptations associated with pregnancy, impose an increased hemodynamic stress on the cardiovascular system, increasing the risk of cardiovascular complications and poorer outcomes for both the mother and fetus. Nevertheless, pregnancy complicated by nonsevere valvular heart disease is generally associated with a favorable prognosis, providing that the risks are managed appropriately. For many patients living in LMICs, however, adequate preconception and prenatal care are not available.

Over the last number of years new data have emerged relating to pregnant women with heart disease and the recently updated European Society of Cardiology (ESC) guidelines on cardiovascular disease in pregnancy have introduced a number of important updates and recommendations.[6] In particular, counseling is stressed as a crucial intervention for all women with heart disease who are contemplating pregnancy or are already pregnant. Moreover, those with moderate or greater risk heart disease should receive counseling

and a full risk assessment by a "pregnancy heart team," ideally in an expert center using modified WHO (mWHO) criteria. Other important new recommendations include the introduction of the Pregnancy and Lactation Labeling Rule (PLLR) drug table, which replaces the FDA's A to X categorial system with a more narrative approach, and the recommendation to consider inducing labor at 40 weeks' gestation for all women with cardiac disease (to reduce obstetric risk).

The 2014 American Heart Association and American College of Cardiology (AHA/ACC) guidelines on the management of valvular heart disease[7] also make important recommendations on the management of pregnant women. It must be stressed however that most of the data on which the ESC and AHA/ACC recommendations are based are not from randomized control trials, so the guidelines' recommendations are mostly level C (expert opinion). Furthermore, these guidelines have been developed by experts in HICs, where resource limitation is usually not an issue.

This chapter will focus on the main issues surrounding preconception evaluation and management of RHD in stable pregnant patients. The medical (Chapter 6), interventional (Chapter 7), surgical (Chapter 8), and emergency (Chapter 16) management of nonpregnant RHD patients is discussed in detail elsewhere, with important differences in the management of pregnant patients discussed here.

EPIDEMIOLOGY OF RHEUMATIC HEART DISEASE IN PREGNANCY

The scarcity of data on RHD in pregnancy is in part due to underdiagnosis as well as a lack of adequate antenatal care in most endemic settings. Although RHD and other cardiac diseases (such as hypertensive diseases and cardiomyopathies) are recognized as a major

Acute Rheumatic Fever and Rheumatic Heart Disease. https://doi.org/10.1016/B978-0-323-63982-8.00009-X

health burden in LMICs, a systematic search for these conditions is usually not performed during pregnancy in these settings.[8]

Prevention and control programs for acute rheumatic fever (ARF) and RHD have not been implemented in many endemic areas.[9] The lower a country's income category, the younger the median age and more advanced the disease is at presentation, and this epidemiological pattern has direct implications for the maternal health of a country's population.[10] Poor countries with a high prevalence of RHD usually have a low human development index, poor provision of family planning, high fertility rates, weak prepregnancy advice for women with heart disease,[11,12] and a 14 times higher maternal mortality ratio than HICs.[8]

The Registry of Pregnancy and Cardiac Disease (ROPAC) data, which aimed to determine the variation in structural heart disease in pregnant patients, is the largest prospective cohort of pregnant women with RHD, and included 390 pregnant women with rheumatic mitral valve disease and no prepregnancy valve replacement.[13] Three quarters of the patients (75%) came from LMICs. MS with or without mitral regurgitation (MR) was present in 273 women, and was moderate to severe in 59.0% of patients. One maternal death occurred during pregnancy in a patient with severe MS.

The first prospective global registry of RHD (REMEDY), which collected data from 12 African countries, India and Yemen, provides a contemporary description of the presentation, complications, and treatment of RHD.[14] Young females were highly represented (median age 28 years, females 66.2%) among the 3343 patients enrolled at the 25 participating hospitals, and had a higher prevalence of major cardiovascular complications. Female predominance was seen across all income groups, varying from 63.0% in lower middle-income countries (Egypt, India, Mozambique, Nigeria, Sudan, and Yemen) to 71.3% in upper middle-income countries (Namibia and South Africa). Among the 1825 women of childbearing age (12–51 years), only 65 (3.6%) were on contraception, which can be explained by low level of education and awareness, poor access to healthcare, culturally inadequate care provision, and health systems that do not meet the needs of pregnant women with RHD.

With current management practices, maternal and fetal mortality can be reduced, and the incidence of complications is predictable based on known risk factors. Available data demonstrate that pregnancy outcomes in RHD patients are determined by the development status of a country and its health system,

and the studies summarized here highlight these health disparities. In a study to determine maternal cardiac complications and obstetric outcomes among the 52 indigenous women of childbearing age in northern Australia with RHD, there were no maternal or neonatal deaths.[15] Despite four patients being first diagnosed with RHD after developing acute pulmonary edema during the peripartum period, this study showed that a very low incidence of cardiac complications and no deaths is possible with expert and skilled care. In comparison, Diao et al.[5] report on maternal and fetal outcomes in 50 Senegalese pregnant women with heart disease, of which 46 had RHD. Pulmonary edema (36), arrhythmias (18), and pulmonary embolism (2) were major complications found on admission among the 39 unoperated females (32 of whom had MS). There were 17 maternal deaths (34%) and the fetal outcomes were also poor: six fetal deaths, five therapeutic abortions, and four stillbirths (neonatal mortality was 7.6%). It is not possible to clearly assess to what extent these results are influenced by differences in the severity of cases at presentation and quality of care in the two countries. However, they do suggest that late presentation of patients and lack of access to specialized care for diagnosis and management might explain the high frequency of pregnancy-related hemodynamic decompensation and poor outcomes in women with rheumatic MS in studies from developing countries. This contrasts with a number of recent series from Western countries, which reported maternal mortality rates below 3%.[16–19]

MATERNAL CARDIAC PHYSIOLOGY

Given that pregnancy is akin to a physiological stress test, the period following conception can unmask previously silent maternal heart disease or exacerbate previously well-controlled preexisting conditions. The major hemodynamic changes that occur in pregnancy are summarized in Fig. 9.1.[20] A 30% increase in stroke volume and 10%–20% increase in heart rate result in a 30%–50% increase in cardiac output above the nonpregnant state. These changes begin in early pregnancy and plateau between the second and third trimesters.[21,22] Systemic vasodilation and the low-resistance utero-placental circulation facilitate a drop in systemic vascular resistance (SVR) by 35%–40%, which helps accommodate for the increase in cardiac output.[23] SVR reaches the nadir by the end of the second trimester and then slowly begins to increase until term. By the sixth week of pregnancy, the plasma volume also begins to increase and by the second trimester is 50% above

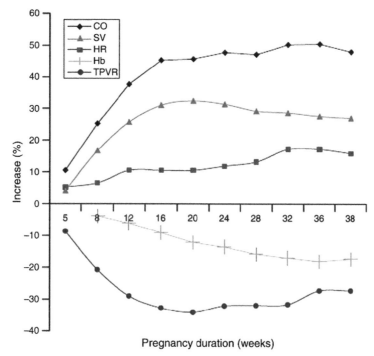

FIG. 9.1 Changes in cardiac output (CO), stroke volume (SV), heart rate (HR), hemoglobin (Hb), and total peripheral vascular resistance (TPVR) during pregnancy. (Reproduced with permission from Karamermer et al.[20])

baseline. Although there is a corresponding rise in red cell mass, this is not in proportion to the plasma volume, resulting in physiological anemia.[24]

Together, each of these changes culminates in a hyperdynamic circulation leading to increased flow, and thus increased gradients, across heart valves.[25] In normal valves, this results in physiological murmurs but in stenotic valves, gradients can increase significantly, particularly at the mitral valve level, and result in heart failure (HF) symptoms. For example, in MS any further elevation of the transmitral gradient is transmitted upstream, increasing both the left atrial and pulmonary venous pressures and resulting in breathlessness on exertion, orthopnea, paroxysmal dyspnea, or even frank pulmonary edema. The increased heart rate associated with pregnancy also decreases the time for diastolic filling, reducing both left ventricular volumes and cardiac output. Because pregnancy is an arrhythmogenic state, in patients with MS any further increase in the ventricular rate and/or loss of atrial filling (in the context of atrial fibrillation (AF)) can also precipitate acute HF (see Chapter 16).[26] In contrast to stenotic lesions, regurgitant valve lesions are typically well tolerated because the fall in SVR compensates for the volume loading conditions of pregnancy.[2]

Pregnancy also results in a highly thrombogenic state. This is in part mediated by an increased concentration of clotting factors, resulting in a 20% reduction of both the prothrombin time and activated partial thromboplastin time (aPTT), but also through increased platelet adhesiveness and decreased fibrinolysis.[27–29] The risk of thrombosis is higher in the puerperium (particularly during the first 6 weeks) than during pregnancy.[30] This increased thrombotic status is clearly a hazard for patients with mechanical heart valves (MHVs), significant MS, and AF. Meticulous management of anticoagulation is therefore particularly important during this period.

Regarding labor and delivery, a 30% increase in cardiac output occurs during the first stage of labor and a 60%–80% increase immediately postdelivery.[31] These changes are driven by an increase in heart rate (due to pain and anxiety) and stroke volume (300–500 mL of blood is "autotransfused" into the systemic circulation with each uterine contraction).[32] When spinal anesthesia is used a significant reduction in SVR also occurs, necessitating compensatory increases in heart rate and stroke volume. At delivery, the baby no longer mechanically compresses the inferior vena cava, resulting in a further increase in preload, unless there has been significant postpartum hemorrhage. Shifts in maternal hemodynamics peak within the first 24–72 h postpartum and are more rapid when delivery is by cesarean section. Therefore, women with heart disease are at increased risk of developing HF within this period, particularly if cesarean section was the mode of delivery.[2,33] The period of increased risk of HF, thrombotic events, and bleeding lasts up to 1 year postpartum leading to late maternal death.[34,35]

PRECONCEPTION EVALUATION

Given the potential for increased risk of cardiovascular complications while pregnant, preconception counseling should be offered to all women with RHD, and is strongly recommended based on current ESC and AHA/ACC guidelines.[6,7] Individualized care and informed decision-making are both central to this process, taking into account the severity of the valvular lesions and cardiac function, as well as emotional, cultural, psychological, and ethical issues.[6]

The reality, however, is that many newly pregnant women with RHD living in LMICs often present after 20 weeks' gestation, and a considerable number are unaware that they have RHD until hemodynamic decompensation occurs due to pregnancy. Delayed diagnosis is a risk factor for maternal death: in a report from the UK, most deaths occurred in those women who had undiagnosed preconception heart disease,[36] a situation that is also true for women in LMICs.[5] Unplanned pregnancies, which are widely acknowledged as both a cause and consequence of socioeconomic inequality,[37,38] are also seen in many women with RHD and are associated with poorer outcomes for both the mother and fetus.

Issues that may be discussed during counseling include helping the woman understand the risk of death during pregnancy, the risk of embryopathy, need to cease or commence medications, the risks of thrombosis, and risks of peripartum bleeding. In more complex cases, interventional or surgical treatment may also be recommended before any planned pregnancy. Women at the highest risk should be counseled against pregnancy.

Risk Stratification

Risk stratification is an important part of preconception evaluation. In addition to a thorough assessment of symptoms and cardiac status, routine booking tests should include chest X-ray, full blood count, urine analysis, and HIV testing. The minimum cardiac investigations for maternal risk stratification for women with RHD are an electrocardiogram (ECG), echocardiogram, and an exercise test.[6] Other tests, such as exercise echocardiography, cardiac computed tomography or

magnetic resonance imaging may also be utilized if further information is required. Exercise testing can objectively estimate functional capacity: favorable outcomes are predicted by a pregnancy exercise capacity >80% (see individual valve lesions section).[6]

The following factors should be considered during pregnancy risk stratification: maternal cardiac and obstetric risk, fetal and neonatal risks, long-term effects of pregnancy on the heart, maternal life expectancy, and modification of cardiac drugs.

Pregnancy risk should be determined using general and lesion-specific risk factors. General risk factors for adverse maternal cardiac events in those with heart disease include baseline New York Heart Association (NYHA) class III/IV (see Chapter 5), cyanosis, previous cardiac event (e.g., pulmonary edema, transient ischemic attack, or stroke), arrhythmia, systemic ventricular ejection fraction (EF) <40%, left heart obstruction (echocardiographic mitral valve area (MVA) <2 cm^2, aortic valve area (AVA) <1.5 cm^2, or peak left ventricular (LV) outflow tract gradient >30 mmHg), pulmonary regurgitation, mechanical heart valve, as well as significant mitral or tricuspid regurgitation.[39–41] It is worth noting that the most frequent complications during pregnancy are HF, arrhythmias, and thromboembolic events.[36] CARPREG (Cardiac Disease in Pregnancy) is an established general risk index based on these predictors and was derived from an observational prospective cohort study of pregnant women with congenital and acquired heart disease (Box 9.1).[39]

Another established risk index is the mWHO classification, which incorporates both general and lesion-specific diagnoses and is considered the most accurate system for risk assessment currently in use (Table 9.1),[2,6] although it is probably better suited to

---

BOX 9.1
The Cardiac Disease in Pregnancy (CARPREG) Risk Score[39]

RISK FACTOR
- Prior cardiac event or arrhythmia
- NYHA Class III or IV or cyanosis
- Left heart obstruction
- Systemic ventricular dysfunction (EF <40%)

SCORE AND RISK OF CARDIAC COMPLICATIONS
- Score 0: 5% risk
- Score 1: 27% risk
- Score >1: 62% risk

NYHA, New York Heart Association; EF, ejection fraction.

TABLE 9.1
Modified World Health Organization (mWHO) classification of maternal cardiovascular risk.[a,2,6]

	mWHO I	mWHO II	mWHO II-III	mWHO III	mWHO IV
Diagnosis (If otherwise well and uncomplicated)	- Trivial MR - Uncomplicated mitral valve prolapse - Trivial AR - Mild TR - Mild PS, PR - Isolated atrial or ventricular ectopic beats	- Mild MS, MR - Mild AS, AR - Mild TS[b] - Moderate TR[b] - Moderate PS, PR - Most arrhythmias (supraventricular arrhythmias)	- Moderate MR - Moderate AS - Moderate AR - Severe PR - Mild LVSD (EF 45-54%)	- Mechanical valve - Moderate MS - Severe MR - Severe, asymptomatic AS - Severe AR - Severe TS[b], TR[b] - Severe PS - Ventricular tachycardia - Moderate LVSD (EF 30-44%)	- Severe MS - Severe symptomatic AS - Critical AS - Pulmonary hypertension[c] - Severe systemic ventricular dysfunction (EF <30% or NYHA class III or IV)
Risk	No detectable increased risk of maternal mortality and no/mild increased risk in morbidity	Small increased risk of maternal mortality or moderate increase in morbidity	Intermediate increased risk of maternal mortality or moderate to severe increase in maternal morbidity	Significantly increased risk of maternal mortality or severe morbidity	Extremely high risk of maternal mortality or severe morbidity
Maternal Cardiac Event Rate	2.5-5%	5.7-10.5%	10-19%	19-27%	40-100%
Counselling	Yes	Yes	Yes	Expert counselling required	Pregnancy is contraindicated. If pregnancy occurs, termination should be discussed
Care During Pregnancy and Delivery	Local hospital	Local hospital	Referral hospital	Expert center for pregnancy and cardiac disease	Expert center for pregnancy and cardiac disease
Minimal Follow-Up Visits During Pregnancy	Once or twice	Once per trimester	Bimonthly	Monthly or bimonthly	Monthly

MS mitral stenosis; MR mitral regurgitation; AS aortic stenosis; AR aortic regurgitation; TS tricuspid stenosis; TR tricuspid regurgitation; PS pulmonary stenosis; PR pulmonary regurgitation; LVSD left ventricular systolic dysfunction; EF ejection fraction; NYHA New York Heart Association
[a] Please see Regitz-Zagrosek[6] for full list of risk factors; only those most relevant to patients with RHD are presented here
[b] Very rare in isolation
[c] Secondary to any cause and of any grade
Adapted from Regitz-Zagrosek et al[6]

patients from HICs rather than LMICs. For example, van Hagen and colleagues recently validated the mWHO classification in advanced and emerging countries and identified additional risk factors for cardiac events during pregnancy using data from ROPAC, which included more than 2500 pregnant women.[13] The mWHO classification showed only a moderate performance of predicting risk between women with or without cardiac events (c-statistic 0.711, 95% CI 0.686—0.735) with a better performance in HICs versus LMICs. Prepregnancy signs of HF, and in HICs, AF, added prognostic value.

When using the mWHO index, it is important to remember that risks are additive. Therefore, risks are higher if, for example, the woman has mixed or multivalve disease (the most common RHD phenotype), concomitant left ventricular dysfunction, or noncardiac risk factors such as hypertension, obesity, or chronic kidney disease.[2]

Women with low-risk valvular heart disease can usually be managed by their local cardiology and obstetric team. It is important to avoid anxiety and overtesting and reassurance plays an important role here.[33] Those at higher risk should be managed within a pregnancy heart team, an important concept highlighted by the 2018 ESC guidelines[6] that emphasizes the importance of expert and individualized care delivered in a specialist center for those women who are at moderate-to-extremely high-risk of complications (mWHO class II—III, III, or IV). Women with RHD that falls within these higher risk classes should ideally be referred to a tertiary centre before pregnancy where they can be appropriately assessed and managed. Centres that perform percutaneous mitral balloon commissurotomy (PMBC) and cardiac surgery, as well as other diagnostic and interventional procedures, should be chosen.

The minimum team requirements within a pregnancy heart team are a cardiologist, obstetrician, and anesthetist, and may include others: a nurse specialist, a cardiothoracic surgeon, pediatric cardiologist, neonatologist, and hematologist. Each of these experts should have experience in the management of high-risk pregnancies in women with heart disease. The pregnancy heart team should be involved in all aspects of care, from preconception evaluation and counseling to management during pregnancy and around delivery.[6] It is recognized, however, that in many LMICs, these resources are simply not available.

In addition to the mWHO index, further considerations are given below regarding valve-specific risk stratification.

Mitral Stenosis
Even with ideal care, 35%—74% of women with rheumatic MS show clinical deterioration with

pregnancy[1,17]. Women with asymptomatic mild MS (MVA >1.5 cm^2) usually do well and are considered low risk (mWHO II), although elevated event rates are still seen in this group.[17,39] Recent ROPAC data showed that although mortality was only 1.9% in those with MS during pregnancy, nearly half of patients with severe MS (<1 cm^2) and one-third of patients with moderate MS (1.0—1.5 cm^2) developed heart failure (HF), even if the patient was asymptomatic before pregnancy. Those with mixed mitral valve disease (moderate-to-severe MS and MR) had adverse pregnancy outcomes similar to those with isolated severe MS.[13] HF due to MS is most likely to occur in the second trimester as cardiac output nears its peak.

Those with severe MS are likely to decompensate and should be advised to avoid pregnancy, at least until they receive successful intervention/surgical treatment. Other predictors of increased maternal complications in MS include NYHA III—IV, systolic pulmonary artery pressure (PAP) >30 mmHg, history of cardiac complications (pulmonary edema, transient ischemic attack, or stroke), reduced left ventricular EF (LVEF), and older age.[13,17—19] Mortality is higher in LMICs (although data is lacking here) compared to HICs, where the death rate is between 0% and 3%.[13,18] Persistent AF may also precipitate HF, although this occurs in <10% of pregnancies.[6] Pulmonary hypertension (pHT), which is a contraindication to pregnancy, may occur secondary to pulmonary venous hypertension (in patients with RHD, this is almost always due to severe left-sided valve disease) and carries a high maternal risk, with mortality rates ranging from 16-30%. pHT is discussed in detail in chapter 5.[43,44]

The rapid fluid shifts and tachycardia associated with labor and the immediate postpartum period can cause pulmonary edema and a low output state.[2] Fetal risks include prematurity (20%—30%), intrauterine growth restriction (5%—20%), and fetal death (1%—5%).[13,17,18] These risks are higher if the mother is NYHA III or IV during pregnancy.[19,39]

Aortic Stenosis
Women with asymptomatic mild or moderate AS or asymptomatic severe AS with a previously normal exercise tolerance usually tolerate pregnancy well, with a low risk of HF (<10%). In contrast, one quarter of patients with symptomatic AS will experience HF[45] and those with severe symptomatic AS should be advised to avoid pregnancy until they undergo valve intervention.[6] Arrhythmias and maternal mortality are now rare, providing high-quality management is offered, although this is not always possible in most LMICs. Obstetric risk may be increased in severe AS. Miscarriage and fetal

death risk are both <5%. Other fetal risks include prematurity, intrauterine growth restriction, and low birth weight, which occur in 20%–25% of those with moderate AS and are increased in severe AS.[45]

Mitral and Aortic Regurgitation

Mild regurgitation is usually well tolerated in pregnancy. Women are at high risk for HF if there is severe regurgitation with associated symptoms, reduced LVEF, severe LV dilatation, or pHT. The risk of developing HF in those with moderate or severe MR is 20%–25%.[13] Women with LVEF <30% or any degree of pHT should be advised to avoid pregnancy.[6] There appears to be no increased obstetric risk associated with regurgitant lesions. Intrauterine growth restriction is seen in 5%–10%.[6,13]

Tricuspid Regurgitation

Maternal risk is usually determined primarily by the severity of left-sided valve lesions or the presence of pHT.[6] Mild or moderate TR is tolerated well during pregnancy. Women with severe TR, although they can do well in pregnancy, are at increased risk for right-sided HF and atrial arrhythmias.[46]

Mixed Valve Lesions

Due to a lack of data, risk stratification is compromised for mixed (e.g., concomitant MR and MS) and multivalve (e.g., concomitant MS and AR) lesions. In general, however, risk and management should be based on the most hemodynamically significant lesion (see also Chapters 5 and 6). As discussed earlier, lesions are additive using the mWHO risk index.

Mitral/Aortic Valve Replacement

Bioprosthetic Valves. Pregnancy is usually well tolerated and the risk of maternal cardiovascular complications is low in women with normal functioning, or minimally dysfunctional, *bioprosthetic valves* and normal LV function.[47] Risk increases significantly if there is significant bioprosthetic dysfunction.[6]

Mechanical valves. In women with MHVs, the risk of complications during pregnancy is very high (mWHO class III) and the chances of an event-free pregnancy with a live birth are only 58%. This is in stark contrast to those with a bioprosthetic valve (79%) and those with cardiovascular disease but no prosthetic valves (78%).[48] The bulk of the risk arises from the need for anticoagulation (hemorrhagic complications) and the consequences of the prothrombotic pregnant state on MHVs (valve thrombosis).[6] Complications associated

with prosthetic valves and anticoagulation are discussed later in the chapter.

CLINICAL EVALUATION DURING NORMAL PREGNANCY

Although it is important to recognize and treat early the signs and symptoms of HF in pregnant patients with RHD, it is also important to understand that normal pregnancy is accompanied by changes to the cardiovascular system that can erroneously be attributed to heart disease. However, with careful history taking and examination, normal pregnancy should be distinguishable from cardiac decompensation (Table 9.2).[2]

In addition to these changes, increased flow through the left or right ventricular outflow tracts is responsible for the ejection systolic murmur (never more than 2/6) that is commonly heard at the left sternal edge in pregnant patients. The hyperdynamic

---

TABLE 9.2

Signs and Symptoms of Normal Pregnancy and Pregnancy With Cardiac Compromise.

Signs and Symptoms that May Occur in Normal Pregnancy	Signs and Symptoms Suggesting Cardiac Decompensation During Pregnancy
Breathlessness on exertion	Marked breathlessness, e.g., minor exertion, talking and eating
Difficulty sleeping due to discomfort	Orthopnea and paroxysmal nocturnal dyspnea
Increased heart rate <100 bpm (10–20 bpm higher than prepregnancy)	Sinus tachycardia persistently >100 bpm
Chest discomfort due to reflux	Exertional, tearing, or pleuritic chest pain
Vasovagal syncope, postural hypotension	Exertional or palpation-related syncope
Palpation due to atrial and ventricular ectopics	Sustained tachyarrhythmias
Jugular venous pulse visible +2 cm	Jugular venous pulse raised >2 cm
3rd heart sound	4th heart sound
Mild peripheral edema	Marked peripheral edema

Reproduced with permission from Thorne S[2]

circulation may also result in a cervical venous hum (best heard over the right supraclavicular fossa) or the mammary soufflé (a continuous or systolic murmur best heard over the breasts in late gestation or during lactation). Diastolic murmurs, which are uncommonly associated with normal pregnancy (e.g., increased flow through the mitral or tricuspid valve), should prompt a search for underlying pathology.[49] Peripheral edema is found in 80% of normal pregnant women and is due to increased venous pressures in the lower extremities.

Increased gradients may be observed across diseased valves on echocardiography and so a valve area calculation may be more accurate. Physiological multivalve regurgitation (predominantly right-sided), four-chamber enlargement, and a small pericardial effusion may also be seen on echocardiography. The left, anterior, and superior rotation of the heart during normal pregnancy can also lead to a 15–20 degree left-axis deviation on ECG and give the illusion of cardiomegaly on chest X-ray. Increased pulmonary markings can also be seen on chest X-ray in normal pregnancy.

MANAGEMENT OF RHEUMATIC HEART DISEASE IN PREGNANCY

General management principles, which apply to all patients with RHD and include regular penicillin prophylaxis and good dental hygiene, are discussed in Chapter 6. ESC guidelines recommend that safety tables should be used before pharmacological therapy in pregnancy is commenced (such a safety table can be found in these guidelines).[6] In the absence of clinical safety data, it is recommended to check the electronic drug table at www.safefetus.com for preclinical safety data. Decision-making based on former FDA categories alone, which have been replaced by PLLR since 2015, is no longer recommended (class III).[6] Fig. 9.2 summaries the safety of selected drugs during pregnancy and breastfeeding. Panel 1 includes those drugs most commonly used during the treatment of ARF and panel 2 details commonly used cardiovascular drugs that might be used in the treatment of HF or specific valvular lesions (see below).

Management of Heart Failure in Pregnancy

The management of HF in pregnancy is challenging because of concerns related to potential adverse effects of standard HF therapies on the mother and the fetus. With some important exceptions however, the components of HF therapy during and after pregnancy reflect current guidelines for nonpregnant patients with

chronic and acute HF,[34,50] both of which are discussed in detail in Chapters 6 and 16, respectively. In general, diuretics are used in pregnancy to treat pulmonary congestion (although spironolactone should be avoided - see Fig 9.2). β-1-selective blockers (e.g., metoprolol and bisoprolol) can be continued into pregnancy in those with established HF (or started during pregnancy), while avoiding unselective β-blockers, like atenolol, which can cause uterine relaxation and intrauterine growth restriction. For those with persistent HF symptoms, the vasodilator of choice in pregnancy is hydralazine plus isosorbide dinitrate,[3,35] given that angiotensin inhibition is contraindicated in all trimesters of pregnancy. Finally, in those with HF and reduced EF who remain symptomatic despite diuretics, β-blockers, and vasodilators, digoxin can be added.

Management of Specific Valve Lesions During and Before Pregnancy

Echocardiographic evaluation of heart valves in RHD is discussed in detail in Chapter 5. The indications for interventional or surgical treatment of valvular lesions are, with few exceptions, no different in women who contemplate pregnancy compared to the general population[6] and are discussed in Chapter 6. The most relevant exception to this rule in the context of RHD relates to women with moderate or severe MS (see later).

Surgery (or PMBC for MS) remain the most effective long-term management options for most advanced rheumatic valvular lesions and ideally should be undertaken before conception. ESC guidelines recommend that the choice of prosthesis is made in consultation with a pregnancy heart team (class I).[6] During pregnancy, maternal mortality rates with cardiopulmonary bypass are now approximately the same as that in nonpregnant women, but fetal mortality remains high (~20%).[51] Therefore, valve operations should not be performed in pregnant patients with valve stenosis or regurgitation in the absence of severe intractable HF symptoms (class III).[7]

Mitral Stenosis

Careful echocardiographic evaluation of the mitral valve and PAP is important in all women with RHD who contemplate pregnancy. Mitral valve morphology and any associated MR are important considerations if PMBC is considered. Prepregnancy exercise testing (to objectively assess exercise tolerance) and exercise echocardiography (to asses MV gradient and presence or absence of pHT in response to effort) may yield useful information. In those with mild MS, clinical evaluation is recommended every trimester and before delivery. Monthly or bimonthly follow-up is required in more significant MS, depending on patient symptoms, and should include both a clinical and echocardiographic evaluation.[6]

β-blockers are the mainstay of medical therapy during pregnancy for those with MS who develop HF symptoms or clinically significant pulmonary hypertension (pulmonary artery systolic pressure ≥50 mmHg on echocardiography).[6] β-blockers are also first line for either rhythm or rate control (the former strategy is favored in pregnancy) in those who develop atrial fibrillation.[6] Physical activity should also be restricted. By reducing the heart rate, these measures reduce the

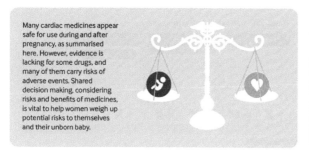

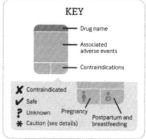

Panel 1: Using Drugs for Acute Rheumatic Fever During Pregnancy

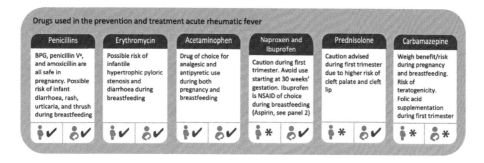

Panel 2: Using Cardiovascular Drugs During Pregnancy

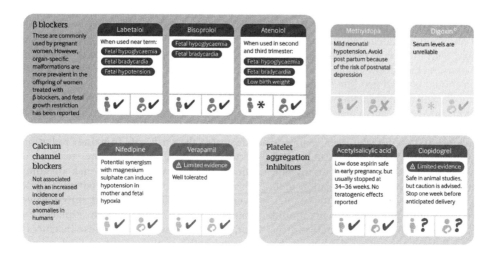

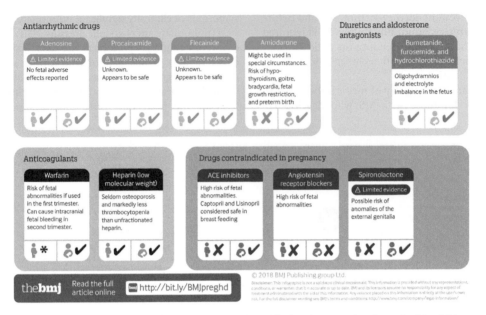

Panel 1 authors' original; panel 2 reproduced and modified with permission from: Cauldwell M et al[2a]

[a]Also known known as penicillin V potassium (PVK) or phenoxymethylpenicillin
[b]Experience with digoxin is extensive and it is considered to be the safest antiarrhythmic drug during pregnancy. A prophylactic antiarrhythmic efficacy has never been demonstrated
[c]There is insufficient clinical experience regarding the use of doses between 100-500 mg/day

BPG benzathine penicillin G; ACE inhibitors angiotensin converting enzyme inhibitors

FIG. 9.2 Treating Acute Rheumatic Fever and Rheumatic Heart Disease During Pregnancy

transvalvular gradient, decompress the left atrium, and reduce pulmonary venous pressure, while increasing diastolic filling time of the left ventricle, thus increasing cardiac output.[26] If HF symptoms persist despite adequate heart rate control, diuretics should be added but must be used with caution to maintain adequate placental circulation and high doses should be avoided. β-Blockers again should be used first line for rate control in those who develop atrial fibrillation but digoxin remains an option, either as an alternative in those patients where β-blockers are contraindicated or not tolerated, or as an adjunct in those for whom adequate rate control is not achieved. Ivabradine, which can be used in those with symptomatic MS who are in sinus rhythm, is contraindicated in pregnancy. Anticoagulation indications and regimens are discussed later in the chapter.

All women with MS and an MVA ≤1.5 cm² should be considered for either PMBC or surgery before pregnancy, even if asymptomatic and particularly if the MVA is <1.0 cm² (Table 9.3). These women should be counseled against pregnancy until the MS has been successfully treated.[6,7] Some women may then be able to complete pregnancy without the need for any cardiovascular medicines.[52] In women with unfavorable anatomy for PMBC or those with mixed MS and MR, the decision is more complex and needs to be individualized (Box 9.2).

There are no class I recommendations for mitral valve intervention during pregnancy.[6,7] PMBC should ideally be performed after 20 weeks' gestation to decrease the risk of ionizing radiation to the fetus[2,53], with similar outcomes to women who are not pregnant. Although the risk of complications from PMBC is low, rarely the patient will develop severe MR necessitating urgent mitral valve replacement. Surgical mitral valve replacement during pregnancy is reserved only those instances when the mother's life is threatened and all other measures

TABLE 9.3

Recommendations for the Management of Mitral Stenosis Before and During Pregnancy.

	EUROPEAN SOCIETY OF CARDIOLOGY 2018 GUIDELINES[6]		AMERICAN HEART ASSOCIATION/ AMERICAN COLLEGE OF CARDIOLOGY 2014 GUIDELINES[7]	
	COR	LOE	COR	LOE
Interventional or Surgical management: before pregnancy				
Recommendations for valve intervention:				
• in patients with MS and MVA <1.0 cm^2	I	C	Not Specified	
• if symptomatic with MS and MVA ≤1.5 cm^2	Not specified		I	C
• in patients with MS and MVA <1.5 cm^2	IIa	C	Not specified	
PMBC for asymptomatic patients with MVA ≤1.5 cm^2	Not specified		I	C
Interventional or Surgical management: during pregnancy				
Recommendations for PMBC (with favorable valve morphology):				
• For patients with HF symptoms (NYHA class III or IV) or PASP >50 mmHg, despite medical therapy	IIa	C	Not specified	
• For patients with severe MS (MVA ≤1.5 cm^2) who remain symptomatic with HF symptoms (NYHA class III or IV) despite medical therapy	Not specified		IIa	B
Valve intervention is reasonable for patients with MS (MVA ≤1.5 cm^2) with unfavorable valve morphology for PMBC who remain symptomatic with HF symptoms (NYHA class IV only) despite medical therapy	Not specified		IIa	C

COR class of recommendation; LOE level of evidence; MS mitral stenosis; MVA mitral valve area; PASP pulmonary artery systolic pressure; PMBC percutaneous mitral balloon commissurotomy; HF heart failure; NYHA New York Heart Association

have failed. Closed mitral commissurotomy, which does not require cardiopulmonary bypass,[6] remains an option for LMICs.

Vaginal delivery, with a shortened second stage of labor, can be attempted for most women with MS,[26] and should be the preferred method of delivery in those with either mild MS or in those with significant MS and NYHA class I or II without pulmonary hypertension (pHT).[6] Cesarean section may be considered in those patients with HF NYHA class III or IV or have pHT. Epidural anesthesia has been shown to reduce cardiac output variability[54] and lower PAP.[55] Postdelivery care is of upmost importance, as increased venous return following delivery can cause a rapid increase in left atrial and PAP.[56] For best management, invasive hemodynamic monitoring is recommended, when available, both during delivery and for up to 24 h postpartum.[26]

Mitral and Aortic Regurgitation

A comprehensive preconception echocardiogram is important to determine baseline regurgitation severity and LV dimensions and function. Patients with mild or moderate regurgitation should be followed up every trimester and more frequently if severe.[6] It is particularly important to monitor MR, which can worsen as the pregnancy progresses owing to physiological LV dilatation. Women with severe aortic regurgitation (AR) plus symptoms or decreased left ventricular function are at substantial risk of HF and arrhythmia. In those with asymptomatic severe MR or AR, preconception exercise testing may help identify those at higher risk of complications during pregnancy, which may be associated with reduced exercise tolerance, exercise-induced pHT, or abnormal symptoms. Those with symptoms precipitated by exercise testing are considered symptomatic (see Chapter 5 for further details on exercising testing).[7]

Preconception surgical intervention is recommended for severe MR or AR with symptoms due to LV dysfunction (COR: I, LOE: C)[6,7] or for asymptomatic severe MR where the valve is suitable for repair (COR: IIb, LOE: C).[7] Treatment decisions are often complex and require an individualistic approach (Box 9.2). During pregnancy, surgical intervention is reasonable only if the patient remains in severe intractable HF (NHYA class IV), despite optimal medical management (COR: IIa, LOE: C).[7]

Preconception surgery is not recommended prophylactically in women with severe MR unless they meet standard criteria, as the management of anticoagulation complicates pregnancy, if a mechanical valve is used.[26] However, intrapartum surgical mitral valve repair and replacement should be avoided—if possible—as they are associated with high rates of fetal loss.[58,59] Vaginal delivery is recommended in all cases with a shortened second stage of labor and epidural anesthesia for pain control.[6]

Aortic Stenosis

Aortic stenosis (AS) rarely occurs in isolation in RHD. For asymptomatic patients, a stress test can be useful to assess functional capacity, blood pressure response, and arrhythmias. The patient should be considered symptomatic if symptoms are provoked during stress testing.[7] Mild and moderate AS is generally well tolerated if the patient is asymptomatic with a normal functional capacity. Those with severe AS and excellent functional capacity with a normal blood pressure response to exercise may also be able to tolerate pregnancy. If the LV size and function as well as stress test are normal, then pregnancy can proceed and should not be counseled against, even in the presence of severe AS. Monthly or bimonthly clinical and echocardiographic evaluation is recommended in severe AS.[6]

Restricted activities, β-blockers, and diuretics can be used if HF develops during pregnancy. Before pregnancy, valve intervention is recommended in those with severe AS if: (1) the patient is symptomatic[6,7]; (2) or LVEF <50%; (3) or if the patient develops symptoms during stress testing (all class I recommendations). A class IIa recommendation is given by the AHA/ACC guidelines for preconception valve intervention in those with asymptomatic severe AS.[7] The recently updated ESC guidelines are more restrictive, recommending preconception intervention in those with severe asymptomatic AS only if there is a drop in blood pressure below baseline during stress testing (class IIa).[6] During pregnancy, AHA/ACC guidelines give a class IIa recommendation for valve intervention (surgical aortic valve replacement or balloon aortic valvuloplasty (BAV)) if there is severe AS with hemodynamic deterioration or advanced HF symptoms (NYHA class III or IV).[7] The ESC guidelines are again more restrictive, limiting their recommendation to BAV only when there is severe AS and severe symptoms (class IIa).[6]

In nonsevere AS, vaginal delivery is preferable with assisted second stage of labor. In severe symptomatic AS, cesarean section is recommended.[6] Epidural anesthesia poses a high risk as hypotension can mediate poor coronary perfusion in the setting of AS and general anesthesia may be preferable if cesarean section is performed.[26]

Anticoagulation in Pregnancy

In general, heparins (subcutaneous low molecular weight heparin (LMWH) or intravenous unfractionated heparin (UFH)) are the anticoagulant of choice for most pregnant women because they do not cross the placenta and so are not teratogenic, whereas vitamin K antagonists (VKAs) are associated with increased risks of embryopathy, fetopathy, fetal hemorrhage, and fetal loss, and should be avoided if possible.[60] One exception to this is MHVs, which are associated with an especially high risk for thrombosis, particularly in the prothrombotic pregnancy state, and in such patients VKAs during pregnancy are a potential option because they have a lower risk of valve thrombosis and maternal death compared to the heparins.

Anticoagulation for Mechanical Prostheses

Anticoagulation for pregnant women with MHVs is controversial and no universal consensus has emerged. A number of major challenges need to be considered, including teratogenic risks, dosing complexities of the various anticoagulation regimens, and anticoagulation management around the time of labor. Potential options include VKAs throughout pregnancy, heparins throughout pregnancy, or sequential treatment involving the use of heparins in the first trimester and VKAs in the second and third trimesters.[61]

None of these regimens are perfect and all entail some risk for the mother and fetus although in general VKAs are safest for the mother and heparins are safest for the fetus. The anticoagulation regimen therefore is the primary determinant of risk for maternal valve thrombosis, but other factors include valve type (newer valves are less thrombogenic than older ones - see Chapter 6), valve position (mitral MHVs carry a higher risk of valve thrombosis than aortic MHVs), and valve function. All pregnant women with MHVs are high risk (mWHO III) and thus ideally should be managed by a pregnancy heart team in a specialist center.[6]

The recently updated ESC recommendations on anticoagulation management for MHVs in pregnancy are summarized in Fig. 9.3.[6] Additional class I recommendations from the ESC guidelines include: i) implementing any changes to the anticoagulant regimen during pregnancy in hospital; ii) anticipating the timing of delivery to ensure safe and effective peripartum anticoagulation; and iii) if delivery starts while on a VKA or less than 2 weeks after discontinuation of a VKA, cesarean section is recommended. These are in broad agreement with the AHA/ACC guidelines, but there are few notable differences. The AHA/ACC guidelines provide no recommendation for VKAs if the baseline warfarin dose is >5 mg/day or for heparin use during the second and third trimesters, where VKAs only are

recommended. AHA/ACC guidelines also recommend that all patients with an MHV, in addition to VKAs, should receive low-dose aspirin (75−100 mg/day) during the second and third trimesters (Class I).[7]

Because there is no consensus on the therapeutic approach to anticoagulation in pregnant women with MHVs, clinicians managing these patients should be aware of the maternal and fetal complications of each treatment option in order to provide effective counseling to women. However, regardless of which anticoagulation regimen is chosen, the mother's strict adherence to dosing and monitoring is essential for successful outcomes.

Vitamin K Antagonists. A meta-analysis by D'Souza et al., which included data from 46 different publications, found that the use of VKAs with standard INR targets (2.5−3.5) throughout pregnancy was associated with the lowest pooled proportions of maternal mortality and thromboembolic complications, followed by sequential treatment and LMWH throughout pregnancy.[61] The risk of thromboembolic complications were lower (1.6% vs. 2.7%) in the studies where warfarin was not changed to peripartum heparin, but continued until 24 h before planned cesarean section.

Warfarin-specific embryopathy includes nasal hypoplasia and stippled epiphyses with the critical exposure occurring between 6 and 9 weeks' gestation.[62] Warfarin risk continues throughout pregnancy and neurological sequelae related to intrauterine exposure includes Dandy-Walker malformation, ventral midline dysplasia with corpus callosum agenesis, and dorsal midline dysplasia with optic atrophy.[62] In structurally normal infants, intrauterine exposure has been further associated with increased incidence of minor neurological dysfunction and IQ scores below 80.[63]

A dose-dependent effect of warfarin-related fetal complications was first reported by Vitale.[64] In their study of 58 pregnancies, 15% of women treated with up to 5 mg warfarin daily had fetal complications compared to 88% in the group receiving >5 mg. However, other studies have reported conflicting results. A prospective cohort of 62 pregnancies from South Africa reported an embryopathy rate of 5% if the warfarin dose was 5 mg or less and 7% for women using >5 mg warfarin per day.[13] Furthermore, this study did not find any significant differences between the miscarriage and live birth rates between the two groups, although the stillbirth rate was significantly higher (3.6% vs. 24.0%, $P = .026$)

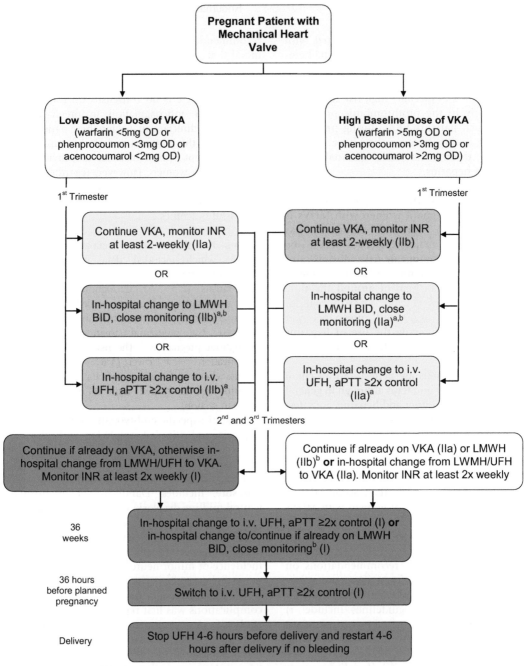

FIG. 9.3 2018 ESC guidelines on anticoagulation for mechanical valves during pregnancy.
[a]Weeks 6–12
[b]Monitoring LMWH: starting dose for LMWH is 1 mg/kg body weight for enoxaparin and 100 IU/kg for dalteparin, twice daily subcutaneously. In-hospital daily anti-Xa levels until target, then weekly (I). Target anti-Xa levels: 1.0–1.2 U/ml (mitral and right-sided valves) or 0.8–1.2 U/ml (aortic valves) 4–6 hours post-dose (I). Pre-dose anti-Xa levels >0.6 U/ml (IIb)
Green boxes represent class I recommendation; yellow boxes class IIa recommendation; orange boxes class IIb recommendation; the classes of recommendation in the white box are individualized and are indicated in brackets VKA vitamin K antagonist, INR international normalized ratio; aPTT activated partial thromboplastin time; OD omne in die (once daily); BID bis in die (twice daily); LMWH low molecular weight heparin; UFH unfractionated heparin; i.v. intravenous" (Adapted from Regitz-Zagrosek et al.[6])

in women receiving >5 mg of warfarin per day. ROPAC also did not demonstrate reduced fetal loss with low-dose VKAs (warfarin <5 mg/day, acenocoumarol <2 mg/day or phenprocoumon <3 mg/day).[65] Therefore, safety of low-dose warfarin still needs to be confirmed and the uncertainties must be discussed with the patient.

Heparins. Both LMWH and UFH are associated with improved fetal outcomes as they do not cross the placenta but are associated with higher rates of maternal thromboembolic complications compared to VKAs. Thromboembolic rates of 9%−33% have been reported in studies where UFH was used throughout pregnancy.[6,60] Although most thromboembolic complications occurred in women on low- or fixed-dose UFH, they also occurred in dose-dependent adjusted subcutaneous UFH regimens with aPTTs within target therapeutic ranges.[66,67] The AHA/ACC guidelines therefore no longer recommend the use of subcutaneous UFH for women with MHVs.[7] The use of dose-adjusted, continuous intravenous UFH is more effective but requires meticulous management of a central line for prevention of infective endocarditis.[68]

The advantage of LMWH over UFH is the superior absorption and bioavailability, 2−4-fold longer half-life, more predictable and stable dose response, less bleeding, and lower risk of heparin-induced thrombocytopenia and osteopenia[4,68]. Unfortunately, it is more expensive and requires close monitoring, and there is a precaution in the label regarding its use in pregnancy for MHVs.[61] Meta-analyses by Steinberg and D'Souza have reported the highest live birth rate if LMWH was used throughout pregnancy but a higher incidence of maternal complications compared with VKAs.[61,69] Most thromboembolic events in these studies were related to subtherapeutic anticoagulation secondary to inappropriate dosing, poor monitoring, or poor patient adherence.[69]

LMWH should therefore not be used in pregnancy unless anti-Xa levels can be monitored weekly and LMWH doses adjusted accordingly given that dosage requirements increase markedly throughout pregnancy because of increased renal clearance.[6,7] When monitoring is available, the valve thrombosis risk is 4.4%−8.7% when LMWH is used throughout pregnancy and 5.8%−7.4% when LMWH is used in the first trimester only.[61,70] However, even with adequate peak anti-Xa levels, valve thrombosis still occurs and there are unresolved questions regarding the safety of LMWH use in pregnancy.[6]

Sequential treatment may be an attractive option in LMICs where the use of UFH and LMWH may be cost prohibitive and continued anticoagulant monitoring may be difficult due to geographical, educational, and financial constraints.[61] In the meta-analysis by D'Souza, sequential treatment was associated with higher maternal mortality and thromboembolic complications than VKAs but lower than LMWH. Additionally, sequential treatment was associated with the lowest numbers of small for gestational age infants, miscarriages, and preterm birth.[61]

In conclusion, the most effective regimen to prevent valve thrombosis appears to be the use of VKAs throughout pregnancy, while LMWH is possibly safer than UFH. It should be emphasized that these conclusions have been made on the basis of low-quality evidence, given the lack of randomized control trials.[6]

Emergency Reversal of Anticoagulation
Local guidelines should be available in the event of unplanned preterm delivery. Rapid reversal of VKAs is usually achieved with fresh frozen plasma. Both oral and intravenous vitamin K takes at least 12 h for reversal.[71] Neither of these measures reverse the anticoagulant effects in the fetus so delivery should be as atraumatic as possible, and fetal scalp electrodes, forceps, and ventouse devices should be avoided. Protamine is used to reverse the anticoagulant effect of UFH but is only partially effective for LMWHs. Fresh frozen plasma does not reverse the effects of UFH or LMWHs. The aPTT may be used to monitor levels of UFH but does not provide reliable information regarding anticoagulation status for women on LMWH. Most laboratories will not provide urgent testing for anti-Xa levels.

Labor and Delivery
A clear delivery plan based on maternal risk analysis should be formulated in advance by the multidisciplinary team. The following strategies will help to reduce risk during labor and delivery:
- Epidural anesthesia—reduces pain response and sympathetic-induced tachycardia
- Strict hemodynamic monitoring for 24−72 h postpartum
- Assisted vaginal delivery
- Avoid bolus dose oxytocin
- Avoid Ergometrine
- Planned elective cesarean section with postpartum ICU care for high risk women

Timing and mode of delivery needs special consideration in women with significant native valve pathology and, in particular, in women with prosthetic valves. Induction and management of labor, delivery, and postpartum monitoring requires specific expertise and joint management by the obstetrician, cardiologist, and anesthesiologist as part of the pregnancy heart team in specialist heart centers for all women who are at moderate-to-high risk.[6]

By week 35, an individualized delivery plan should be created, which should also be available outside of normal working hours. Due to lack of prospective data for pregnant women with RHD and the influence of individual patient and healthcare characteristics, standard guidelines do not exist and management should therefore be individualized. In general, the preferred mode of delivery is vaginal, with a delivery plan that includes information on the timing of delivery (spontaneous vs. induced), method of induction, type of analgesia, level of intensity of monitoring, need for postpartum surveillance, and subacute bacterial endocarditis prophylaxis.[72]

A new recommendation by the recent ESC guidelines is that induction of labor should be considered at 40 weeks' gestation in all women with cardiac disease (class IIa).[6] In women without heart disease, induction of labor reduces the risk of emergency Cesarian section by 12% and risk of stillbirth by 50%, and both risks are likely to be reduced further in the pregnant women with heart disease, where obstetric complications are higher.[73,74]

When applicable, specific instructions for type of anticoagulation should be clearly documented. An algorithmic approach to anticoagulation in those with MHVs is recommended (for example, Fig. 9.3). At 36 weeks' gestation, most patients are converted to either LMWH or UFH. Delivery is usually planned allowing an UFH infusion to be started 36 h before induction/Cesarean section and for it to be discontinued 4−6 h before planned delivery. When labor is being induced with prostaglandins, it will mean in practical terms to continue with the infusion until contractions are becoming regular (>2 times in 10 min) or until it is possible to perform an artificial rupture of membranes. If there are no bleeding complications during the delivery, then the UFH infusion can be restarted 4−6 h after delivery. However, in case of signs of vaginal tears or a hematoma, delaying restarting the UFH infusion could be considered depending on the clinical situation and the risk of valve thrombosis (higher risk for mitral position or double valve replacement).

Cesarean delivery should be considered for patients with RHD presenting in preterm labor on oral anticoagulants, in patients with symptomatic severe stenotic lesions (AS, MS), severe pHT,[43] or presenting with signs of acute HF.

If labor starts or an emergency delivery should be carried out while the patient is taking warfarin, then Cesarean section should be performed under general anesthesia with fresh frozen plasma cover and prothrombin complex concentrate added if necessary to reverse anticoagulation. If the patient is on a UFH infusion, where possible stopping the infusion and waiting as long as possible is the best approach as the half-life of UFH is 60−90 min. Where delivery has been by cesarean section and early reintroduction of anticoagulation is planned due to high risk of thrombosis, placing a uterine compression suture and the insertion of pelvic and subrectus drains should be considered.[75]

Peripartum and postpartum obstetric complications are common in patients with valvular heart disease and can include postpartum hemorrhage (PPH), defined as blood loss >500 mL (vaginal delivery) or >1000 mL (Cesarian section), which required transfusion or is accompanied by a reduction in hemoglobin by >2.0 g/L. The impact of PPH in the context of valvular heart disease is greater than in the normal population. In the context of women with MHVs or other needs for anticoagulation, such as AF, this problem is compounded by the need for anticoagulation.

Therapy with ergometrine is relatively contraindicated due to its effects on blood pressure and potential to cause coronary artery spasm. Oxytocin can also have adverse effects, inducing vasodilatation in the subcutaneous vessels, vasoconstriction in the splanchnic bed and coronary arteries, with the overall effect of hypotension, tachycardia, and myocardial ischemia.[76,77] Low-dose oxytocin infusions are most commonly used although the benefit of this approach is not clear.[78] In the case of PPH, oxytocin should be given and prostaglandins are generally well tolerated. However, early intervention is key with a greater emphasis on mechanical approaches including an intrauterine balloon and uterine compression sutures.

Infective endocarditis in pregnancy is rare, with an estimated incidence of 3−12 per 1000 in patients with prosthetic valves.[79] The use of antibiotics is controversial and at present antibiotic prophylaxis is not routinely recommended during vaginal or cesarian delivery by the current ESC guidelines.[6] The Australian Guidelines on the management of RHD do however recommend antibiotic prophylaxis for all patients with prosthetic valves and for those with a history of infective endocarditis. In these patients, antibiotics should be given before delivery and for 24−48 h after delivery. Antimicrobial prophylaxis should also be

TABLE 9.4
WHO Classification of Risk From Contraception in Cardiovascular Disease.

WHO Class	Risk for Contraceptive Method by Cardiac Condition
WHO 1 **A**lways useable	Risk no higher than general population
WHO 2 **B**roadly useable	Small increased risk; advantages of method generally outweigh risks
WHO 3 **C**aution in use	Risks usually outweigh advantages of method. Other methods preferable. Exceptions if: 1. Patient accepts risks and rejects alternatives 2. Risk of pregnancy very high and other methods less effective
WHO 4 **D**o not use	Method contraindicated represents unacceptable health risk

WHO, World Health Organization

given during prolonged labor or in the event of premature rupture of the membranes.[80] However, in some underresourced settings prophylaxis may be recommended with any mode of delivery other than an uncomplicated vaginal delivery, especially in patients with a MHV or women who previously had infective endocarditis. Infective endocarditis is discussed in more detail in Chapter 16.

CONTRACEPTIVE CHOICES IN WOMEN WITH RHEUMATIC HEART DISEASE

For most women with RHD living in LMICs, the risks associated with pregnancy are far greater than a carefully chosen contraceptive method. Contraceptive advice for women with RHD should be given before the patient is sexually active. The contraceptive selected should pose a minimal risk to the specific disease but should still be efficacious and suited to the patient's lifestyle and reproductive history. Contraceptive efficacy is paramount for the women with serious cardiovascular pathology in whom pregnancy may be life threatening. The risk of maternal death ranges from up to 50% for pHT to almost the same as the general population for minor lesions such as mild MR.[12] Treating physicians may be overcautious denying women appropriate contraception, leading to unwanted pregnancies.[81] A recent audit of maternal deaths in South Africa has identified the need to establish specialized contraceptive clinics for women with medical diseases.[82] The following points should be considered before selecting a contraceptive agent:

- Efficacy of each contraceptive method. Table 9.6 summarises the failure rates of different contraceptive methods. Failure rates are highly dependent on correct patient usage and are therefore described using data for "typical use" and "perfect use".[89]
- The thrombotic and hypertensive risks of estrogen-containing contraceptives. Table 9.4 summarises the WHO risk stratification scale when using contraceptives in cardiovascular disease and Table 9.5 compares the risk associated with each contraceptive method in the presence of specific pathology.[83]
- Vagal stimulation and infective risks with the insertion of intrauterine contraceptive devices
- Bleeding risks in patients on warfarin therapy
- The effect of drug interaction on contraceptive metabolism

Contraceptive Methods

Combined oral contraceptives: Combined estrogens and progestogens are available as oral preparations, vaginal ring, injection, or transdermal patch. The estrogen component increases the risk of venous thromboembolism 2−7-fold.[84] The absolute risk, however, is small (8−10/10,000 women-years exposure) and the risk of pregnancy must be balanced against the risk of the combined oral contraceptive.[85,86] Additional risks associated with combined oral contraceptives are arterial and cardiac thrombosis, atherosclerosis, hyperlipidemia, and hypertension. The risks of ischemic stroke and ischemic heart disease are increased in women with additional risk factors such as age >40 years, smoking, diabetes mellitus, and obesity. Cardiac thrombosis is a risk in women with atrial fibrillation or MHVs. Warfarin interacts with the metabolism of estrogens and progestogens and may not be protective if combined hormonal contraception is used.[87]

TABLE 9.5
WHO Class for Contraceptive Methods in Specific Clinical Conditions.[a]

Clinical condition	Combined hormonal methods (estrogen containing)	POP[b] ("minipill")	Cerazette®	Implanon®	Depo-Provera®	Mirena® IUS	Copper IUD[c]	Emergency hormonal contraception
Physiological murmur	1	1	1	1	1	1	1	1
Uncomplicated valvular heart disease	2	1	1	1	1	1	1	2
Complicated valvular heart disease (risk of pHT, risk of AF, history of sub-acute bacterial endocarditis)	4	1	1	1	1	2	2	2
Moderate aortic stenosis	2	1	1	1	1	2	3	1
Bjork Shiley mitral valve replacement[d]	4	1	1	1	3	3	4	1
Bileaflet mitral valve replacement[d]	3	1	1	1	3	3	4	1

IUD, Intrauterine device; *IUS*, Intrauterine system; *POP*, Progestogen-only pill; *WHO*, World Health Organization; *pHT*, pulmonary hypertension; *AF*, atrial fibrillation.

[a] See sections of text on specific contraceptive methods for more information.

[b] Although safe, the limited efficacy of the progestogen-only pill limits its use to women in whom pregnancy carries a particular risk (WHO Class 3 or 4- see Tables 9.4 and 9.6).

[c] May be used if no other method suitable and risk of pregnancy outweighs risk of insertion.

[d] Warfarin: care with monitoring the international normalized ratio (INR), which may alter with both estrogen and progestogen hormone therapy. With Depo-Provera there is a specific risk of local hematoma (see text).

TABLE 9.6
Failure Rates of Different Contraceptive Methods.

PERCENTAGE OF WOMEN WITH UNINTENDED PREGNANCY WITHIN THE FIRST YEAR OF USE		
Contraceptive Method	Typical Use	Perfect Use
No method	85	85
Barriers	15–32	2–26
Standard POP	5–10	0.5
COC	3–8	0.1
• Cerazette	0.4	0.1
Depo Provera	3	0.3
Copper IUD	0.8	0.6
Mirena IUS	0.1	0.1
Implanon	0.05	0.05
Female sterilisation	0.5	0.5
Male sterilisation	0.15	0.15

COC, Combined oral contraceptive (estrogen and progestogen); IUD, Copper intrauterine device; IUS, Levonorgestrel intrauterine system; POP, Progestogen-only pill.
The data on the new POP, Cerazette, are from a different source than the other contraceptive methods in this table and may not therefore be directly comparable. Being from a single study, the Cerazette data are more likely to represent ideal use than typical use. Nonetheless, the efficacy of Cerazette may prove to be greater than both the COC and Depo Provera, because it is taken continuously, without a break, and does not rely on remembering to start a new pack after a week's break or on returning every 12 weeks for a repeat injection.
Adapted from Trussell.[89]

Progestogen-only methods

These methods are available in a variety of formulations and are considered the contraceptives of choice for women with severe cardiac disease, as they are not associated with an increased risk of arterial or venous thrombosis.[87] They sometimes interact with warfarin affecting the INR so additional anticoagulation monitoring is advised during early use and following discontinuation.[88]

Progestogen only pills (POPs) are safe but are generally not recommended in women where pregnancy is contraindicated (mWHO IV) and maximum efficacy is needed[5,6,89]. POPs are also contraindicated in women receiving bosentan for pHT as it is an enzyme inducer that reduces the efficacy of POPs.[88]

Depot-Provera is an effective contraception that is especially attractive with 12-weekly injections and a quick return to fertility when its use is stopped. Hematomas at the injection site may pose a risk for women on anticoagulants.

Levonorgestrel-containing intra-uterine system (Mirena®) is effective for 5 years. In patients with pHT, it may cause a vasovagal response during insertion, which may lead to life-threatening arrhythmias or acute right-sided HF. In these patients, intrauterine device (IUD) insertion should therefore occur in hospital, although many clinicians avoid the use of IUDs in such patients. Women at risk of infective endocarditis must be given prophylactic antibiotics before insertion.

Implanon is a subdermal implant that is effective for 3 years. There are no cardiac contraindications to its use, but prolonged irregular bleeding may pose a problem for some women.

Copper IUD

This method is popular in LMICs due to its cost-effectiveness and low thrombogenic risk.

Emergency contraception

Emergency contraception may be used in cases of unprotected intercourse. A single dose of 1.5 mg of levonorgestrel has a 1.1% failure rate if taken within 72 h of unprotected intercourse.[90] A single dose of mifepristone (25 mg) and ulipristal (30 mg) is equally effective and may be used up to 120 h after intercourse.[84] The copper intrauterine device has a 0.09% failure rate and can be used within 120 h of intercourse. Interaction between high-dose levonorgestrel and warfarin has been reported in case-series, thus necessitating the need for close INR monitoring for a few days after levonorgestrel ingestion.[91]

CONCLUSION

Valvular heart disease due to RHD remains an important contributor to the burden of maternal disease globally. In LMICs where RHD is endemic, this condition accounts for 50%–90% of maternal cardiac complications. Mortality has been as high as 34% in LMICs when RHD is first diagnosed in pregnancy. Conversely, with early recognition and good antenatal care, good maternal outcomes can be achieved. New data has recently been published on pregnant women with heart disease, including the recently updated ESC guidelines on cardiovascular disease in pregnancy, which contain a number of important updates and recommendations. Counseling is a crucial intervention for all women with heart disease who are contemplating pregnancy or are already pregnant. Women with moderate or severe risk heart conditions should receive counseling, full risk assessment and—if deciding to plan a pregnancy—be managed by a "pregnancy heart team", ideally in an expert center using mWHO criteria.

REFERENCES

1. Cirelli JF, Surita FG, Costa ML, Parpinelli MA, Haddad SM, Cecatti JG. The burden of indirect causes of maternal morbidity and mortality in the process of obstetric transition: a cross-sectional multicenter study. *Rev Bras Ginecol Obstet.* 2018;40(3):106–114.
2. Thorne S. Pregnancy and native heart valve disease. *Heart.* 2016;102(17):1410–1417.
2a. Cauldwell M, Dos Santos F, Steer PJ, Swan L, Gatzoulis M, Johnson MR. Pregnancy in women with congenital heart disease. *BMJ.* 2018;360. k478.
3. European Society of G, Association for European Paediatric C, German Society for Gender M, et al. ESC guidelines on the management of cardiovascular diseases during pregnancy: the task force on the management of cardiovascular diseases during pregnancy of the European society of cardiology (ESC). *Eur Heart J.* 2011;32(24):3147–3197.
4. Haththotuwa HR, Attygalle D, Jayatilleka AC, Karunaratna V, Thorne SA. Maternal mortality due to cardiac disease in Sri Lanka. *Int J Gynaecol Obstet.* 2009;104(3):194–198.
5. Diao M, Kane A, Ndiaye MB, et al. Pregnancy in women with heart disease in sub-Saharan Africa. *Arch Cardiovasc Dis.* 2011;104(6–7):370–374.
6. Regitz-Zagrosek V, Roos-Hesselink JW, Bauersachs J, et al. 2018 ESC Guidelines for the management of

cardiovascular diseases during pregnancy. *Eur Heart J.* 2018;39(34):3165–3241.
7. Nishimura RA, Otto CM, Bonow RO, et al. 2014 AHA/ACC guideline for the management of patients with valvular heart disease: a report of the American College of cardiology/American heart association task force on practice guidelines. *J Am Coll Cardiol.* 2014;63(22). e57-185.
8. Mocumbi AO, Sliwa K, Soma-Pillay P. Medical disease as a cause of maternal mortality: the pre-imminence of cardiovascular pathology. *Cardiovasc J Afr.* 2016;27(2):84–88.
9. Dougherty S, Beaton A, Nascimento BR, Zuhlke LJ, Khorsandi M, Wilson N. Prevention and control of rheumatic heart disease: overcoming core challenges in resource-poor environments. *Ann Pediatr Cardiol.* 2018;11(1):68–78.
10. French KA, Poppas A. Rheumatic heart disease in pregnancy: global challenges and clear opportunities. *Circulation.* 2018;137(8):817–819.
11. Mocumbi AO, Sliwa K. Women's cardiovascular health in Africa. *Heart.* 2012;98(6):450–455.
12. Thorne S, MacGregor A, Nelson-Piercy C. Risks of contraception and pregnancy in heart disease. *Heart.* 2006;92(10):1520–1525.
13. van Hagen IM, Thorne SA, Taha N, et al. Pregnancy outcomes in women with rheumatic mitral valve disease: results from the registry of pregnancy and cardiac disease. *Circulation.* 2018;137(8):806–816.
14. Zuhlke L, Engel ME, Karthikeyan G, et al. Characteristics, complications, and gaps in evidence-based interventions in rheumatic heart disease: the Global Rheumatic Heart Disease Registry (the REMEDY study). *Eur Heart J.* 2015;36(18), 1115-22a.
15. Sartain JB, Anderson NL, Barry JJ, Boyd PT, Howat PW. Rheumatic heart disease in pregnancy: cardiac and obstetric outcomes. *Intern Med J.* 2012;42(9):978–984.
16. Marijon E, Iung B, Mocumbi AO, et al. What are the differences in presentation of candidates for percutaneous mitral commissurotomy across the world and do they influence the results of the procedure? *Arch Cardiovasc Dis.* 2008;101(10):611–617.
17. Hameed A, Karaalp IS, Tummala PP, et al. The effect of valvular heart disease on maternal and fetal outcome of pregnancy. *J Am Coll Cardiol.* 2001;37(3):893–899.
18. Silversides CK, Colman JM, Sermer M, Siu SC. Cardiac risk in pregnant women with rheumatic mitral stenosis. *Am J Cardiol.* 2003;91(11):1382–1385.
19. Lesniak-Sobelga A, Tracz W, KostKiewicz M, Podolec P, Pasowicz M. Clinical and echocardiographic assessment of pregnant women with valvular heart diseases–maternal and fetal outcome. *Int J Cardiol.* 2004;94(1):15–23.
20. Karamermer Y, Roos-Hesselink JW. Pregnancy and adult congenital heart disease. *Expert Rev Cardiovasc Ther.* 2007;5(5):859–869.
21. Sanghavi M, Rutherford JD. Cardiovascular physiology of pregnancy. *Circulation.* 2014;130(12):1003–1008.
22. Ouzounian JG, Elkayam U. Physiologic changes during normal pregnancy and delivery. *Cardiol Clin.* 2012;30(3):317–329.

23. Mahendru AA, Everett TR, Wilkinson IB, Lees CC, McEniery CM. A longitudinal study of maternal cardiovascular function from preconception to the postpartum period. *J Hypertens.* 2014;32(4):849−856.

24. Sifakis S, Pharmakides G. Anemia in pregnancy. *Ann N Y Acad Sci.* 2000;900:125−136.

25. Samiei N, Amirsardari M, Rezaei Y, et al. Echocardiographic evaluation of hemodynamic changes in left-sided heart valves in pregnant women with valvular heart disease. *Am J Cardiol.* 2016;118(7):1046−1052.

26. Elkayam U, Bitar F. Valvular heart disease and pregnancy part I: native valves. *J Am Coll Cardiol.* 2005;46(2):223−230.

27. Walker MC, Garner PR, Keely EJ, Rock GA, Reis MD. Changes in activated protein C resistance during normal pregnancy. *Am J Obstet Gynecol.* 1997;177(1):162−169.

28. Toglia MR, Weg JG. Venous thromboembolism during pregnancy. *N Engl J Med.* 1996;335(2):108−114.

29. McColl MD, Ramsay JE, Tait RC, et al. Risk factors for pregnancy associated venous thromboembolism. *Thromb Haemost.* 1997;78(4):1183−1188.

30. Kamel H, Navi BB, Sriram N, Hovsepian DA, Devereux RB, Elkind MS. Risk of a thrombotic event after the 6-week postpartum period. *N Engl J Med.* 2014;370(14):1307−1315.

31. Robson SC, Dunlop W, Boys RJ, Hunter S. Cardiac output during labour. *Br Med J.* 1987;295(6607):1169−1172.

32. Lee W, Rokey R, Miller J, Cotton DB. Maternal hemodynamic effects of uterine contractions by M-mode and pulsed-Doppler echocardiography. *Am J Obstet Gynecol.* 1989;161(4):974−977.

33. Windram JD, Colman JM, Wald RM, Udell JA, Siu SC, Silversides CK. Valvular heart disease in pregnancy. *Best Pract Res Clin Obstet Gynaecol.* 2014;28(4):507−518.

34. Yancy CW, Jessup M, Bozkurt B, et al. 2013 ACCF/AHA guideline for the management of heart failure: executive summary: a report of the American College of Cardiology Foundation/American Heart Association Task Force on practice guidelines. *Circulation.* 2013;128(16):1810−1852.

35. Sliwa K, Hilfiker-Kleiner D, Petrie MC, et al. Current state of knowledge on aetiology, diagnosis, management, and therapy of peripartum cardiomyopathy: a position statement from the Heart Failure Association of the European Society of Cardiology Working Group on peripartum cardiomyopathy. *Eur J Heart Fail.* 2010;12(8):767−778.

36. Malhotra S, Yentis SM. Reports on confidential enquiries into maternal deaths: management strategies based on trends in maternal cardiac deaths over 30 years. *Int J Obstet Anesth.* 2006;15(3):223−226.

37. Logan C, Holcombe E, Manlove J, Ryan S. *The Consequences of Unintended Childbearing.* Vol. 28. Washington, DC: Child Trends and National Campaign to Prevent Teen Pregnancy; 2007:142−151.

38. Sonfield A, Hasstedt K, Kavanaugh ML, Anderson R. *The Social and Economic Benefits of Women's Ability to Decide whether and when to Have Children.* New York: Guttmacher Institute; 2013.

39. Siu SC, Sermer M, Colman JM, et al. Prospective multicenter study of pregnancy outcomes in women with heart disease. *Circulation.* 2001;104(5):515−521.

40. Khairy P, Ouyang DW, Fernandes SM, Lee-Parritz A, Economy KE, Landzberg MJ. Pregnancy outcomes in women with congenital heart disease. *Circulation.* 2006;113(4):517−524.

41. Drenthen W, Boersma E, Balci A, et al. Predictors of pregnancy complications in women with congenital heart disease. *Eur Heart J.* 2010;31(17):2124−2132.

42. van Hagen IM, Boersma E, Johnson MR, et al. Global cardiac risk assessment in the registry of pregnancy and cardiac disease: results of a registry from the European society of cardiology. *Eur J Heart Fail.* 2016;18(5):523−533.

43. Sliwa K, van Hagen IM, Budts W, et al. Pulmonary hypertension and pregnancy outcomes: data from the registry of pregnancy and cardiac disease (ROPAC) of the European society of cardiology. *Eur J Heart Fail.* 2016;18(9):1119−1128.

44. Mandalenakis Z, Rosengren A, Skoglund K, Lappas G, Eriksson P, Dellborg M. Survivorship in children and young adults with congenital heart disease in Sweden. *JAMA Intern Med.* 2017;177(2):224−230.

45. Orwat S, Diller GP, van Hagen IM, et al. Risk of pregnancy in moderate and severe aortic stenosis: from the multinational ROPAC registry. *J Am Coll Cardiol.* 2016;68(16):1727−1737.

46. Connolly HM, Warnes CA. Ebstein's anomaly: outcome of pregnancy. *J Am Coll Cardiol.* 1994;23(5):1194−1198.

47. Sadler L, McCowan L, White H, et al. Pregnancy outcomes and cardiac complications in women with mechanical, bioprosthetic and homograft valves. *Br J Obstet Gynaecol.* 2000;107:245−253.

48. van Hagen IM, Roos-Hesselink JW, Ruys TP, et al. Pregnancy in women with a mechanical heart valve: data of the European society of cardiology registry of pregnancy and cardiac disease (ROPAC). *Circulation.* 2015;132(2):132−142.

49. Cutforth R, MacDonald CB. Heart sounds and murmurs in pregnancy. *Am Heart J.* 1966;71(6):741−747.

50. Ponikowski P, Voors AA, Anker SD, et al. 2016 ESC Guidelines for the diagnosis and treatment of acute and chronic heart failure: the Task Force for the diagnosis and treatment of acute and chronic heart failure of the European Society of Cardiology (ESC)Developed with the special contribution of the Heart Failure Association (HFA) of the ESC. *Eur Heart J.* 2016;37(27):2129−2200.

51. Kapoor MC. Cardiopulmonary bypass in pregnancy. *Ann Card Anaesth.* 2014;17(1):33−39.

52. Bhatla N, Lal S, Behera G, et al. Cardiac disease in pregnancy. *Int J Gynaecol Obstet.* 2003;82(2):153−159.

53. Routray SN, Mishra TK, Swain S, Patnaik UK, Behera M. Balloon mitral valvuloplasty during pregnancy. *Int J Gynaecol Obstet.* 2004;85(1):18−23.

54. Clark SL, Cotton DB, Lee W, et al. Central hemodynamic assessment of normal term pregnancy. *Am J Obstet Gynecol.* 1989;161(6 Pt 1):1439−1442.

55. Hemmings GT, Whalley DG, O'Connor PJ, Benjamin A, Dunn C. Invasive monitoring and anaesthetic management of a parturient with mitral stenosis. *Can J Anaesth.* 1987;34(2):182–185.

56. Clark SL, Phelan JP, Greenspoon J, Aldahl D, Horenstein J. Labor and delivery in the presence of mitral stenosis: central hemodynamic observations. *Am J Obstet Gynecol.* 1985; 152(8):984–988.

57. Shotan A, Widerhorn J, Hurst A, Elkayam U. Risks of angiotensin-converting enzyme inhibition during pregnancy: experimental and clinical evidence, potential mechanisms, and recommendations for use. *Am J Med.* 1994;96: 451–456.

58. Weiss BM, von Segesser LK, Alon E, Seifert B, Turina MI. Outcome of cardiovascular surgery and pregnancy: a systematic review of the period 1984–1996. *Am J Obstet Gynecol.* 1998;179:1643–1653.

59. de Souza JA, Martinez Jr EE, Ambrose JA, et al. Percutaneous balloon mitral valvuloplasty in comparison with open mitral valve commissurotomy for mitral stenosis during pregnancy. *J Am Coll Cardiol.* 2001;37:900–903.

60. McLintock C. Anticoagulant therapy in pregnant women with mechanical prosthetic heart valves: no easy option. *Thromb Res.* 2011;127(suppl 3):S56–S60.

61. D'Souza R, Ostro J, Shah PS, et al. Anticoagulation for pregnant women with mechanical heart valves: a systematic review and meta-analysis. *Eur Heart J.* 2017;38(19): 1509–1516.

62. Hall JG, Pauli RM, Wilson KM. Maternal and fetal sequelae of anticoagulation during pregnancy. *Am J Med.* 1980; 68(1):122–140.

63. Goland S, Elkayam U. Anticoagulation in pregnancy. *Cardiol Clin.* 2012;30(3):395–405.

64. Vitale N, De Feo M, De Santo LS, Pollice A, Tedesco N, Cotrufo M. Dose-dependent fetal complications of warfarin in pregnant women with mechanical heart valves. *J Am Coll Cardiol.* 1999;33(6):1637–1641.

65. Soma-Pillay P, Nene Z, Mathivha TM, Macdonald AP. The effect of warfarin dosage on maternal and fetal outcomes in pregnant women with prosthetic heart valves. *Obstet Med.* 2011;4(1):24–27.

66. Meschengieser SS, Fondevila CG, Santarelli MT, Lazzari MA. Anticoagulation in pregnant women with mechanical heart valve prostheses. *Heart.* 1999;82(1):23–26.

67. Kawamata K, Neki R, Yamanaka K, et al. Risks and pregnancy outcome in women with prosthetic mechanical heart valve replacement. *Circ J.* 2007;71(2):211–213.

68. Elkayam U. Anticoagulation therapy for pregnant women with mechanical prosthetic heart valves: how to improve safety? *J Am Coll Cardiol.* 2017;69(22):2692–2695.

69. Steinberg ZL, Dominguez-Islas CP, Otto CM, Stout KK, Krieger EV. Maternal and fetal outcomes of anticoagulation in pregnant women with mechanical heart valves. *J Am Coll Cardiol.* 2017;69(22):2681–2691.

70. Xu Z, Fan J, Luo X, et al. Anticoagulation regimens during pregnancy in patients with mechanical heart valves: a systematic review and meta-analysis. *Can J Cardiol.* 2016; 32(10), 1248 e1–e9.

71. Gallus AS, Baker RI, Chong BH, Ockelford PA, Street AM. Consensus guidelines for warfarin therapy. Recommendations from the australasian society of thrombosis and haemostasis. *Med J Aust.* 2000;172(12):600–605.

72. Sliwa K, Anthony J. Risk assessment for pregnancy with cardiac disease-a global perspective. *Eur J Heart Fail.* 2016;18(5):534–536.

73. Mishanina E, Rogozinska E, Thatthi T, Uddin-Khan R, Khan KS, Meads C. Use of labour induction and risk of cesarean delivery: a systematic review and meta-analysis. *Can Med Assoc J.* 2014;186(9):665–673.

74. Roos-Hesselink JW, Ruys TP, Stein JI, et al. Outcome of pregnancy in patients with structural or ischaemic heart disease: results of a registry of the European Society of Cardiology. *Eur Heart J.* 2013;34(9):657–665.

75. Sliwa K, Johnson MR, Zilla P, Roos-Hesselink JW. Management of valvular disease in pregnancy: a global perspective. *Eur Heart J.* 2015;36(18):1078–1089.

76. Langesaeter E, Rosseland LA, Stubhaug A. Haemodynamic effects of oxytocin in women with severe preeclampsia. *Int J Obstet Anesth.* 2011;20(1):26–29.

77. Pinder AJ, Dresner M, Calow C, Shorten GD, O'Riordan J, Johnson R. Haemodynamic changes caused by oxytocin during caesarean section under spinal anaesthesia. *Int J Obstet Anesth.* 2002;11(3):156–159.

78. Davies GA, Tessier JL, Woodman MC, Lipson A, Hahn PM. Maternal hemodynamics after oxytocin bolus compared with infusion in the third stage of labor: a randomized controlled trial. *Obstet Gynecol.* 2005;105(2): 294–299.

79. Habib G, Lancellotti P, Antunes MJ, et al. 2015 ESC guidelines for the management of infective endocarditis: the task force for the management of infective endocarditis of the European society of cardiology (ESC). Endorsed by: European association for cardio-thoracic surgery (EACTS), the European association of nuclear medicine (EANM). *Eur Heart J.* 2015;36(44):3075–3128.

80. RHDAustralia (ARF/RHD writing group). National heart foundation of Australia and the cardiac society of Australia and New Zealand. In: Carapetis JR, Brown A, Maguire G, Walsh W, Noonan S, Thompson D, eds. *Australian Guideline for Prevention, Diagnosis and Management of Acute Rheumatic Fever and Rheumatic Heart Disease.* 2nd ed.; 2012. Available online at: http://www.rhdaustralia.org.au/resources/arf-rhd-guideline.

81. Leonard H, O'Sullivan JJ, Hunter S. Family planning requirements in the adult congenital heart disease clinic. *Heart.* 1996;76(1):60–62.

82. *Saving Mothers: Seventh Report on Confidential Enquiries into Maternal Deaths in South Africa. 2014–2016.* Pretoria: Department of Health; 2017.

83. World Health Organisation. *Medical Eligibility Criteria for Contraceptive Use: A WHO Family Planning Cornerstone,* 2013/06/07 ed Geneva. 2010.

84. Roos-Hesselink JW, Cornette J, Sliwa K, Pieper PG, Veldtman GR, Johnson MR. Contraception and cardiovascular disease. *Eur Heart J.* 2015;36(27):1728–1734, 34a-34b.

85. Lidegaard O, Lokkegaard E, Svendsen AL, Agger C. Hormonal contraception and risk of venous thromboembolism: national follow-up study. *BMJ.* 2009;339:b2890.
86. Dinger J, Bardenheuer K, Heinemann K. Cardiovascular and general safety of a 24-day regimen of drospirenone-containing combined oral contraceptives: final results from the International Active Surveillance Study of Women Taking Oral Contraceptives. *Contraception.* 2014; 89(4):253—263.
87. Soma-Pillay P. Contraception for women with a medical disease. In: Dreyer G, ed. *Contraception, A South African Perspective.* Van Schaik Publishers; 2012.
88. Thorne S, Nelson-Piercy C, MacGregor A, et al. Pregnancy and contraception in heart disease and pulmonary arterial hypertension. *J Fam Plan Reprod Health Care.* 2006;32(2): 75—81.
89. Trussell J. Contraceptive efficacy. In: Hatcher R, Trussell J, Stewart F, et al., eds. *Contraceptive Technology.* 18th ed. New York: Ardent Media; 2004.
90. Cheng L, Che Y, Gulmezoglu AM. Interventions for emergency contraception. *Cochrane Database Syst Rev.* 2012;8: CD001324.
91. Ellison J, Thomson AJ, Greer IA, Walker ID. Drug points: apparent interaction between warfarin and levonorgestrel used for emergency contraception. *BMJ.* 2000; 321(7273):1382.

CHAPTER 10

Primary Prevention of Acute Rheumatic Fever and Rheumatic Heart Disease

SULAFA K.M. ALI • MARK E. ENGEL • LIESL ZÜHLKE • SUSAN J. JACK

PRIMORDIAL PREVENTION

Acute rheumatic fever (ARF) and rheumatic heart disease (RHD) are predominantly diseases of social, environmental, and economic poverty. Primordial prevention, defined as improving socioeconomic and living conditions, and having well-organized, effective health systems, is arguably the most important and effective population-based strategy for prevention of both ARF and RHD.

Even before the introduction of penicillin in the 1940s and 1950s, the incidence of ARF was declining and largely disappeared from countries as they developed economically.[1,2] The best recorded data come from Denmark, where a dramatic decline in ARF incidence over a 100 year period from 200 per 100,000 population in 1862, to 11 per 100,000 in 1962 was documented, with the decline largely occurring before the introduction of penicillin (Fig. 10.1).[3]

Deaths from ARF similarly declined in the United States between 1910 and 1977, the steepest decline seen before penicillin was introduced (Fig. 10.2).[4]

Early in the 20th century, researchers recognized the link between improved housing and hygiene, less household crowding, improved nutrition, and declining rates of many infectious diseases including ARF—although the specific environmental and/or host factors contributing to the decline in ARF remain elusive.[5-7] Social and economic improvements coupled with better healthcare systems and access to effective antibiotic treatment for group A streptococcus (GAS) infections have led to ARF becoming a rare disease in almost all high-income countries, although remaining endemic and significant in many low- and middle-income countries.[6] In more recent years, case-control and cohort studies have provided some empirical evidence of an association between poor housing conditions and household crowding and ARF, as described in Chapter 1. However, as noted, although poverty and social deprivation are strong predictors of developing ARF, it is difficult to identify what are the most important modifiable proximal risk factors where preventive actions could be focused.

EFFECTIVENESS OF PRIMARY PREVENTION

Primary prevention of ARF/RHD is defined as early diagnosis and prompt treatment of GAS infections to prevent the first episode of ARF.[1] Vaccination against GAS will be an important primary prevention intervention, once developed (see Chapter 14).

To be implemented as a primary healthcare policy, primary prevention needs to be effective in reducing the incidence of ARF. A simple, reliable, affordable, and sensitive method for diagnosis, and available treatment of primary GAS infections, the most common of which is GAS pharyngitis, is required. In recent years, evidence of the contribution of GAS skin infections to the development of ARF in some countries such as Australia, New Zealand, and Fiji has become stronger (see Box 10.1 for clinical features).[8-10] Although the role of skin infections is less clear in other countries, consideration of GAS skin infection management as a preventive measure for ARF may need to be evaluated in certain settings.

Acute Rheumatic Fever and Rheumatic Heart Disease. https://doi.org/10.1016/B978-0-323-63982-8.00010-6

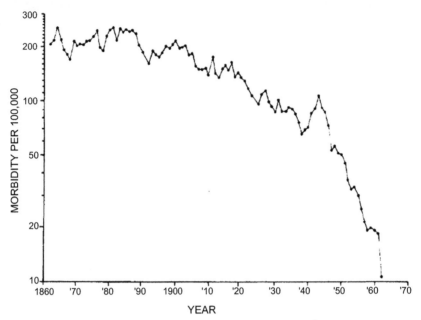

FIG. 10.1 Decline in Rheumatic Fever Incidence in Denmark, 1862–1962.[3] (Reproduced with permission from DiSciascio and Taranta[3].)

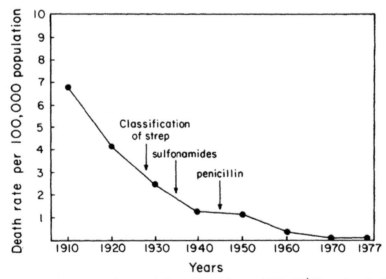

FIG. 10.2 Crude Death Rates from Rheumatic Fever, United States, 1910–77.[4] (Reproduced with permission from Gordis[4].)

Prompt use of antibiotics is effective in reducing the incidence of ARF following an episode of suspected GAS pharyngitis. A systematic review and meta-analysis comprising studies mainly conducted among US Military personnel in the 1950s showed a protective effect of 68% (RR = 0.32; 95% CI = 0.21–0.48) when using antibiotics to reduce the incidence of ARF following a GAS throat infection. The absolute risk reduction was 1.67% with a number-to-treat (NNT) of 53. Penicillin alone, assessed in a subgroup analysis, had a protective effect of 80% (fixed effect RR = 0.20, 95% CI = 0.11–0.36) with an NNT of 60.[11]

> **BOX 10.1**
> **Clinical Features of Group A Streptococcal infection**
>
> **GAS PHARYNGITIS**
> Viral infections are the most common cause of acute pharyngitis but GAS is the most common bacterial cause. There is significant overlap between the clinical features of streptococcal and nonstreptococcal throat infections and no single sign or symptom readily identifies GAS pharyngitis. Abrupt onset of fever, malaise, and sore throat are, however, common initial symptoms of GAS pharyngitis.
>
> The clinical features used within clinical predictive rules (see text for further details) include (i) fever, (ii) presence of tonsillar exudates, (iii) presence of tender anterior cervical lymphadenopathy, (iv) absence of rhinorrhoea and cough.
>
> **GAS IMPETIGO**
> Impetigo (or pyoderma) is an infection of the superficial keratin layer of the skin. The vast majority of cases are caused by β-hemolytic streptococci (usually GAS), *Staphylococcus aureus*, or both. Impetigo shares many of the same risk factors for ARF, including poverty, overcrowding, poor hygiene, and scabies. It is usually found in warm, humid areas, is highly contagious, and usually occurs in children. It mostly affects the face or lower extremities and presents clinically as papules, vesicles, and pustules. The pustules break down to form sores and characteristic thick, golden adherent crusts. Lesions are usually well localized but may appear in small groups and there is usually no systemic upset, although regional lymphadenitis may occur.

GAS, Group A streptococcus.

Experience from several regions of the world has shown that widespread use of antibiotics to treat GAS pharyngitis led to a decrease in ARF and RHD. In Cuba (1986–2002) and the French Caribbean islands, primary prevention was integrated into comprehensive programs that included public awareness, training of health personnel and establishment of ARF/RHD registries, which was associated with a dramatic decline in the ARF rate.[12,13] In Costa Rica, prompt clinical diagnosis of GAS pharyngitis without doing throat cultures and using a single penicillin injection was also associated with a decrease in ARF incidence.[14] Similarly, in Tunisia, an RHD control program based on early notification, early treatment of GAS pharyngitis using a single penicillin injection, and a strong secondary prevention program was associated with a decline in ARF from 8.7 (1985) to 1.5 per 100,000 population (2001).[15] Consequently, RHD is shown to have declined significantly over the corresponding period.[16,17]

Of course, ecological studies such as these do not provide definitive evidence for efficacy of the intervention itself, given that other factors such as economic development, improved housing or health systems strengthening may also have contributed to the decline in ARF and RHD. However, collectively, these reports suggest that integration of multiple approaches including education of the public and health personnel, and active management of GAS pharyngitis successfully contributed to the prevention of ARF in these settings.[12–14] However, other similar attempts at primary prevention through school-based programs did not demonstrate a reduction in ARF in Hawaii[18] and had only a modest effect among Navajo Indian communities in the 1960s and 1970s,[19] suggesting there are other contributing factors and that the specific context factors including the incidence of ARF and health system delivery mechanisms are important to consider.

A meta-analysis that included six studies investigated the role of treatment of GAS throat infection at the community and school levels to prevent ARF reported a relative risk of 0.41 (95% CI: 0.23–0.70) and concluded that treatment of GAS pharyngitis in school children could reduce the cases of ARF by 60%.[20] However, many of the studies included were noted to be of poor quality.[20] In New Zealand, a randomized controlled trial assessing the efficacy of school-based clinics for the primary preventions of ARF implemented from 1998 to 2001 reported a nonsignificant 21% ($P = .47$) to 28% ($P = .27$) reduction in ARF cases.[21] New Zealand recently implemented a national Rheumatic Fever Prevention Programme with several facets of primary prevention for ARF among high-risk populations. These included school-based sore throat clinics, where children self-identified as having a sore throat, had a throat swab, and any children whose swabs cultured GAS were given a 10-day course of oral amoxicillin. An evaluation of the school-based sore throat clinic component reported an overall effectiveness of 23% (95% CI: −6%–44%) (rate ratio (RR) 0.77 (95% CI: 0.56–1.06)).[22] In one high-risk area with high coverage of the program, effectiveness was greater (46%, 95% CI: 16%–66%; RR 0.54 (95% CI: 0.34–0.84)) with this finding supported by other evaluations.[22,23] The authors concluded that population-based primary prevention of ARF through sore throat management in schools where high-risk populations are geographically concentrated may be effective in well-resourced settings. However, where high-risk populations are dispersed, a school-based primary prevention approach appears ineffective and is expensive.[22]

Taken together, these findings suggest that incorporation of a strategy of primary antibiotic prophylaxis into a comprehensive program working in concert for disease control, including awareness and surveillance, may reduce the incidence of ARF and RHD but requires careful consideration of costs and feasibility.

This provides support for the efforts of the Pan African Society of Cardiology (PASCAR), which is convening a series of meetings with the World Health Organization: Africa region (WHO Region) to develop and endorse an action plan to implement a control program for RHD that includes primary and secondary prevention in African countries with a policy of "treat all" sore throats with one injection of benzathine penicillin G (BPG).[24]

DIAGNOSIS OF GROUP A STREPTOCOCCAL PHARYNGITIS

Given that the signs and symptoms of GAS pharyngitis are difficult to distinguish from viral causes of sore throat, microbiological culture of a throat swab is the gold standard for diagnosing GAS pharyngitis.[25] Given the necessary delay between the swab being taken and culture results becoming available, rapid antigen diagnostic tests (RADTs) are an alternative method for diagnosing GAS pharyngitis, although are associated with variable sensitivity (70%–90%) that depends on the clinical likelihood of GAS infection is an identified drawback.[25–27] However, the need for an accurate and specific test that is affordable and validated in low-resource settings is clear. More recent progress in this area include newer tests such as the nucleic acid amplification tests that have much better sensitivity and specificity and are now being increasingly used in low-resource settings for other diagnoses. We anticipate that this need will generate new data in the near future, hopefully with applicability to low-resource but endemic areas of the world.

A third alternative for diagnosing GAS pharyngitis is using clinical predictive rules (Box 10.2). Various clinical decision or predictive rules have been developed over the years.[28–32] Systematic reviews and meta-analyses have concluded that symptoms alone are not sufficient to rule in or rule out GAS pharyngitis diagnosis and only the rule of Joachim et al. was clinically useful to exclude GAS pharyngitis.[33–35] However, in low-resource settings where the use of laboratory facilities or RADTs may not be available or feasible, there is recent evidence that clinical diagnosis of GAS pharyngitis using clinical predictive rules can be reliably implemented in RHD endemic countries, obviating the need for more expensive bacteriological diagnostic

> **BOX 10.2**
> **Features of the Best Clinical Predictive Rule**
>
> 1. Utilizes few, well-defined criteria
> 2. Has maximum sensitivity with acceptable specificity
> 3. Can be easily used by primary healthcare workers
> 4. Evidence-based
> 5. Does not require laboratory confirmation

methods.[36] See Chapter 3 for a more detailed discussion of the diagnosis of GAS infection.

The American Heart Association (AHA) guidelines indicate that clinical and epidemiological findings have to be considered before deciding on using a microbiological test and only if these findings suggest GAS then throat culture or RADTs should be performed. It is stated that if there is evidence of viral infection (coryza, cough) then bacteriological investigations should not be performed.[37] Therefore, clinical rules may be applied even in high-resource settings, emphasizing their usefulness alongside bacteriological investigations.

The WHO included sore throat in the Integrated Management of Childhood Illness (IMCI) Program, which has been implemented in many developing countries. The diagnosis of GAS pharyngitis in IMCI is based on the presence of fever or sore throat and two of the following: red congested throat, white or yellow pharyngeal exudates, or enlarged anterior cervical lymph nodes. Of note, the algorithm suggested by the WHO did not perform well when applied to children in Brazil, Croatia, and Egypt, missing up to 96% of children with positive cultures.[38] This indicates that this clinical predictive rule is too specific to be utilized in areas with a high incidence of ARF. Tailoring decision rules to a specific population allows for improvement in performance characteristics such as the Turkish experience where less strict criteria were used.[39]

The New Zealand ARF Guidelines recommend the protocol depicted in Fig. 10.3. The most important features of this protocol are the considerations given to the ethnic/geographical and socioeconomic background of the patient (risk stratification), where less strict criteria are used for high-risk populations and if any criteria is positive then either empiric treatment is started immediately or bacteriological tests are performed and patients followed with treatment as indicated.[40]

In South Africa, a "treat-all" strategy, where all children presenting with pharyngitis were treated

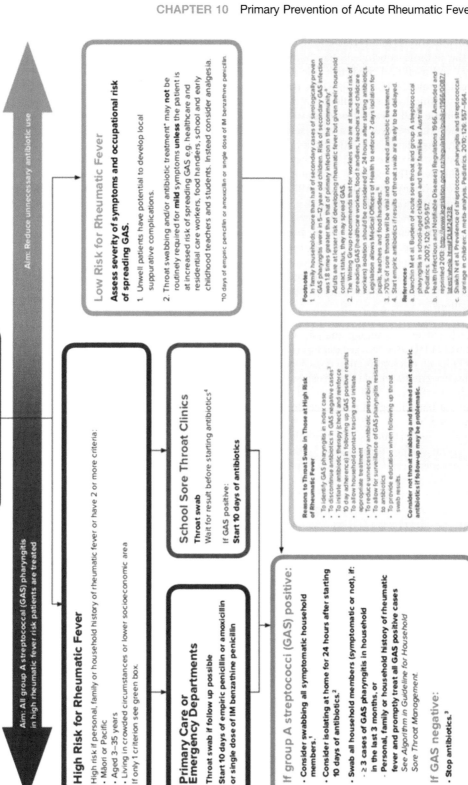

FIG. 10.3 New Zealand Protocol for Sore Throat Management. (Reproduced with permission from the New Zealand Heart Foundation.)

with penicillin, was found to be cost-effective and affordable.[41] The authors concluded that both the treat-all strategy and a clinical predictive rule called the clinical decision rule 2+ (CDR2+), where two or more criteria in a clinical decision rule are met, are affordable and simple and missed few cases of GAS pharyngitis at the primary level of care. In settings with a similar GAS prevalence and ARF attack rate in the Cape Town study area, the CDR2+ strategy was the most cost-effective. The authors recommended that a strategy for primary prevention of ARF and RHD in urban South Africa should be adopted to complement strategies to improve primordial prevention (better housing and hygiene) and secondary prevention (regular penicillin for those with a history of ARF). This strategy recommends that all patients complaining of a sore throat should receive antibiotics in the form of injectable BPG without requiring bacteriological investigations.[42]

In Sudan, a protocol for the management of pharyngitis was based on a mapping analysis, which showed clustering of RHD in certain geographical areas. Similar to New Zealand, risk stratification is used and in high-risk patients two criteria are taken to diagnose GAS pharyngitis (age 3−18 years and absence of viral symptoms) without bacteriological tests. One dose of BPG is recommended.[43]

Steinhoff et al. tested a clinical predictive rule that utilizes two points (sore throat with either a pharyngeal membrane or cervical lymphadenopathy) and found that it has a sensitivity of 80% and specificity of 40%.[44] This rule was reviewed for the Cape Town setting and found to have a higher than acceptable missed diagnosis (MDx) to wrong diagnosis (WDx) ratio, whereas the locally developed Cape Town prediction rule (used in the primary prevention cost-effectiveness study) had a MDx/WDx ratio closest to 0.044, which met the target parameters of a sensitivity of $\geq$90% and a specificity of $\geq$40%.[36]

In settings with research infrastructure, an approach may be to consider local investigation into clinical findings of sore throat parameters and a review of suitable clinical prediction rules and treat-all policies in line with local findings. However, it may be more feasible and cost-effective to consider likely similarities with other similar or nearby geographical settings and adapt a recommendation from one of those settings. The AFRO*Strep* registry is seeking to define the clinical, microbiological, epidemiological, and molecular characteristics of GAS infection in Africa.[45] An active surveillance component will collect comprehensive data on GAS in African settings and may define locally accurate and adaptable clinical predictive rules in the future.

Streptococcal Antibody Tests

As there is a time lag between infection and a serological response, antistreptococcal antibody titers (e.g., antistreptolysin O and antideoxyribonuclease (B)) reflect past and not current GAS infection. Therefore, they cannot be used to diagnose GAS pharyngitis in a sufficiently timely manner to guide treatment decisions that aim to prevent subsequent ARF (but are very useful as part of the diagnostic work-up of ARF - see Chapter 3).[46]

TREATMENT OF GROUP A STREPTOCOCCAL PHARYNGITIS

Penicillin is the drug of choice for treatment of GAS pharyngitis. To date, there have been no reports of penicillin-resistant GAS. Although treatment with oral penicillin for a duration of 10 days is effective in preventing ARF, it is less efficacious than BPG and adherence with this treatment in RHD endemic areas is expected to be suboptimal. Therefore, a single injection of BPG is preferred. Table 10.1 summarizes the treatment options. The treatment of GAS infection in patients who develop ARF is similar to that for GAS pharyngitis and is discussed in Chapter 4 (the main difference is that patients with ARF should receive long-term antibiotic prophylaxis).

Serious allergy (anaphylaxis) to BPG is rare. In a study including 32,000 injections and 2736 patient-years of follow-up, anaphylaxis occurred in 1.2/10,000 and death in 0.3/10,000 injections (see Chapter 11 for a detailed discussion on the epidemiology, diagnosis, and management of anaphylaxis due to penicillin prophylaxis).[47]

Delivery of Benzathine Penicillin G: Barriers and Potential Solutions

Many health workers hesitate to use BPG due to inherent problems of constitution and administration and fear of anaphylaxis. Table 10.2 lists the most common problems with BPG administration and potential solutions.

A common practice in many developing countries is to use dilute BPG to perform a skin test for allergy before injection. This practice is not evidence-based; penicillin skin testing should only be performed using a standard kit that contains benzylpenicilloyl polylysine such as Pre-Pen®.[49]

TABLE 10.1				
Antibiotics for Group A Streptococcal Pharyngitis.[a,48]				
Agent	Dose	Route	Duration	Rating
PENICILLINS				
Penicillin V (phenoxymethyl penicillin)	**Children** ($\leq$27 kg ($\leq$60 lbs)) 250 mg 2–3 times daily **Children** (>27 kg (>60 lb)), **adolescents**, and **adults**: 500 mg 2–3 times daily	Oral	10 days	IB
Amoxicillin	50 mg/kg once daily (maximum 1 g)	Oral	10 days	IB
Benzathine penicillin G	600,000 U for patients $\leq$27 kg ($\leq$60 lb); 1,200,000 U for patients >27 kg (>60 lb)	Intramuscular	Once	IB
FOR INDIVIDUALS ALLERGIC TO PENICILLIN				
Narrow-spectrum cephalosporin[b] (cephalexin, cefadroxil)	Variable	Oral	10 days	IB
Clindamycin	20 mg/kg per day divided in three doses (maximum 1.8 g/d)	Oral	10 days	IIaB
Azithromycin	12 mg/kg once daily (maximum 500 mg)	Oral	5 days	IIaB
Clarithromycin	15 mg/kg per day divided BID (maximum 250 mg BID)	Oral	10 days	IIaB

Rating indicates classification of recommendation and LOE (e.g., IB indicates class I, LOE B); BID bis in die (twice per day).
[a] For other acceptable alternatives, see text. The following are not acceptable: sulfonamides, trimethoprim, tetracyclines, and fluoroquinolones.
[b] To be avoided in those with immediate (type I) hypersensitivity to penicillin.

An important barrier to the use of BPG is pain. To overcome this, investigators have shown that mixing BPG powder with a local anesthetic like lidocaine can alleviate the pain without affecting the drug efficacy. It was shown that the serum concentration of penicillin was not affected when lidocaine is used instead of water for injection.[50] This practice is now well established in both powder and liquid forms of BPG. In the latter form, lidocaine is drawn into the same BPG syringe and injected first followed by BPG. The safe preparation of BPG with lidocaine is discussed in detail in Chapter 11.

Safe Administration of Benzathine Penicillin G

Special precautions: BPG should *not* be given to those with history of a severe reaction to previous injection or to other penicillins or cephalosporins

In addition, extreme caution should be exercised with patients with decompensated heart failure as it can lead to collapse and death, mimicking an "anaphylactic reaction." Because of poor cardiac function, these patients are more susceptible to vasovagal reactions (which may be precipitated as a result of intramuscular

BPG administration) and are at higher risk of life-threatening arrhythmias.[51] Patients with critical mitral stenosis, especially if dehydrated or in atrial fibrillation, may also be at risk of life-threatening arrhythmias secondary to vasovagal reactions.

There is currently little evidence to confirm the pathophysiology of nonanaphylactic deaths in severe RHD,[52] until such time we suggest caution and vigilance under these circumstances. These concepts are discussed further in Chapter 11.

Future Directions in the Treatment of Group A Streptococcal Infections

Although BPG is effective and affordable, it has the aforementioned inherent problems. Deaths related to BPG are unforgettable and have been reported,[47,53] although most of these are unlikely to be due to anaphylaxis. Therefore, it is desirable to develop better formulations or alternatives to BPG that are affordable, effective, and have minimal side effects. Oral penicillin needs to be continued for 10 days, which poses the risk of nonadherence, especially in RHD endemic communities. Shorter durations of later generation antibiotics have been evaluated in a

TABLE 10.2
Barriers to Benzathine Penicillin G Administration and Potential Solutions.

Problem	Solution
The drug is viscous and can block the needle	- Use appropriate amount of diluents - Use a large-bore needle - Do not use cold diluent
Pain upon administration	- Use lidocaine 2% as a diluent or with the premixed injection - Use thumb pressure for 10 seconds - Inject slowly
Fear of allergy	- Training of health workers to follow local protocols - Prepare items required for allergy management (BPG Kit) - Monitoring of side effects
Fear of inadvertent deaths	- Strictly avoid intravenous administration - Avoid giving to patients with decompensated heart failure
BPG shortage and quality	- Health systems and World Health Organization need to make BPG kits available and ensure the quality of BPG

BPG, benzathine penicillin G.

meta-analysis and although the clinical parameters were comparable with standard duration protocols, the overall bacteriological recurrence rates were higher in the shorter duration protocols, and none has been evaluated for its prevention of ARF.[54] There has been limited research into alternatives to BPG; this will remain a major obstacle for primary prevention and management of ARF/RHD, and global efforts in this regard are urgently needed.

COST-EFFECTIVENESS OF PRIMARY PREVENTION

Following an assessment of the costs of different strategies for primary prevention in South African urban settings, which included treating all sore throats, performing throat cultures and treating only those with a positive culture, and using a clinical predictive rule with two or three points (see later), it was found that treating all children with pharyngitis with intramuscular penicillin is the least costly.[41] A strategy of using a clinical predictive rule without culture is preferred as culturing throat swabs from all children presenting with sore throat is extremely expensive.[41] Similarly, an Indian study compared the cost effectiveness of primary and secondary prevention and concluded that in low-resource settings, primary prevention, even with a culture confirmation and BPG treatment strategy, is a viable economic option.[55]

WHO acknowledges primary prevention as an important tool for ARF/RHD control.[56] However, the need for bacteriological confirmation of GAS infection was emphasized, resulting in unacceptably high costs of implementing this strategy. This has recently been revisited after the growing evidence that clinical predictive rules could replace bacteriological diagnosis in certain settings (see later).

Yet, it is well recognized that up to two-thirds of patients with ARF do not recall any symptoms of sore throat, a real obstacle when instituting such primary prevention programs in isolation.[57] This could partly be overcome by education of the public about the importance of health-seeking behavior relating to sore throat and subsequent early detection of GAS pharyngitis (see Chapter 15). Another concern about adopting clinical predictive rules for diagnosis of bacterial pharyngitis is the overuse of antibiotics or fear of developing antimicrobial resistance. To date there have been no reports of penicillin-resistant GAS, although the contribution of antibiotic use for sore throats to antimicrobial resistance in other pathogens (e.g., *Streptococcus pneumoniae*) is not clear. In fact, the decline in ARF in developed countries was attributed to the increasing use of antibiotics, alongside the improvement in living conditions.[58] Fig. 10.4 depicts the strengths and limitations of primary prevention of ARF/RHD.

DELIVERY OF PRIMARY PREVENTION STRATEGIES

Primary prevention can be instituted at different levels (Fig. 10.5).

Population-Based Strategies

More focused population-based strategies can be implemented to improve the uptake of primary prevention

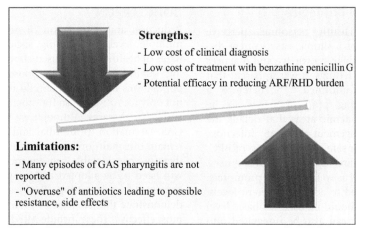

FIG. 10.4 Strengths and Limitations of Primary Prevention of Acute Rheumatic Fever. ARF, acute rheumatic fever; RHD, rheumatic heart disease; GAS, group A streptococcal.

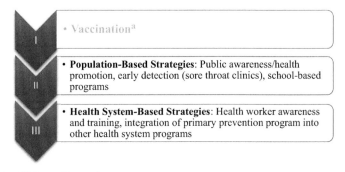

FIG. 10.5 Levels of Primary Prevention.
[a]Yet to be developed, although there is now a coordinated global effort to overcome roadblocks to GAS vaccine development - see Chapter 14.

interventions for ARF, especially if these are integrated into existing primary healthcare programs.

However, as mentioned, it is well documented that many patients with ARF/RHD will not recall an episode of sore throat. This could be attributed to the following causes:

- The episode was asymptomatic (i.e., subclinical): in this situation, it is not feasible to prevent the disease by antibiotics and the only feasible primary prevention measure will ultimately be improving the social determinants of health or by vaccination.
- The episode was clinically apparent, but the family did not seek medical attention either because it was self-limiting, or it was treated with home remedies. This situation is commonly encountered as some people do not give much consideration to a sore

throat, particularly if they have more pressing concerns. There is potential for improved early diagnosis and treatment using the following measures aiming to improve health-seeking behaviors:

1. Public awareness through media, schools, and other approaches using consistent and simple messages such as follows: "sore throat can lead to serious heart disease." Posters, pamphlets, and songs can be effective when the messages are clearly indicated, and social media is an increasingly effective method for health promotion messaging.[59]

2. Sore throat clinics: can be instituted in schools and primary healthcare centers in target areas. These programs can be led by trained nurses. Although this approach is feasible, its costs might prohibit its implementation in resource-limited countries.[60]

Health System-Based Strategies

- Health Personnel: Health personnel perceive bacterial pharyngitis as a simple, easy to treat disease; however, when their knowledge and practices were tested, in many settings, it was apparent that they were not well informed.[61,62] Therefore, a comprehensive training program needs to be instituted in RHD endemic areas that details the diagnosis and management of GAS infection, including methods for safe administration of BPG. Training needs to be directed to physicians, nurses, and medical assistants as well as health promoters. Training modules need to address different levels, and local languages should be used for basic level health workers. These can also be integrated into existing training programs for maximum impact.
- Health System Level: Training programs for primary prevention can be integrated at many levels within the departments of the Ministries of Health such as noncommunicable disease, IMCI, and school health programs (Fig. 10.6).

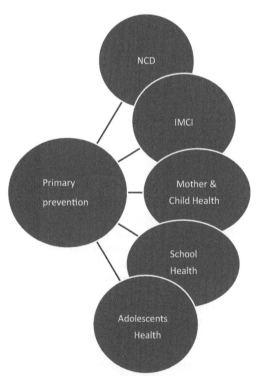

FIG. 10.6 Integration of Primary Prevention of Acute Rheumatic Fever into Different Health System Programs. NCD, non-communicable disease; IMCI, integrated management of childhood illness.

CONCLUSION

Reduction and elimination of ARF require efforts at multiple levels. Addressing socioeconomic determinants of health with a focused effort on improved housing quality and reducing household crowding for populations most at risk should reap positive benefits not only for ARF but also for other common respiratory and other diseases. Although we wait for an effective GAS vaccination, primordial and primary prevention remain our main options to reduce the incidence and therefore considerable consequences of ARF. Strategies will need to be adopted and adapted to best suit the context of each setting. Positive country examples demonstrate that strategies working in concert are the most effective. These include ARF/RHD health information promoted to populations and health staff showing the link between sore throats and ARF/RHD, and effective delivery services to diagnose and treat GAS infections that are available, accessible, affordable, and acceptable to the populations most at risk.

REFERENCES

1. Denny FW, Wannamaker LW, Brink WR, Rammelkamp Jr CH, Custer EA. Prevention of rheumatic fever; treatment of the preceding streptococcic infection. J Am Med Assoc. 1950;143(2):151−153.
2. Quinn RW. Comprehensive review of morbidity and mortality trends for rheumatic fever, streptococcal disease, and scarlet fever: the decline of rheumatic fever. Rev Infect Dis. 1989;11(6):928−953.
3. DiSciascio G, Taranta A. Rheumatic fever in children. Am Heart J. 1980;99(5):635−658.
4. Gordis L. The virtual disappearance of rheumatic fever in the United States: lessons in the rise and fall of disease. T. Duckett Jones memorial lecture. Circulation. 1985;72(6):1155−1162.
5. Markowitz M. The decline of rheumatic fever: role of medical intervention. Lewis W. Wannamaker memorial lecture. J Pediatr. 1985;106(4):545−550.
6. Bisno AL. Landmark perspective: the rise and fall of rheumatic fever. J Am Med Assoc. 1985;254(4):538−541.
7. Steer AC, Carapetis JR. Prevention and treatment of rheumatic heart disease in the developing world. Nat Rev Cardiol. 2009;6(11):689−698.
8. McDonald M, Currie BJ, Carapetis JR. Acute rheumatic fever: a chink in the chain that links the heart to the throat? Lancet Infect Dis. 2004;4(4):240−245.
9. Parks T, Smeesters PR, Steer AC. Streptococcal skin infection and rheumatic heart disease. Curr Opin Infect Dis. 2012;25(2):145−153.
10. O'Sullivan L, Moreland NJ, Webb RH, Upton A, Wilson NJ. Acute rheumatic fever after group A Streptococcus pyoderma and group G Streptococcus pharyngitis. Pediatr Infect Dis J. 2017;36(7):692−694.

11. Robertson KA, Volmink JA, Mayosi BM. Antibiotics for the primary prevention of acute rheumatic fever: a meta-analysis. *BMC Cardiovasc Disord.* 2005;5(1):11.

12. Nordet P, Lopez R, Duenas A, Sarmiento L. Prevention and control of rheumatic fever and rheumatic heart disease: the Cuban experience (1986−1996−2002). *Cardiovasc J Afr.* 2008;19(3):135−140.

13. Bach JF, Chalons S, Forier E, et al. 10-year educational programme aimed at rheumatic fever in two French Caribbean islands. *Lancet.* 1996;347(9002):644−648.

14. Arguedas A, Mohs E. Prevention of rheumatic fever in Costa Rica. *J Pediatr.* 1992;121(4):569−572.

15. Ben Romdhane H, Haouala H, Belhani A, et al. [Epidemiological transition and health impact of cardiovascular disease in Tunisia]. *Tunis Med.* 2005;83(Suppl 5):1−7.

16. Houda Ben Ayed SY, Ben Hmida M, Ben Jemaa M, et al. Is rheumatic heart disease still endemic in Tunisia? A review of 14-year period and future projections. *CPQ Cardiol.* 2018;1:1−11.

17. Sriha Belguith A, Koubaa Abdelkafi A, El Mhamdi S, et al. Rheumatic heart disease in a developing country: incidence and trend (Monastir; Tunisia: 2000−2013). *Int J Cardiol.* 2017;228:628−632.

18. Chun LT, Reddy V, Rhoads GG. Occurrence and prevention of rheumatic fever among ethnic groups of Hawaii. *Am J Dis Child.* 1984;138(5):476−478.

19. Coulehan J, Grant S, Reisinger K, Killian P, Rogers KD, Kaltenbach C. Acute rheumatic fever and rheumatic heart disease on the Navajo reservation, 1962−77. *Public Health Rep.* 1980;95(1):62−68.

20. Lennon D, Kerdemelidis M, Arroll B. Meta-analysis of trials of streptococcal throat treatment programs to prevent rheumatic fever. *Pediatr Infect Dis J.* 2009;28(7): e259−e264.

21. Lennon D, Stewart J, Farrell E, Palmer A, Mason H. School-based prevention of acute rheumatic fever: a group randomized trial in New Zealand. *Pediatr Infect Dis J.* 2009; 28(9):787−794.

22. Jack SJ, Williamson DA, Galloway Y, et al. Primary prevention of rheumatic fever in the 21st century: evaluation of a national programme. *Int J Epidemiol.* 2018;47(5):1585−1593.

23. Lennon D, Anderson P, Kerdemilidis M, et al. First presentation acute rheumatic fever is preventable in a community setting: a school-based intervention. *Pediatr Infect Dis J.* 2017;36(12):1113−1118.

24. Mayosi BM, Gamra H, Dangou JM, Kasonde J, 2nd all-Africa workshop on rheumatic F, rheumatic heart disease participants. Rheumatic heart disease in Africa: the Mosi-o-Tunya call to action. *Lancet Glob Health.* 2014;2(8): e438−e439.

25. Lean WL, Arnup S, Danchin M, Steer AC. Rapid diagnostic tests for group a streptococcal pharyngitis: a meta-analysis. *Pediatrics.* 2014;134(4):771−781.

26. Edmonson MB, Farwell KR. Relationship between the clinical likelihood of group a streptococcal pharyngitis and the sensitivity of a rapid antigen-detection test in a pediatric practice. *Pediatrics.* 2005;115(2):280−285.

27. Tanz RR, Gerber MA, Kabat W, Rippe J, Seshadri R, Shulman ST. Performance of a rapid antigen-detection test and throat culture in community pediatric offices: implications for management of pharyngitis. *Pediatrics.* 2009;123(2):437−444.

28. Centor RM, Witherspoon JM, Dalton HP, Brody CE, Link K. The diagnosis of strep throat in adults in the emergency room. *Med Decis Mak.* 1981;1(3):239−246.

29. McIsaac WJ, White D, Tannenbaum D, Low DE. A clinical score to reduce unnecessary antibiotic use in patients with sore throat. *CMAJ Can Med Assoc J.* 1998;158(1): 75−83.

30. Organization WH. *The Management of Acute Respiratory Infections in Children: Practical Guidelines for Outpatient Care.* 1995.

31. Smeesters PR, Campos Jr D, Van Melderen L, de Aguiar E, Vanderpas J, Vergison A. Pharyngitis in low-resources settings: a pragmatic clinical approach to reduce unnecessary antibiotic use. *Pediatrics.* 2006;118(6): e1607−e1611.

32. Joachim L, Campos Jr D, Smeesters PR. Pragmatic scoring system for pharyngitis in low-resource settings. *Pediatrics.* 2010;126(3):e608−e614.

33. Le Marechal F, Martinot A, Duhamel A, Pruvost I, Dubos F. Streptococcal pharyngitis in children: a meta-analysis of clinical decision rules and their clinical variables. *BMJ Open.* 2013;3(3).

34. Shaikh N, Swaminathan N, Hooper EG. Accuracy and precision of the signs and symptoms of streptococcal pharyngitis in children: a systematic review. *J Pediatr.* 2012; 160(3):487−493 e3.

35. Cohen JF, Cohen R, Levy C, et al. Selective testing strategies for diagnosing group A streptococcal infection in children with pharyngitis: a systematic review and prospective multicentre external validation study. *CMAJ Can Med Assoc J.* 2015;187(1):23−32.

36. Engel ME, Cohen K, Gounden R, et al. The Cape Town clinical decision rule for streptococcal pharyngitis in children. *Pediatr Infect Dis J.* 2017;36(3):250−255.

37. Gerber MA, Baltimore RS, Eaton CB, et al. Prevention of rheumatic fever and diagnosis and treatment of acute streptococcal pharyngitis: a scientific statement from the American heart association rheumatic fever, Endocarditis, and Kawasaki disease committee of the council on cardiovascular disease in the young, the interdisciplinary council on functional genomics and translational biology, and the interdisciplinary council on quality of care and outcomes research: endorsed by the American academy of pediatrics. *Circulation.* 2009;119(11):1541−1551.

38. Rimoin AW, Hamza HS, Vince A, et al. Evaluation of the WHO clinical decision rule for streptococcal pharyngitis. *Arch Dis Child.* 2005;90(10):1066−1070.

39. Sahin F, Ulukol B, Aysev D, Suskan E. The validity of diagnostic criteria for streptococcal pharyngitis in Integrated Management of Childhood Illness (IMCI) guidelines. *J Trop Pediatr.* 2003;49(6):377−379.

40. The National Heart Foundation of New Zealand. *Group A Streptococcal Sore Throat Management Guideline.*

2014 Update. Auckland: The National Heart Foundation of New Zealand; 2014.

41. Irlam J, Mayosi BM, Engel M, Gaziano TA. Primary prevention of acute rheumatic fever and rheumatic heart disease with penicillin in South African children with pharyngitis : a cost-effectiveness analysis. *Circ-Cardiovasc Qual.* 2013; 6(3):343−351.

42. Irlam JH, Mayosi BM, Engel ME, Gaziano TA. A cost-effective strategy for primary prevention of acute rheumatic fever and rheumatic heart disease in children with pharyngitis. *S Afr Med J.* 2013;103(12):894−895.

43. Ali SKM, Al Khaleefa MS, Khair SM. *Acute Rheumatic Fever and Rheumatic Heart Disease: Sudan's Guidelines for Diagnosis.* Management and Prevention; 2017.

44. Steinhoff MC, Abd el Khalek MK, Khallaf N, et al. Effectiveness of clinical guidelines for the presumptive treatment of streptococcal pharyngitis in Egyptian children. *Lancet.* 1997;350(9082):918−921.

45. Barth DD, Engel ME, Whitelaw A, et al. Rationale and design of the African group a streptococcal infection registry: the AFROStrep study. *BMJ Open.* 2016;6(2):e010248.

46. Wessels MR. Clinical practice. Streptococcal pharyngitis. *N Engl J Med.* 2011;364(7):648−655.

47. International rheumatic fever study group Markowitz M, Kaplan E, Cuttica R, et al. Allergic reactions to long-term benzathine penicillin prophylaxis for rheumatic fever. International rheumatic fever study group. *Lancet.* 1991; 337(8753):1308−1310.

48. Organization WH. *WHO Model Prescribing Information: Drugs Used in the Treatment of Streptococcal Pharyngitis and Prevention of Rheumatic Fever. Geneva.* 1999.

49. Bernstein IL, Li JT, Bernstein DI, et al. Allergy diagnostic testing: an updated practice parameter. *Ann Allergy Asthma Immunol.* 2008;100(3 Suppl 3):S1−S148.

50. Amir J, Ginat S, Cohen YH, Marcus TE, Keller N, Varsano I. Lidocaine as a diluent for administration of benzathine penicillin G. *Pediatr Infect Dis J.* 1998; 17(10):890−893.

51. WHO model prescribing information. Streptococcal pharyngitis and prevention of rheumatic fever. *WHO Drug Inf.* 2000;14(2):99−104.

52. Marantelli S, Hand R, Carapetis J, Beaton A, Wyber R. Severe adverse events following benzathine penicillin G injection for rheumatic heart disease prophylaxis: cardiac compromise more likely than anaphylaxis. *Heart Asia.* 2019;11(2):e011191.

53. Organization WH. Benzathine penicillin: three fatal reports following mega unit injections. *Drug Inf Bull.* 2000; 4:2000.

54. Altamimi S, Khalil A, Khalaiwi KA, Milner RA, Pusic MV, Al Othman MA. Short-term late-generation antibiotics versus longer term penicillin for acute streptococcal pharyngitis in children. *Cochrane Database Syst Rev.* 2012;(8): CD004872.

55. Soudarssanane MB, Karthigeyan M, Mahalakshmy T, et al. Rheumatic fever and rheumatic heart disease: primary prevention is the cost effective option. *Indian J Pediatr.* 2007; 74(6):567−570.

56. Strategy for controlling rheumatic fever/rheumatic heart disease, with emphasis on primary prevention: memorandum from a joint WHO/ISFC meeting. *Bull World Health Organ.* 1995;73(5):583−587.

57. Carapetis JR, McDonald M, Wilson NJ. Acute rheumatic fever. *Lancet.* 2005;366(9480):155−168.

58. Seckeler MD, Hoke TR. The worldwide epidemiology of acute rheumatic fever and rheumatic heart disease. *Clin Epidemiol.* 2011;3:67−84.

59. Society. SCH. New Training and Awareness Tools: Sudanese Children Heart Society.; [Available from:: http://www.sudankidsheart.org/index.php/component/content/article/90-home/148-new-training-and-awareness-tools.html.

60. Gray S, Lennon D, Anderson P, Stewart J, Farrell E. Nurse-led school-based clinics for skin infections and rheumatic fever prevention: results from a pilot study in South Auckland. *N Z Med J.* 2013;126(1373):53−61.

61. Osman GM, Abdelrahman SMK, Ali SKM. Evaluation of physicians' knowledge about prevention of rheumatic fever and rheumatic heart disease before and after a teaching session. *Sudan J Paediatr.* 2015;15(2):37−42.

62. Robertson KA, Volmink JA, Mayosi BM. Lack of adherence to the national guidelines on the prevention of rheumatic fever. *S Afr Med J.* 2005;95(1):52−56.

CHAPTER 11

Secondary Prevention of Acute Rheumatic Fever and Rheumatic Heart Disease

JESSICA L. DE DASSEL • DIANA LENNON • SCOTT DOUGHERTY • ANNA P. RALPH

INTRODUCTION

Definition of Secondary Prevention

Individuals within a vulnerable age group who have had an episode of acute rheumatic fever (ARF), or already have established rheumatic heart disease (RHD), are at high risk of recurrence of ARF if further episodes of group A streptococcal (GAS) infection occur. Secondary prevention of ARF and RHD is therefore warranted (Box 11.1). A holistic view of secondary prevention comprises both secondary prophylaxis with an antibiotic (discussed here), plus enhanced primordial and primary preventive activities targeted for individuals and households affected by ARF and/or RHD (discussed in Chapter 10).

Enhanced primordial and primary prevention for individuals and households affected by ARF and/or RHD includes activities to tackle the socioeconomic drivers of RHD, such as infrastructure support for households to mitigate crowding and ensure access to washing facilities. Health literacy support and other educational activities described in Chapters 10 and 15 can enable early health seeking behavior for syndromes consistent with potential GAS infection (e.g., sore throat, impetigo), which may help ensure timely receipt of antibiotic treatment (Box 11.2).

Historical Background

Before the introduction of antibiotics, ARF and RHD resulted in significant morbidity and premature mortality, particularly for children. One study in the preantibiotic era followed 588 children for 10 years after their initial episode of ARF: 58% had a recurrence in the first 5 years; 23% progressed to RHD and 24% died from ARF or bacterial endocarditis.[1] One of the largest prepenicillin cohorts included 1000 patients who were followed for 20 years: 19% had recurrences in the first 5 years after admission to hospital with ARF or RHD, and the vast majority (89%) who had RHD at baseline had persistent evidence of valvular disease at the 10 years follow-up review.[2]

Historically, implementation of antibiotic secondary prophylaxis has been the only medical intervention to have altered the course of disease for individuals after an initial ARF diagnosis. The risk of ARF after the first attack of GAS is approximately 0.3%–3%, but with

---

BOX 11.1
Definition of Secondary Prophylaxis

- Secondary prophylaxis of acute rheumatic fever (ARF) and rheumatic heart disease (RHD) comprises long-term antibiotic therapy for individuals diagnosed with ARF or RHD, to prevent ARF recurrences triggered by recurrent group A streptococcal (GAS) infection, and therefore prevent the development of RHD or worsening of existing RHD.
- International guidelines differ slightly on recommendations for antibiotic choice, duration, and patient groups in whom it is indicated.
- Key standard recommendations usually include use of parenteral (intramuscular) benzathine penicillin G (BPG) every 4 weeks in individuals diagnosed with ARF and/or RHD, for a minimum 5–10 year period after diagnosis of the most recent ARF episode, or to the age of 21, whichever comes later. In some countries, duration for severe cases is lifelong.

Acute Rheumatic Fever and Rheumatic Heart Disease. https://doi.org/10.1016/B978-0-323-63982-8.00011-8

BOX 11.2
Key Points on Secondary Prevention of Acute
Rheumatic Fever and Rheumatic Heart Disease

- The standard secondary prophylaxis regimen is benzathine penicillin G (BPG) administered every 4 weeks
- It is essential to ensure that the correct form of penicillin is prescribed: long-acting intramuscular BPG, not short-acting intramuscular procaine penicillin G
- Accurate diagnosis of acute rheumatic fever (ARF) to allow the instigation of secondary prophylaxis is a cornerstone for rheumatic heart disease (RHD) control
  - Failure to recognize ARF represents a missed opportunity to provide secondary prevention
- Secondary prophylaxis reduces the risk of ARF recurrences and the risk of RHD development or progression. Secondary prophylaxis is also associated with regression of the severity of RHD in a proportion of cases
- If ARF recurrence occurs despite excellent adherence (i.e. no days at risk - no gaps, with needles being received every 28 days) with a 4-weekly BPG regimen, a 3-weekly regimen should be adopted
- The severity of RHD does not influence the recommended frequency of BPG dosing but does influence the duration of secondary prophylaxis
- Adherence to secondary prophylaxis schedules can be highly challenging, due to the frequency of injections, requirement for long-term engagement with health services, and pain of the injections
- Adherence support must be provided using innovative, culturally responsive approaches that are tailored to engage children and adolescents
- Secondary prophylaxis is cost-effective

subsequent infection this risk rises to 25%–75%,[3] emphasizing the critical importance of secondary prophylaxis.

Evidence of Effectiveness

The following section and Table 11.1 review the data on the effectiveness of secondary prophylaxis with penicillin, showing that it is effective in reducing ARF recurrences, reducing RHD progression, increasing the likelihood of regression of existing RHD, and reducing overall mortality.[4] Emerging data from Africa also suggests that high adherence (>80% of scheduled injections) is associated with reduced mortality from RHD.[5] Secondary prophylaxis with penicillin has also been shown to be the most cost-effective RHD prevention strategy.[6] In early studies of ARF prophylaxis using sulfonamides, 1.5% of treated cases developed ARF recurrences, compared to 20% of untreated cases. Subsequently, penicillin was found to be more efficacious

than sulfonamides in preventing ARF recurrences (Level I evidence).[7,8] A Cochrane meta-analysis[9] concluded that penicillin, compared to no therapy, significantly reduces the rate of ARF recurrences, and that intramuscular BPG is superior to oral penicillin.

There is strong evidence that secondary prophylaxis also reduces the severity of RHD by preventing RHD progression.[2,3,10,11] Data on the extent to which RHD can regress with secondary prophylaxis are mixed. In people receiving secondary prophylaxis with good adherence, some studies indicate that RHD severity improves in up to 50%–70% of people, with higher regression rates in mild RHD than in moderate or severe disease,[12–14] and a mortality reduction has also been noted.[15] Tompkins et al. reported in 1972 that acute mitral regurgitation resolved in 70% of patients with ARF who were adherent to 4-weekly BPG for at least 5 years.[11] These early studies used auscultation to determine disease severity rather than echocardiography,[16] so these are less accurate than more recent work using echocardiography to grade RHD severity. A more recent study measured changes in valve lesion severity and all patients prescribed secondary prophylaxis ($n = 6$) had regression of mild lesions.[17] A further study used valvular regurgitation as an indication of disease severity; regurgitation improved in 7 of the 13 people who received ≥75% of doses and did not improve in any of the people who were not adherent ($n = 4$).[18]

Numerous studies have reported that in nontrial (programmatic) settings, adherence to secondary prophylaxis reduces the likelihood of ARF recurrence and can prevent progression of RHD (Table 11.1). Many of these studies have also reported rare recurrences occurring despite high adherence to secondary prophylaxis. In one study from New Zealand, which closely examined the circumstances of apparent "breakthrough" episodes, it was shown that there had been "days at risk" due to an injection being administered late by several days or more.[19] In another from Australia's Northern Territory, while nearly all ARF recurrences occurred due to nonreceipt of BPG, some genuine "breakthrough" episodes did occur despite absence of "days at risk."[20]

Limitations and Challenges in Delivery of Secondary Prophylaxis

Secondary prophylaxis can only prevent RHD if implemented before RHD has developed, yet most RHD diagnoses are made in individuals with no prior diagnosed episodes of ARF. In Australia's Northern Territory, for example, approximately 75% of people diagnosed with RHD have not had a documented prior ARF diagnosis. This group of patients represents the missed opportunities for prevention. However, if the person

TABLE 11.1
English Language Studies Which Have Reported on the Clinical Outcomes Associated With Secondary Prophylaxis.

Country (Region)	Study Design	Participants	Follow up	SP Type and Frequency	Definition of Adherence	Sample Size for Adherence Data	"Break-through" ARF Recurrences Reported?	Findings
Australia (Northern Territory)[23]	Prospective cohort	Children with RHD	Mean: 10.6 years	Not stated	Not stated	25	No	- 11 recurrences (7 people) - 1 person had 4 recurrences, all 4 of these recurrences were due to "nonadherence"
Australia (Kimberley and Far North Queensland)[24]	Retrospective record review	People with ARF or RHD	12 months	3–4-weekly BPG	Not stated	293	No	- 12 recurrences - None of the people who had a recurrence had "adequate" adherence in the 2 months before their recurrence
Australia (Townsville)[18]	Prospective cohort	Children with first episode of ARF or RHD	Up to 4 yrs	4-weekly BPG	≥75% doses	23 (6 ARF only, 17 RHD at baseline)	No	- 70% were "compliant" in 2014 - Four people progressed from ARF to RHD, two of them were adherent - RHD improved in 7 people, all were adherent - RHD progressed in 3 people, 1 was adherent
Australia (Northern Territory)[4]	Case control	People with ARF or RHD	Up to 6 years	3–4-weekly BPG	≥80% doses	ARF recurrences: 97 cases; all-cause mortality: 69 cases	No	- ARF recurrence risk did not decrease until ≈40% of doses had been administered. - Receiving <80% was associated with a fourfold increase in the odds of ARF recurrence - Receiving <80% appeared to be associated with increased all-cause mortality
Brazil (Rio Branco, Acre)[25]	Cross section	People with ARF	Not reported	BPG, frequency not stated	Not stated	99	Yes	- 38% of the participants were "regular" with their SP - 71% of ARF recurrences were in people who were "regular"
Brazil (Sao Paulo)[26]	Retrospective record review	Children <16 with chorea at first ARF episode	Mean: 3.6 years	3-weekly BPG	Not stated	86	Yes	- 17 children had recurrences of chorea - 9 of the children who had ARF recurrences used "regular" SP

Continued

TABLE 11.1
English Language Studies Which Have Reported on the Clinical Outcomes Associated With Secondary Prophylaxis.—cont'd

Country (Region)	Study Design	Participants	Follow up	SP Type and Frequency	Definition of Adherence	Sample Size for Adherence Data	"Break-through" ARF Recurrences Reported?	Findings
Brazil (Rio de Janeiro)[27]	Retrospective record review	People with ARF	Not reported	BPG, frequency not stated	≤1 delayed or missed dose in 6 months	536	Yes	- 88 ARF recurrences - 40 ARF recurrences in people who were adherent - Being adherent was associated with a reduced risk of ARF recurrence ($P < .0001$)
Chile (Santiago)[28]	Prospective cohort	People with Sydenham's chorea	Not stated	Monthly BPG	Not stated	31	Yes	- 17 ARF recurrences (10 people) - 15 ARF recurrences in people who had received monthly BPG for at least the 7 months before recurrence - 2 recurrences occurred 5 months after the previous episode, SP had been given "continuously" between episodes - No doses were more than 4 days late
China (Guangzhou)[29]	Prospective cohort	People with ARF	Range 5–10 years	Not stated	Not stated	35	Yes	- 30 ARF recurrences (22 people) - 4 ARF recurrences in people on "regular" SP - "Regular" adherence associated with reduced risk of a recurrence ($P < .05$)
Egypt (Alexandria)[30]	Cross section	Children with RHD	6–12 months	Oral, 2- and 4-weekly BPG	2-weekly BPG: ≥11 doses in 6 months or ≥22 doses in 12 months (4-weekly not stated)	2-weekly BPG: 104 4-weekly BPG: 14	Yes	- 28% of "compliant" patients had an ARF recurrence - Being "irregular" with SP increased the risk of a recurrence (AOR: 2.45 [95% CI1.04–5.17]) (logistic regression included nine people on oral SP)

Setting	Study type	Population	Duration	Regimen	Adherence	N		Results
Ethiopia (Addis Ababa)[31]	Retrospective record review	Children with RHD	Range: 7–126 months	Monthly BPG	No missed doses	211	Yes	- 188 adherent people, 23 nonadherent people - 22 ARF recurrences - 10 ARF recurrences in adherent people - 12 ARF recurrences in people who were not adherent - Nonadherent people were more likely to have a recurrence (OR: 19.42 [95% CI: 6.89–54.77], $P < .001$)
India (rural villages near Vellore)[32]	Surveillance study	Children with ARF or RHD	3.5 years	4-weekly BPG then 3-weekly BPG	Not stated	24	Unclear	- 22 were "regular" with SP, none of them had "rheumatic reactivation" - No comment on outcomes for nonadherent children
India (Haryana state)[33]	Prospective cohort study	People with ARF or RHD	3 years	Oral, monthly BPG	≥11 doses per year	110	No	- 2 ARF recurrences (1 person) - No recurrences in people on penicillin prophylaxis - Recurrences were in a boy who was not adherent to sulfadiazine (prescribed due to sensitivity to penicillin) - 4 deaths, none of these people were on "regular prophylaxis"
India (New Delhi)[12]	Prospective cohort study	Children with first episode ARF	5 years	Monthly BPG	"Regular prophylaxis without omission"	85	Yes	- 22 ARF recurrences - 2 recurrences in compliant patients - Recurrence rate: 0.006/ patient year
Kuwait[13,34]	Prospective cohort	Children with a first episode of ARF who were "regular" with SP	Mean: 12.3 years	Monthly BPG	Not stated	64	Yes	- 2 ARF recurrences - Recurrence rate: 0.003/ person year - Carditis resolved at 12-year follow-up in 51% of patients who had carditis at initial ARF episode - No patient developed aortic stenosis

Continued

TABLE 11.1
English Language Studies Which Have Reported on the Clinical Outcomes Associated With Secondary Prophylaxis.—cont'd

Country (Region)	Study Design	Participants	Follow up	SP Type and Frequency	Definition of Adherence	Sample Size for Adherence Data	"Break-through" ARF Recurrences Reported?	Findings
New Zealand (Auckland)[35]	Retrospective record review	People with ARF	1428 person-yrs for people with an ARF recurrence	4-weekly BPG	Nonadherence: missing >3 months of BPG	360	Yes	- 20 ARF recurrences (19 people) - 10 ARF recurrences due to nonadherence - 1 ARF recurrence in a "fully adherent" person - 9 ARF recurrences occurred when people were not prescribed SP
New Zealand (Auckland)[36]	Retrospective record review	Children with ARF	1062 person-years	Oral or 4-weekly BPG	Not stated	288	Yes	- 49 ARF recurrences (41 people) - 43 ARF recurrences in people on oral SP - 3 ARF recurrences in people adherent to 4-weekly BPG - 1 ARF recurrence after improper storage of BPG; 1 ARF recurrence in a nonadherent person; 1 ARF recurrence after underdosing of a child
Pakistan Rahimyar Khan Tehsil[17]	12-year follow-up of survey participants	People diagnosed with RHD during community survey	12 years	Not stated	Not stated	21	Yes	- 5 people had ARF recurrences - Recurrence rate for people on "continuous" SP: 0.01/patient year - 6 people were prescribed SP, all had regression of mild lesions - 15 people were not prescribed SP, 6 had new lesions, 6 had more severe lesions
Saudi Arabia (Al Baha)[37]	Retrospective record review	People with a first episode of ARF or moderate or severe mitral stenosis	Range: 1 to >11 yrs	Not stated	Not stated	190 with ARF	Unclear	- 44 of the 190 people with ARF developed an ARF "exacerbation" - 46% of "exacerbations" occurred in people who were "not on antibiotic prophylaxis"

Saudi Arabia (Riyadh)[38]	Prospective cohort	Children with ARF	5 yrs	Not stated	Not stated	67	No	- 22 recurrences - 14 recurrences in people who were not adherent to SP - 8 recurrences in people not prescribed SP
Taiwan (Taipei)[39]	Randomized controlled trial	Children with ARF or RHD	1569 person-years	3- and 4-weekly BPG	"Stay in compliance": missed ≤1 dose per year. "Stay in noncompliant": missed 2–3 doses per year. "Drop out": missed ≥4 doses	249	Yes	- 9 recurrences in 3-weekly group (2 children were "compliant") - 16 recurrences in 4-weekly group (10 children were "compliant") - Breakthroughs more common in 4-weekly group (risk ratio: 5.15, 95% CI: 1.13 to 23.49)
Taiwan (Taipei)[40]	Prospective cohort	Children with ARF or RHD	Mean: 4.4 years Total: 462 person-yrs	Monthly BPG	See above	105	Yes	- 21 recurrences (19 people) - 3 recurrences in "compliant" patients - Recurrence rate in adherent patients was lowest when compared with other groups (χ^2: 19.109, $P < .001$)
Turkey (Ankara)[41]	Case study	13 years old girl	n/a	3-weekly BPG	Not stated	1	Yes	- 4 recurrences - "Continuous regular BPG" maintained from first episode - Authors recommend 2-weekly BPG for people with at least one ARF recurrence
Turkey (Ankara)[42]	Retrospective record review	Children with ARF and carditis	Mean: 44 months	3-weekly BPG (lifelong)	Not stated	74	Yes	- 9 recurrences - 5 recurrences in people who received SP "regularly"
Turkey (Ankara)[43]	Retrospective record review	People with chorea during first ARF episode	Range: 1–10 years	3-weekly BPG	No missing or late doses	63	Yes	- 17 recurrences (13 people) - 20% of adherent people had a recurrence (56 people were adherent) - 29% of nonadherent people had a recurrence - No significant difference in likelihood of recurrence between the adherent and nonadherent groups ($P = .44$)

Continued

TABLE 11.1

English Language Studies Which Have Reported on the Clinical Outcomes Associated With Secondary Prophylaxis.—cont'd

Country (Region)	Study Design	Participants	Follow up	SP Type and Frequency	Definition of Adherence	Sample Size for Adherence Data	"Break-through" ARF Recurrences Reported?	Findings
Turkey (Ankara)[44]	Retrospective chart review	People with chorea	Range: 6 months to 9 yrs	3-weekly BPG	Not stated	85	Yes	- 14 people had ARF recurrences - 12% of adherent patients had a recurrence - 63% of nonadherent patients had a recurrence. - Adherent patients were less likely to have a recurrence ($P < 0.001$)
Turkey (Konya)[45]	Prospective cohort	People with ARF	3.0 ± 1.5 years	3-weekly BPG	Not stated	236	No	- 2 people had ARF recurrences, both were nonadherent
Uganda (Kampala)[5]	Prospective cohort	People with RHD	12 months	4-weekly BPG	$\geq$80% doses	331	Not reported	- 21 people had ARF recurrences - Nonadherent people were more likely to have a recurrence (OR: 33.9 [95%CI 7.58–151.3]; $P = 0.001$)
USA (New York City, New York)[46]	Retrospective record review	People with ARF	Not stated	4-weekly BPG	Not stated	115 ARF episodes	Yes	- 11 ARF recurrences (10 people) - 9 people who had a recurrence were "totally noncompliant" for several months before recurrence - 1 person had been adherent
USA (Nashville, Tennessee)[47]	Prospective cohort	People with ARF	Median: 55 months	Oral or injection (frequency not stated)	Not stated	269	Yes (oral SP only)	- 16 ARF recurrences - No recurrences in people adherent to SP injections - 6 recurrences in people adherent to oral SP - 10 recurrences in people who took SP irregularly

| USA (Cleveland, Ohio)[11] | Retrospective record review | Children with a first episode of ARF who maintained "regular" SP | ≥5 yrs | 4-weekly BPG | Not stated | 115 | Yes | - 1 recurrence, the patient was adherent
- 70% with acute mitral regurgitation during their initial episode lost this murmur
- No increase in mitral regurgitation severity
- No development of aortic stenosis
- No development of bacterial endocarditis
- No deaths |

AOR, Adjusted odds ratio, CI, confidence interval, OR, odds ratio, SP, secondary prophylaxis, ARF, acute rheumatic fever, RHD, rheumatic heart disease, BPG, benzathine penicillin G.
Reproduced with permission: de Dassel, J.L. (2019) Adherence to prophylactic penicillin and clinical outcomes for people with acute rheumatic fever and/or rheumatic heart disease in the Northern Territory of Australia (Doctoral dissertation).

is still in an age group vulnerable to recurrent GAS infection and ARF (Table 11.3), implementation of secondary prophylaxis is still of high value to reduce the chance of further RHD progression.

A second limitation is that high adherence to secondary antibiotic prophylaxis long term is very challenging. Programmatic approaches to support adherence, including register-based recall systems and use of pain minimization techniques, are detailed later.

The potential for "breakthrough" ARF recurrences is another potential limitation—that is, ARF that occurs despite high adherence to the 4-weekly BPG regimen. This is very uncommon but has been noted,[19,20] in which case a switch to a 3-weekly regimen is recommended. Details on the pharmacokinetics and pharmacodynamics of penicillin underpinning this decision-making are discussed later. A final challenge is that people with penicillin allergy are usually recommended a macrolide antibiotic regimen. In many settings, macrolides are prescribed in the absence of proven penicillin allergy, bringing with it difficulties in ensuring oral adherence, which is potentially even more challenging and difficult to measure. Furthermore, the proportion of GAS isolates resistant to macrolides is as high as 30% in some settings.[21,22]

PENICILLIN FOR SECONDARY PROPHYLAXIS

Penicillins and Pharmacokinetics

Fortunately, GAS remain fully susceptible to penicillin. This is likely to be because the organism lacks capacity to express β-lactamase or low-affinity penicillin-binding proteins; an alternative hypothesis is that expression of either is toxic to the organism.[48] Resistance does, however, readily develop to non β-lactam antibiotics, as mentioned earlier in relation to macrolides such as erythromycin.

BPG is the first-line antibiotic for secondary prophylaxis. BPG is a fusion of two penicillin G molecules, characterized by very low solubility and low hydrolysis in vivo.[49] These features allow for slow absorption from a depot intramuscular injection, producing low but adequate serum concentrations for streptococcal prophylaxis, for a number of weeks. There are two main formulations of BPG: a low-cost lyophilized powder (produced by many brands) and a high-cost cold-chain-dependent premixed suspension (produced by Pfizer alone).[50] It is important to note that Pfizer has recently changed the naming and expression of product strength regarding BPG (Box 11.3). Powdered BPG may suffer from variable quality and efficacy compared to the suspension form. Moreover, significant

pharmacokinetic differences were found between two brands of powdered BPG, with no clear explanation found.[51] Where available, the premixed suspension is preferred over powdered BPG.

Anecdotes are commonly heard about doctors mistakenly prescribing other forms of penicillin, such as procaine penicillin G. This form is also administered intramuscularly, but achieves high blood concentrations for only 24 h and is therefore ineffective as a form of secondary prophylaxis against ARF.

In cases where BPG is refused, oral penicillin V (phenoxymethylpenicillin) may be prescribed, although this is associated with a higher risk of ARF recurrence.[9] Although the lower effectiveness of oral administration may be partly attributable to greater difficulty in adhering to such a regimen compared with a 4-weekly supervised injection regimen, the half-life of oral penicillin V is only around 1 h, so even full adherence to a twice-daily oral penicillin V regimen has been considered to be inferior to intramuscular BPG in preventing recurrent ARF.[52]

Although the standard secondary prophylaxis BPG regimen comprises administration every 4 weeks (28 days), serum penicillin levels may be low or undetectable much earlier than 28 days, often within 14 days, following a standard BPG dose of 1.2 million units (900 mg).[53] Indeed, fewer streptococcal infections and ARF recurrences have been reported among individuals receiving 3-weekly BPG compared with a 4-weekly regimen.[9,54,55] Moreover, the 3-weekly regimen resulted in greater resolution of mitral regurgitation in a long-term randomized study in Taiwan (66% vs. 46%).[39]

As noted earlier, prospective data from New Zealand, and other analyses from Australia, show that recurrences are extremely rare among people who are fully adherent to a 4-weekly BPG regimen.[19,20] 3-weekly as opposed to four-weekly penicillin has important workforce implications. It is likely that with a four-weekly regimen, any streptococcal infection acquired after serum penicillin concentrations have dropped below the protective level would be treated early by the next administered BPG dose. Historical work suggested that treating GAS infection within 9 days was likely to reduce most ARF episodes,[56] but these data derive from a small cohort, and are somewhat immunologically implausible, especially in highly immunologically primed hosts in whom the abnormal immune response causing ARF would likely be triggered early after onset of symptomatic disease. Nevertheless, despite the pharmacokinetic data and uncertainty about the "grace period" in which to treat GAS to avoid ARF, 4-weekly

- The name and strength description for the premixed suspension of benzathine penicillin G (BPG), otherwise known as benzathine benzylpenicillin or Bicillin® LA, has recently been changed by Pfizer, following changes in international practice
- The expression of the name of the product will now be benzathine benzylpenicillin tetrahydrate (see images later)
- The expression of product strength will now be 1,200,000 units/2.3 mL

	New Labeling	Old Labeling
Product name	Benzathine benzylpenicillin tetrahydrate Alternative name: benzathine penicillin tetrahydrate	Benzathine benzylpenicillin
Strength expression	1,200,000 units/2.3 mL	900 mg/2.3 mL

Reproduced with permission from the Health Quality and Safety Commission New Zealand

- There are no other changes: the active ingredient, the strength of the active ingredient, the product information, the dosing, and administration all remain the same
- **Do not confuse** long-acting intramuscular benzathine benzylpenicillin tetrahydrate with:
  - Rapidly acting benzylpenicillin (otherwise known as penicillin G), which is administered via the intravenous route
  - Short-acting intramuscular procaine penicillin G

New syringe artwork introduced in January 2019:

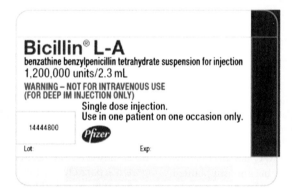

New carton artwork introduced in January 2019:

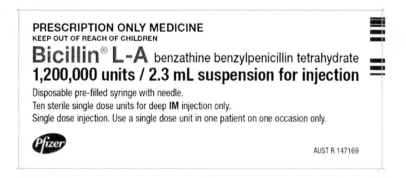

Reproduced (and modified) with permission from Pfizer and the Health Quality and Safety Commission, New Zealand.[131]

regimens work very effectively, even in environments where GAS transmission is very high.

A pharmacokinetic study in Aboriginal children and adolescents in Australia has recently been undertaken to better understand serum concentrations after intramuscular dosing in children of a variety of ages and weights.[57] Serum concentration of penicillin was tested using liquid chromatography—mass spectroscopy assay on dried blood spots.[58] Counterintuitively, the study found that blood concentrations of penicillin remained above the minimum inhibitory concentration (protective level) for only 9.8 days on average in normal weight children (body mass index <25 kg/m^2) after administration of a BPG dose intended to provide protection for 4 weeks. The authors concluded that more knowledge is therefore needed to reconcile this finding with the observed protectiveness conferred by 4-weeks dosing regimens of BPG.

Penicillin reformulation, for instance as an implant or long-acting depot that could provide slow release of penicillin over months, has been under investigation in recent years. Despite technical challenges, there is optimism that reformulated penicillin may be a reality in the coming years,[59,60] which would dramatically improve the ability to deliver effective secondary prophylaxis for ARF.

Penicillin Supply

BPG is an off-patent, generally inexpensive antibiotic. Stock-outs occur repeatedly in both low- and high-income settings, posing major challenges to ARF prevention. As recently noted,[49] attention to the supply, manufacture, and accessibility of BPG has declined as its use in high-income settings has become supplanted by newer, broader-spectrum antibiotics. Attention must be given to BPG availability and quality in low-resource settings. Although BPG is included in the World Health Organization's Essential Medicines List, practitioners in many countries lack access. In 2011, a survey of healthcare providers who manage patients with ARF or RHD was undertaken by the World Heart Federation in African countries, the Asia—Pacific region, and Central and South America.[61] Responses indicated that many settings had minimal or no access to BPG. Supply of the preferred formulation of BPG (premixed liquid formulation) has been precarious in many settings, with stock-outs documented in Australia in 2001, 2004, and 2006.[52] The problem is far more pronounced in low-income settings.[49]

Penicillin Adverse Reactions

BPG should **not** be given to patients with a documented allergy to penicillins or cephalosporins. **Extreme** **caution** should be exercised in giving BPG to patients with decompensated heart failure, as this can lead to collapse and death, mimicking an "anaphylactic reaction" (discussed later and also chapter 10).

Global experience with long-acting penicillin administration is extensive. As well as being administered for ARF and RHD prophylaxis, BPG is used for treatment of streptococcal infections, syphilis, and yaws. Anaphylaxis to BPG is rare. This section provides reported rates of adverse reactions, and concerns about increased risk for adverse reactions in low-resource settings; the following section details the diagnosis and clinical management of anaphylaxis.

Hypersensitivity reactions to BPG have been reported after multiple monthly injections, and anaphylaxis has been reported to occur in patients who have previously tolerated the injection for months and years without incident.[62] In a prospective international study after 32,430 injections (given specifically for secondary prevention of ARF and RHD) during 2736 patient years of observation, 57 (3.2%) of the 1790 patients had an allergic reaction and four (0.2% or 1.2 per 10 000 injections) developed anaphylaxis.[63] A meta-analysis of 13 studies that reported on adverse reactions after BPG administration (for any indication; the study referred to above was included) found that the risk of death across studies was 0 (there were 4 deaths in a sample of 2,108,117 patients) and the absolute risk of serious adverse events including anaphylaxis was 0.17%.[64] The authors indicated that the risk of adverse reactions was higher for people who received multiple BPG injections; however, the results for this group were not reported separately.

A recent review documented that alongside rising concerns about the quality of available BPG internationally, anecdotal reports of adverse reactions appear to have increased in recent years. The review[49] cites three deaths occurring in Zimbabwe in 2000 associated with BPG from three different manufacturers.[65] In the World Heart Federation's BPG survey,[61] 26% of 39 clinicians surveyed internationally reported being involved in at least 1 anaphylactic reaction, and 21% of providers reported that they had had a patient die due to anaphylaxis after BPG injection.

This clinical experience has not been replicated in other high-use settings, including Australia and New Zealand. Indeed, the more commonly recognized problem in these settings is erroneous labeling of individuals as being penicillin allergic when in fact they are not—when investigated, only around 10% of individuals with a penicillin allergy label in fact are allergic.[66] Reports of anaphylaxis occurring after BPG in Australian and New Zealand ARF/RHD registers are vanishingly rare.

It is impossible to determine whether the adverse drug reactions reported in Zimbabwe and in the World Heart Federation survey can be attributed to penicillin, reactions to other components that might be present in the vial (such as contaminants), or incorrect classification of reactions. Indeed, patients with underlying cardiac conditions may experience fatal or near-fatal reactions (with no clinical features of anaphylaxis) seconds to minutes after BPG administration.[64,67,68] Fatal cases have included young patients (10–12 years old) with severe mitral regurgitation who were receiving BPG for secondary prophylaxis of ARF.[67] The mechanism for death in these circumstances remains obscure. A suggested hypothesis is that some reactions could represent vasovagal reactions ($\pm$ bradycardia) to intramuscular injection in general, not related to penicillin specifically, which may precipitate cardiovascular collapse in patients with significant valvular heart disease.[68] For example, mitral stenosis is a preload-dependent state and any reduction in blood pressure from vasovagal syncope may precipitate a cardiac arrest[68]; or in patients with pulmonary hypertension (secondary to left-sided valve disease), a vasovagal reaction may result in life-threatening arrhythmias or acute right heart failure. The vasovagal hypothesis is supported by the observation that almost all severe adverse reactions appear to be in cases with significant valvular heart lesions, whereas anaphylaxis should be equally common in people with mild or no RHD. It is important that systems are in place for the reporting of adverse drug reactions to better understand safety of BPG and potentially, as a proxy guide to BPG quality.[49]

At the time of writing, a consensus guideline for delivery of secondary prophylaxis in cases of moderate or severe RHD was being prepared, highlighting the extreme care needed in these cases, and that in some circumstances oral penicillin prophylaxis may be preferred to BPG.

Care should also be taken to ensure that BPG is **not** inadvertently given by the intravascular route (FDA black-box warning). Intravenous administration has been associated with hyperkalemia, arrhythmias, and cardiac arrest,[69] whereas intraarterial administration has also been associated with cardiac arrest (attributed to emboli after injection) and life-threatening pulmonary edema.[70]

Other forms of adverse reaction to penicillin have also been noted. In qualitative work in Australia's Northern Territory, most individuals receiving regular BPG did not experience side effects, but a small number described taking to bed for several days afterward and feeling generally unwell.[71]

CLINICAL EVALUATION AND MANAGEMENT OF ANAPHYLAXIS

Definition and Diagnosis

Anaphylaxis is a severe, systemic allergic reaction that can cause death. It is most often triggered by IgE allergic antibodies directed against a specific allergen, but can also be due to direct mast cell activation.[72] The diagnosis of anaphylaxis is based primarily on a constellation of signs and symptoms. Diagnostic criteria were published by a multidisciplinary group of experts in 2005/2006, which reflect the variable presentations of anaphylaxis (Table 11.2).[72]

In some patients, the diagnosis may be difficult to recognize clinically, although it is usually clear in the case of recent exposure to BPG. Because BPG is administered intramuscularly, presentation is usually within seconds to minutes following exposure (whereas ingested allergens more often precipitate symptoms within minutes to 1–2 hours later). Skin and mucosal signs and symptoms, as defined in Table 11.2, are the most frequent manifestations of anaphylaxis (occurring in up to 90% of episodes), followed by respiratory (up to 70%), gastrointestinal (up to 45%), and cardiovascular (up to 45%) manifestations. It is worth emphasizing that neither hypotension nor shock is required for the diagnosis of anaphylaxis.

The clinical course of anaphylaxis is highly variable, from mild symptoms that resolve spontaneously to severe respiratory and/or cardiovascular deterioration and death. Fatal anaphylaxis can develop very quickly. In a series of 164 cases of death from anaphylaxis, 55 were iatrogenic due to medications (including 16 due to antibiotic administration), with the median time interval from symptom onset to respiratory/cardiac arrest being 5 min.[73]

Management of anaphylaxis

A suggested approach to the initial evaluation and management of suspected anaphylaxis is summarized in Fig. 11.1.[74] However, where available, local clinical policies for guidance on the management of anaphylaxis should be referred to as there may be considerable variability between sites. The ABC principles used in the assessment of the unwell patient are discussed in detail in Chapter 16.

Early recognition and treatment of anaphylaxis is critical. Prompt administration of intramuscular epinephrine (adrenaline) is the single most important treatment for anaphylaxis, and delayed administration is associated with increased mortality.[75–77] Epinephrine should also be given if clinical suspicion of anaphylaxis is high, even if the patient does not meet

---

TABLE 11.2
Clinical Criteria for Diagnosing Anaphylaxis.

Anaphylaxis is highly likely when any **one** of the following three criteria are fulfilled:

1. Acute onset of an illness (minutes to several hours) with involvement of the skin, mucosal tissue, or both (e.g., generalized hives, pruritus or flushing, swollen lips—tongue—uvula)
   AND AT LEAST ONE OF THE FOLLOWING:
   a. Respiratory compromise (e.g., dyspnea, wheeze-bronchospasm, stridor, reduced PEF, hypoxemia)
   b. Reduced BP or associated symptoms of end-organ dysfunction (e.g., hypotonia [collapse], syncope, incontinence)

2. Two or more of the following that occur rapidly after exposure *to a **likely** allergen for that patient* (minutes to several hours):
   a. Involvement of the skin-mucosal tissue (e.g., generalized hives, itch-flush, swollen lips—tongue—uvula)
   b. Respiratory compromise (e.g., dyspnea, wheeze-bronchospasm, stridor, reduced PEF, hypoxemia)
   c. Reduced BP or associated symptoms (e.g., hypotonia [collapse], syncope, incontinence)
   d. Persistent gastrointestinal symptoms (e.g., crampy abdominal pain, vomiting)

3. Reduced BP after exposure to ***known*** *allergen for that patient* (minutes to several hours):
   a. Infants and children: low-systolic BP (age specific) or greater than 30% decrease in systolic BP[a]
   b. Adults: systolic BP of less than 90 mmHg or greater than 30% decrease from that person's baseline

PEF, peak expiratory flow, *BP*, Blood pressure.
[a] Low-systolic blood pressure for children is defined as less than 70 mmHg from 1 month to 1 year, less than (70 mmHg + [2 × age]) from 1 to 10 years, and less than 90 mmHg from 11 to 17 years. Reproduced with permission from Sampson et al.[72]

---

diagnostic criteria. There are no absolute contraindications to epinephrine when used to treat anaphylaxis.[75,76] Most patients respond to the first dose. The ideal site for intramuscular injection of epinephrine is the anterolateral thigh, where skin to muscle depth is least. A second dose of epinephrine is required in 12%—36% of cases and further doses are occasionally needed.[78—80] If a second dose is required, it should be given at a different site (e.g., contralateral thigh). In cases where the response to a single dose of epinephrine is inadequate, intravenous inotropes may be needed and may be lifesaving.

High-flow oxygen (15 L via reservoir mask) should be given initially to all patients, with a target S_pO_2 of 94%—98%.[81] In the event of respiratory distress, early discussion with an anesthetist is essential as the patient may require endotracheal intubation due to upper airway obstruction (from edema of the larynx or epiglottis). Adjunctive medications, such as antihistamines, glucocorticoids, and bronchodilators should also be considered as part of the overall management of anaphylaxis but are not lifesaving.[73] Glucagon, which has inotropic and chronotropic effects not mediated through β-receptors, may be required for patients taking β-blockers who are resistant to epinephrine.[82] Administration and dosing information of epinephrine and glucagon are summarized in Table 11.3.[83,84]

Up to 23% of anaphylactic reactions can be biphasic, with return of symptoms which can be of greater severity than the initial symptoms. All patients with anaphylaxis need a period of close observation.[85] Patients in whom the symptoms resolved rapidly and completely following treatment should be observed for a minimum of 4—6 hours,[86] whereas those with more severe symptoms, or those needing multiple doses of epinephrine, should ideally be observed for at least 12—24 hours.

Assessment of possible penicillin allergy
It is recommended that monitoring and screening for adverse reactions be completed at each BPG injection, and adverse reactions should be notified through the standard channels for adverse reaction reporting. Up to 10% of the population may report drug allergy, in particular to penicillin-based antibiotics, with true drug allergy much less common. A careful drug allergy history may indicate a low likelihood of drug allergy[87] and depending on the clinical history, allergy testing may not be required, in which case patients may be considered for supervised test dosing of a penicillin-based antibiotic. Other patients will need referral to allergy services for consideration of penicillin testing (with interim erythromycin until evaluation is complete), which involves graded skin prick and then intradermal allergy tests, to help determine allergic status. If there has been an allergic reaction to an injection of BPG then referral for specialist allergy evaluation should be made to define the cause of the allergic reaction (penicillin, medication excipient, or rarely lidocaine). Appropriate alerts need to be in place

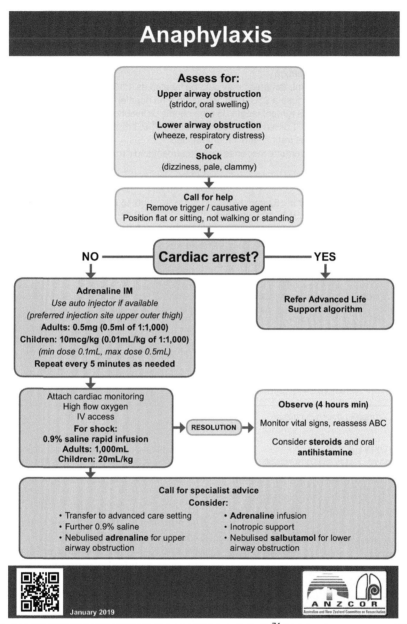

FIG. 11.1 Assessment and management of suspected anaphylaxis.[74] *IV*, intravenous access; *ABC*, airway, breathing, circulation. (Reproduced with permission from the Australian and New Zealand Committee on Resuscitation.[74])

to prevent further inadvertent use of the implicated medication. Temporary desensitization for drug allergy is possible, but there is no data to show that regular use of BPG can safely maintain desensitization.

Overall, the long-term benefits of prophylaxis far outweigh the potential risk of a serious allergic reaction.[63] The first BPG injection should be given in a supervised medical setting with ready access to epinephrine and resuscitation equipment. Subsequent injections may then be given in the home or school environment, depending on local program structures and family choices.

TABLE 11.3
Therapeutic Management of Anaphylaxis in Adults and Children.[83,84]

EPINEPHRINE (ADRENALINE)

- Administration by intramuscular (IM) injection
- Dilution for IM injection contains 1 mg/mL (ampules may also be labeled as 1:1000)
- IM injection site: midanterolateral thigh (use a 23G (blue, length 25 mm) needle)
- If morbidly obese, consider using a 21G (green, length 38 mm) needle or injection into the calf
- Epinephrine autoinjectors may be used (EpiPen Jr® 0.15 mg or EpiPen® 0.3 mg)
- Subcutaneous or deltoid muscle administration NOT recommended
- Consider intravenous epinephrine if inadequate response to IM treatment and if appropriate monitoring and resources are available

Route	Weight or Age Group (if weight unknown)[a]	Dose
Intramuscular	10–25 kg (or if <5 years old) 26–50 kg (or if 5–12 years old) >50 kg (or if >12 years old) and all adults	0.15 mg (0.15 mL of 1:1000) 0.3 mg (0.3 mL of 1:1000) 0.5 mg (0.5 mL of 1:1000)
Intravenous infusion	Children and adults	Start at 0.1 µg/kg/minute and titrate according to response

GLUCAGON

- Given intravenously; in children, bolus dose is weight-based but infusion dose is not
- Has a very short half-life (around 5 min); may cause severe nausea at high doses

Age Group	Dose
Adults	Bolus: 1–5 mg IV over 5 min Infusion: 5–15 µg/min
Children	Bolus: 20–30 µg/kg (maximum 1 mg) over 5 min Infusion: 5–15 µg/min

[a] May also refer to Fig. 11.1 for mcg/kg dosing in children.

SECONDARY PROPHYLAXIS RECOMMENDATIONS AND REGIMENS

Efficient register-based delivery of secondary prophylaxis (along with early diagnosis of ARF) is an essential component of ARF and RHD control programs. BPG is the first-line antibiotic for secondary prophylaxis. A macrolide antibiotic, usually oral erythromycin, is the first-line recommendation in cases of proven penicillin allergy. Organizational approaches to secondary prevention should seek to ensure consistent medication supply at the national, regional, and local levels. When BPG is unavailable, oral penicillin can be given, noting the caveats regarding lesser effectiveness as described earlier.

Antibiotic Dosing and Frequency

The recommended doses for secondary prophylaxis vary. A summary of different international guidelines is provided in Table 11.4. Without exception, these guidelines recommend intramuscular BPG as the first choice for secondary prophylaxis. The merits of 3-weekly versus 4-weekly BPG[88] are discussed in the section earlier. The choice of frequency may be influenced by the resources available to deliver secondary prophylaxis and the acceptability of a more frequent regimen to the patient and their families.

Duration of Secondary Prophylaxis

The appropriate duration of secondary prophylaxis depends on age, severity of RHD, the estimated likelihood of future GAS exposure, and time elapsed since the last ARF episode. It is also critical to determine patient preferences, and to ensure that decisions to continue or cease prophylaxis are made in agreement between the treating physician and the patient. Age is relevant since ARF recurrences become less common with increasing age, as a result either of greater immunity to GAS over time,[96] or of increasing immunological maturity such that the abnormal immune response after GAS infection becomes less likely, or a combination of both factors. Overall, ARF is uncommon after the age of 25,[19,89] but continues to be seen in older people occasionally in highly endemic settings. In an audit from northern Australia of 343 older individuals who were receiving secondary prophylaxis for ARF, 32 clients were documented to have an ARF episode after the age of 40.[97]

TABLE 11.4
Recommended Doses of Benzathine Penicillin G for Acute Rheumatic Fever Prophylaxis According to Different Guidelines.

Guidelines	IM BPG Doses	Interval of BPG Doses	Oral Alternatives
WHO (2004)[89]	<30kg: 0.6 million units[a] ≥30 kg: 1.2 million units[b]	4-weekly for low risk 3-weekly for high risk	Penicillin V 250 mg twice daily
Australia (2012)[90]	<20 kg: 0.6 million units ≥20 kg: 1.2 million units	4-weekly[c]	Penicillin V 250 mg twice daily
India (2008)[91]	<27 kg: 0.6 million units ≥27 kg: 1.2 million units		Penicillin V Children: 250 mg twice daily Adults: 500 mg twice daily
South Africa (2003)[92]	<30 kg: 0.6–0.9 million units[d] ≥30 kg: 1.2 million units		Penicillin V <30 kg: 125 mg twice daily ≥30 kg: 250 mg twice daily
New Zealand (2014)[93]	<30 kg: 0.6 million units ≥30 kg: 1.2 million units	4-weekly[c]	Penicillin V <20 kg: 250 mg 2–3 times daily ≥20 kg: 500 mg 2–3 times daily
America (AHA 2009)[94]	≤27 kg: 0.6 million units >27 kg: 1.2 million units	4-weekly[c]	Penicillin V 250 mg twice daily Sulfadiazine[e] ≤27 kg: 500 mg daily >27 kg: 1000 mg daily

[a] 0.6 million units is equivalent to 450 mg BPG.
[b] 1.2 million units is equivalent to 900 mg BPG.
[c] 3-weekly injections if ARF recurrence occurs despite full adherence to 4-weekly injections.
[d] 0.9 million units is equivalent to 675 mg BPG.
[e] For people allergic to penicillin.
Adapted from Wyber et al.[95]

In addition to age, the number of years elapsed since the last episode of ARF is also an important determinant of the risk of ARF recurrence, with the risk falling with each year, and becoming significantly less common after 5 years.[19,89,98]

Estimating an individual's future risk of exposure to GAS is difficult. In highly endemic settings, the risk is evident, but in settings with low background GAS rates, the organism is readily able to reemerge unpredictably in individuals or in outbreaks.[99] Therefore, the conservative option as advised by most guidelines is to provide secondary prophylaxis for any individual after ARF, rather than withholding it where infection rates are estimated to be low.

In some guidelines, the clinical pattern of ARF may be taken into account in recommendations made, due to the assumption that ARF is "mimetic" in recurrent presentations—that is, if carditis is absent in the first episode, it is less likely to be present subsequently than in those with carditis during the first episode. Indeed, those who suffer carditis during their initial attack are significantly more likely to develop further carditis with subsequent streptococcal throat

infections.[100] However, the conservative approach is to assume that any manifestation of ARF can occur in recurrence (a well-documented phenomenon), and therefore to recommend the same secondary prophylaxis regimen regardless of clinical manifestations, to ensure protection against RHD even in those initially presenting with noncarditis manifestations. A summary of the recommended durations of secondary prophylaxis in different national guidelines is provided in Table 11.5.

Stopping Secondary Prophylaxis

Before stopping prophylaxis, the patient's physician should discuss with both the patient and with a physician knowledgeable in ARF, for example, internal medicine physician with a special interest in ARF/RHD, infectious diseases pediatrician/physician or cardiologist. Recipients who are known to have had carditis should undergo an echocardiogram before planned cessation, to determine whether cessation is appropriate. The anticipated and actual dates of cessation should be documented in the medical

TABLE 11.5
Recommended Durations of Secondary Prophylaxis for Acute Rheumatic Fever According to Major International Guidelines.

Guideline	Recommended Secondary Prophylaxis Duration
Australia (2012)[90]	• In all patients for at least 10 years after previous ARF • Severe RHD: until age 40 or indefinitely per physician discretion • Moderate RHD or RHD without prior documented ARF: until age 35 • Mild RHD or ARF without RHD diagnosis: until age 21 or for 10 years after last ARF (whichever is longer)
New Zealand (2014)[93]	• After definite/probable ARF: continue prophylaxis for at least 10 years, consider 5 years of prophylaxis after ARF in patients with mild or no carditis over 21 years or in patients with ARF classified as "possible" • Severe RHD: generally until age 40, with review at age 30[a] • Moderate RHD: until age 30[a] • Mild RHD or ARF without RHD diagnosis: until age 21 or for 10 years after last ARF (whichever is longer)
America (AHA 2009)[94]	• ARF with carditis and residual heart disease: until age 40 or for 10 years after last ARF (whichever is longer), lifetime prophylaxis may be needed • ARF with carditis but no residual heart disease: until age 21 or for 10 years after last ARF (whichever is longer) • ARF without carditis: until age 21 or for 5 years after last ARF (whichever is longer)
India (2008)[91]	• Lifelong in severe disease or postintervention patients, may opt for secondary prophylaxis until age 40 • ARF with healed, mild or moderate carditis: until age 25 or for 10 years after last ARF (whichever is longer) • ARF without carditis: until age 18 or for 5 years after last ARF (whichever is longer)
WHO Expert Consultation Geneva (2001)[89]	• Lifelong if severe valvular disease or after valve surgery • For 10 years after last ARF or until age 25 in patients with previous diagnosis of carditis • For 5 years after last ARF or until age 18 in patients without proven carditis
South Africa[101]	• Lifelong if severe valvular disease or after valve surgery • For 10 years after last ARF or until age 25 in patients with previous diagnosis of carditis • For 5 years after last ARF or until age 18 in patients without proven carditis
Sudan[102]	• Lifelong if any rheumatic heart disease • For 10 years after last ARF or until age 25 in all patients after ARF

[a] For severe RHD at age 40 or moderate RHD at age 30, cessation of prophylaxis is still at the physician's discretion based on the individual patient risk.

records and on the ARF register where possible. The date of cessation may be reviewed if there is a change in clinical or echocardiographic severity, specialist recommendation, a change in environmental exposure to GAS, or a recurrence of ARF.

Unnecessary continuation of prophylaxis in older individuals with no or mild RHD and no recent ARF has been documented.[97] Adherence to guidelines by clinicians is important to ensure that patients and health systems are not unnecessarily overburdened.

IMPROVING ADHERENCE TO SECONDARY PROPHYLAXIS

The persistence of recurrent ARF internationally highlights the continued failure of secondary prevention.

Adherence is required at two levels: by clinicians to guidelines, and by patients to their treatment regimen. The responsibility for adherence should be seen as belonging to health systems, and therefore, systems approaches are required, which will be discussed in this section.

Reasons for Nonadherence

A study undertaken in New Zealand sought to identify reasons for failures to prevent recurrent ARF. Factors identified included prescriber factors (e.g., a lack of recognition of the efficacy of parenteral BPG compared to oral regimens), patient factors (inadequate adherence), and system factors (unreliable data collection and the lack of long-term continuity of care).[103] In remote Aboriginal communities in Northern Australia, qualitative studies have identified that the cultural responsiveness of health services is a key factor underpinning adherence. Aboriginal patients in one community reported the need to feel nurtured by their local clinic in order for a trusting relationship to develop which supports adherence.[104] In another setting, the pain of injections and staff not listening to patients about how they would like their injection to be delivered served as important disincentives for some—although others reported that they had either grown used to the pain of injections, or did not experience pain.[71] Lack of knowledge about the importance of secondary prophylaxis, due to health literacy information not being provided in a digestible way and in the correct language, appears to play a critical role in some settings.[105]

Methods to Support Adherence

Adherence-support strategies lack evidence of effectiveness in general and are context-specific, but concepts that may be applicable to many settings are summarized in Table 11.6 and Fig. 11.2.

PROGRAMMATIC APPROACHES TO SECONDARY PROPHYLAXIS DELIVERY

Although ARF is an acute condition, it is managed as a chronic disease, with long-term engagement with health services required over many years. Use of the "Chronic Care Model" has therefore been proposed as a way to address health system approaches to the management of this condition.[110,111] The "Chronic Care Model" was proposed in 2001 as a way to bridge the gulf between patient needs and the healthcare system.[112] It describes key domains that should be addressed to deliver quality care for patients with chronic conditions; namely: health systems, delivery system design, decision support, clinical information systems, self-management support, and community linkages.

ARF and RHD cause particular burdens of disease in Indigenous populations in high-income countries, and other marginalized populations who are not well represented within mainstream medical services. Often, there is a mismatch between the world views and cultural beliefs about disease causation and management between patients and healthcare providers. ARF and RHD are exemplars of the need for health services to be highly responsive to cultural needs and to engage vulnerable, young individuals in medical care over many years. Healthcare providers themselves need to be culturally respectful, but moreover, so do health systems, supporting approaches such as outreach, a nurturing attitude,[104] and engagement of community members such as Indigenous Health Practitioners.[113]

In some settings, it may be appropriate and effective to deliver secondary prophylaxis at schools, the workplace or in the home. When BPG injections are administered outside the clinical setting, appropriate medical equipment to manage adverse reactions must be available. Secondary prophylaxis should also be available in primary, secondary, and tertiary healthcare settings. Local protocols should be developed at public health units and in healthcare pathways in general practice (where these are available).

Delivery of secondary prophylaxis should be supported by a rheumatic fever register, and it is also recommended that provision is made to allow nurses to administer BPG once a physician has authorized the initial prescription. In some programmatic settings, especially remote nurse-run services where nurses can deliver but not prescribe penicillin, another requirement is for prescriptions to be long-term, to avoid the problem of a dose being due, but no prescription being available.

INDIVIDUAL APPROACHES TO SECONDARY PROPHYLAXIS DELIVERY

Health education is critical at all levels.[89] Information that should be provided to patients and families is summarized in Box 11.4. However, provision of education is ineffective if the style of communication is inappropriate, or if it is only done once. Effective awareness-raising needs to be culturally appropriate,

TABLE 11.6

Examples of Adherence Support Approaches that May be Useful in Supporting Adherence to Benzathine Penicillin G for Acute Rheumatic Fever and Rheumatic Heart Disease Secondary Prophylaxis.

Categories of Adherence Support	Examples of Strategies
Health center-related approaches	• Use of register-based recall systems to ensure patients are recalled for their next dose and given adequate notice (e.g., up to 1 week) to avoid late delivery of next dose • Engagement with local schools to deliver BPG dosing in the school environment • Where doing is administered in a clinic, fast-tracking patients to reduce waiting time to receive BPG • Ensuring that clinics are respectful and provide culturally appropriate care where relevant (where patients and staff are from different cultural backgrounds) • Ensure that staff have high-level training in the importance of secondary prophylaxis • Use of continuous quality improvement methods to track adherence rates and thereby measure the progress of a clinic over time[106] • Ensure good communication between clinics to track patients who are mobile
Community-level approaches	• Collaboration with community groups to encourage adherence through rewards or incentives systems • Community awareness-raising events, such as education evenings and maternal health events incorporating ARF/RHD education • Peer support groups • Outreach and transport services to allow easier access to clinics, including collaboration with community members to assist patients in getting to the clinic

Patient approaches	• Use of self-management support approaches[107] to help patients understand and participate in their disease management, and have "agency" in being able to articulate their needs (e.g., how and where they would like their injection to be delivered; who administers the injection). Ensure family engagement.
	• Ensuring that ARF and RHD educational materials are used which are suitable for the target audience, for example, in the patient's local language; provided in audio or video format for people who are illiterate
	• Use of BPG dose reminder systems, such as:
	  • Smart phone application
	  • Electronic or paper calendar
	• Incentives

Condition and therapy-specific approaches	• Understand the profound consequences of a chronic disease diagnosis in childhood; use validated methods such as "transition care" to support chronic care management from childhood through to adolescence and adulthood[108]
	• Use of physical methods to reduce injection pain, including:
	  • Lidocaine
	  • Ice, pressure or vibration at injection site
	• Use of distracting techniques such as play therapy for children

ARF, acute rheumatic fever; *RHD*, rheumatic heart disease; *BPG*, benzathine penicillin G.

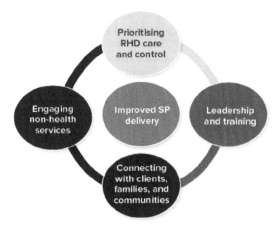

FIG. 11.2 Important elements for improving delivery of secondary prophylaxis (SP). This figure was developed in consultation between Rosemary Wyber, Anna Ralph, Catalina Lizama, and Jonathan Carapetis, based on findings from the RHDSP trial.[109]

BOX 11.4
Information to Cover When Providing Acute Rheumatic Fever and Rheumatic Heart Disease Health Literacy

- The cause and complications of ARF and RHD
- The reason for secondary prophylaxis
- Signs and symptoms of ARF recurrence
- Signs and symptoms of worsening RHD
- Understanding that RHD is asymptomatic until severe
- Importance of conception planning for women of childbearing age with RHD
- Measures that could be implemented in the home or community to reduce risk of exposure to group A streptococcus (e.g., tackling household crowding)
- The prevention of endocarditis and the differences between this and secondary prophylaxis of ARF
- Sore throat management (for the person with ARF as well as their family/household members)
- The importance of medical and dental follow-up
- How to contact the relevant people or agencies should they require further information or assistance.

ARF, acute rheumatic fever; *RHD*, rheumatic heart disease.

respectful, consistent, and repeated. It also needs to be delivered in the patient's first language, and in a culturally appropriate environment. Lack of parental awareness of the causes and consequences of ARF/RHD was a key contributor to poor adherence among children

on long-term prophylaxis in Egypt.[30] In a number of regions in India, comprehensive health education has improved community awareness of sore throat, ARF, and RHD[114] and assisted case identification.[115] Comprehensive health education and promotion was also a key component in the successful control of RHD in the French Caribbean.[116] Improved healthcare provider awareness of the diagnosis and management of ARF and RHD is necessary to improve case findings, encourage compliance with prophylaxis and to improve the quality and delivery of health education delivered to cases and their families. Awareness, education, and advocacy in relation to ARF and RHD are discussed in detail in Chapter 15.

There are various education packages available worldwide and many have been translated into several languages. There are several applications for smartphones that remind patients when their next BPG dose is due, for example, the Treatment Tracker developed for Indigenous Australians. Many resources can be found at the RHD Action Resource Hub (http://rhdaction.org/resource-hub) and on the Wired International website (http://www.wiredhealthresources.net/mod-rheumatic-heart-disease.html).

In summary, methods to support adherence should be tailored to the patient's age, level of family support, and whether the patient is adept with technology (such as owning a smartphone to track injections).

REDUCING THE PAIN OF BENZATHINE PENICILLIN G INJECTIONS

Intramuscular BPG injections can cause local pain and discomfort. The pain of BPG injections is usually not a critical factor in determining adherence to secondary prophylaxis; however, in some settings, it has contributed to poor adherence in those requiring ongoing prophylaxis.[117,118] Regardless of whether patients or their carers have expressed concerns about the pain of the injections, techniques that safely reduce injection pain (Box 11.5) should be promoted. Pain has been significantly reduced when 1% lidocaine (lignocaine) was used to reconstitute BPG for injection, and there is evidence that serum penicillin levels are not affected.[117] The manufacturer of the prefilled liquid formulation recommends against drawing up lidocaine into the prefilled syringe due to the risk of biohazard injury; however, this can be undertaken carefully and safely if staff are adequately trained.

A New Zealand study of ARF patients receiving monthly BPG demonstrated a reduction in the

Measures that may Reduce the Pain of Benzathine Penicillin G Injections

- Use a 23-gauge needle[39]
- Provide oral analgesia, for example, paracetamol or NSAID medication before the injection and during subsequent days if the injection site remains painful. Avoid NSAIDS if symptoms of an ARF recurrence are present, until clarification of the diagnosis.
- Use 2% lidocaine to reconstitute BPG for injection[117] or draw up into a prefilled syringe to allow administration of lidocaine first before the remainder of the syringe contents
- Apply pressure with thumb for 10 s before inserting needle[120]
- Apply a cold pack before inserting needle[36]
- Temperature of syringe contents:
  - Guidelines have traditionally recommended warming the syringe to room temperature before using, but there are no data to support this practice
  - A recent randomized study found that self-reported pain was lower after chilling the needle[a,121]
- Allow alcohol from swab to dry before inserting needle[b]
- Use ethylchloride spray before injection[c]
- Deliver injection very slowly (preferably over at least 2–3 min)[b]
- Use distraction techniques during injection (e.g., with conversation)
- Develop good rapport with the patient, assisted by having a designated nurse for each case, is a significant aid to injection comfort, compliance, and understanding[b]
- Use lidocaine and vibrating device

NSAID, non-steroid anti-inflammatory drug; *BPG*, benzathine penicillin G.
[a]The 21-gauge needle was cooled to 0–2°C in the chiller chamber of a refrigerator, packed in an impermeable plastic packet to maintain sterility and prevent it from getting wet.
[b]As these measures are logical and benign they are recommended, despite the lack of evidence.
[c]Although merely a topical agent, some cases have reported reduced pain and bruising following the appropriate use of ethylchloride spray.

subjective experience of pain when two analgesic interventions were offered: intramuscular delivery of BPG with either 0.25 mL of 2% lidocaine alone or 0.25 mL of 2% lidocaine with a vibrating device with cold pack.[119] Lidocaine and the vibrating cold pack together resulted in a greater reduction in pain than lidocaine alone, but only in children aged 13 years or younger. In this age group, the fear of injection was also reduced.

In many areas, the vibrating device may not be available but the use of lidocaine should still be considered. The addition of 0.25 mL of 2% lidocaine has become standard practice in New Zealand. This is optional for the patient and informed consent is required before administration.

Procedure for Preparation and Delivery of Benzathine Penicillin G Injection With Lidocaine

Before preparing BPG, it is important to ask the patient **and** check the medical chart for any history of penicillin allergy. A careful history is usually sufficient to exclude true allergy, but if there is any doubt the patient should be prescribed oral erythromycin and referred for allergy testing (see anaphylaxis section discussed earlier).

It is also important to ensure that healthcare providers administering BPG are adequately trained in (i) intramuscular injection (particularly when identifying anatomical landmarks, which minimizes the risk of intravascular administration—see later) and (ii) diagnosis and management of anaphylaxis (full resuscitation facilities should ideally be available, including dosed prefilled syringes of epinephrine).

Addition of 2% lidocaine to benzathine penicillin G pre-filled syringe

There are two procedures for mixing lidocaine with BPG due to there being two BPG dose options (which are weight-dependant—see Table 11.4):

Full doseBPG: 1,200,000 units (2.3mL)

1. Draw 0.25 mL of 2% lidocaine into a sterile 1 mL syringe using a sterile filter needle
2. Remove cap of prefilled BPG syringe and draw back to allow space (0.5 mL) at the needle end
3. Add lidocaine from 1 mL syringe to prefilled BPG syringe through syringe tip
4. Push plunger up gently to expel air from the syringe
5. Attach IM luer lock needle to syringe
6. Attach medication added label to syringe with correct details

Half doseBPG: 600,000 units (1.15mL)

1. Use a sterile 3 mL syringe
2. Pull the plunger back to 1.15 mL
3. Decant the BPG from the prefilled syringe into the 3 mL syringe using a sharp sterile drawing-up needle
4. Insert the needle through the 3 mL syringe tip and fill from the plunger end (being careful not to cause an air bubble)

5. Draw 0.25 mL of 2% lidocaine into a 1 mL syringe using a filter needle
6. Add lidocaine to the 3 mL syringe in the same way as you added the BPG
7. Gently push plunger up to expel air from the syringe
8. Add IM luer lock needle to 3 mL syringe
9. Attach medication added label to syringe with correct details

It is important to note that:
- Filter needles are required for glass ampoules only
- The viscosity of the BPG prevents the lidocaine mixing
- Medication labels for added medication must be applied

ADMINISTERING THE INTRAMUSCULAR INJECTION

1. Obtain necessary equipment for the procedure
2. Keep the injection needle cool (see Box 11.5)
3. Locate site on upper outer quadrant of the gluteus maximus (dorsogluteal site) or the ventrogluteal site
   a. Important neurovascular structures are found near the dorsogluteal site; injection into the ventrogluteal site is therefore likely to be safer, as it avoids these structures
4. Use distraction while administering the injection
5. Clean site with alcohol wipe
6. Use pressure and/or ice and/or vibration and other pain minimization techniques described earlier
7. Insert needle and aspirate first (to ensure not in a blood vessel), then inject the BPG slowly
8. Ask for a pain rating on faces scale 0−10
9. Observe for 15 min following injection
10. Give advice (to caregiver or adolescent) on the use of paracetamol at home if the child or young person is experiencing pain later that day or the following day

SECONDARY PROPHYLAXIS IN SPECIAL CIRCUMSTANCES

Secondary Prophylaxis During Pregnancy

Penicillins and erythromycin are considered safe for use in pregnancy (see also Chapter 9).[122]

Low-dose lidocaine is safe in pregnancy. Therefore, correctly administered intramuscular BPG with lidocaine as described earlier is safe in pregnancy. A large number of pregnant women and women of childbearing age have been exposed to lidocaine.[123,124] Lidocaine crosses the placenta, but there is no evidence of an association with fetal malformations, cardiac rhythm disturbances, or other significant side effects in pregnant women or their babies.[122,124]

Secondary Prophylaxis while Breastfeeding

Penicillins are excreted into breast milk in low concentrations and are considered safe for use in breastfeeding.[122,125] Erythromycin is also excreted into breastmilk but has been considered safe while breastfeeding.[122,125] There have been reports of a correlation between the use of erythromycin in breastfeeding mothers and infantile hypertrophic pyloric stenosis in newborns.[125]

Monitor infants for vomiting, diarrhea, and rash while breastfeeding mothers are on amoxicillin and erythromycin courses.[125]

Lidocaine can be administered to breastfeeding women.[123] Lidocaine is excreted into breast milk in small amounts[122–126]; however, the oral bioavailability of lidocaine is very low (35%).[125] Given the small amount of lidocaine used with BPG, the amount excreted into breast milk to which the infant is therefore exposed is minimal. Lidocaine is unlikely to cause adverse effects in breastfeeding infants.[122–126]

Secondary Prophylaxis while on Oral Contraceptive

Oral contraceptives are still recommended for women of childbearing age while on BPG prophylaxis. Progesterone-only oral contraceptives do not interact with BPG therapy.[127–130] An interaction between BPG and the combined oral contraceptive is possible, although this interaction is suggested to only be of significance for short courses of antibiotic therapy (less than 3 weeks). Pregnancy- and contraceptive-related issues in patients with RHD are discussed in detail in Chapter 9.

Secondary Prophylaxis in Anticoagulated Patients

Administration of intramuscular injection is not contraindicated in anticoagulated patients, and is not reported to be associated with local bleeding or bruising. Thus, BPG injections should be continued for those who are anticoagulated, unless there is evidence of uncontrolled bleeding or the international normalized ratio (INR) is greater than 4.5, in which instance oral penicillin should be used instead until the INR has decreased sufficiently. The INR level should be monitored monthly as a minimum for adults, more frequently in children. Patients discharged from hospital on oral penicillin following valve surgery should recommence BPG as soon as is practical.

REFERENCES

1. Ash R. The first ten years of rheumatic infection in childhood. *Am Heart J.* 1948;36(1):89−97.
2. Bland EF, Duckett Jones T. Rheumatic fever and rheumatic heart disease; a twenty year report on 1000 patients followed since childhood. *Circulation.* 1951;4(6):836−843.
3. Taranta A, Kleinberg E, Feinstein AR, et al. Rheumatic fever in children and adolescents: a long-term epidemiologic study of subsequent prophylaxis, streptococcal infections, and clinical sequelae: v. relation of the rheumatic fever recurrence rate per streptococcal infection to pre-existing clinical features of the patients. *Ann Intern Med.* 1964;60(2_Part_2):58−67.
4. de Dassel JL, de Klerk N, Carapetis JR, Ralph APJJAHA. How many doses make a difference? An analysis of secondary prevention of rheumatic fever and rheumatic heart disease. *Circulation.* 2018;7(24):e010223.
5. Okello E, Longenecker CT, Beaton A, Kamya MR, Lwabi P. Rheumatic heart disease in Uganda: predictors of morbidity and mortality one year after presentation. *BMC Cardiovasc Disord.* 2017;17(1):20.
6. Michaud C, Rammohan R,JN. Cost-effectiveness analysis of intervention strategies for reduction of the burden of rheumatic heart disease. In: Narula J, Reddy KS, Tandon R, eds. *Rheumatic Fever.* Washington, D.C: American Registry of Pathology; 1999.
7. Wood HF, Feinstein AR, Taranta A, Epstein JA, Simpson R. Rheumatic fever in children and adolescents: a long-term epidemiologic study of subsequent prophylaxis, streptococcal infections, and clinical sequelae: iii. comparative effectiveness of three prophylaxis regimens in preventing streptococcal infections and rheumatic recurrences. *Ann Intern Med.* 1964;60(2_Part_2):31−46.
8. Stollerman G. *Rheumatic Fever and Streptococcal Infection.* New York: Grune & Stratton; 1975.
9. Manyemba J, Mayosi BM. Penicillin for secondary prevention of rheumatic fever. *Cochrane Database Syst Rev.* 2002;3:CD002227.
10. Wilson MG, Lubschez R. Recurrence rates in rheumatic fever: the evaluation of etiologic concepts and consequent preventive therapy. *JAMA, J Am Med Assoc.* 1944;126(8):477−480.
11. Tompkins DG, Boxerbaum B, Liebman J. Long-term prognosis of rheumatic fever patients receiving regular intramuscular benzathine penicillin. *Circulation.* 1972;45(3):543−551.
12. Sanyal SK, Berry AM, Duggal S, Hooja V, Ghosh S. Sequelae of the initial attack of acute rheumatic fever in children from north India. A prospective 5-year follow-up study. *Circulation.* 1982;65(2):375−379.
13. Majeed HA, Batnager S, Yousof AM, Khuffash F, Yusuf AR. Acute rheumatic fever and the evolution of rheumatic heart disease: a prospective 12 year follow-up report. *J Clin Epidemiol.* 1992;45(8):871−875.

14. Feinstein AR, Stern EK, Spagnuolo M. The prognosis of acute rheumatic fever. *Am Heart J.* 1964;68:817−834.
15. Lue HC, Tseng WP, Lin GJ, et al. Clinical and epidemiological features of rheumatic fever and rheumatic heart disease in Taiwan and the Far East. *Indian Heart J.* 1983;35(3):139−146.
16. Remenyi B, Wilson N, Steer A, et al. World Heart Federation criteria for echocardiographic diagnosis of rheumatic heart disease–an evidence-based guideline. *Nat Rev Cardiol.* 2012;9(5):297−309.
17. Rizvi SF, Kundi A, Naveed A, Faiz A, Samad A. Natural history of rheumatic heart disease, a 12 years observational study "penicillin bites the muscle but heals the heart". *J Ayub Med Coll Abbottabad.* 2014;26(3):301−303.
18. Haran S, Crane N, Kazi S, Axford-Haines L, White A. Effect of secondary penicillin prophylaxis on valvular changes in patients with rheumatic heart disease in Far North Queensland. *Aust J Rural Health.* 2018;26(2):119−125.
19. Spinetto H, Lennon D, Horsburgh M. Rheumatic fever recurrence prevention: a nurse-led programme of 28-day penicillin in an area of high endemnicity. *J Paediatr Child Health.* 2011;47(4):228−234.
20. de Dassel JL, Malik H, Ralph AP, et al. Four-weekly benzathine penicillin G provides inadequate protection against acute rheumatic fever in some children. *Am J Trop Med Hyg.* 2019;100(5):1118−1120.
21. Kim S, Lee NY. Epidemiology and antibiotic resistance of group A streptococci isolated from healthy schoolchildren in Korea. *J Antimicrob Chemother.* 2004;54(2):447−450.
22. Lamagni TL, Efstratiou A, Vuopio-Varkila J, et al. The epidemiology of severe Streptococcus pyogenes associated disease in Europe. *Euro Surveill.* 2005;10(9):179−184.
23. Carapetis JR, Kilburn CJ, MacDonald KT, Walker AR, Currie BJ. Ten-year follow up of a cohort with rheumatic heart disease (RHD). Australian and New Zealand. *J Med.* 1997;27(6):691−697.
24. Remond MG, Severin KL, Hodder Y, et al. Variability in disease burden and management of rheumatic fever and rheumatic heart disease in two regions of tropical Australia. *Intern Med J.* 2013;43(4):386−393.
25. Borges F, Barbosa MLA, Borges RB, et al. [Clinical and demographic characteristics of 99 episodes of rheumatic fever in Acre, the Brazilian Amazon]. *Arq Bras Cardiol.* 2005;84(2):111−114.
26. Terreri MT, Roja SC, Len CA, et al. Sydenham's chorea–clinical and evolutive characteristics. *Sao Paulo Med J.* 2002;120(1):16−19.
27. Pelajo CF, Lopez-Benitez JM, Torres JM, de Oliveira SK. Adherence to secondary prophylaxis and disease recurrence in 536 Brazilian children with rheumatic fever. *Pediatr Rheumatol Online J.* 2010;8:22.
28. Berrios X, Quesney F, Morales A, et al. Are all recurrences of "pure" Sydenham chorea true recurrences of acute rheumatic fever? *J Pediatr.* 1985;107(6):867−872.

29. Chen L, Xie X, Gu J, et al. Changes of manifestations of 122 patients with rheumatic fever in South China during last decade. *Rheumatol Int.* 2009;30(2):239–243.

30. Bassili A, Zaher SR, Zaki A, et al. Profile of secondary prophylaxis among children with rheumatic heart disease in Alexandria, Egypt. *East Mediterr Health J.* 2000;6(2–3): 437–446.

31. Dagmawi F. *Factors Determining Rheumatic Fever Recurrence Among Rheumatic Heart Disease Patients Who Are Taking Monthly Benzanthine G Penicillin Prophylaxis Addis.* Ababa University; 2014.

32. Koshi G, Benjamin V, Cherian G. Rheumatic fever and rheumatic heart disease in rural South Indian children. *Bull World Health Organ.* 1981;59(4):599–603.

33. Grover A, Dhawan A, Iyengar SD, et al. Epidemiology of rheumatic fever and rheumatic heart disease in a rural community in Northern India. *Bull World Health Organ.* 1993;71:59–66.

34. Majeed HA, Yousof AM, Khuffash FA, Yusuf AR, Farwana S, Khan N. The natural history of acute rheumatic fever in Kuwait: a prospective six year follow-up report. *J Chronic Dis.* 1986;39(5):361–369.

35. Spinetto H, Lennon D, Horsburgh M. Rheumatic fever recurrence prevention: a nurse-led programme of 28-day penicillin in an area of high endemnicity. *J Paediatr Child Health.* 2011;47(4):228–234.

36. Newman J, Lennon D, Wong-Toi W. Patients with rheumatic fever recurrences. *N Z Med J.* 1984;97:678–680.

37. Andy JJ, Soomro RM. The changing incidence of juvenile mitral stenosis and natural history of rheumatic mitral valvulitis in Al Baha, Saudi Arabia. *Ann Trop Paediatr.* 2001;21(2):105–109.

38. al-Eissa YA. Acute rheumatic fever during childhood in Saudi Arabia. *Ann Trop Paediatr.* 1991;11(3):225–231.

39. Lue HC, Wu MH, Wang JK, Wu FF, Wu YN. Long-term outcome of patients with rheumatic fever receiving benzathine penicillin G prophylaxis every three weeks versus every four weeks. *J Pediatr.* 1994;125(5 Pt 1): 812–816.

40. Lue HC, Chen CL, Wei H. Some problems in long term prevention of streptococcal infection among children with rheumatic heart disease in Taiwan. *JPN Heart J.* 1976;17(5):550–559.

41. Çetin II , Bikmaz YE, Varan B, Tokel K. A case of rheumatic fever with multiple recurrences of carditis. *Turk J Pediatr.* 2008;50(2):186–188.

42. Pekpak E, Atalay S, Karadeniz C, Demir F, Tutar E, Uçar T. Rheumatic silent carditis: echocardiographic diagnosis and prognosis of long-term follow up. *Pediatr Int:* 2013; 55(6):685–689.

43. Ekici F, Cetin II, Cevik BS, et al. What is the outcome of rheumatic carditis in children with Sydenham's chorea? *Turk J Pediatr.* 2012;54(2):159–167.

44. Gurkas E, Karalok ZS, Taskin BD, et al. Predictors of recurrence in Sydenham's chorea: clinical observation from a single center. *Brain Dev.* 2016.

45. Karaaslan S, Oran B, Reisli I, Erkul I. Acute rheumatic fever in Konya, Turkey. *Pediatr Int.* 2000;42(1):71–75.

46. Griffiths SP, Gersony WM. Acute rheumatic fever in New York City (1969 to 1988): a comparative study of two decades. *J Pediatr.* 1990;116(6):882–887.

47. Quinn RW, Federspiel CF, Lefkowitz LB, Christie AU. Recurrences and sequelae of rheumatic fever in Nashville. A follow-up study. *J Am Med Assoc.* 1977;238(14): 1512–1515.

48. Horn DL, Zabriskie JB, Austrian R, et al. Why have group A streptococci remained susceptible to penicillin? Report on a symposium. *Clin Infect Dis.* 1998;26(6):1341–1345.

49. Wyber R, Taubert K, Marko S, Kaplan EL. Benzathine penicillin G for the management of RHD: concerns about quality and access, and opportunities for intervention and improvement. *Glob Heart.* 2013;8(3):227–234.

50. Wyber R. reportGlobal Status of BPG Report AhrosdfRAGSoBROVp.

51. Kassem AS, Zaher SR, Abou Shleib H, et al. Rheumatic fever prophylaxis using benzathine penicillin G (BPG): two- week versus four-week regimens: comparison of two brands of BPG. *Pediatrics.* 1996;97(6 Pt 2):992–995.

52. Currie B. Benzathine penicillin – down but not out. *NT Dis Control Bulletin.* 2006;13(2):1–3.

53. Broderick MP, Hansen CJ, Russell KL, et al. Serum penicillin G levels are lower than expected in adults within two weeks of administration of 1.2 million units. *PLoS One.* 2011;6(10):e25308.

54. Kaplan EL, Berrios X, Speth J, et al. Pharmacokinetics of benzathine penicillin G: serum levels during the 28 days after intramuscular injection of 1,200,000 units. *J Pediatr.* 1989;115(1):146–150.

55. Lue HC, Wu MH, Hsieh KH, Lin GJ, Hsieh RP, Chiou JF. Rheumatic fever recurrences: controlled study of 3-week versus 4-week benzathine penicillin prevention programs. *J Pediatr.* 1986;108(2):299–304.

56. Catanzaro FJ, Stetson CA, Morris AJ, et al. The role of the streptococcus in the pathogenesis of rheumatic fever. *Am J Med.* 1954;17(6):749–756.

57. Hand RM, Salman S, Newall N, et al. A population pharmacokinetic study of benzathine benzylpenicillin G administration in children and adolescents with rheumatic heart disease: new insights for improved secondary prophylaxis strategies. *J Antimicrob Chemother.* 2019; 74(7):1984–1991.

58. Page-Sharp M, Coward J, Moore BR, et al. Penicillin dried blood spot assay for use in patients receiving intramuscular benzathine penicillin G and other penicillin preparations to prevent rheumatic fever. *Antimicrob Agents Chemother.* 2017;61(8).

59. Montagnat OD, Webster GR, Bulitta JB, et al. Lessons learned in the development of sustained release penicillin drug delivery systems for the prophylactic treatment of rheumatic heart disease (RHD). *Drug Deliv Transl Res.* 2018;8(3):729–739.

60. Sika-Paotonu D, Tiatia R, Sung YK, et al. The benzathine penicillin G (BPG) reformulation preferences study – towards a new pencillin for rheumatic fever and rheumatic heart disease. *J Immunol.* 2017;198(1 supplement), 213.2-.2.

61. Taubert K, Marko SB. Access to essential medicines: illuminating disparities in the global supply of benzathine penicillin G in the context of rheumatic fever/rheumatic heart disease prevention. *J Am Coll Cardiol*. 2013;61(10 Supplement):E2004.

62. Markowitz M, Lue HC. Allergic reactions in rheumatic fever patients on long-term benzathine penicillin G: the role of skin testing for penicillin allergy. *Pediatrics*. 1996;97(6 Pt 2):981−983.

63. International Rheumatic Fever Study Group. Allergic reactions to long-term benzathine penicillin prophylaxis for rheumatic fever. International Rheumatic Fever Study Group. *Lancet*. 1991;337(8753):1308−1310.

64. Galvao TF, Silva MT, Serruya SJ, et al. Safety of benzathine penicillin for preventing congenital syphilis: a systematic review. *PLoS One*. 2013;8(2):e56463.

65. World Health Organization. Benzathine penicillin - three fatal reports following mega-unit injections. *Drug Inf Bull*. 2000;4(2).

66. Knezevic B, Sprigg D, Seet J, et al. The revolving door: antibiotic allergy labelling in a tertiary care centre. *Intern Med J*. 2016;46(11):1276−1283.

67. Berkovitch M, Ashkenazi-Hoffnung L, Youngster I, et al. Fatal and near-fatal non-allergic reactions in patients with underlying cardiac disease receiving benzathine penicillin G in Israel and Switzerland. *Front Pharmacol*. 2017;8:843.

68. Marantelli S, Hand R, Carapetis J, Beaton A, Wyber R. Severe adverse events following benzathine penicillin G injection for rheumatic heart disease prophylaxis: cardiac compromise more likely than anaphylaxis. *Heart Asia*. 2019;11(2):e011191.

69. Levetan BN, Conradie EA, Linton DM. Inadvertent intravenous administration of a long-acting depot penicillin preparation. *S Afr Med J*. 1988;74(8):427−428.

70. Lelubre CLP, Lheure P. Acute paraplegia and pulmonary edema after benzathine penicillin injection. *Am J Emerg Med*. 2008;26:250.e1−250.e5.

71. Mitchell AG, Belton S, Johnston V, et al. Aboriginal children and penicillin injections for rheumatic fever: how much of a problem is injection pain? *Aust N Z J Public Health*. 2018;42(1):46−51.

72. Sampson HA, Munoz-Furlong A, Campbell RL, et al. Second symposium on the definition and management of anaphylaxis: summary report–second national institute of allergy and infectious disease/food allergy and anaphylaxis network symposium. *Ann Emerg Med*. 2006;47(4):373−380.

73. Pumphrey RS. Lessons for management of anaphylaxis from a study of fatal reactions. *Clin Exp Allergy*. 2000;30(8):1144−1150.

74. Anaphylaxis. Australian and New Zealand Committee on Resuscitation. Available from: https://www.nzrc.org.nz/assets/Uploads/ANZCOR-Anaphylaxis-2019.pdf.

75. Simons KJ, Simons FE. Epinephrine and its use in anaphylaxis: current issues. *Curr Opin Allergy Clin Immunol*. 2010;10(4):354−361.

76. Sheikh A, Shehata YA, Brown SG, Simons FE. Adrenaline for the treatment of anaphylaxis: cochrane systematic review. *Allergy*. 2009;64(2):204−212.

77. McLean-Tooke AP, Bethune CA, Fay AC, Spickett GP. Adrenaline in the treatment of anaphylaxis: what is the evidence? *BMJ*. 2003;327(7427):1332−1335.

78. Korenblat P, Lundie MJ, Dankner RE, Day JH. A retrospective study of epinephrine administration for anaphylaxis: how many doses are needed? *Allergy Asthma Proc*. 1999;20(6):383−386.

79. Kelso JM. A second dose of epinephrine for anaphylaxis: how often needed and how to carry. *J Allergy Clin Immunol*. 2006;117(2):464−465.

80. Manivannan V, Campbell RL, Bellolio MF, Stead LG, Li JT, Decker WW. Factors associated with repeated use of epinephrine for the treatment of anaphylaxis. *Ann Allergy Asthma Immunol*. 2009;103(5):395−400.

81. O'Driscoll BR, Howard LS, Earis J, Mak V, British Thoracic Society Emergency Oxygen Guideline G, Group BTSEOGD. BTS guideline for oxygen use in adults in healthcare and emergency settings. *Thorax*. 2017;72(Suppl 1):ii1−ii90.

82. Lieberman P, Nicklas RA, Oppenheimer J, et al. The diagnosis and management of anaphylaxis practice parameter: 2010 update. *J Allergy Clin Immunol*. 2010;126(3):477−480 e1-42.

83. Sicherer SH, Simons FER, Section On A, Immunology. Epinephrine for first-aid management of anaphylaxis. *Pediatrics*. 2017;139(3).

84. https://www.nzrc.org.nz/assets/Uploads/Dosage-of-IM-Adrenaline-for-Anaphylaxis-2019-Large.pdf.

85. Stark BJ, Sullivan TJ. Biphasic and protracted anaphylaxis. *J Allergy Clin Immunol*. 1986;78(1 Pt 1):76−83.

86. Cox L, Platts-Mills TA, Finegold I, et al. American academy of allergy, asthma & immunology/American college of allergy, asthma and immunology joint task force report on omalizumab-associated anaphylaxis. *J Allergy Clin Immunol*. 2007;120(6):1373−1377.

87. Blumenthal KG, Shenoy ES, Varughese CA, et al. Impact of a clinical guideline for prescribing antibiotics to inpatients reporting penicillin or cephalosporin allergy. *Ann Allergy Asthma Immunol*. 2015;115(4):294−300 e2.

88. Lue HC, Wu MH, Wang JK, Wu FF, Wu YN. Three- versus four-week administration of benzathine penicillin G: effects on incidence of streptococcal infections and recurrences of rheumatic fever. *Pediatrics*. 1996;97(6 Pt 2):984−988.

89. World Health Organization. *Rheumatic Fever and Rheumatic Heart Disease : Report of a WHO Expert Consultation*. WHO Technical Report Series. Geneva: WHO Expert Consultation; 2004. Available from: http://apps.who.int/iris/bitstream/10665/42898/1/WHO_TRS_923.pdf.

90. RHDAustralia (ARF/RHD writing group). The Australian guideline for prevention, diagnosis and management of acute rheumatic fever and rheumatic heart disease. In: *National Heart Foundation of Australia and the Cardiac*

Society of Australia and New Zealand. 2nd ed.; 2012 [cited August 29]:Available from: https://www.rhdaustralia.org. au/node/950/attachment.

91. Working Group on Pediatric Acute Rheumatic F, Cardiology Chapter of Indian Academy of P, Saxena A, et al. Consensus guidelines on pediatric acute rheumatic fever and rheumatic heart disease. *Indian Pediatr.* 2008;45(7): 565–573.

92. South African National Department of Health. *National Guidelines on Primary Prevention and Prophylaxis of Rheumatic Fever (RF) and Rheumatic Heart Disease (RHD) for Health Professionals at Primary Level.* Pretoria, South Africa: Western Cape Government; 2003.

93. Heart Foundation of New Zealand. *New Zealand Guidelines for Rheumatic Fever: Diagnosis, Management and Secondary Prevention of Acute Rheumatic Fever and Rheumatic Heart Disease: 2014 Update;* 2014 [cited 2017 Dec 10](Available from: www.heartfoundation.org.nz.

94. Gerber MA, Baltimore RS, Eaton CB, et al. Prevention of rheumatic fever and diagnosis and treatment of acute streptococcal pharyngitis: a scientific statement from the American heart association rheumatic fever, endocarditis, and Kawasaki disease committee of the council on cardiovascular disease in the young, the interdisciplinary council on functional genomics and translational biology, and the interdisciplinary council on quality of care and outcomes research: endorsed by the American academy of pediatrics. *Circulation.* 2009;119(11): 1541–1551.

95. Wyber R, Grainger Gasser A, Thompson D, et al. *Tools for Implementing RHD Control Programmes (TIPS) Handbook.* Australia: World Heart Federation and RhEACH. Perth; 2014.

96. Brandt ER, Yarwood PJ, McMillan DJ, et al. Antibody levels to the class I and II epitopes of the M protein and myosin are related to group A streptococcal exposure in endemic populations. *Int Immunol.* 2001;13(10): 1335–1343.

97. Holland JV, Hardie K, de Dassel J, Ralph AP. Rheumatic heart disease prophylaxis in older patients: a register-based audit of adherence to guidelines. *Open Forum Infect Dis.* 2018 (accepted).

98. Lawrence JG, Carapetis JR, Griffiths K, Edwards K, Condon JR. Acute rheumatic fever and rheumatic heart disease: incidence and progression in the Northern Territory of Australia, 1997 to 2010. *Circulation.* 2013;128(5): 492–501.

99. Lamagni T, Guy R, Chand M, et al. Resurgence of scarlet fever in England, 2014–16: a population-based surveillance study. *Lancet Infect Dis.* 2018;18(2): 180–187.

100. Guasch J, Vignau A, Mortimer Jr EA, Rammelkamp Jr CH. Studies of the role of continuing or recurrent streptococcal infection in rheumatic valvular heart disease. *Am J Med Sci.* 1962;244:290–297.

101. Department of Health (Government of South Africa). *National Guidelines on Primary Prevention and Prophylaxis of Rheumatic Fever (RF) and Rheumatic Heart Disease (RHD)*

for Health Professionals at Primary Level; 2009. Available from: https://www.westerncape.gov.za/sites/www.western cape.gov.za/files/documents/2003/rheuma.pdf.

102. Ali SKM, Khaleefa MSA, Khair SM. *Acute Rheumatic Fever and Rheumatic Heart Disease: Sudan's Guidelines for Diagnosis, Management and Prevention;* 2017. Available from: http://rhdaction.org/sites/default/files/Sudan_RHD%20 Guidelines_Jan%2017.pdf.

103. Frankish JD. Rheumatic fever prophylaxis: gisborne experience. *N Z Med J.* 1984;97(765):674–675.

104. Harrington Z, Thomas DP, Currie BJ, Bulkanhawuy J. Challenging perceptions of non-compliance with rheumatic fever prophylaxis in a remote Aboriginal community. *Med J Aust.* 2006;184(10):514–517.

105. Mitchell AG, Belton S, Johnston V, Read C, Scrine C, Ralph AP. "That heart sickness": young Aboriginal people's understanding of rheumatic fever. *Med Anthropol.* 2018. accepted).

106. McCalman J, Bailie R, Bainbridge R, et al. Continuous quality improvement and comprehensive primary health care: a systems framework to improve service quality and health outcomes. *Front Public Health.* 2018;6:76.

107. Harris MF, Williams AM, Dennis SM, Zwar NA, Davies GP. Chronic disease self-management: implementation with and within Australian general practice. *Med J Aust.* 2008;189(10):17–20.

108. Mitchell AG, Belton S, Johnston V, Ralph AP. Transition to adult care for aboriginal children with rheumatic fever: a review informed by a focussed ethnography in northern Australia. *Aust J Prim Health.* 2018;24(1):9–13.

109. Ralph AP, Read C, Johnston V, et al. Improving delivery of secondary prophylaxis for rheumatic heart disease in remote Indigenous communities: study protocol for a stepped-wedge randomised trial. *Trials.* 2016;17(1): 51.

110. Ralph AP, Read C, Johnston V, et al. Improving delivery of secondary prophylaxis for rheumatic heart disease in remote Indigenous communities: study protocol for a stepped-wedge randomised trial. *Trials.* 2016;17:51.

111. Katzenellenbogen JM, Ralph AP, Wyber R, Carapetis JR. Rheumatic heart disease: infectious disease origin, chronic care approach. *BMC Health Serv Res.* 2017; 17(1):793.

112. Wagner EH, Austin BT, Davis C, Hindmarsh M, Schaefer J, Bonomi A. Improving chronic illness care: translating evidence into action. *Health Aff.* 2001;20(6): 64–78.

113. de Dassel JL, Ralph AP, Cass A. A systematic review of adherence in Indigenous Australians: an opportunity to improve chronic condition management. *BMC Health Serv Res.* 2017;17(1):845.

114. Arya RK. Awareness about sore-throat, rheumatic fever and rheumatic heart disease in a rural community. *Indian J Public Health.* 1992;36(3):63–67.

115. Iyengar SD, Grover A, Kumar R, Ganguly NK, Anand IS, Wahi PL. A rheumatic fever and rheumatic heart disease control programme in a rural community of North India. *Nat Med J India.* 1991;4(6):268–271.

116. Bach JF, Chalons S, Forier E, et al. 10-year educational programme aimed at rheumatic fever in two French Caribbean islands. *Lancet.* 1996;347(9002):644–648.

117. Amir J, Ginat S, Cohen YH, Marcus TE, Keller N, Varsano I. Lidocaine as a diluent for administration of benzathine penicillin G. *Pediatr Infect Dis J.* 1998; 17(10):890–893.

118. Morsy M-MF, Mohamed MA, Abosedira MM, et al. Lidocaine as a diluent for benzathine penicillin G reduces injection pain in patients with rheumatic fever: a prospective, randomized double-blinded crossover study. *Aust JBasic Appl Sci.* 2012;6(5):236–240.

119. Russell K, Nicholson R, Naidu R. Reducing the pain of intramuscular benzathine penicillin injections in the rheumatic fever population of Counties Manukau District Health Board. *J Paediatr Child Health.* 2014;50(2): 112–117.

120. Barnhill BJ, Holbert MD, Jackson NM, Erickson RS. Using pressure to decrease the pain of intramuscular injections. *J Pain Symptom Manage.* 1996;12(1):52–58.

121. Thomas NAR, Kaur S, Juneja R, Saxena A. Needle temperature and pain perception in the treatment of rheumatic heart disease. *Br J Card Nursing.* 2019;14(3).

122. Briggs G, Freeman RK, Yaffe SJ. *Drugs in Pregnancy and Lactation.* 9th ed. Philadelphia: Lippincott Williams & Wilkins; 2011.

123. Schaefer C. 4.1 – analgesics, antiphlogistics and anesthetics. In: Schaefer C, Peters PWJ, Miller RK, eds. *Drugs during Pregnancy and Lactation.* 2nd ed. London: Elsevier BV; 2007:623–638.

124. AstraZenica Ltd. *Lignocaine Hydrochloride New Zealand Data Sheet. Information for Health Professionals.* Wellington: Medsafe; 2017. Available from: http://www.medsafe.govt.nz/profs/datasheet/x/XylocaineAndAdrenalineinj.pdf.

125. Hale T, Rowe H. *Medications and Mother's Milk.* 16th ed. USA; 2014.

126. Loke YC, In M, Vo-Tran H, Wong S, eds. *The Women's Pregnancy and Breastfeeding Medicines Guide.* Parkville, Victoria: Royal Women's Hospital; 2014.

127. Sweetman S, ed. *Martindale: The Complete Drug Reference.* 34th ed. London; Chicago: Pharmaceutical Press; 2005.

128. Baxter K, ed. *Stockley's Drug Interactions: A Source Book of Interactions, Their Mechanisms, Clinical Importance and Management.* 7th ed. London: Pharmaceutical Press; 2006.

129. Szarewski A, Guillebaud J. *Contraception: A User's Handbook.* 2nd ed. Oxford; New York: Oxford University Press; 1998.

130. Mehta D, ed. *British National Formulary.* 49th ed. London: British Medical Association & Royal Pharmaceutical Society of Great Britain; 2005.

131. Health Quality and Safety Commission New Zealand, 2019. Available from: https://www.medsafe.govt.nz/safety/DHCPLetters/BicillinLAAugust2018.pdf.

132. Greenway K. Using the ventrogluteal site for intramuscular injection. *Nursing Standard.* 2004;18(29):39–42.

CHAPTER 12

Rheumatic Heart Disease Control Programs, Registers, and Access to Care

ROSEMARY WYBER • JOSEPH KADO

RHEUMATIC HEART DISEASE CONTROL PROGRAMS

Disease control is the "reduction in the incidence, prevalence, morbidity, or mortality of an infectious disease to a locally acceptable level."[1] Efforts to control acute rheumatic fever (ARF) and rheumatic heart disease (RHD) have been underway for nearly a century and are entering a new era with passing of the resolution on rheumatic fever and RHD at the 71st World Health Assembly.[2] Indeed, a growing focus on the potential of RHD control programs has led to calls for elimination of the disease entirely.[3] This chapter traces the development of RHD control initiatives and identifies common themes to inform development of new programs in the postresolution era. It is intended as a primer on key lessons in RHD control worldwide.

The terms control program and control initiatives are used interchangeably in this chapter and are broadly defined, spanning all activities intended to reduce the burden of group A *Streptococcus* (GAS), ARF, and RHD. Burden is considered to be both epidemiologic impact (on incidence and prevalence of disease) and human impact (on the lived experience of RHD and experience of people, families, and communities). Few of the RHD control programs described are discrete, planned, and continuously funded initiatives; almost all span years of mixed funding sources, research activities, and clinical care delivery. This approach can lead to fragmentation and is heavily reliant on individual "champions" to persevere with RHD activities. However, case studies—particularly from Sudan, Uganda, and Fiji—highlight how combinations of different activities can contribute to increasingly comprehensive and well-developed programs over a number of years. This overview is not exhaustive and is limited by underrepresentation of programs from low-resource settings in the published literature. Ensuring that results and outcomes from RHD control programs worldwide are evaluated, published, and acted upon is a shared global priority for improving service delivery and achieving equitable gains in reducing RHD.

1900 − 1950s

RHD was a leading cause of childhood morbidity and hospital admission in the United Kingdom and United States in the early part of the 20th century.[4,5] This considerable disease burden prompted interest in improving clinical outcomes and exploring opportunities for prevention. In the absence of disease-altering therapies, early RHD control programs focused on research to understand etiology, case notification, and systems to improve medical management.[6] Social determinants of health—including household crowding, lack of hygiene facilities and poverty—had been identified as risk factors for ARF. Strategies to address social determinants of health were a feature of this early period, and include efforts to improve housing for people at risk of ARF recurrences.[6,7] For example, a 1930s program in Dublin, Ireland was established to identify children with symptoms of ARF in schools and refer them to hospital clinics for assessment. ARF education was provided for parents, and public health authorities were engaged to improve living conditions, particularly overcrowding, where necessary.[8]

1950s−2000

The discovery of sulfonamides and penicillin in the 1940s and 1950s offered the first therapeutic opportunity to prevent ARF and progression of RHD.[9] As evidence for primary and secondary prevention emerged, systems to deliver these disease-altering interventions were needed and RHD control programs assumed a new remit.

Acute Rheumatic Fever and Rheumatic Heart Disease. https://doi.org/10.1016/B978-0-323-63982-8.00012-X

Registers to facilitate prophylaxis delivery began in the 1940s and 1950s in North America. In Toronto, Canada, a register was established in 1948 to facilitate care for children with congenital heart disease and RHD, including provision of prophylaxis.[10] In the United States, the Maryland Register was developed in the mid-1950s to supply low cost oral penicillin and record medication adherence to prophylaxis.[11] As the Maryland Register developed and became automated with punch cards, the role of the register expanded to include clinical review and advice to referring clinicians. Indeed, a system of community-based efforts to reduce ARF risk, supported by cardiology management of symptoms and prevention of recurrences, was a hallmark of this period.[12]

Expansion of RHD registers and increasing access to disease-altering antibiotics spurred research interest, leading to a "cooperative investigative project" coordinated by the World Health Organization from 1972 to 1980.[13] One of the goals of this formative program was "demonstration of the feasibility of community control of rheumatic heart disease in pilot programmes."[13] Nearly 3000 people were enrolled across seven sites with reasonable evidence of enhanced delivery of secondary prophylaxis over this time (see Table 12.1).[13] One of the participating project sites in Delhi published an independent overview suggestive of increased engagement with RHD control and general support for register-based secondary prophylaxis.[14]

Evidence for primary prevention and primary care programs grew in the 1960s and 1970s. A number of studies of comprehensive care programs in Baltimore suggested that primary care services may reduce ARF incidence.[23,24] Similarly, an ARF program in Costa Rica in the 1970s focused on improving primary prevention through changes to clinical guidelines: healthcare workers could treat sore throats without microbiological confirmation of GAS infection and with injectable penicillin instead of oral medication.[19] This focus on primary prevention and increased use of benzathine penicillin G (BPG) seemed to accelerate the decline in ARF incidence in Costa Rica, although the introduction of a nationalized healthcare system and other social policies makes it difficult to identify the impact of individual interventions. By 1978, a detailed WHO Memorandum called for community RHD control projects, incorporating both primary and secondary prevention of ARF.[25]

The success of early RHD control programs led to the creation of the WHO Global Programme for the Prevention of RF/RHD in Sixteen Developing Countries in 1984.[16] Supported by external development funding, this program focused on secondary prevention, with

elements of active case finding, health worker training, and health education.[26] Growing interest in incorporating primary prevention elements emerged at a 1994 expert meeting.[27] By 1999, all 16 countries had completed a pilot phase and over 15 million school children had been auscultated to screen for RHD. An unpublished review of this program suggested that it was highly efficient to run, costing less that $US 1 million, while raising awareness and generating new data about the burden of disease.[28]

In some WHO regions, this work was amplified by guidelines for program standardization and implementation.[29,30] Alongside this momentum, RHD control programs emerged organically in a number of locations (outlined in Table 12.1), including landmark programs in Cuba and the French Caribbean.[18,21] Collectively, these formative control initiatives formed a template of how RHD control programs have been conceived and delivered worldwide.

A number of the RHD programs seeded by the WHO Global Programme have endured and transitioned to new funding models. For example, an ARF/RHD National Control Program began in Jamaica in 1985 as part of the WHO Global Programme following preliminary burden of disease assessments.[31] A pilot phase was initiated in two regions, expanding in 1991 to provide coverage to the whole country through the Ministry of Health.[20] The program focused on primary prevention and development of an RHD register. A secondary prophylaxis program is ongoing in Jamaica and notifications of ARF are provided to the Ministry of Health National Surveillance Unit.[20] Despite these efforts, a significant burden of RHD persists and cardiac surgery for RHD is frequently necessary.[32]

Outside the auspices of the WHO Global Programme, the Division of Pediatric Cardiology at the Federal University of Minas Gerais in Brazil established the Prevention Program for Rheumatic Fever in 1986.[22] Since 1988, the program has been delivered by the Reference Centre for Rheumatic Fever focusing on secondary prophylaxis and encompassing an innovative package of service delivery and support services including standardized clinical protocols, transport provided to biannual clinical review, centralized appointment scheduling, free access to BPG, and accommodation for parents of inpatients.[22] Statistically significant improvements in recurrence rates and severity and surgical demand have been recorded as the program began, though secondary prophylaxis adherence is not provided in published reports.[22] Evidence from echocardiography screening studies demonstrates a persistently high burden of RHD in Minas Gerais.[33] This may be indicative of an ongoing need

	Program Reporting Dates[a]	Register for Secondary Prevention	Health Worker Education	Community Education or Engagement	Primary Prevention	Clinical Guidelines	Concurrent Research Activities	Notifications/ Disease Surveillances	Community Screening	Notes	Reported Outcomes
WHO study "community control of RF/RHD"— community level projects in the following countries: Egypt, Cyprus, Jamaica, Lagos, India, Iran, Mongolia.[13,15]	1972 –1980	Yes	Yes	Yes	Not addressed	Not addressed	Yes	Yes	Yes—auscultation	Observational study. No control or comparison data.	In aggregated analysis across seven study sites with 50% response rate, delivery of secondary prophylaxis injections improved from 38.3% of people receiving 10-12 scheduled injections in year 1 to 76% receiving 10-12 scheduled injections in year 6.[13] Increasing number of injections each year associated with reduced hospital admissions. Many practical difficulties noted in delivering the program. One positive report from project site.[14]
WHO Global Programme in the following countries: Mali, Zambia, Zimbabwe, Bolivia, El Salvador, Jamaica, Egypt, Iraq, Pakistan, Sudan, India, Sri Lanka, Thailand, China, Phillippines, Tonga.[16,17]	1984 –2001	Yes	Yes	Yes	Yes	Not addressed	Yes	Not addressed	Yes—auscultation	Over 200,000 children screened through auscultation.[17] Observational study. No control or comparison data.	Reports of improved adherence with secondary prophylaxis but baseline data or temporal changes not clearly reported.[16,17]
Martinique and Guadeloupe[18]	1981 –1992	Yes	Yes	Yes	Yes [including treatment of skin infections]	Not addressed	Yes	Not addressed	Yes—pharyngeal swabbing	Term used to describe the disease was changed to help public education campaign. Full time pediatrician dedicated to RHD in each island. Observational study. No control or comparison data.	Reduced total ARF incidence (78% reduction in Martinique, 74% reduction in Guadeloupe). Reports of reduction in need for open heart surgery
		Yes	Yes						Not addressed		

Continued

TABLE 12.1
Selected 20th Century Control Programs for Rheumatic Heart Disease.—cont'd

Program	Program Reporting Dates[a]	Register for Secondary Prevention	Health Worker Education	Community Education or Engagement	Primary Prevention	Clinical Guidelines	Concurrent Research Activities	Notifications/ Disease Surveillances	Community Screening	Notes	Reported Outcomes
Costa Rica[19]	1985–1990			Not addressed	Yes [changed clinical criteria for treatment of GAS pharyngitis]	Yes [changed clinical criteria for treatment of GAS pharyngitis]	Not addressed	Not addressed		Observational study. No control or comparison data.	Reduced total ARF incidence (7.8/100,000 in 1985 to 1/100,000 in 1990)
Jamaica[20]	1985–1995	Yes	Yes	Yes	Yes	Yes	Yes	Yes	Not addressed		Description of different clinical presentations at beginning and end of reporting period presented but no clear epidemiologic data.
Pinar del Rio, Cuba[21]	1986–1996	Yes	Yes	Yes	Yes	Not addressed	Yes	Yes	No	Observational study. No control or comparison data.	Reduced total ARF incidence (28.4/100,000 to 2.7/100,000) Reduced proportion of recurrent ARF (5/100,000 to 0.9/100,000) Improved adherence to SP from (n = 52) 50% "regular" adherence in 1986 to (n = 193) 93.8% regular SP in 1996
Minas Gerais, Brazil[22]	1988–2000	Yes	Yes	Yes	Not addressed	Yes	Yes	Not addressed	No	Financial support for people with RHD and their families. Dedicated ARF clinic. Observational study. No control or comparison data.	Statistically significant decline in recurrences, severity of carditis, hospitalization, surgery and deaths over the time period 1977/1978 – 1988–2000. Declines attributed to improved adherence though this was not quantified. *Changes in adherence rates to secondary prophylaxis not provided.

ARF, acute rheumatic fever; RHD, rheumatic heart disease; GAS, group A streptococcus; SP, secondary prophylaxis

[a] Many programs continued to operate beyond specified reporting dates.

for primary prevention activities to reduce disease incidence in similar settings.[34]

RHD control programs in the 1970s and 1980s generally began as pragmatic responses to the high burden of RHD. Hospital records and data collection of that period were not usually intended for rigorous epidemiologic analysis or research outcomes. Observational data published in a number of papers indicated some evidence of impact—particularly in reducing the incidence of ARF[18,35] and, perhaps, reduced progression of RHD.[36] However, it was not possible to assess whether these changes were causally associated with the activities of control programs. Indeed, the incidence of ARF began to fall before the advent of antibiotics, a change widely attributed to reduction of overcrowding and improved living standards.[37] This decline continued throughout the latter half of the 20th century, even in places without a control program, including Slovakia,[38] Denmark and Sweden.[39] Conversely, in the United States rates of ARF declined more dramatically at about the time penicillin became widely used for the management of pharyngitis.[39] The contribution of control program activities to changes in RHD epidemiology was, and remains, empirically unproven. However, the etiologic complexity of GAS, ARF, and RHD meant that multimodal interventions would be needed for many people, over many years, to detect changes in critical endpoints. This would be ethically and financially challenging, particularly given that biologically plausible recommendations for reducing the burden of disease have already been adopted by WHO.

At the end of the century, it was largely accepted that RHD control programs could accelerate the decline in incidence and severity of ARF and RHD by improving access to disease-altering penicillin.[40,41] Emerging evidence of cost-effectiveness of RHD control programs strengthened this assessment.[42] Therefore, in settings with a high burden of RHD, control programs were considered an appropriate intervention to improve outcomes of people already living with disease and to reduce the incidence of new cases. This rationale remains important, particularly in places where persistent social and economic disparity contributes to ongoing disease.[42]

2000–2005

By the turn of the millennium, new cases of ARF and RHD were rare in most high-income countries. In association with this decline, register-based control programs had largely ceased throughout the United States and were even closing in parts of New Zealand.[43,44] New global health priorities emerged, including a marked increase in noncommunicable cardiovascular disease burden and HIV. In 2001, the WHO Global Programme in RHD disbanded in the face of competing health priorities.[45] At around this period, WHO held a technical meeting on RHD, producing a document that summarized the lessons of RHD control programs of the 20th century. This WHO Technical Report Series identified six main components of national RHD control programs: secondary prevention, primary prevention, health education activities, training of healthcare providers, epidemiological surveillance, and community involvement.[46] However, the discontinuation of the WHO Global Programme meant that these recommendations were not systematically adopted into practice or evaluated. Relatively few RHD control programs were initiated in the early 2000s.

2005–2018

Clinician-led research in low-resource settings in the early 2000s highlighted the persistent burden of RHD and very poor clinical outcomes.[47,48] This work indicated an ongoing unmet need for RHD control activities in many regions of the world, including in Fiji (Box 12.1) and Australia and New Zealand (Box 12.2). In 2005, the First All Africa Workshop on ARF and RHD and the resulting Drakensberg Declaration became a call to action. The Drakensberg Declaration promulgated the A.S.A.P (Awareness, Surveillance, Advocacy, Prevention) approach and called for "establishment of national primary and secondary prevention programmes for RF and RHD" in conjunction with international partners.[49]

In many places, the initiation of new RHD control programs was further catalyzed by echocardiographic screening. Auscultation screening for RHD had been a part of some formative RHD control initiatives and had been endorsed in the 2001 WHO technical guidelines.[46] In 2007, a landmark study found almost 10 times as many cases of RHD detectable on echocardiographic screening of school children in Cambodia and Mozambique than were detectable by auscultation screening alone.[50] Echocardiography screening was rapidly and widely adopted as a new approach to addressing RHD and many thousands of young people were screened around the world over the next few years.[51] Outstanding questions remain about the clinical utility of echocardiography screening, and whether it satisfies accepted public health criteria for diseases warranting population-based screening (see Chapter 9), but the increasingly accessible modality has been critical to growing awareness of the need for action on RHD.[52]

Other events in the 2000s challenged established thinking about best practice in control programs. Long-standing debate about the most appropriate balance of

BOX 12.1
Rheumatic Heart Disease Control in Fiji

Other rheumatic heart disease (RHD) control initiatives have evolved outside the auspices of the formative WHO program and can provide instructive lessons about priorities and sustainability. For example, RHD control activities have been underway in Fiji for over 50 years spanning different projects and funding agencies. The first Rheumatic Fever Control Program in Fiji was established in 1964 by the Fiji Medical Department to tackle the growing concern about the increasing numbers of young "cardiac cripples" resulting from acute rheumatic fever (ARF).[76] ARF control included making "*Acute rheumatism*" a notifiable disease, regional ARF registers based at divisional hospitals and the primary care level responsible for delivery of secondary prevention, and ensuring timely attendance at specialist clinics. In 1967, concerns about overdiagnosis led to all suspected cases of ARF being referred to the Consultant Physician for confirmation and provision of medical literature about ARF.[77]

Within 5 years of establishing the control program, there were reports that the incidence rates of both ARF and RHD were showing a declining trend, though these were based on hospital admissions, and there was evidence of underreporting.[76,78] This downward trend from 35 - 37/100,000 in 1960s seemed to be confirmed up to 1984 with a reported incidence for ARF of 9.6/100,000, with the greatest decrease noted among the ethnic Indians (who previously represented over 80% of admissions) and among women.[77,79]

By the turn of the century, there were growing concerns from the medical fraternity about the number of young people presenting for the first time with ARF but already with established RHD and heart failure and occasionally atrial fibrillation [Tikoduadua, personal communication Kado, 2018]. This gave impetus to the formation of a revamped Fiji RHD Control Program in 2005 with 3-year funding support from the World Heart Federation (WHF). The program was register-based (stand-alone, health services research-based) and focused on improving secondary prophylaxis, standardizing diagnosis and management of ARF/RHD, improving health worker knowledge and providing support to the community. The program established the role of the National Coordinator for RHD whose activities were governed by a Technical Advisory Committee.

In 2006, the Fiji Group A Streptococcal Project (GrASP) was established to determine the burden of GAS disease in Fiji as a fore-runner to establish a potential vaccine trial site. Studies from this project highlighted the high burden of underdiagnosis and the estimated cost of illness of ARF and RHD.[80–82] GrASP also established the normal ranges of GAS antibody tests for Fiji,[83] burden of subclinical RHD diagnosed by echocardiographic screening and explored task-shifting the role of echocardiography to briefly trained, less-skilled cadres of health workers,[84] and development of a standard curriculum for training.[85,86] The project also quantified the poor adherence to secondary prophylaxis and clinical outcomes of screening detected RHD in Fiji.[87–89]

Funding for the RHD program lapsed but a concept paper prepared by the Fiji RHD Control Program formed the basis for the development of the Acute Rheumatic Fever and Rheumatic Heart Disease Policy of the Fiji Ministry of Health in 2014. This policy and the ground work of the GrASP team helped leverage funding from partners Cure Kids and the New Zealand Ministry of Foreign Affairs and Trade and ushered in the third iteration of the Fiji RHD Prevention and Control Program in 2015.

Aligned to the Fiji RF and RHD Policy with global guidance from the published Tools for Implementing RHD Control Programmes (TIPs)[70] resource, the program aims to be integrated rather than siloed and has four major components:

1. National register (RF information system [RFIS]) linked to the national patient information system (PATIS): This is both a patient-care and public health register custom-built to allow national, divisional, health clinic and hospital staff to effectively monitor and manage the national register-based prevention program with the explicit focus of improving secondary prophylaxis adherence and clinical management and to facilitate timely reporting.
2. Clinical care for patients: to help clinical care providers deliver effective comprehensive ARF/RHD related services through development of best practice guidelines for ARF and sore throat management [under development], clinical pathways, and capacity building for all cadres of health staff including preservice training modules for delivery in training institutions. This includes the employment of divisional RHD coordinators and liaison nurses at all health centers.
3. Early case detection: to develop a model for RHD early case detection for the Ministry of Health that includes improved surveillance and notification of newly diagnosed cases of ARF and RHD; pilot of utility and cost effectiveness of school health nurses conducting RHD screening in primary schools and expanded notification to include both incident cases of ARF and newly diagnosed RHD.
4. Primary prevention, health promotion, and advocacy: to improve community awareness and engagement in ARF and RHD and destigmatize ARF/RHD.

The new control program has focused on involvement of people living with ARF/RHD, and this is reflected in the terms of reference for the RHD Technical Advisory Committee with representation of people living with RHD, health center-based RHD working groups and the popular peer-support groups, and the parallel parent/career support meetings. An off-shoot of the early peer support group formation has been the identification of RHD Champions. In particular, a young woman diagnosed with RHD through school screening participated in the Fiji Hibiscus Pageant to raise the profile of RHD. She has become the face of RHD in Fiji and has represented people living with RHD (PLWRHD) in three international forums, including a side-event organized by the WHF at the 71st World Health Assembly (WHA) in Geneva in 2018.[90]

Advocacy work by the program and a technical advisory committee has seen Fiji's senior health executives engage in both local and international spheres relating to RHD. Fiji played a key role in supporting the New Zealand-led RHD resolution that was endorsed at the 71st WHA.

There are some indications that awareness of ARF and RHD and adherence to secondary prophylaxis has improved.[91] Assessment is ongoing, and the impact of these interventions will form part of the program evaluation. Interim lessons from the Fiji experience include the need to deliver care through primary care clinics, to address both primary and secondary prevention and the important role of PLWRHD to amplify program outcomes.

primary and secondary prevention was revisited on the basis of new empiric data about primary prevention focused programs.[53-55] Additionally, slight growth in cardiac surgical capacity in low-resource settings necessitated improved systems for preoperative triage and waiting list management.[56] In parallel, new challenges in RHD control emerged including widespread stockouts of BPG, which stymied the options for effective control programs.[57] In the absence of global clinical guidelines for RHD control, local guideline development took increasing precedence in some places.[58-60] Changes in funding sources and the role of nongovernment organizations evolved, necessitating increased collaboration and a practical role for the World Heart Federation (WHF).[61] These technical and programmatic evolutions have driven a new era of systematic national and international efforts to tackle RHD.

Contemporary RHD control programs are necessarily more complex and comprehensive than programmatic examples of the 20th century. This is well demonstrated by the experience of Sudan where a historic secondary prevention program provided the foundation for a modern RHD program with expanded scope. The Ministry of Health in Sudan participated in the WHO Global Programme on RHD from 1986 to 2000.[16] Over 13,000 children underwent auscultation screening for RHD. The program focused on delivery of secondary prophylaxis, reportedly achieving prophylaxis coverage of 72%.[16] In the absence of ongoing funding, the initiative ended in the year 2000. A Sudanese review of the program identified three key outstanding needs from the WHO program: increased primary prevention alongside secondary prevention, increased advocacy by nongovernment organizations, public and patients, and increased cooperation with regional partners.[62]

In 2012 a new RHD control program began as a partnership between the Sudan Heart Society and Sudan Ministry of Health.[63] The new program includes primary prevention, secondary prevention, and awareness raising. A National RHD Awareness Day is held in July each year to raise awareness of the burden of RHD.[64] New clinical guidelines were developed in 2012 and updated in 2017.[65] A National Registry for RHD was developed, initially enrolling patients into tertiary clinics with echocardiography facilities.[64,66] Over 2 years, 370 patients were added to the register, the vast majority of whom had severe RHD.[66] Echocardiography screening has been used to better understand the burden and distribution of RHD and amplify key messages about RHD.[67] Secondary prophylaxis and access to ongoing care is limited. Adherence to secondary prophylaxis is low and compounded by shortages of BPG.[68] Only a third of people receive ongoing follow-up and less than one in 10 people who need cardiac surgery can access it.[66,69] Multiple sources of funding support the RHD control program in Sudan, including from WHO Sudan Country Office, Sudanese Children's Heart Society and the Sudanese American Medical Association.[70]

Zambia was also part of the WHO global program for RHD control from 1986, including large-scale auscultation screening.[71] In 2014, a new "BeatRHD Zambia" initiative began as part of a "multifaceted public–private effort" with a particular focus on primary prevention. The new program raises awareness about sore throats to influence health seeking behavior. This has included a partnership with the Ministries of Health and Education to deliver education in nearly 50 schools and through an RHD Week.[72] Research initiatives have demonstrated a high burden of pharyngitis.[73] Service responses have included training for health professionals on administering BPG injections safely and management of anaphylaxis.[74] People living with RHD have been involved in delivering some activities and trainings associated with the program.[75]

In Nepal, a program of RHD prevention and control was initiated in 2007 as a partnership between the Nepal Heart Foundation and the Government of Nepal.[92] This comprehensive program focuses on early detection and registration of ARF/RHD patients and establishing centers for safe administration of BPG. An

---

BOX 12.2
Rheumatic Heart Disease Control in Australia and New Zealand

Alongside the renaissance of RHD control programs in endemic low-resource settings, RHD control has continued to evolve in a small number of high-income countries with a high burden of ARF/RHD in Indigenous communities. The development of RHD control programs in Australia and New Zealand is somewhat anomalous to global experience and provides some unique insights.

Research and programmatic initiatives began early in New Zealand, including an early control program in 1974, political engagement with the Maori Women's Welfare League, and local clinical guidelines in 1984.[44,102] Throughout New Zealand, RHD registers evolved organically, some with an epidemiologic surveillance focus and others addressing clinical management and program delivery.[44] For example, the Auckland Rheumatic Fever register was developed in 1981 to support delivery of monthly secondary prophylaxis injections. The program evolved to be a nurse-led service with in–home injection delivery, very high rates of adherence and ARF recurrence rates of less than 5%.[103,104] Although significant progress was achieved in secondary prophylaxis delivery, the incidence of first episode of ARF remained high in Māori and Pacific Island people in New Zealand. Between 1998 and 2001, a large randomized clinical trial of 22,000 school children in South Auckland was conducted to explore improving primary prevention through nurse-led, school-based sore throat services.[54] Results from this study did not meet statistical significance but a subsequent meta-analysis suggested that ARF incidence could potentially be reduced by school-based sore throat programs.[55]

The increasing disparity in ARF incidence for Maori and Pacific Island people in New Zealand made ARF a political issue in 2011.[105] In 2012, the government of New Zealand set a Better Public Service Target to reduce the incidence of ARF by two thirds by 2017.[106] Implemented through the Rheumatic Fever Prevention Program, this included the largest school-based sore throat program ever developed—a peak intensity it included 251 schools, covering 53,998 children in high-risk communities with regular access to throat swabs and oral antibiotics.[107] By December 2017, the rate of ARF had fallen by 23%, but this increased subsequently.[108] Detailed evaluation has not found a statistically significant association in areas participating in the school sore throat program, although it did reach statistical significance in the highest-incidence region.[109]

Other initiatives in New Zealand included focused efforts to improve housing quality for people at high risk of ARF and considerable investment in public education and health literacy campaigns.[110,111] Overall, reduction in ARF rates in New Zealand was likely to be multifactorial, including the impact of widespread community education, changes in health seeking behavior and primary care management of ARF.[112]

In Australia, a high burden of ARF in urban children was documented in the 1930s – 1950s.[113] This early study did not report the Indigenous ethnicity of participants but did demonstrate that incidence of ARF in low-income locations was triple that of high-income locations.[113] New cases in nonIndigenous people became rare in the latter half of the 20th century but systematic case record reviews in new locations identified a very high burden of RHD for Aboriginal and Torres Strait Islander people in the 1980s.[114,115] These audits provided the basis for an RHD register and control program in the Northern Territory in 1997.[116] RHD control efforts expanded in a number of Australian states with increasing register coverage, and ARF became notifiable in a number of settings. Evaluation of register data in some locations suggested a reduction in rates of ARF.[116] National clinical guidelines for the management of ARF and RHD were first developed in 2006 and updated in 2012.[117]

Interest and understanding about RHD in Australia was spurred by echocardiography screening studies.[118] In 2009, Australian government support amplified this work by providing funding for a national coordinating unit (RHDAustralia) and support to jurisdictional control programs in a number of states. An extensive review of this program in 2017 identified a number of successes, particularly improved adherence to secondary prophylaxis and epidemiologic data. The review identified future opportunities around a strengthened role for primary care, improved community education, improving automation and strengthening capacity for primary and primordial intervention.[119] A national research initiative is now underway in Australia to develop an evidence-based strategy to eliminate RHD (the "RHD Endgame Strategy").[120] Community models of care, primary prevention, and comprehensive primary healthcare are likely to be part of this strategy.

The resources of Australia and New Zealand and the sharp ethnic disparities in ARF/RHD make control programs different from the rest of the world. However, the evolution in both countries to pivot from register-based secondary prophylaxis to primary prevention and an increased focused on community-based care has some parallels with international experience.

---

overarching goal is to develop a national strategy for ARF/RHD prevention and control with an RHD control toolkit. A national computer register is centrally maintained, in addition to paper registers at hospitals and health centers. The program includes primary and

secondary prophylaxis with a major focus on staff training and addressing provider fears about adverse drug reactions to BPG.[92]

In Uganda, an RHD register was initiated in 2010 as a partnership between the Uganda Heart Institute and the Ministry of Health.[93] Echocardiography screening in 2011 provided new evidence about the burden of disease and spurred an active research collaboration with international partners.[94] With ongoing research and philanthropic funding, the RHD control program in Uganda has expanded from the capital Kampala to three new sites. This allows increased access to secondary prophylaxis clinics, echocardiography services, and referrals for surgical evaluation.[95] Ongoing research efforts have elucidated determinants of secondary prophylaxis adherence, offered new insights into the treatment cascade for patients retained in ongoing care, and explored the role of peer support groups.[96–98] Mortality for people with RHD in the control program is high (1 year mortality rate of 17.8%) with optimal care available to only about a third of patients.[99]

In Tunisia, an RHD control program was established in 1978.[100,101] The program entailed core elements of primary prevention, secondary prevention, and making ARF a notifiable disease.[101] Economic development supported improvements in the social determinants of health over this time. By 2015, the incidence of ARF had fallen from a peak of 900 cases of ARF annually in the late 1970s to 9.[101] This reduction in new cases has paralleled a reduction in new cases of RHD.[100]

Contemporary recommendations for RHD control programs

In 2013, the WHF reemphasized the importance of control programs by identifying them as one of five targets to achieve the goal of a 25% reduction in premature deaths from ARF and RHD in people under 25 years by the 2025. Specifically, the WHF sought to "ensure that 90% of countries with endemic RHD have integrated and comprehensive control programmes by 2025."[45] However, the constituent parts of a "comprehensive" RHD control program were not defined.

A review of RHD control programs attempted to address this gap by analyzing WHO, WHF, and published evaluations of existing initiatives. This review informed development of a conceptual framework for describing comprehensive RHD control programs.[121] The conceptual framework included the traditional program elements (primary and secondary prevention, community education and health worker training) alongside emerging issues in RHD control (the role of echocardiography screening, access to BPG, clinical guidelines, government engagement and advocacy). This framework is reproduced in Fig. 12.1 and underpins the RHD Action resource, Tools for Implementing RHD Control Programmes (TIPS).[70] TIPs, in turn, articulates with the RHD Action Needs Assessment Tool.[122]

The TIPs framework helps codify a "typical" pathway in developing RHD control programs that has evolved in recent decades.[70] A generalized trajectory often includes the following elements:

- Concerned clinicians identify that the burden of RHD is high in a given location and often become champions for tackling the condition. This sometimes occurs in conjunction with visiting surgical teams or humanitarian outreach programs.
- Clinicians and collaborators work to document the burden of disease through clinical record audits or active echocardiography screening.
- The process of identifying cases of RHD catalyzes the creation of an RHD register that can be used to facilitate improved delivery of secondary prophylaxis.
- Register development, prophylaxis delivery, community, and health worker education generally begin in a relatively defined geographic region, the location of which is often influenced by disease champions.
- Governments or other funding agencies become engaged in RHD control and may provide some resourcing for scale up to new areas.
- Research activities engage more people in the nascent RHD control program and can provide additional funding sources.

Therefore, the TIPs document is structured so the first five boxes reflect and support these priority areas, in addition to providing a foundation for future development. These first five priority areas are addressed in more detail in Table 12.2.

Longitudinal narrative review of RHD control activities also identifies common programmatic risks. In particular:

- Individual champions who are passionate about RHD control often spearhead program development and are critical to engaging others. Programs can falter if these lynchpin individuals are no longer available. This risk can be mitigated by the formation of an RHD Committee to provide a mechanism for engaging and educating a larger number of RHD champions.
- The protracted causal path of RHD means that activity needs to be sustained for a decade before changes in disease outcomes can be demonstrated. Impetus for program delivery may fade or be crowded out by competing priorities before an impact on disease metrics has been achieved. Using interim measures in primary and secondary prevention, health-seeking behavior can help minimize this risk and demonstrate early evidence of efficacy.

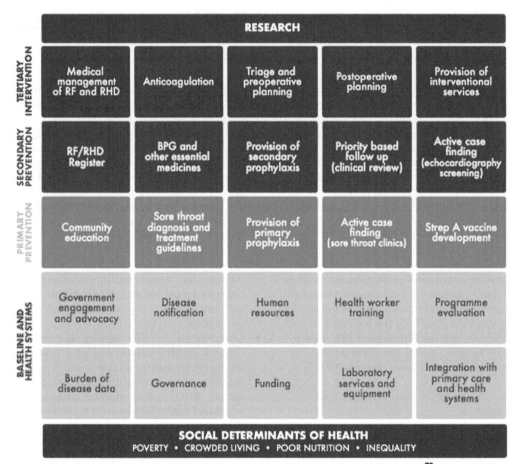

FIG. 12.1 **Conceptual Framework for Rheumatic Heart Disease Control Programs[70].** A conceptual framework for comprehensive rheumatic heart disease control programs. Components are arranged in approximate order of priority, working from left to right, bottom to top, in each row. *RF*, rheumatic fever; *RHD*, rheumatic heart disease; *BPG*, benzathine penicillin G.

- Monitoring and evaluation are not embedded into the design of RHD control programs, which makes it difficult to demonstrate success or identify areas for improvement.
- Almost all measurable successes in RHD control have occurred in relatively small, defined geographic/administrative areas. Effective systems for scale up and expansion have not yet been defined, reflecting a shared challenge with other health interventions in low-resource settings.[123]
- Medically and technically advanced approaches (echocardiography screening and cardiac surgical services) may be valued more highly than "basic" innovations in primary healthcare delivery. There is reasonable evidence for focusing on primary healthcare, community education, community

health workers, clinical guidelines, and penicillin delivery as first priorities in RHD control.

The 2018 WHO resolution on ARF and RHD represents a new era in RHD control. The resolution calls for support in *"identifying disease burden and, where appropriate, in developing and implementing rheumatic heart disease programmes and strengthening health systems in order to improve disease surveillance, increase the availability and training of the community and primary health care workforce, and ensure reliable access to affordable prevention, diagnostic and treatment tools."*[2] Additionally, increased rigor in monitoring and evaluation will be needed so that best practice can be identified and refined. New systems, leadership and institutions will be needed to meet this need. As technical support capacity grows some interim key lessons can be extracted

TABLE 12.2
Priority Activities for New Rheumatic Heart Disease Control Programs.

Burden of disease data	Some measure of ARF or RHD incidence, recurrence, or prevalence has been needed in almost all RHD control initiatives. This information can be used to established baseline burden (to assess the impact of subsequent intervention), engage governments and funding agencies to support control programs, and predict demand. Determining burden of RHD through echocardiography screening projects has catalyzed RHD control programs in many countries in recent years. Good use of routinely collected data or focused audits is also appropriate.
Government engagement and advocacy	Governments generally control access to health resources and are critical stakeholders in the success of RHD control programs. Ensuring that governments are aware of the local burden of RHD and are taking action to ensure the disease is included in National Action Plans for noncommunicable and health benefits packages is an important role for control programs.
Community education	Almost all RHD control programs have included some element of community education or awareness raising around GAS, ARF, or RHD. Ensuring that people at risk of ARF present for medical evaluation of relevant symptoms is a critical element of disease control—particularly to enable primary prevention of new cases. A further discussion on raising awareness of GAS, RHD, and RHD is included in Chapter 15.
RHD register	RHD registers have an essential role in supporting prophylaxis delivery, facilitating ongoing care delivery for people living with RHD and program evaluation. They may also be used for research, for managing surgical waiting lists and for providing focused education support to people with a history of ARF or living with RHD. Many registers also provide a focus point for healthcare workers seeking advice on how to manage RHD through a lead clinician.
Medical management of ARF and RHD	RHD control initiatives have a humanitarian imperative to support care delivery for people already living with ARF and RHD, alongside activities to prevent new cases of disease. In some places this means facilitating access to surgical services but even in the absence of surgical capacity, medical care can include accurate diagnosis, management of complications and comorbidities.

ARF, acute rheumatic fever; *RHD*, rheumatic heart disease; *GAS*, group A streptococcus

from existing program experience, outlined in Box 12.3. These pragmatic suggestions closely parallel the six recommended control program elements of the 2001 WHO Technical Report on ARF and RHD (secondary prevention, primary prevention, health education, health worker training, epidemiologic surveillance, and community involvement).[124] The challenge now, as it was then, is to support countries to implement these elements in high quality, scalable and replicable ways.

INTRODUCTION TO DISEASE REGISTERS WITH A FOCUS ON RHEUMATIC HEART DISEASE

Registers of people with a history of ARF or established RHD underpin the idea of contemporary RHD control programs. Early registers provided critical information about the natural history of RHD and supported delivery of evolving secondary prophylaxis regimes.[125] However, the definition, goals, and utility of ARF/RHD registers have evolved in conjunction with increasing complexity of RHD control programs and clinical care delivery. Some registers have expanded to incorporate echocardiography screening studies, others as clinical research initiatives or surgical waiting lists. This section introduces issues related to disease specific registers and identifies priorities for register-based RHD control worldwide.

Introduction to Registers

Registers of people diagnosed with specific infectious diseases began in the late 1800s. These registers evolved and accelerated as treatments for these diseases emerged.[126] For example, from 1905 doctors in Denmark were required to notify cases of pulmonary

> **BOX 12.3**
> **Ten Key Lessons for Rheumatic Heart Disease Control Programs**
>
> 1. A mix of primary prevention activities (community awareness, healthcare worker training) and register-based secondary prevention is needed to reduce the incidence of ARF and slow progression of RHD.
> 2. RHD control activities should be embedded into comprehensive primary healthcare programs wherever possible—and it is usually possible.
> 3. The RHD register can be used to support service delivery in primary care and can be used to provide clinical and administrative advice. A register coordinator and a lead clinician help ensure these roles are fulfilled and can be champions for the program.
> 4. Sustained effort and investment are needed for at least a decade to have a measurable impact on ARF and RHD outcomes.
> 5. Government funding and administrative support is a prerequisite for sustainability and scale up in almost all settings. Efforts to engage governments and transition to their operational management of programs should begin as early as possible.
> 6. Community engagement, education, and capacity building are important to increase access to healthcare for primary prevention and to ensure that people at greatest risk of RHD have a voice in tackling the disease.
> 7. Healthcare worker training is necessary to support the use of clinical guidelines for diagnosis and management of ARF and RHD.
> 8. It is generally more feasible to address these issues in smaller geographic and administrative areas before scaling up to state or national levels. The science of scale up needs to be further refined.
> 9. Research activities can be an important way to engage, amplify, and upskill people in RHD control and to augment funding sources. Epidemiologic research using echocardiographic screening can catalyze RHD control programs but is not a prerequisite for program development.
> 10. Action on household crowding and other social determinants of health was a mainstay of early RHD control programs but is rare in contemporary initiatives. Addressing social determinants of health remains a valid target for research, advocacy, and potential intervention.

ARF, acute rheumatic fever; *RHD*, rheumatic heart disease

tuberculosis to the National Health Service. From the 1920s onwards, these notified cases were monitored by the Danish Tuberculosis Index, tracking movement of individuals between jurisdictions, recording disease relapses and mortality data by cross-referencing with death certificates.[127] The number of disease-specific registers grew dramatically in the 1950s, encompassing noncommunicable and rare diseases. Many of these midcentury registers were intended primarily as epidemiologic tools to describe the prevalence of disease in a given population. This was reflected in a focus on complete coverage of a geographic population, commonly described as a "population-based registry."[128] With increased computing power came increased capacity for data collection and analysis, dramatically expanding the role of disease-specific registers.

The organic expansion of disease registers has led to an unstructured nomenclature with many overlapping terms and an expanding range of register types. This has generated a large number of definitions and

classification systems for disease registers.[129,130] Many of these grew from early definitions of a disease register, including from WHO in 1974 as "the unique identification of each person who presents with a case of the disease, the establishment of a permanent record of all such people, including the recording of all such data as are necessary for identification purposes, the collection of subsequent data for each individual in relation to the course of the disease or to the prevention of relapses."[131] Additionally, important defining characteristics of registers include the following: the ability to merge data from different sources into a single record, that data collection is standardized, that data collection rules are established prospectively, that each patient has a continuous record for data storage, and that follow-up data are recorded.[129]

Different types of registers fulfill different functions that leads to further confusion in terminology. An overview of different types of registers is presented in Table 12.3 with reference to how these different types relate to ARF and RHD.

TABLE 12.3
Types of Registers and Sample Application to Rheumatic Heart Disease.

Types or Roles of Registers	Rationale	Example from Other Disease Registers	Relevance to ARF and RHD Registers
Public health	Primarily an epidemiologic tool to facilitate measures of incidence, prevalence or for disease surveillance. Burden of disease data rely on the register being "population-based" and reflecting a defined community	Population-based cancer registers are used in both high- and low-resource settings to monitor trends in cancer epidemiology.[132]	Population level RHD registers are those that record cases from a defined geographic area with high levels of reporting—for example, in the Northern Territory of Australia[133]
Patient care	Intended to improve or facilitate clinical care	An increasing number of noncommunicable disease registers are used in low-resource settings to facilitate high-quality, guideline-based care[134,135]	RHD registers can be used to support delivery of secondary prophylaxis, follow-up plans and potentially also for management of waiting lists for surgical procedures
Health services research	Intended for evaluation of healthcare delivery, audits and assessment of healthcare quality. These are often hospital-based registers	Tuberculosis registers are widely used in low-resource settings to assess treatment outcomes and service delivery.[136]	RHD registers may be used for services research, for example, in Australia to assess adherence to national RHD guidelines[137] and in Uganda to assess the proportion of people on the RHD register needing surgical evaluation.[138]
Health promotion tools and education	Intended to facilitate outreach education	The National Gestational Diabetes Register in Australia is used to send reminders about diabetes screening and lifestyle to women who have been identified as having diabetes during pregnancy[139]	RHD registers may be used to collect contact data and engage people living with RHD in health education and secondary prophylaxis reminders, including text messages
Clinical research	Registration of people with a disease to understand the natural history of disease or evaluate interventions	Congenital pediatric cardiac surgery databases are used to monitor operative outcomes in high- and low-resource settings[140]	Collection of research data to answer outstanding questions about diagnosis and management of ARF/RHD, for example the REMEDY and VALVAFRIC studies.[141,142] Other registers explore pregnancy outcomes, including for women with RHD[143]
Regulatory	Intended to assess safety of new drugs or devices after they are approved for marketing use	Registers are commonly established to evaluate outcomes from new technologies in cardiology, for example the national Transcatheter Valve Therapy Registry established in the United States[144]	New therapeutic agents for RHD may emerge, potentially including new valve devices or new medications. For example, the INVICTUS study will form a register of people with RHD to explore the use of new anticoagulation agents[145]

ARF, acute rheumatic fever; *RHD*, rheumatic heart disease
Adapted from Richesson and Vehik.[126]

Issues Specific to Rheumatic Heart Disease Registers

The natural history of ARF/RHD means that ARF/RHD registers have a constellation of unique features and challenges. First, RHD is one of few diseases in which register enrollment is generally intended to facilitate clinical care over a period of years—decades for the delivery of secondary prophylaxis. Although registers for other diseases are used to facilitate clinical care, register enrollment is usually only for a defined period of relatively timely treatment (for example, tuberculosis). Additionally, in RHD, the period of register enrollment also tends to span pediatric and adult services that can be associated with fragmentation of care in some countries. Second, the inclusion of people with a history of ARF or early-stage disease detected on echocardiographic screening is novel—in that, people in the "latent" subclinical phase of disease are often included. Third, ARF and/or RHD is a notifiable condition in some endemic locations. However, in the absence of a clear diagnostic test, laboratory notification is not possible and links are needed between clinicians notifying notification systems and ARF/RHD registers. Finally, the inclusion of people who have had cardiac surgical procedures for RHD may introduce additional data domains that would usually be confined to a surgical outcomes database. These unique features coexist in a disease that is neglected by funders and occurs almost exclusively in low-resource populations. Therefore, the challenge of developing and deploying best practice and standards for RHD registers is considerable.

Variations in the primary role of RHD registers have made it difficult to establish and disseminate data definitions and standards. A global registry was first launched in 2008 in conjunction with the WHF and the A.S.A.P program to combine clinical and research goals.[146] Paper data collection forms and a Microsoft Access database were made available online and formed the basis of national register development in some countries. This project has evolved into the development of an electronic CommCare database, used as a register in Zambia and planned for expansion through the PASCAR program.[147] A large number of other research initiatives have used customized REDCap databases for data collection, including projects in Uganda, Nepal, and Brazil.[33,96,148] Other countries have established their own data collection instruments and standards—ranging from simple spreadsheet software in Timor-Leste[149] to a customized web-based register in Fiji[150] and detailed recommended dataset standards in Australia.[151] Many of these approaches to collecting and recording data show promise, but there is yet to

be overwhelming global consensus on how ARF and RHD are best defined, documented, and recorded.

The absence of data standardization for ARF/RHD care is a missed opportunity to deliver better quality care and to enhance global understanding of the disease. For example, without a standardized nomenclature for RHD, transfers of people between different control program areas may result in data loss if data fields do not align. This has real world implications given many of the communities with a high burden of RHD are geographically mobile, including refugee and migrant populations.[152] Similarly, there is no agreed definition of "lost to follow-up" or how to record people who have been prescribed, but are not receiving, secondary prophylaxis. This leads to inconsistencies in reporting of secondary prophylaxis adherence—a critical measure of program success. For example, removing people who have been lost to follow-up from register analysis can artificially inflate the proportion of people receiving adequate secondary prophylaxis.[153] Inconsistencies in terms and recording therefore have the potential to cloud or confound evidence of program effect. This kind of variation in data collection and recording is in stark contrast to other control programs for diseases of global public health significance. For example, global tuberculosis guidelines have had a highly standardized nomenclature making it possible to record suspected/confirmed cases, screening status and a small number of treatment outcomes.[154] Similarly, a modular rare disease registry framework has been developed and uses "base modules" (patient details, diagnosis information) as a foundation for customization to different projects and outcomes of interest.[155] The TIPs handbook proposes some similar standards for RHD, but, in the absence of definitive global clinical guidelines, agreement and adoption of data standards is challenging.[70]

The last WHO clinical guidelines for ARF and RHD were developed in 2001, preceding widespread echocardiography screening projects, updated Jones Criteria for ARF diagnosis and the resurgence of control programs in the late 2000s. A comprehensive global clinical guideline for management of ARF and RHD in resource-limited settings is urgently needed to inform data standards for register development. The issue of data standardization has been faced by other disease communities. For example, in 1966 the International Association of Cancer Registries was formed to develop standardized procedures for a growing number of cancer registers worldwide.[156] A similar approach is needed for RHD including development of a data dictionary and recommendations about a minimum essential dataset. Some countries have established their own data standards but these have not been adopted internationally, and considerable variation in terminology and definitions remains a barrier to international progress.[151] Establishing global RHD register standards should be a priority to measure progress following the 2018 WHA resolution on RHD. In the interim, researchers and register developers should work together to maximize the interoperability of existing terms and resources.

Trade-offs between feasibility of data collection and data utility for clinical and research purposes are inevitable.[157] It is not possible for register-based programs to maintain an entire medical record on every person with a history of ARF or RHD. Judicious selection of relevant data is needed, and this is underpinned by the core goals of the register. People living with RHD around the world have persistently poor clinical outcomes. The medical ethics principle of beneficence means that RHD registers should have capacity to improve delivery of healthcare, particularly the delivery of secondary prophylaxis. Research databases in the absence of mechanisms to enhance care delivery risk compounding global inequalities in RHD, especially in populations that are overresearched and underserved. This is particularly pertinent for registers initiated following echocardiography screening studies.

Recent data from New Zealand illustrate the ongoing value of register-based delivery of secondary prophylaxis. Young people receiving secondary prophylaxis injections through a register-based program received 94% of their scheduled injections. In contrast, those who received their injections through an unstructured primary care program received only 37% of their scheduled injections.[158] Therefore, all registers should have capacity to record adherence with secondary prophylaxis for people who have been prescribed prophylaxis. Additionally, registers should have a mechanism to share this information with usual care providers, ideally through integrating with clinical record systems. In practice, this kind of integration is enormously challenging in low-resource settings and advocacy for health system resourcing and strengthening may be the first useful step toward integration. For example, a recent study of South African primary care clinics found that each clinic was attempting to maintain more than 20 different paper-based registers (spanning tuberculosis to pap smears) in addition to two kinds of electronic registers.[159] New register developers should consider ways to minimize this kind of administrative burden, acknowledging that electronic medical records systems in developing countries are

probably necessary to substantively address these issues.[160]

To support longitudinal care delivery and improved epidemiologic understanding, registers should also be as demographically and clinically inclusive as possible, including pediatric and adult patients and the full spectrum of disease severity.[161] For example, registers should have capacity to record data about history of ARF, screening-detected asymptomatic RHD, people actively receiving secondary prophylaxis or who have completed secondary prophylaxis, people who are awaiting or have undergone surgery. Opportunities to link to vital statistic data and death records may provide an important epidemiologic function in understanding disease outcomes.

In addition to improving secondary prevention, an RHD register should have adaptable modular elements to meet specific research or follow-up objectives. For example, in Australia, a priority-based system is incorporated into RHD registers to specify follow-up needs for individual patients.[162] Other opportunities may include recording adverse reactions to secondary prophylaxis injections. It may be helpful to collect sufficient information to be able to track the newly developed cascade of care and retention for RHD.[96] Collecting a small number of standardized socioeconomic indicators may also be a valuable way to compare data between jurisdictions and could potentially map to Sustainable Development Goal indicators to avoid excessive data collection. There is also a growing movement for people living with a specific disease to contribute to register development and data collection for that disease.[163] Engaging people living with RHD in register design and utilization may be an opportunity to build shared values between control programs and consumers.

Maintaining a functional disease register requires staffing support. For example, a survey of 23 cancer registries in sub-Saharan Africa found that approximately one full time equivalent staff member was employed per 300 registered cases.[132] Staffing roles included registration, administration, medical, programming, and statistician/epidemiologists. Regular training is required for people in these roles to maintain and develop skills.[164] Anecdotally, most RHD registers include database managers or program officers to review data fidelity, follow-up on missing information and extract reports.[92] In some settings, the ARF/RHD register is used to actively follow-up people who are due for secondary prophylaxis injections. This active outreach role necessitates additional staffing resources. Finally, registers should be associated with a lead clinician to have oversight and provide clinical support to other people managing ARF/RHD cases. The register provides a vehicle for this kind of collegiality and can be an important positive externality to support collaboration and education.[11,165]

Collection and retention of personal and medical information for ARF/RHD registers necessitates careful consideration of privacy and data governance. Confidentiality expectations are often enshrined in law in developed countries but less commonly in developing settings. Confusion about when and how information can be shared between agencies is common and has been reported by cancer registers in South Africa and Nigeria.[164,166] For data storage, some best practice examples have evolved from cancer register programs in Africa, including a register in Ghana that uses confidentiality agreements with staff and password-limited access to the register.[167] Similar standards should be developed by RHD registers and shared to assist others to establish similar practices. In some settings, strict regulatory standards may mean that patients need to sign formal consent to be enrolled in an RHD register.[168,169] Decisions about consent to be enrolled on a register are probably best made at a local level after consultation with a wide range of stakeholders and any relevant regulatory bodies.

When RHD register data are going to be (or may be) used for research, informed consent for research participation also needs to be considered. Some authors believe that the Declaration of Helsinki on ethical principles for medical research requires informed consent for data collection from individuals in population registers.[170] Others believe that this is unnecessarily onerous.[171] Much of this debate has focused on implications for high-resource settings though there has been some exploration of relevant issues in South Africa.[172] Where ethics bodies exist they should be consulted about local standards of consent for research. In the absence of local standards, consultation with peer countries and experts is recommended.

The structure of ARF/RHD registers varies worldwide, and different models are appropriate in various settings.[70] Some locations have a centralized (hospital or health department-based) register that often has an epidemiologic function. Others have local registers that are more often used to facilitate active case management at a community level. Electronic registers tend to be used centrally and offer benefits in accurate data collection and extraction. Paper-based records are often used at a local level. Although these have disadvantages in accuracy, they may offer reasonable functionality at low cost and greater acceptance by frontline staff.[157]

RHD registers are central to improving clinical care, providing clinical support for RHD, research, and improved epidemiologic understanding of the disease. Achieving these goals at a global scale remains an unmet challenge; too often, emerging RHD control programs have to work from first principles to develop local protocols and register standards. Addressing this gap will be integral to responding to the World Health Assembly RHD resolution—priorities for this work and for register developers are summarized in Box 12.4.

ACCESS TO CARE

Healthcare for GAS, ARF, and RHD is grossly insufficient in almost all settings with a high burden of disease. These are diseases of disparity that reflect the social determinants of health in which people live and work. This disparity extends to inadequate access to healthcare.

Inadequate access to care reflects challenges in almost all of the WHO Health System building blocks, impacting all levels of care for RHD, outlined in Table 12.4.[173] This population-level framework

---

BOX 12.4
Priorities for Rheumatic Heart Disease Registers

- Registers should be used to support secondary prophylaxis delivery, be a conduit for clinical advice services and be underpinned by adequate administrative support. Other register roles can be added to meet identified needs in different contexts.
- Agreed international minimum datasets for RHD registers should be established with clear case and data definitions.
- Maximum benefits can be accrued when the RHD register communicates with health records and with disease notification systems. Systems to facilitate this communication are needed in a variety of different settings.
- Resources should be developed so that this dataset can be recorded in different formats for different settings, including paper-based register and secure electronic registers.
- Protocols for sharing deidentified register data should be developed to help monitor progress toward RHD control goals globally and identify best practice in care delivery.
- In addition to data governance standards established in different countries, people and communities living with RHD should have input into the governance and management of RHD registers.

RHD, rheumatic heart disease

TABLE 12.4

Access to Care for Group A Streptococcus, Acute Rheumatic Fever, and Rheumatic Heart Disease by the WHO Health System Building Blocks.

	Service Delivery	Health Workforce	Health Information Systems	Access to Essential Medicines	Financing	Leadership/Governance
Primary prevention	Guidelines for management of sore throat are not available in many countries making consistent delivery of high-quality care very difficult.	Community health workers and nurses are often responsible for managing common childhood illnesses like sore throat but this is limited by a global shortage of frontline healthcare workers.[174]	Decision support resources to help identify that sore throats should be treated with antibiotics are rarely embedded into health information systems.	Access to essential medicines stymies effective management of RHD, particularly stockouts of the essential antibiotic BPG. [57,68]	Primary and secondary prevention of ARF are usually delivered in primary care settings. However, financing for primary care in endemic countries is often limited and cost-effective access to preventative care is frequently delayed or unavailable.[175]	Assessment, diagnosis, and management of sore throats are rarely prioritized—it may erroneously be considered a benign condition and not an opportunity to prevent a fatal noncommunicable disease.[176]
Secondary prevention	Clinical follow-up and adherence to secondary prophylaxis is often limited by resources and infrastructure constraints. Difficulties in delivering high-quality secondary prophylaxis are a missed opportunity to change the course of disease.	Dedicated staffing is needed to deliver register-based secondary prophylaxis but resourcing and training is often lacking when registers are established.	RHD registers and medical record infrastructure is essential for delivering secondary prophylaxis over many years.			Guidelines and governance on register formation and data use are often lacking, making it difficult to establish high quality secondary prophylaxis programs.
Tertiary intervention	Humanitarian surgical programs offer the only access to surgical services in most endemic settings—raising concerns about access sustainability and capacity development.[177]	Shortages of medical specialists limits diagnosis and management of advanced RHD	Safe and sustained pre- and postoperative care requires medial information to be transferred between different levels of the health service. Without health information systems, this process is often delayed or impossible.[70]	Medications to prevent and address the complications of RHD—including heart failure and arrhythmias are often not available in low resource settings. Diuretics, antiarrhythmics, anticoagulants and contraceptives are all needed.	Health financing in many RHD endemic, low-resource countries is insufficient to meet basic healthcare needs.[178] Financial costs for people with advanced RHD can be a catastrophic cause of medical bankruptcy.	Access to heart surgery is sometimes prioritized over preventative care. Leadership and good governance are needed to ensure that surgical services enhance local capacity and articulate with preventative activities

ARF, acute rheumatic fever; *RHD*, rheumatic heart disease; *BPG*, benzathine penicillin G

highlights the intersect between RHD care and the architecture needed to deliver health services—including essential medicines, information systems, financing and governance. Reviewing the WHO health systems building blocks illustrates the importance of health system strengthening to make reliable, high quality care available for people living with RHD.

RHD is a sentinel condition for health system strengthening because it spans infectious diseases, child health, adolescent health, maternal health, and adult chronic disease. Services are needed to treat sore throat in the most isolated clinics, in addition to providing open heart surgery in quaternary centers of excellence. The prolonged period of follow-up required for secondary prevention necessitates good health information systems, and the disease-altering antibiotic BPG is an

essential medicine that should be widely available. Therefore, RHD encompasses the gamut of priorities in low and middle-income countries and can be used to illustrate common issues across the life course using a single unifying disease. This approach may prove a useful lens for describing complex, interrelated issues in tangible ways to decision and policy makers.

At an individual level, access to care can be considered across five dimensions of healthcare access in the Levesque et al. model, outlined in Table 12.5.[179] This model highlights barriers to seeking and engaging in ongoing healthcare. It has been expanded and adapted by some authors to reflect unique challenges of Indigenous people seeking healthcare, a framework that may be useful for control programs in countries with an Indigenous burden of RHD.[180]

TABLE 12.5
Determinants of Healthcare Access and Relationship to Rheumatic Heart Disease.

Domain	Relationship to RHD Care
Approachability Knowledge that services exist	People with symptoms of GAS infection, ARF, and RHD need to know that health services are reachable and relevant to access them. In low-resource settings, where health literacy is low, this may be a major barrier. Additionally, awareness about specialty and surgical services in remote locations may be poor.
Affordability Capacity of people to spend time and money seeking health services	Out of pocket costs can be a barrier to all levels of prevention and care for RHD. For example, the cost of medication or clinic visits demonstrably reduces secondary prevention in Ethiopia.[181]
Availability and accommodation The geographic and temporal location of healthcare services	Geographic distance can be a barrier to accessing care. For example, in Tanzania and Ethiopia, cost, transport problems, and time away from home have been identified as barriers to primary prevention.[176,181] similarly, in New Zealand lack of access to health services outside of working hours made primary prevention more challenging.[182] these issues are amplified in secondary prevention when regular visits to healthcare facilities are needed over a period of many years.
Appropriateness The services provided meet the medical needs of people seeking care	Primary care for primary and secondary prevention of ARF is generally available, in that clinics and some health staff exist. However, quality of care and access to essential medicines is variable. Surgical services are rarely available in endemic settings. For example, in Uganda a review of register data indicated that over 3 years only 8% of the people needing surgical intervention for RHD received the necessary surgery.[138] similarly, the VALVAFRIC register study recruited from tertiary cardiac clinics in Cameroon, Cote d'Ivore, Gabon Guinea, Mali, Nigeria, Senegal and Togo between 2004 and 2008. Here, 1334 people with RHD were identified and 1200 (89.9%) had an indication for heart surgery. However, only 27 (2.3%) of people who needed an operation received surgery.[142]
Acceptability Social and cultural factors that determine whether people present for treatment and engage with medical care	Services to prevent and treat may not be acceptable to the people who are intended to use them. For example, some people preferentially visit traditional healers for management of sore throat.[183] experiences with racism and stigma may also be barriers to acceptable care, including in Australia and New Zealand.[184,185] Language, gender, and cultural barriers to care may also occur in other settings

GAS, group A streptococcus; ARF, acute rheumatic fever; RHD, rheumatic heart disease

The WHO building blocks and Levesque models both illustrate the complex individual, economic and systems factors that constrain access to care for RHD. It is not feasible or sensible for endemic countries to address these issues in isolation. Rather, a system is needed to address barriers to care for all conditions— and for GAS, ARF, and RHD to be included within that system. Efforts to achieve Universal Health Coverage (UHC) offer the most promising and effective opportunity to improve healthcare access and equity.

UHC addresses the belief that all people should be able to access health services of reasonable quality without financial hardship.[186] Achieving this necessarily involved trade-offs about the kinds of services covered, and the financial proportion of services covered.[187] The magnitude of UHC and trade-offs about coverage differ between various countries and communities. In some low-income settings, the choices are made explicit by defining a health benefits package—the services provided by the healthcare system.[188] This provides an important opportunity to embed RHD prevention and control in routine clinical services, particularly including diagnosis and management of childhood sore throat, secondary prophylaxis for people with a history of ARF and medical management of the consequences of RHD (including reproductive health services for women with RHD, anticoagulation, management of arrhythmia, and heart failure). Access to cardiac surgical services can also be addressed as part of a decision-making process on minimum health benefits package choices.

CONCLUSION

Reductions in the burden of RHD can be achieved without focused control programs when improvements in the social determinants of health are driven by sustained, substantive, and equal economic development. However, in settings where equity and economic development are not rapidly improving, active disease control measures are needed to reduce the burden of RHD. This remains the case in most of the developing world and some marginalized populations in high-income countries. The WHO Resolution on Rheumatic Fever and Rheumatic Heart Disease marks the beginning of a new era in RHD control activities.

The challenge is to shift RHD control programs from an intervention that can be delivered in smaller, scattered locations to a packaged approach that can be provided at scale.

The complexities of delivering high quality secondary prophylaxis still requires a dedicated register and register staffing in most places. Efficiencies and improvements are possible if an established minimum dataset and data dictionary for RHD registers can be defined. Primary prevention and basic clinical management are appropriately within the remit of comprehensive primary care services. The need for robust primary care services dovetails the broader health systems strengthening agenda and UHC. Indeed, RHD offers a tangible framework for addressing some of these critical issues.

REFERENCES

1. Dowdle WR. The principles of disease elimination and eradication. *Bull World Health Organ*. 1998;76(Suppl 2): 22–25.
2. WHO. . *Rheumatic Fever and Rheumatic Heart Disease*. WHA71.14. Geneva, Switzerland: World Health Organization; 2018. Available from: http://apps.who.int/gb/ebwha/pdf_files/WHA71/A71_R14-en.pdf.
3. Yacoub M, Mayosi B, ElGuindy A, Carpentier A, Yusuf S. Eliminating acute rheumatic fever and rheumatic heart disease. *Lancet*. 2017;390(10091):212–213.
4. Richie W. Rheumatic heart disease: its nature, course and prevention. *Edinb Med J*. 1935;42(7):T117–T128.
5. Markowitz M. Rheumatic fever—a half-century perspective (mm ref 1009). *Pediatrics*. 1998;102:272–274.
6. Richie W. The crusade against acute rheumatism. *Br Med J*. 1936;1(3926):679–683.
7. White G. The role of the medical social worker in the management and control of rheumatic fever and rheumatic heart disease. *Am J Med*. 1947;2(6):618–629.
8. Holland Clarke P. The clinical and public health aspects of juvenile rheumatism in Dublin. *Ir J Med Sci*. 1940; 171:98–118.
9. Wyber R, Carapetis J. Evolution, evidence and effect of secondary prophylaxis against rheumatic fever. *J Prac Cardiovasc Sci*. 2015;1(1):9–14.
10. Rose V, Boyd A, Ashton T. Incidence of heart disease in the children in the city of Toronto. *Can Med Assoc J*. 1964;91(3):95–100.
11. Gordis L, Lilienfeld A, Rodriguez R. An evaluation of the Maryland rheumatic fever registry. *Public Health Rep*. 1969;84:333–339.
12. Rutstein D. The role of the cardiac clinic in the rheumatic program. *JAMA*. 1944;126:484–486.
13. Strasser T, Dondog N, Kholy A, et al. The community control of rheumatic fever and rheumatic heart disease: report of a WHO international cooperative project. *Bull World Health Organ*. 1981;59(2):285–294.
14. Padmavati S, Sharma KB, Jayaram O. Epidemiology and prophylaxis of rheumatic fever in Deli – a five year follow-up. *Singap Med J*. 1973;14(3):457–461.
15. Nordet P. *Rheumatic Fever/Rheumatic Heart Disease Prevention: Lessons Learned 1999*. Available from: http://www.fac.org.ar/cvirtual/cvirteng/cienteng/sweng/swc6002i/inordet/inordet.htm.

16. Nordet P. WHO programme for the prevention of rheumatic fever/rheumatic heart disease in 16 developing countries: report from Phase I (1986-90). WHO cardiovascular diseases unit and principal investigators. *Bull World Health Organ*. 1992;70(2):213–218.

17. Organization WH. WHO Global Programme for the prevention of rheumatic fever/rheumatic heart disease in sixteen developing countries (AGFUND supported). In: *Meeting of National Programme Managers Geneva: 4–6 November, 1986*. 1986.

18. Bach JF, Chalons S, Forier E, et al. 10-year educational programme aimed at rheumatic fever in two French Caribbean islands. *Lancet*. 1996;347:644–648.

19. Arguedas A, Mohs E. Prevention of rheumatic fever in Costa Rica. *J Pediatr*. 1992;121(4):569–572.

20. Millard-Bullock D. The rheumatic fever and rheumatic heart disease control programme—Jamaica. *West Indian Med J*. 2012;61(4):361–364.

21. Nordet P, Lopez R, Duenas A, Sarmiento L. Prevention and control of rheumatic fever and rheumatic heart disease: the Cuban experience (1986–1996–2002). *Cardiovasc J Afr*. 2008;19(3):135–140.

22. Mota C, Meira Z, Graciano R, Graciano F, Araujo F. Rheumatic fever prevention program: long-term evolution and outcomes. *Front Paediatr*. 2014;2:141. https://doi.org/10.3389/fped.2014.00141.

23. Gordis L. Effectiveness of comprehensive-care programs in preventing rheumatic fever. *N Engl J Med*. 1973;289:331–335.

24. Durham J, Kljakovic M. *Primary Prevention of Rheumatic Fever: Is There a Role for General Practice*. Wellington, New Zealand: General Practice Department, Wellington School of Medicine and New Zealand Ministry of Health; 1997.

25. El Kholy A, Rotta J, Wannamaker L, et al. Recent advances in rheumatic fever control and future prospects: a WHO Memorandum. *Bull World Health Organ*. 1978;56(6):887–912.

26. WHO. *The WHO Global Programme for the Prevention of Rheumatic Fever and Rheumatic Heart Disease. Report of a Consultation to Review Progress and Develop Future Activities*. Geneva: World Health Organization; 1999. Contract No.: WHO/CVD00.1.

27. World Health Organization. Strategy for controlling rheumatic fever/rheumatic heart disease, with emphasis on primary prevention: memorandum from a joint WHO/ISFC meeting. *Bull World Health Organ*. 1995;73:583–587.

28. JR C. In: Wyber R, ed. *Review of the WHO 1980s/1990s RHD Program*. 2019.

29. PAHO. *Prevention and Control of Rheumatic Fever in the Community. Manual of Operational Standards for a Progam to Extend Coverage at Different Levels of Care*. Scientified Publication No. 399. Washington, D.C.: Pan American Health Organization.; 1985.

30. ISFC, WHO, UNESCO. *ISFC/WHO/UNESCO Joint Project on RF/RHD Prevention and Health Promotion in School Children*. Guidelines for the Plan of Operation for Phase I. 1995 17. August 1995.

31. Wilson W, Hughes G. Rheumatic disease in Jamaica. *Ann Rheum Dis*. 1970;38:320–325.

32. Little SG. The challenges of managing rheumatic disease of the mitral valve in Jamaica. *Cardiol Young*. 2014;24(6):1108–1110.

33. Nascimento BR, Beaton AZ, Nunes MC, et al. Echocardiographic prevalence of rheumatic heart disease in Brazilian school children: data from the PROVAR study. *Int J Cardiol*. 2016;219:439–445.

34. Karthikeyan G, Mayosi BM. Letter by Karthikeyan et al regarding article, "Acute rheumatic fever and rheumatic heart disease: incidence and progression in the Northern Territory of Australia, 1997 to 2010. *Circulation*. 2014;129(11):e396.

35. Nordet P, Lopez R, Duenas A, Luis S. Prevention and control of rheumatic fever and rheumatic heart disease: the Cuban experience (1986–1996–2002). *Cardiovasc J Afr*. 2008;19(3):135–140.

36. Tompkins D, Boxerbaum B, Liebman J. Long-term prognosis of rheumatic fever patients receiving regular intramuscular benzathine penicillin. *Circulation*. 1972;45:543–551.

37. Markowitz M. The decline of rheumatic fever: role of medical intervention. Lewis W. Wannamaker Memorial Lecture. *J Pediatr*. 1985;106:545–550.

38. Sitaj S, Urbanek T, Bosmansky K. Some aspects of epidemiology and surveillance of rheumatic fever. *Scand J Rheumatol*. 1987;16(1):30–39.

39. Ekelund H, Enocksson E, Michaelsson M, Voss H. The incidence of acute rheumatic fever in Swedish children 1952–1961. A survey from four hospitals. *Acta Med Scand*. 1967;181(1):89–92.

40. Massell B, Chute C, Walker A, Kurland G. Penicillin and the marked decrease in the morbidity and mortality from rheumatic fever in the United States. *N Engl J Med*. 1988;1988(318):280–286.

41. Michaud C, Gutierrez J, Cruz C, Pearson T. Rheumatic heart disease. In: Jamison DT, Mosley WH, Measham AR, Bobadilla JL, eds. *Disease Control Priorities in Developing Countries*. New York: World Bank; 1993:221.

42. Strasser T. Cost-effective control of rheumatic fever in the community. *Health Policy*. 1985;5(2):159–164.

43. Kaplan EL. Current status of rheumatic fever control programs in the United States (mm ref 2160). *Public Health Rep*. 1981;96(3):267–268.

44. Thornley C, McNicholas A, Baker M, Lennon D. Rheumatic fever registers in New Zealand. *N Z Public Health Rep*. 2001;8(6):41–44.

45. Remenyi B, Carapetis J, Wyber R, Taubert K, Mayois B. Position statement of the world heart federation on the prevention and control of rheumatic heart disease. *Nat Rev Cardiol*. 2013;10:284–292.

46. WHO. *WHO Expert Consultation on Rheumatic Fever and Rheumatic Heart Disease*. Geneva: World Health Organisation; 2001, 29 October–1 November, 2001. Report No: WHO Technical Report Series;923.

47. Oli K, Asmera J. Rheumatic heart disease in Ethiopia: could it be more malignant. *Ethiop Med J*. 2004;41(1):1–8.

48. Danbauchi S, Alhassan M, David S, Wammanda R, Oyati I. Spectrum of rheumatic heart disease in Zaria, Northern Nigeria. *Ann Afr Med.* 2004;3(1):17−21.

49. Mayosi B, Robertson K, Volmink J, et al. The Drakensberg declaration on the control of rheumatic fever and rheumatic heart disease in Africa. *S Afr Med J.* 2006; 96(3):246.

50. Marijon E, Ou P, Celermajer DS, et al. Prevalence of rheumatic heart disease detected by echocardiographic screening. *N Engl J Med.* 2007;357(5):470−476.

51. Rothenbuhler M, O'Sullivan CJ, Stortecky S, et al. Active surveillance for rheumatic heart disease in endemic regions: a systematic review and meta-analysis of prevalence among children and adolescents. *Lancet Glob Health.* 2014;2(12):e717−e726.

52. Saxena A, Zuhlke L, Wilson N. Echocardiographic screening for rheumatic heart disease: issues for the cardiology community. *Glob Heart.* 2013;8(3):197−202.

53. Karthikeyan G, Mayosi B. Is primary prevention of rheumatic fever the missing link in the control of rheumatic heart disease in Africa? *Circulation.* 2009;120(8). https://doi.org/10.1161/CIRCULATIONAHA.108.836510.

54. Lennon D, Stewart J, Farrell E, Palmer A, Mason H. School-based prevention of acute rheumatic fever: a group randomized trial in New Zealand. *Pediatr Infect Dis J.* 2009;28(9):787−794.

55. Lennon D, Kerdemelidis M, Arroll B. Meta-analysis of trials of streptococcal throat treatment programs to prevent rheumatic fever. *Pediatr Infect Dis J.* 2009;28(7):e259−e264.

56. Robinson O, Kwang G, Romain J, Crapanzo M, Wilentz J. A national coordinated cardiac surgery registry in Haiti: the Haiti cardiac alliance experience. *Lancet Glob Health.* 2016;4(S31). http://www.thelancet.com/pdfs/journals/langlo/PIIS2214-109X(16)30036-5.pdf.

57. Wyber R. *Global Status of BPG Report: RHD Action;* 2016. Available from: https://rhdaction.org/sites/default/files/RHD%20Action_Global%20Status%20of%20BPG%20Report_Online%20Version.pdf.

58. Carapetis J, Brown A, Wilson NJ, Edwards K. An Australian guideline for rheumatic fever and rheumatic heart disease: an abridged outline. *Med J Aust.* 2007;186(11):581−586.

59. Atatoa-Carr P, Lennon D, Wilson N, New Zealand Rheumatic Fever Guidelines Writing Group. Rheumatic fever diagnosis, management, and secondary prevention: a New Zealand guideline. *N Z Med J.* 2008;121(1271):59−69.

60. Working Group on Pediatric Acute Rheumatic Fever. Consensus guidelines on pediatric acute rheumatic fever and rheumatic heart disease. *Indian Pediatr.* 2008;45:565−573.

61. *World heart federation regional reports.* In: *CVD Prevention and Control.* vol. 2. 2008:103−113.

62. Ali SKM, Al Khaleefa MS, Khair SM. *Acute Rheumatic Fever and Rheumatic Heart Disease: Sudan's Guidelines for Diagnosis.* Management and Prevention; 2017.

63. Kheir SM, Ali SKM. The control of rheumatic fever and rheumatic heart disease: a call to raise the awareness. *Sudan J Paediatr.* 2014;14(1):21.

64. Markbreiter J. *RHD Global Status Report: People, Policy, Programmes, Progress.* Geneva, Switzerland: RHD Action; 2016.

65. Ali SKM, Al Khaleefa MS, Khair SM. *Acute Rheumatic Fever and Rheumatic Heart Disease: Sudan's Guidelines for Diagnosis, Management and Prevention.* Sudan's Federal Ministry of Health, Sudan's Heart Society-Working Group on Paediatric Cardiology, Sudanese Association of Paediatricians and Sudanese Children's Heart Society. 2017.

66. Khalid E, El Banna H, Mahmoud R, Hassan H, El Mahdi L, Ali S. Clinical and echocardiographic features of 370 children with rheumatic heart disease seen in Khartoum. *Sudan Med J.* 2014;11(2256):1−8.

67. Ali S, Domi S, Abbo B, et al. Echocardiographic screening for rheumatic heart disease in 4 515 Sudanese school children: marked disparity between two communities. *Cardiovasc J Afr.* 2018;29:1−5.

68. Nurse-Findlay S, Taylor MM, Savage M, et al. Shortages of benzathine penicillin for prevention of mother-to-child transmission of syphilis: an evaluation from multi-country surveys and stakeholder interviews. *PLoS Med.* 2017;14(12):e1002473.

69. Ali A, Domi S, Elfaki A, et al. The echocardiographic prevalence of rheumatic heart disease in Northern Kodofan and initation of a control program. *Sudan Med J.* 2017; 53(2):63−68.

70. Wyber R, Johnson T, Perkins S, Watkins D, Mwangi J, La Vincente S. *Tools for Implementing Rheumatic Heart Disease Control Programmes (TIPs) Handbook.* 2nd ed. Geneva, Switzerland: RHD Action; 2018.

71. WHO. WHO programme for the prevention of rheumatic fever/rheumatic heart disease in 16 developing countries: report from Phase I (1986−90). *Bull World Health Organ.* 1992;70(2):213−218.

72. Musuku J, Chipili J, Machila E, et al. Fostering public awareness for rheumatic heart disease in Zambia: progress and lessons learned. *Pediatrics.* 2018;141(1).

73. Musuku J, Lungu JC, Machila E, et al. Epidemiology of pharyngitis as reported by Zambian school children and their families: implications for demand-side interventions to prevent rheumatic heart disease. *BMC Infect Dis.* 2017;17(1):473.

74. Long A, Lungu JC, Machila E, et al. A programme to increase appropriate usage of benzathine penicillin for management of streptococcal pharyngitis and rheumatic heart disease in Zambia. *Cardiovasc J Afr.* 2017;28(4):242−247.

75. RHD Action. *RHD Action Small Grant Update: Zambia;* 2018. Available from: http://rhdaction.org/news/rhd-action-small-grant-update-zambia.

76. Beckett D. Rheumatic carditis in Fiji. *Fiji Sch Med J.* 1970; 5(1):14−15.

77. Varea S, Ram P. Acute rheumatic fever and rheumatic heart disease in Fiji. *Fiji Med J.* 1986;14(3&4):66−70.

78. Randall G. Rheumatic fever and rheumatic heart disease in Labasa. *Fiji Sch Med J.* 1970;5(1):10−11.

79. Negus R. Rheumatic fever in Western Fiji, the female preponderance. *Med J Aust.* 1971;2:251−254.

80. Steer AC, Kado J, Wilson N, et al. High prevalence of rheumatic heart disease by clinical and echocardiographic screening among children in Fiji. *J Heart Valve Dis.* 2009; 18(3):327–335. Discussion 36.

81. Parks T, Kado J, Colquhoun S, Carapetis J, Steer A. Underdiagnosis of acute rheumatic fever in primary care settings in a developing country. *Trop Med Int Health.* 2009;14(11):1407–1413.

82. Heenan R, Barnighausen T, O'Brien J, et al. The cost-of-illness of rheumatic heart diseases: a national estimation in Fiji. *Glob Heart.* 2014;9(1):e30–e31.

83. Steer AC, Vidmar S, Ritika R, et al. Normal ranges of streptococcal antibody titers are similar whether streptococci are endemic to the setting or not. *Clin Vaccine Immunol.* 2009;16(2):172–175.

84. Colquhoun SM, Carapetis JR, Kado JH, et al. Pilot study of nurse-led rheumatic heart disease echocardiography screening in Fiji—a novel approach in a resource-poor setting. *Cardiol Young.* 2013;23(4):546–552.

85. Engelman D, Kado JH, Remenyi B, et al. Focused cardiac ultrasound screening for rheumatic heart disease by briefly trained health workers: a study of diagnostic accuracy. *Lancet Glob Health.* 2016;4(6):e386–e394.

86. Engelman D, Kado J, Remenyi B, et al. Teaching focused echocardiography for rheumatic heart disease screening. *Ann Pediatr Cardiol.* 2015;8(2):118–121.

87. Ward A, Erbas B, Taiot R, et al. PW353 the Fiji acute rheumatic fever prophylaxis adherence study. *Glob Heart.* 2014;9(S1):e331.

88. Engelman D, Wheaton GR, Mataika RL, et al. Screening-detected rheumatic heart disease can progress to severe disease. *Heart Asia.* 2016;8(2):67–73.

89. Engelman D, Mataika RL, Ah Kee M, et al. Clinical outcomes for young people with screening-detected and clinically-diagnosed rheumatic heart disease in Fiji. *Int J Cardiol.* 2017;240:422–427.

90. Buli AR. *Wainiqolo Strong Advocate for Rheumatic Fever Prevention in Fiji: RHD Action;* 2017. Available from: http://rhdaction.org/news/buli-wainiqolo-strong-advocate-rheumatic-fever-prevention-fiji.

91. Kennedy E, Naiceru E, Ramaka A, Matatolu L, Silai M, Boladuadua S, et al. Innovations in delivery of secondary prophylaxis treatment for people living with RHD in the Fiji Islands. In: *20th Lancefield International Symposium on Streptococci and Streptococcal Disases; Suva, Fiji.* 2017.

92. Regmi P. Comprehensive approach to rheumatic fever and rheumatic heart disease prevention and control: the Nepalese model. *Nepalse Heart J.* 2016;13(2):3–10.

93. Omagino J. Rheumatic heart disease in Uganda. Treatment and prevention. In: *Uganda RHD Stakeholders Meeting; Kampala, Uganda.* 2017.

94. Beaton A, Okello E, Lwabi P, Mondo C, McCarter R, Sable C. Echocardiography screening for rheumatic heart disease in Ugandan schoolchildren. *Circulation.* 2012; 125(25):3127–3132.

95. Okello E, Longenecker C, Scheel A, et al. Impact of regionalization of a national rheumatic heart disease registry: the Ugandan experience. *Heart Asia.* 2018;10(1). https://doi.org/10.1136/heartasia-2017-010981.

96. Longenecker CT, Morris SR, Aliku TO, et al. Rheumatic heart disease treatment cascade in Uganda. *Circ Cardiovasc Qual Outcomes.* 2017;10(11).

97. Huck D, Nalubwama H, Longenecker C, Frank S, Okello E, Webel A. A qualitative examination of secondary prophylaxis in rheumatic heart disease: factors influencing adherence to secondary prophylaxis in Uganda. *Glob Heart.* 2015;10(1):63–69.

98. Scheel A, Beaton A, Okello E, et al. The impact of a peer support group for children with rheumatic heart disease in Uganda. *Patient Educ Couns.* 2018;101(1):119–123.

99. Okello E, Longenecker CT, Beaton A, Kamya MR, Lwabi P. Rheumatic heart disease in Uganda: predictors of morbidity and mortality one year after presentation. *BMC Cardiovasc Disord.* 2017;17(1):20.

100. Sriha Belguith A, Koubaa Abdelkafi A, El Mhamdi S, et al. Rheumatic heart disease in a developing country: incidence and trend (Monastir; Tunisia: 2000–2013). *Int J Cardiol.* 2017;228:628–632.

101. Yusuf S, Narula J, Gamra H. Can we eliminate rheumatic fever and premature deaths from RHD. *Glob Heart.* 2017; 12(1):3–4.

102. Lennon D. Rheumatic fever as an indicator of child health. *N Z Med J.* 2018;130(1460).

103. Grayson S, Horsburgh M, Lennon D. An Auckland regional audit of the nurse-led rheumatic fever secondary prophylaxis programme. *N Z Med J.* 2006;119(1243): U2255.

104. Webb R, Wilson N. Rheumatic fever in New Zealand. *J Paediatr Child Health.* 2011. https://doi.org/10.1111/j.1440-1754.2011.02218.x.

105. Grigg M, McDuff I. *RFPP Implementation and Formative Evaluation Report.* New Zealand: Litmus Limited; 2013.

106. MoHN Z. *Progress on the Better Public Services Rheumatic Fever Target: Ministry of Health New Zealand;* 2017. Available from: http://www.health.govt.nz/about-ministry/what-we-do/strategic-direction/better-public-services/progress-better-public-services-rheumatic-fever-target.

107. Jack S, Williamson D, Galloway Y, Pierse N, Milne R. *Interim Evaluation of the Sore Throat Management Component of the New Zealand Rheumatic Fever Prevention Program - Quantitative Findings.* Porirua, New Zealand: The Institue of Environmental Science and Research; 2015.

108. *Previous BPS Target: Reduce Rheumatic Fever Wellington, New Zealand.* New Zealand: Ministry of Health; 2017. Available from: https://www.health.govt.nz/about-ministry/what-we-do/better-public-services/previous-bps-target-reduce-rheumatic-fever.

109. Jack SJ, Williamson DA, Galloway Y, et al. Primary prevention of rheumatic fever in the 21st century: evaluation of a national programme. *Int J Epidemiol.* 2018;47(5): 1585–1593.

110. *Kids at Risk of Rheumatic Fever Top Priority in Housing Policy New Zealand: New Zealand Herald.* 2013. Available from: https://www.nzherald.co.nz/nz/news/article.cfm?c_id=1&objectid=11131054.

111. Vermillion P, Akroyd S, Tafuna P, et al. *Evaluation of the 2015 Rheumatic Fever Awareness Campaign.* Wellington, New Zealand: Allen + Clarke; 2015.

112. Jack SJ, Williamson DA, Galloway Y, Pierse N, Zhang J, Oliver J, et al. *Primary Prevention of Rheumatic Fever in the 21st Century: Evaluation of a National Programme.* 1464-3685. (Electronic).

113. Holmes MC, Rubbo SD. A study of rheumatic fever and streptococcal infection in different social groups in Melbourne. *J Hyg.* 1953;51(4):450−457.

114. Patten B. Rheumatic fever in the west Kimberly. *Med J Aust.* 1981;1:11−15 (Special suppliment).

115. MacDonald K, Walker A. Rheumatic heart disease in aboriginal children in the northern territory. *Med J Aust.* 1989;(150):9.

116. Lawrence JG, Carapetis JR, Griffiths K, Edwards K, Condon JR. Acute rheumatic fever and rheumatic heart disease: incidence and progression in the Northern Territory of Australia 1997−2010. *Circulation.* 2013;128(5):492−501.

117. National Heart Foundation of Australia. *Cardiac Society of Australia and New Zealand. Diagnosis and Management of Acute Rheumatic Fever and Rheumatic Heart Disease in Australia: An Evidence-Based Review.* Melbourne: National Heart Foundation of Australia; 2006.

118. Roberts KV, Maguire GP, Brown A, et al. Rheumatic heart disease in Indigenous children in northern Australia: differences in prevalence and the challenges of screening. *Med J Aust.* 2015;203(5):221 e1−7.

119. Analysis HP. *Evaluation of the Commonwealth Rheumatic Fever Strategy Final Report.* Canberra, ACT: Primary Healthcare Branch, Commonwealth Department of Health.

120. Carapetis J. END RHD CRE: developing an endgame for rheumatic heart disease in Australia. *Prospectus.* 2015. Available from: https://www.rhdaustralia.org.au/system/files/fileuploadsend_rhd_cre_prospectus_2015_1.pdf.

121. Wyber R. A conceptual framework for comprehensive rheumatic heart disease control programs. *Glob Heart.* 2013;8(3):241−246.

122. Zuhlke LJ, Watkins DA, Perkins S, et al. A comprehensive needs assessment tool for planning RHD control programs in limited resource settings. *Glob Heart.* 2017;12(1):25−31.

123. Yamey G. Scaling up global health interventions: a proposed framework for success. *PLoS Med.* 2011;8(6):e1001049.

124. WHO. *Rheumatic Fever and Rheumatic Heart Disease.* Geneva: World Health Organization; 2001.

125. McDonald M, Brown A, Noonan S, Carapetis JR. Preventing recurrent rheumatic fever: the role of register based programmes. *Heart.* 2005;91(9):1131−1133.

126. Richesson R, Vehik K. Patient registries: utility, validity and inference. *Adv Exp Med Biol.* 2010;686:87−104.

127. Groth-Petersen E, Knudsen J, Wilbek E. Epidemiological basis of tuberculosis eradication in an advanced country. *Bull World Health Organ.* 1959;21:5−49.

128. Cavero-Carbonell C, Gras-Colomer E, Guaita-Calatrava R, et al. Consensus on the criteria needed for creating a rare-disease patient registry. A Delphi study. *J Public Health.* 2016;38(2):e178−e186.

129. Drolet BC, Johnson KB. Categorizing the world of registries. *J Biomed Inform.* 2008;41(6):1009−1020.

130. Solomon DJ, Henry RC, Hogan JG, Van Amburg GH, Taylor J. Evaluation and implementation of public health registries. *Public Health Rep.* 1991;106(2):142−150.

131. Brooke E. *The Current and Future Use of Registers in Health Information Systems.* Geneva, Switzerland: World Health Organization; 1974.

132. Gakunga R, Parkin DM, African Cancer Registry Network. Cancer registries in Africa 2014: a survey of operational features and uses in cancer control planning. *Int J Cancer.* 2015;137(9):2045−2052.

133. Cannon JRK, Milne C, Carapetis J. Rheumatic heart disease severity, progression and outcomes: a multi-state model. *J Am Heart Assoc.* 2017;6(3). https://doi.org/10.1161/JAHA.116.003498.

134. Lakshminarayanan S, Kar SS, Gupta R, Xavier D, Bhaskar Reddy SV. Primary healthcare-based diabetes registry in puducherry: design and methods. *Indian J Endocrinol Metab.* 2017;21(3):373−377.

135. Hoque DME, Kumari V, Hoque M, Ruseckaite R, Romero L, Evans SM. Impact of clinical registries on quality of patient care and clinical outcomes: a systematic review. *PLoS One.* 2017;12(9):e0183667.

136. Mlotshwa M, Smit S, Williams S, Reddy C, Medina-Marino A. Evaluating the electronic tuberculosis register surveillance system in Eden District, Western Cape, South Africa, 2015. *Glob Health Action.* 2017;10(1):1360560.

137. Remond M, Severin K, Hodder Y, et al. Variability in disease burden and management of rheumatic fever and rheumatic heart disease in two regions of tropical Australia. *Intern Med J.* 2013;43(4):386−393.

138. Zhang W, Okello E, N W, Lwabi P, Mondo C. Proportion of patients in Uganda rheumatic heart disease registry with advanced disease requiring urgent surgical interventions. *Afr Health Sci.* 2015;15(4):1182−1188.

139. NDSS. *The National Gestational Diabetes Register*; 2013. Available from: https://static.diabetesaustralia.com.au/s/fileassets/diabetes-australia/ba4ab34d-aa38-469d-9f20-a116091120c1.pdf.

140. Hickey PA, Connor JA, Cherian KM, et al. International quality improvement initiatives. *Cardiol Young.* 2017;27(S6):S61−S68.

141. Zuhlke L, Karthikeyan G, Engel ME, et al. Clinical outcomes in 3343 children and adults with rheumatic heart disease from 14 low- and middle-income countries: two-year follow-up of the global rheumatic heart disease registry (the REMEDY study). *Circulation.* 2016;134(19):1456−1466.

142. Kingue S, Ba SA, Balde D, et al. The VALVAFRIC study: a registry of rheumatic heart disease in Western and Central Africa. *Arch Cardiovasc Dis.* 2016;109(5):321−329.

143. van Hagen IM, Thorne SA, Taha N, et al. Pregnancy outcomes in women with rheumatic mitral valve disease: results from the registry of pregnancy and cardiac disease. *Circulation.* 2018;137(8):806−816.

144. Grover FL, Vemulapalli S, Carroll JD, et al. 2016 annual report of the society of thoracic surgeons/American college of cardiology transcatheter valve therapy registry. *J Am Coll Cardiol.* 2017;69(10):1215−1230.

145. *Investigation of RheumatiC AF Treatment Using Vitamin K Antagonists, Rivaroxaban or Aspirin Studies, Superiority (INVICTUS-ASA)*. ClinicalTrials.gov; 2016 [Available from: https://clinicaltrials.gov/ct2/show/NCT02832531.

146. Engel M, Zuhlke L, Robertson K. Rheumatic fever and rheumatic heart disease: where are we now in South Africa. *SA Heart*. 2009;6(1):20−23.

147. PASCAR. *African Union Communique on Eradication of ARF and RHD. Action Group 1 Meeting Minutes*; December 6, 2016. Available from: http://www.pascar.org/uploads/files/PASCAR_RHD_Task_Force_Action_Group_1_-_December_2016_Minutes.pdf.

148. *Rheumatic Heart Disease School Project*; 2017. Available from: https://rhedproject.org/program/research.

149. Davis K, Remenyi B, Draper AD, et al. Rheumatic heart disease in Timor-Leste school students: an echocardiography-based prevalence study. *Med J Aust*. 2018;208(7):303−307.

150. Government TF. *Health Ministry Launches Rheumatic Fever Information System*; 2016. Available from: http://www.fiji.gov.fj/Media-Center/Press-Releases/HEALTH-MINISTRY-LAUNCHES-RHEUMATIC-FEVER-INFORMATI.aspx.

151. RHDAustralia. National heart foundation of Australia and the cardiac Society of Australia and New Zealand. In: *Australian Guidelines for Prevention, Diagnosis and Management of Acute Rheumatic Fever and Rheumatic Heart Disease*. 2nd ed. 2012.

152. Rossi G, Lee VS. Assessing the burden of rheumatic heart disease among refugee children: a call to action. *J Glob Health*. 2016;6(2):020305.

153. Culliford-Semmens N, Tilton E, Webb R, et al. Adequate adherence to benzathine penicillin secondary prophylaxis following the diagnosis of rheumatic heart disease by echocardiographic screening. *N Z Med J*. 2017;130(1457):50.

154. Treatment WHO. *Of Tuberculosis Guidelines*. 4th ed. Geneva, Switzerland: World Health Organization.; 2009.

155. Bellgard M, Beroud C, Parkinson K, et al. Dispelling myths about rare disease registry system development. *Source Code Biol Med*. 2013;8(1):21.

156. Saracci R, Wild C. *International Agency for Research on Cancer: The First 50 Years. 1965−2015*: World Health Organization.

157. Westley EW, Greene SA, Tarr GA, Ryman TK, Gilbert SS, Hawes SE. Strengthening paper health register systems: strategies from case studies in Ethiopia, Ghana, South Africa and Uganda. *J Glob Health*. 2016;6(2):020303.

158. Culliford-Semmens N, Tilton E, Webb R, et al. Adequate adherence to benzathine penicillin secondary prophylaxis following the diagnosis of rheumatic heart disease by echocardiographic screening. *N Z Med J*. 2017;130(1457):50−57.

159. HE2RO. *Can Routine Data Be Used to Assess Integration of HIV and Other Primary Healthcare Services in South Africa's Public Health Sector? An Assessment from Three Johannesburg Clinics: Health Economics and Epidemiology Research Office*. 2018. Available from: http://www.heroza.org/wp-content/uploads/2018/05/Policy-Brief-22-Routine-data-February-2018.pdf.

160. Jawhari B, Ludwick D, Keenan L, Zakus D, Hayward R. Benefits and challenges of EMR implementations in low resource settings: a state-of-the-art review. *BMC Med Inf Decis Mak*. 2016;16:116.

161. Beaton A, Sable C. Health policy: reducing rheumatic heart disease in Africa−time for action. *Nat Rev Cardiol*. 2016;13(4):190−191.

162. RHDAustralia. *The Australian Guideline for Prevention, Diagnosis and Management of Acute Rheumatic Fever and Rheumatic Heart Disease*. 2nd ed. 2012.

163. Nelson EC, Dixon-Woods M, Batalden PB, et al. Patient focused registries can improve health, care, and science. *BMJ*. 2016;354:i3319.

164. Jedy-Agba EE, Oga EA, Odutola M, et al. Developing national cancer registration in developing countries − case study of the Nigerian national system of cancer registries. *Front Public Health*. 2015;3:186.

165. MacQueen JC. State registries and the control of rheumatic fever. *Am J Public Health*. 1979;69(8):761−762.

166. Singh E, Ruff P, Babb C, et al. Establishment of a cancer surveillance programme: the South African experience. *Lancet Oncol*. 2015;16(8):e414−e421.

167. Laryea DO, Awwittor F. Ensuring confidentiality and safety of cancer registry data in Kumasi, Ghana. *Online J Public Health Inform*. 2017;9(1):e130.

168. Gliklich R, Dreyer N, Leavy M. *Informed Consent for Registries. Registries for Evaluating Patient Outcomes: A User's Guide*. 3rd ed. Rockville, USA: Agency for Healthcare Research and Quality (US); 2014.

169. *SA Rheumatic Heart Disease (RHD) Register: SA Health*. Available from: http://www.sahealth.sa.gov.au/wps/wcm/connect/da0dce804d627b8d9614b7d08366040b/RHD+Register+consent+form_final_amended+version+for+DCS_FINAL.pdf?MOD=AJPERES&CACHEID=ROOTWORKSPACE-da0dce804d627b8d9614b7d08366040b-l-WK-ro.

170. Illman J. Cancer registries: should informed consent be required? *J Natl Cancer Inst*. 2002;94(17):1269−1270.

171. Sankila R, Martinez C, Parkin DM, Storm H, Teppo L. Informed consent in cancer registries. *Lancet*. 2001;357(9267):1536.

172. Goga Y. *The Cancer Registry in South Africa − Exploring Some of the Ethical and Legal Considerations*. University of Witwatersrand; 2011.

173. WHO. *Everybody Business: Strenghtening Health Systems to Improve Health Outcomes: WHO's Framework for Action*. Geneva, Switzerland: World Health Organization; 2007.

174. Dublin, Ireland. *Dublin Declaration on Human Resources for Health: Building the Health Workforce of the Future Fourth Global Forum on Human Resources for Health*; November 13−17, 2017 [Available from: http://who.int/hrh/events/Dublin_Declaration-on-HumanResources-for-Health.pdf?ua=1.

175. Rao M, Pilot E. The missing link−the role of primary care in global health. *Glob Health Action*. 2014;7:23693.

176. Bergmark R, Bergmark B, Blander J, Fataki M, Janabi M. Burden of disease and barriers to the diagnosis and treatment of group a beta-hemolytic streptococcal pharyngitis for the prevention of rheumatic heart disease in Dar Es

Salaam, Tanzania. *Pediatr Infect Dis J.* 2010;29(12): 1135−1137.

177. Hewitson J, Zilla P. Children's heart disease in sub-Saharan Africa: challenging the burden of disease: children's heart disease. *SA Heart.* 2010;7(1):18−29.

178. Jowett M, Brunal M, Flores G, Cylus J. *Spending Targets for Health: No Magic Number.* World Health Organization; 2016.

179. Levesque JF, Harris MF, Russell G. Patient-centred access to health care: conceptualising access at the interface of health systems and populations. *Int J Equity Health.* 2013;12:18.

180. Davy C, Harfield S, McArthur A, Munn Z, Brown A. Access to primary health care services for Indigenous peoples: a framework synthesis. *Int J Equity Health.* 2016;15(1):163.

181. Petricca K, Mamo Y, Haileamlak A, Seid E, Parry E. Barriers to effective follow-up treatment for rheumatic heart disease in Jimma, Ethiopa: a grounded theory analysis of the patient experience. *Ethiop J Health Sci.* 2009;19(1): 39−44.

182. Mathan JJ, Ekart J, Houlding A, Payinda G, Mills C. Clinical management and patient persistence with antibiotic course in suspected group A streptococcal pharyngitis

for primary prevention of rheumatic fever: the perspective from a New Zealand emergency department. *N Z Med J.* 2017;130(1457):58−68.

183. Allen LB, Allen M, Lesa RF, Richardson GE, Eggett DL. Rheumatic fever in Samoa: education as prevention. *Pac Health Dialog.* 2011;17(1):107−118.

184. Anderson A, Leversha A, Ofanoa M, et al. *Māori and Pacific Whānau Experiences of Recurrent Rheumatic Fever and Unexpected Rheumatic Heart Disease in New Zealand. Auckland.* New Zealand: The University of Auckland; 2018.

185. Askew D, Brady J, Brown A, et al. *To Your Door: Factors that Influence Aboriginal and Torres Strait Islander People Seeking Care.* 2014.

186. Markbreiter J. *Integration, Integration, Integration: Why Rheumatic Heart Disease Must Be Incorporated in Universal Health Coverage. Geneva.* Switzerland: RHD Action; 2015.

187. Abiiro GA, De Allegri M. Universal health coverage from multiple perspectives: a synthesis of conceptual literature and global debates. *BMC Int Health Hum Right.* 2015;15: 17.

188. Glassman A, Giedion U, Sakuma Y, Smith P. Defining a health benefits package: what are the necessary processes. *Health Syst Reform.* 2016;2(1):39−50.

CHAPTER 13

Echocardiographic Screening for Rheumatic Heart Disease

ANDREA BEATON • DANIEL ENGELMAN • MARIANA MIRABEL

INTRODUCTION

Over the past decade, echocardiographic screening for rheumatic heart disease (RHD) has emerged as a *potentially* transformative strategy for global RHD control. School-aged children from nearly every continent have been screened under the premise of epidemiology or research. New Caledonia has established a national echocardiographic screening program[1–3] and several other countries (including Tonga and Samoa) have embraced population-based screening. Echocardiographic screening has revealed a large burden of undiagnosed RHD, broadened our understanding of the spectrum of RHD within endemic communities, and inspired increased research and advocacy that has refocused global attention on RHD. However, many questions remain before echocardiographic screening can be endorsed as an effective strategy in a global RHD control program. In this chapter, we review the rationale behind echocardiographic screening for RHD, what we have learned from screening, provide a review of research in this area, and outline future directions and important outstanding questions.

THE RATIONALE FOR RHEUMATIC HEART DISEASE SCREENING

Despite the importance of the recognition and treatment of streptococcal infection and the recognition of acute rheumatic fever (ARF) and initiation of secondary prophylaxis, RHD cannot be entirely prevented through these strategies. Up to one-third of children with ARF cannot recall a preceding sore throat[4,5] and up to three quarters of children with RHD cannot recall an episode consistent with ARF.[6] In many resource-limited settings, RHD is frequently diagnosed at a late stage, for example, in Uganda, 85% of newly diagnosed RHD patients presented with severe valvular involvement and cardiovascular complications.[7]

This is particularly unfortunate, as severe RHD carries a high risk of morbidity and mortality[8,9] and can only be treated through cardiac surgical or catheterization procedures, which are often cost prohibitive and unavailable in the vast majority of RHD endemic areas. In contrast, when mild RHD is identified following ARF, initiation of secondary prophylaxis can prevent disease progression and, in some cases, allow for resolution of valvular damage.[10] RHD is most typically the manifestation of a cumulative disease process. It stands to reason then, that strategies that improve early detection of RHD may improve outcomes.

Screening aims to identify RHD before an individual develops clinical disease, to intervene to improve health outcomes. The pathogenesis of RHD means that there is often time after an initial ARF episode and the development of advanced cardiac disease, which can occur as late as decades later.[11,12] Screening for RHD by auscultation has been undertaken in various parts of the world from the 1960s to the 1980s. Examples are reports from Pakistan,[13] South Africa,[14] Tonga,[15] India,[16] Samoa,[17] and New Zealand.[18] Active case finding was championed in the 1980s by the World Health Organization as part of the Global Programme for the Prevention of Rheumatic Fever and Rheumatic Heart Disease in 16 countries, utilizing cardiac auscultation to identify pathological heart murmurs; however, case detection was low[19] and scale-up of screening outside of pilot sites was not achieved before the program being discontinued in 2001.

THE EVOLUTION OF RHEUMATIC HEART DISEASE SCREENING

The first study on echocardiographic screening for RHD was published in 1996 by Anabwani and Bonhoeffer. They demonstrated that the use of echocardiography detected more children with RHD than auscultation.[20]

Acute Rheumatic Fever and Rheumatic Heart Disease. https://doi.org/10.1016/B978-0-323-63982-8.00013-1

At that time, the technological capacities of portable echocardiograms were limited. The team needed to carry a generator to provide power in remote villages in Kenya. Nearly a decade later, a collaborative study led in Mozambique and Cambodia demonstrated that echocardiography detected 10–20 times more valvular lesions in schoolchildren in these two endemic countries.[5] This landmark study by Marijon and colleagues, reported in 2007,[5] heralded the beginning of widespread interest in echocardiographic screening of RHD. Within 2 years of publication, several teams, using various diagnostic criteria, showed similar results across different epidemiological settings.[21–23]

Terminology

Cases of RHD detected through echocardiographic screening have been termed *latent* RHD. There has been inconsistent use of vocabulary in the literature (Table 13.1). Latent RHD includes both previously undiagnosed clinical RHD and subclinical RHD, that is, where there is no audible murmur on auscultation. However, latent RHD is most often mild. Although most children with latent RHD on echocardiographic screening have subclinical disease, between 1/3 (Uganda[24]) and 2/3 (Fiji[8]) of children with latent, definite RHD (using 2012 World Heart Federation (WHF) criteria, see later) already have moderate or severe mitral or aortic regurgitation or mitral stenosis. Conversely, the vast majority of children with latent RHD had subclinical disease in higher income countries

TABLE 13.1
Proposed Rheumatic Heart Disease Definitions.

Latent RHD	All cases of RHD diagnosed through echocardiographic screening, to include previously unrecognized clinical RHD and subclinical RHD.
Clinical RHD	All cases of RHD that have clinical signs or symptoms including heart murmur[a] diagnosed either through echocardiographic screening or clinical evaluation. Clinical RHD is typically more advanced than subclinical RHD.
Subclinical RHD	All cases of RHD that do not have clinical signs or symptoms including heart murmur[a]. Subclinical RHD is typically less advanced than clinical RHD.

RHD, rheumatic heart disease.
[a] It is important to again point out that detection of a pathological heart murmur without echocardiography has been shown to be poorly sensitive and specific in echocardiographic screening studies for RHD.

such as New Caledonia[1] and New Zealand[25] (both before WHF criteria). This heterogenous mix of early and advanced disease detected through echocardiographic screening is important when assessing the value of an echocardiography-based screening program.

Accuracy of Auscultation for Rheumatic Heart Disease

The advent of echocardiography has shown auscultation to be unreliable for RHD screening. Specificity is consistently low, as first reported by the sentinel study by Marijon et al., who confirmed rheumatic valvular lesions in only 1 out of 9 children with a murmur.[5] In context, low specificity in screening would result in many false positive RHD diagnoses, which could overwhelm resource-limited health systems and lead to inappropriate use of secondary prophylaxis. Sensitivity is also low, as consistently supported in studies comparing echocardiography and auscultation from several countries.[26–29] A meta-analysis of screening in endemic regions showed a pooled prevalence of RHD by auscultation of 2.9 per 1000 compared to 12.9 per 1000 by echocardiography.[30] Low sensitivity means that auscultatory screening cannot be used even in a two-step design with echocardiographic confirmation, as many cases would be missed in the first screening round. As noted below, these powerful data on the poor performance of auscultation led to modifications in the criteria to removal of the presence or absence of "heart murmur" from the decision around RHD diagnostic certainty.

Standardization of Echocardiographic Criteria

At the time the first studies were designed and published, there were no published guidelines or recommendations on echocardiographic criteria for the diagnosis of subclinical RHD and thus different criteria were used.[31,5,22] Standardization of criteria for RHD became a key issue. A research group was formed and agreed on the diagnostic criteria based on the best level of evidence based on available echocardiographic, surgical, and pathologic descriptions of RHD. These WHF endorsed guidelines allow classification of an echocardiogram in a patient without a history of ARF into three groups: (1) normal; (2) borderline RHD; (3) definite RHD.[32] The WHF criteria include Doppler criteria for the diagnosis of pathological mitral stenosis, mitral regurgitation, and aortic regurgitation. Additional morphological changes of the mitral and aortic valves were introduced. The combination of pathological left-sided regurgitation and morphological changes allows the diagnosis of definite RHD; whereas, if found in isolation, borderline RHD may be diagnosed (see Table 5.1, Chapter 5).

Technical Considerations and Interpretation of the Guidelines

Although the 2012 WHF criteria represent a significant advancement from previous guidelines, there remain important limitations and practical issues to consider for those contemplating or participating in echocardiographic screening. First, the WHF criteria do not include a borderline category in adults. Although there is a solid rationale for this within the details of the guidelines, an unintended consequence has been that, in research studies assessing change in echocardiography over time, transition to adulthood has been recorded as an "improvement" from borderline RHD to normal, when the functional mitral or aortic findings are actually unchanged, with only age causing the change in categorization. This issue should be carefully considered with expert consensus to standardize reporting.

Second, the distinction between physiological and pathological regurgitation is more nuanced than the WHF criteria are able to describe. For example, the length of a mitral regurgitation jet, a critical component of the WHF definition of pathological regurgitation, is fraught with complications. Length can vary substantially based on cardiac loading conditions and blood pressure, resulting in rapid differences within the same individual over short time periods, most important for those "on the edge" of the 2 cm cut-off point. These individuals then waver between a normal and borderline RHD diagnosis despite no clinically significant cardiac change. There is also no provision within the WHF criteria for age- or height-standardized measurement (z-scores) of regurgitation, which are used as standard practice for other pediatric measurements. A jet length of 2 cm in a small child represents a considerably higher mitral regurgitation to left atrial ratio than in an adult, and shorter jets, that may be pathological, are excluded from classification as RHD. Further, the proportion of mitral regurgitation that is physiological is age dependent. Of those aged 10-12 years, 15% have physiological mitral regurgitation,[33] with central, thin jets of mitral regurgitation, irrespective of length, more likely to be physiologic. Conversely, eccentric, posterior jets of mitral regurgitation, a classical finding of RHD, may not measure 2 cm as the jets hit the back of the left atrium. Table 13.2 summaries the differential diagnosis of pathological regurgitation of the mitral and aortic valves.

Despite these issues, jet direction is not incorporated into the guidelines. Caution must also be exercised when interpreting freeze-frame color images of mitral or aortic regurgitation, as these often appear more substantial than those in moving loops. High quality reporting and interreviewer reliability necessitates

---

TABLE 13.2
Differential Diagnosis of Mitral Valve and Aortic Valve Abnormalities Found in Rheumatic Heart Disease Screening[a].

A. Mitral Regurgitation and Structural Nonrheumatic Mitral Valve Abnormalities

1. Upper limit physiological MR

2. Congenital heart disease with MR, for example, secundum ASD or primum ASD

3. Isolated congenital abnormalities of the mitral valve: Double orifice MV, parachute MV, hammock MV, cleft MV

4. Congenital mitral valve prolapse associated with Marfan's syndrome; other connective tissue disorders

5. Interscallop separations of the posterior mitral valve leaflet[35,b]

B. The Differential Diagnosis of Pathological Aortic Regurgitation

1. Bicuspid (also termed bicommissural) aortic valves[c]

2. Dilated aortic root

3. Subaortic membrane (which can be very subtle and challenging to detect in field-based screening)

MR, mitral regurgitation; MV, mitral valve; ASD atrial septal defect; WHF, World Heart Federation; RHD, rheumatic heart disease; AR, aortic regurgitation.
[a] The WHF criteria are designed for diagnosis and interpretation by cardiologists or echocardiographers with specialized training and expertise in RHD evaluation. It is important to avoid over and underdiagnosis of RHD.
[b] Not specifically investigated in an RHD-endemic population, but reported in other studies of the mitral valve.
[c] Both bicuspid aortic valves and dilated aortic root are easily identifiable. Their exclusion make the finding of pathological AR more likely rheumatic.

provision of cine loops and avoidance of bias through still-frame images. Finally, it can be subjective whether a jet of regurgitation is pan-systolic or pan-diastolic. Image gain, equipment, and both regurgitation and Doppler angle can result in suboptimal Doppler signals, even in the presence of otherwise pathological regurgitation. Provision for these considerations should be discussed in research and guideline revisions.

Those interpreting echocardiograms must also consider age-related normal for abnormal thickening of the anterior mitral valve leaflet defined as follows: ≥3 mm for individuals aged ≤20 years[34]; ≥4 mm for individuals aged 21–40 years; ≥5 mm for individuals aged >40 years. Valve thickness measurements obtained using harmonic imaging should be cautiously interpreted and a thickness up to 4 mm should be considered normal in those aged >20 years. Normal mitral and aortic valve thickness data in health children have been published.[32–34] In practice, reproducibly measuring anterior mitral valve leaflet (AMVL) thickness, in particular in the hands of nonexperts, has been challenging. AMVL thickness should be measured during diastole at full excursion. Measurement should be taken at the thickest portion of the leaflet, including focal thickening, beading, and nodularity. Measurement should be performed on a frame with maximal separation of chordae from the leaflet tissue. Valve thickness should only be assessed if the images were acquired at optimal gain settings without harmonics.[32] Further work is needed to improve reliability of this measurement across populations and practitioners.

CONTRIBUTION OF ECHOCARDIOGRAPHIC SCREENING FOR RHEUMATIC HEART DISEASE EPIDEMIOLOGY

Echocardiographic screening has dramatically improved our understanding of the global epidemiology of RHD. The most recent estimates from The Global Burden of Disease 2015 study included a systematic review of all RHD estimates, including echocardiography-based screening studies.[36] Borderline RHD cases were not included in the model, thereby restricting estimates to patients with clinical RHD and definite echocardiographic RHD. Importantly, in the lowest resource settings, where medical records are often sparse or nonexistent, echocardiographic screening studies filled in a major gap of disease estimates. In Africa, only 15 of 54 countries had any fatal or nonfatal RHD estimates. Of the 15 countries with at least some data, eight were based on echocardiographic screening studies. These new estimates placed the prevalence of RHD at 33.4 million people. RHD-related death of 319,400 deaths per annum remained unchanged compared to previous estimates. The novelty in the latest estimates is the computation of the number of years lived with disability. Watkins and coworkers demonstrated the burden that RHD puts on developing countries, including the potentially negative economic impact of RHD (see Chapter 1).[36]

The advent of echocardiography-led active surveillance has also changed the epidemiological concept of RHD.[37] As mentioned earlier, the use of echocardiography unveiled a large number of asymptomatic individuals who are potentially at risk of developing severe RHD. Currently the epidemiology of RHD may be considered as a pyramid of increasing severity, with a smaller number of individuals with severe, symptomatic RHD at the top and a larger base of individuals with borderline, asymptomatic RHD (Fig. 13.1).[37,38] Contemporary data originating both from population- and hospital-based studies in a captive island-bound population reinforced this model, showing a 2- to 3-fold incidence/prevalence ratio in active screening compared to symptomatic cases admitted to the hospital.[39] The authors appropriately concluded that significant numbers of patients with subclinical disease never become symptomatic. Important questions remain regarding the chance of progression up the RHD pyramid, at what rate advancement occurs, risk factors, and finally whether early diagnosis can prevent such progression (discussed further later, *Future Directions*).

Echocardiographic screening has also, to a lesser extent, improved our epidemiological understanding of RHD in populations outside of the school ages. A community-based study in Ethiopia examined 987 children and young adults, revealing a peak prevalence (60 per 1000 cases of definite RHD) in those between 16 and 20 years. These data confirm Nicaraguan community data, which demonstrated a higher prevalence of RHD among teens and young adults, when compared to schoolchildren, though utilizing old guidelines.[21] A community-based study in Uganda, including a house-to-house echocardiographic survey of those between 5 and 50 years, demonstrated a lifetime prevalence of 2.45%, but showed a substantial portion of adults with mild forms of latent RHD, the implications of which will require additional follow-up.[40] Finally, in what could be considered a pilot study, a community-based screening of women presenting for antenatal care in Uganda demonstrated a

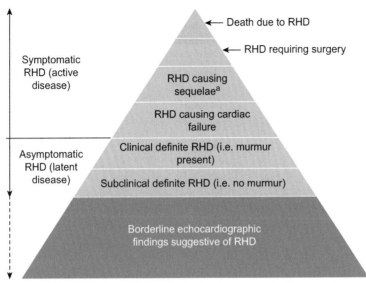

FIG. 13.1 A new model for assessing and reporting the burden of RHD that incorporates asymptomatic and symptomatic disease.
aSequelae include atrial fibrillation, infective endocarditis, and stroke. RHD, rheumatic heart disease.
Reproduced with permission from Zühlke and Steer.[37]

1.5% prevalence of RHD among pregnant women, with significant adverse maternal and neonatal outcomes.[41]

INNOVATIONS IN ECHOCARDIOGRAPHIC SCREENING

Screening by Nonexpert Operators

Screening surveys or population-based screening programs require considerable organization and human resources. Echocardiographic screening requires personnel with specialized skills. The WHF criteria are designed for diagnosis, not as a screening test, and include specialized imaging modalities, intended to be performed and interpreted by cardiologists or echocardiographers with specialized training and expertise. However, in most settings where RHD remains prevalent, there are inadequate numbers of expert operators to perform echocardiograms. Standard training in echocardiography requires considerable time,[42,43] and it is unlikely to be feasible to train a sufficient workforce to screen at mass scale.

Therefore, shorter, focused training programs have been developed, to reallocate a simplified cardiac ultrasound test to nonexpert health workers, known as "task shifting".[63,64]

In parallel, focused cardiac ultrasound protocols, rather than standard comprehensive echocardiography, have been increasingly implemented.[44–46] The

technical requirements for RHD echocardiography screening are competence in basic two-dimensional and color-Doppler imaging in limited views. Initial pilot studies found that training nonexpert nurses or medical students to perform echocardiography for RHD screening was feasible.[47–49] Four subsequent studies have examined this in more detail, with larger sample sizes (Table 13.3).[50–53] Heterogeneity of study design and methods precludes direct comparison of the results of these studies. However, consistent themes have emerged from these studies. There is now convincing evidence that nonexpert health workers can be trained to perform focused echocardiography and measure regurgitation as a risk marker for RHD. The accuracy of this screening strategy is in the range of 80% sensitivity and 85% specificity. Nurses have been trained most commonly, but other cadres of health workers also show proficiency after brief training.[52–55]

Innovative Technologies for Screening

Most of the screening prevalence studies were conducted using portable echocardiography machines, around the size of a large laptop computer, weighing 5–12 kg. Although these are much cheaper and more portable than traditional large-platform hospital-based echocardiography equipment, newer developments in ultrasound technologies offer even greater portability at much lower cost.

TABLE 13.3
Nonexpert Rheumatic Heart Disease Screening Studies.

Setting, Year	Fiji, 2012–13		New Caledonia, 2013	Uganda, 2014	Brazil, 2015
Reference	Engelman et al. 2016.[53]		Mirabel et al. 2015.[50]	Ploutz et al. 2015.[51]	Beaton et al. 2016.[52]
Operators	7 nurses		2 nurses	2 nurses	2 nurses 2 medical students 2 biotechnicians
Previous echocardiography experience	None		None	6 months	6 weeks (4 operators) 12 months (2 operators)
Sample	2004 students 5–15 y		1217 students 9–10 y	956 students 5–17 y	397 students 5–18 y
RHD prevalence	2.8%		4%	4.5%	13% (artificially high sample)
Duration of screening	12 months		5 months	3 months	4 days
Ratios	1–2 trainers to 7 students 2 machines to 7 students		1 trainer to 1–2 students Machine each	1 trainer to 1–2 students Machine each	n/a
Overview of training	1 week theoretical 6 weeks supervised practice No hurdle assessment		3 days theoretical 30 h practical Further 1 to 1 training to address specific issues	4 h theoretical 2 days practical	3 weeks interpretation only Computer-based Weekly hurdle assessments
Machine	Portable (Sonosite M-Turbo)		Handheld (GE Vscan)	Handheld (GE Vscan)	Handheld (GE Vscan)
Screen-positive criteria	Any MR or any AR	MR ≥1.5 cm or any AR	MR ≥2 cm or any AR	MR ≥1.5 cm or any AR	MR ≥1.5 cm or any AR
Screen-positive proportion	16%	9%	11%–12%	24%	n/aᵃ
Sensitivity (95% CI)	84% (72–92)	77% (64–87)	Operator A: 84% Operator B: 78%	74% (59–86)	83% (76–89)
Specificity (95% CI)	85% (84–87)	93% (92–94)	Operator A: 91% Operator B: 92%	79% (76–81)	85% (82–87)
Positive predictive value	15%	25%	29%–39%	14%	n/aᵃ
Negative predictive value	99%	99%	99%	98%	n/aᵃ

RHD, rheumatic heart disease; MR, mitral regurgitation; AR, aortic regurgitation.
ᵃ Study did not use a population sample.

Handheld ultrasound has been investigated as a tool for RHD screening. When used by experienced cardiologists in Uganda, Beaton and colleagues found that diagnosis using handheld machines and modified WHF criteria had encouraging accuracy compared to standard portable echocardiography.[56,57] The same research group reported that handheld echocardiography is more sensitive than auscultation.[27] Another study from South Africa found moderate sensitivity (81% for any RHD) using the Vscan (General Electric

Healthcare) in a highly abbreviated protocol on a small sample of adolescents, performed by an expert.[58] Three of the previous studies of nonexpert operators also used handheld machines.[50-52]

Current handheld ultrasound machines, such as the GE VScan and the Philips Lumify, lack the spectral Doppler imaging capabilities needed to make a diagnosis using the WHF criteria. Further disadvantages include short battery life and a tendency to overheat.[57,59] Newer models or alternate systems using smartphones may offer greater reach for screening teams at reduced cost,[60] but validation and standardization will be required.

Another use of innovative technologies for RHD screening was investigated in Brazil, where the research team used a remote reporting system. Images acquired from handheld and portable machines were uploaded to the internet, and then successfully reported by research cardiologists in Brazil and the United States.[61]

Abbreviated Protocols and Agreed Cut-Off Points

Several recent RHD screening studies have examined RHD screening tests using brief, abbreviated imaging protocols, in comparison to the reference standard of a comprehensive echocardiogram. Lu and colleagues found that criteria combining MR ≥1.5 cm or any aortic regurgitation (AR) to be the best balance of sensitivity and specificity for handheld ultrasound.[62] Mirabel and colleagues, also using handheld ultrasound, concluded that a combination of MR ≥2 cm or any AR was the best strategy, although a shorter MR cut-off was more sensitive.[50] The same group previously proposed a cut-off point of MR ≥2 cm, based on a retrospective analysis,[63] and this 2 cm cut-off point was used in a study from South Africa.[58] However, increasing the MR cut-off point from 1.5 to 2 cm would have unacceptably reduced sensitivity from 83% to 44% in a Brazilian study.[52] The New Caledonian screening program refers all children with any abnormality (regurgitation, stenosis, or other abnormality) on screening; however, the referral rate (5.4%) suggests that the cardiologists performing the screening are likely not referring all cases of trivial regurgitation.[3]

Test protocols that use only regurgitation face the simultaneous challenges of overdiagnosis (physiological mitral regurgitation, which is common finding in children[33]) and underdiagnosis (borderline RHD due to isolated morphological abnormalities). However, these studies suggest that it may be possible to develop a feasible test strategy that can balance sensitivity and

specificity. A formal reassessment of the WHF criteria and potential simplification as a screening test is now timely.

Training Procedures

Variation between nonexperts learning cardiac ultrasound for RHD indicates the need for educational refinement, in line with the WHO guidelines for task-sharing that recommend continuous monitoring and evaluation during implementation.[64] Standardized training is central to this endeavor,[65] and computer-learning modules have been developed and made freely available in three languages[66] that show good performance and acceptability among nurses and other healthcare providers in low- and middle-income countries.[52,67,68] Telemedicine support for early learners has shown promise as a useful adjunct.[52,69] Further research is needed to determine best strategies for scaling up training, including developing standard competency assessments and accreditation processes.

FUTURE DIRECTIONS AND UNANSWERED QUESTIONS

Disease Progression of Latent (Subclinical) Rheumatic Heart Disease

The importance of echocardiographic screening as a public health strategy for global RHD reduction remains to be determined. It remains unclear what proportion of those with latent RHD may progress to clinically significant disease, and at what rate, and if early detection leads to improved outcomes. There have been 10 longitudinal cohorts of children with latent RHD, with between 2 and 7 years median follow-up, reported to date. These data clearly show that latent RHD is a heterogeneous diagnosis with varied outcomes.[8,21,24,70-76] Rates of disease progression are challenging to compare across studies due to inconsistent definitions of progression, use of different binomial outcomes (i.e., stable and progression), and variable inclusion of children with advanced RHD.[24,77] Standardization of reporting outcomes for children with latent RHD is therefore of high priority.

In the largest cohort of latent RHD to date, describing 227 children from Uganda, 10% of children with borderline RHD showed progression, while 25% of children with mild, definite RHD showed progression over a median of 2.3 years.[24] Children with moderate-to-severe RHD (labeled "missed clinical RHD") at time of screening did substantially worse.[24] In Fiji, worse health outcomes, though not increased mortality (not assessed independently in the Uganda study), was seen for those detected through screening than matched controls.[8] All cohorts have consistently reported heterogeneity in progression and outcomes, with no consistent risk or protective factors emerging from analysis to date. Importantly, there appears to be a small subset of children with latent RHD, including those with borderline RHD, who are at risk of progression,[8,21,24,70–76] recurrent ARF,[71] and worse outcomes than their screen negative peers.[8]

Does Identification of Latent Rheumatic Heart Disease Improve Outcomes?

Despite the evidence of efficacy following episodes of ARF,[10] the ability of secondary penicillin prophylaxis to improve outcomes in latent RHD remains unclear. Interestingly, an Australian cohort showed increased risk of progression with penicillin prescription.[71] There was a similar strong trend in Uganda, despite efforts to remove differences between penicillin treated and untreated children.[24] These concerning results may be explained by methodological bias. In both observational studies, allocation to secondary prophylaxis was at the physician's discretion. Penicillin use was associated with disease progression, suggesting that physicians may have prescribed secondary prophylaxis in children with either more severe valve disease or at higher risk (e.g., due to the social and economic environment).

A large, randomized controlled trial of secondary prophylaxis in children with latent RHD is needed and ethically justified to provide further evidence on this critical question. A 2-year randomized controlled trial comparing secondary antibiotic prophylaxis with active surveillance for patients with latent, subclinical RHD (The GOAL trial, Clinicaltrials.gov: NCT03346525) commenced in 2018 to answer this question.

Is Echocardiographic Screening Cost-Effective in Low Resource Areas?

It is not yet known if echocardiographic screening for RHD is cost-effective. There have been three studies to date assessing the cost-effectiveness.[78–80] All studies have necessarily used broad assumptions, particularly as the impact of secondary prophylaxis on latent RHD (see earlier discussion) is not known. However, all three concluded that active case finding utilizing echocardiography could be cost-effective, by assuming RHD can be detected ≥2 years earlier through screening,[80] and showing slight incremental cost savings and gain of quality adjusted life years through screening.[79] Further research is needed as more data are gathered around outcomes for latent RHD and the impact of secondary

prophylaxis, which can more precisely inform the investment case for RHD screening. These assessments need to be conducted in a range of settings due to the wide variation in healthcare costs and utility informing the assumptions.

What Would it Take to Scale-Up Echocardiographic Screening to a National/Global Level?

Scaling up echocardiographic screening to a national or global level requires broad considerations. In broad terms, echocardiographic screening for RHD meets the three main requirements for screening for a disease. First, there is a suitable condition (RHD); second, the condition is detectable by a suitable test (echocardiography); and third, the condition is treatable (by long-acting penicillin).[38] However, as has been discussed in this chapter, there remain unanswered questions. Table 13.4 outlines the principles of screening as outlined by Wilson and Jungner in 1968[81] and the current evidence for each criterion pertaining to echocardiographic screening for RHD.

As screening is only properly established as a program in one country at present (New Caledonia, population 280,000), there is limited evidence to assess these criteria, although experiences of research activities (which are generally more highly resourced than health programs) provide some insights. For example, Roberts described difficulties with enrollment, consent, and timely and appropriate follow-up following RHD screening in Australia.[82] Challenges of community engagement, consent, participation, follow-up, and workforce restrictions for nonexpert operators were reported in Brazil.[83] It is evident the human, infrastructure, and financial resources required for testing, diagnosis, follow-up, monitoring, and quality assurance will be considerable, and are likely to be a major challenge in resource-limited settings.[84]

A New Zealand study found that prescreening education, in the context of a major public health initiative, contributed to high levels of awareness around sore throat and ARF.[85] A Ugandan study found that the screening activity was well accepted by teachers and school students, but identified opportunities to improve prescreening education.[86] Refinement of prescreening information, consent procedures, and education resources for those with positive tests are needed.[87] Given the complexity of the information, and uncertainty surrounding the accuracy of the test and the effectiveness of the intervention, the use of decision aids may be helpful.[88]

TABLE 13.4 Suitability of Echocardiography as a Population Screening Test for Rheumatic Heart Disease.		
Criteria	**Criteria Met?**	**Outstanding Issues**
The condition should be an important health problem	Yes[36]	
There should be a recognizable latent or early symptomatic stage	Yes[11,12]	
The natural history of the condition, including development from latent to declared disease, should be adequately understood	No	Data 2–7 years postscreening shows heterogeneity in outcomes with identifiable risk factors. Long-term follow-up and larger cohorts required.
There should be an accepted treatment for patients with recognized disease	Yes. Recommendations for secondary prophylaxis already exist for patients with ARF and RHD.[89]	Variable and often poor adherence to secondary prophylaxis is due to multiple factors, which may include poor acceptability by patients.
There should be a suitable test or examination that has a high level of accuracy	Yes, with limitations - Echocardiography is highly accurate - WHF criteria for diagnosis[32] partly validated	WHF guidelines need updating Agreed protocols and case definitions for screening required.
The test should be acceptable to the population	Yes[86,90]	Further studies of the harms of screening are required
There should be an agreed policy on whom to treat as patients	No	One RCT is in progress

ARF, acute rheumatic fever; RHD, rheumatic heart disease; WHF, World Heart Federation; RCT, randomised control trial.

If echocardiographic screening proves to be an effective tool for prevention of RHD progression, implementation research to address these and other key considerations will become a needed top priority.

Other criteria of screening programs recommended by Wilson and Jungner are dependent on the local infrastructure of the region and of the country. These include (A) facilities for diagnosis and treatment should be available, (B) the cost of screening (including diagnosis and treatment of patients diagnosed) should be economically balanced in relation to possible expenditure on medical care as a whole,[78–80] and (C) screening should be a continuing process and not a "once and for all" project. All of these factors need full consideration before a decision about implementation of a screening program. Some may be very challenging to ensure in low-income countries with fragile health system structures.

What are the Harms of a Screening Program?

Acknowledging that all screening programs inevitably cause some harm, efforts are also being made to understand the impact of RHD screening on patients, families, and communities. Strong support for RHD screening has been voiced by parents of screened

children in New Zealand[90] and screened children and their teachers in Uganda.[86] However, while a negative screening result seems to have no negative impact,[91] a positive result has been shown to cause increased anxiety,[92] decreased physical activity,[92] and decreased parental[93] and child quality of life.[91,93] A single study on the impact of peer support showed a promising normalization of quality of life and improved social connectedness when youth were linked to a peer support group.[94] Further community-engaged research is needed to minimize negative impacts of RHD screening on children and communities.

Two studies from New Zealand reported the effects of an abnormal screening result. In the first study, 62% of parents reported that they would treat their child differently after an abnormal screening result.[95] The second study found long-standing anxiety and changes in physical activity in 20% of those with positive screening tests, again based on parental reports. There were no harms documented for those with normal results.[92] A Ugandan study found that a diagnosis of latent RHD led to a reduction in health-related quality of life scores, even though the cohort was largely asymptomatic.[91] An Australian study found no overall difference in quality of life scores after screening, but children with positive screening tests had lower scores in some subscale areas.[93] The potential harms of screening, raised by these studies, need to be considered in the broader framework of screening appropriateness.[96]

What is the Ideal Model/Test Strategy for Echocardiographic Screening?

Despite the large advances in RHD screening knowledge, there is still uncertainly about the optimal model for a screening program, including use of nonexperts, models for diagnostic review, follow-up, and the optimal target screening population.

Most RHD prevalence surveys have screened school-aged children, mainly for logistic reasons but also because ARF incidence peaks in this age group. School screening may not be appropriate in areas where school enrollment and attendance are lower.

Screening of older adolescents has shown a higher prevalence,[97] consistent with the known epidemiology of clinical RHD, but targeting this population needs to be balanced against the reduced "window period" for intervention, lower school attendance, increased need for privacy, and technical challenges of echocardiography in adolescents. Several studies have also included young adults.[21,58,98,99] A Ugandan study screened first-degree relatives of latent RHD cases, including adult parents.[100] A single study from Eritrea screened pregnant women and reported a high RHD prevalence, although the sample size was small and low-specificity diagnostic criteria were used.[101] Combining screening for RHD with an antenatal obstetric ultrasound is opportunistic and may be logistically achievable. Selective screening of only highest-risk populations (for example, by ethnicity) may be scientifically justifiable, but culturally sensitive. Screening in New Caledonia, Australia, and New Zealand has thus far included low and high-risk ethnic groups. If echocardiographic screening is elevated on public health agendas in the future, further work will be needed to identify and personalize the ideal model for different, high-risk environments. These issues are summarized in Table 13.5.

CONCLUSIONS

Echocardiographic screening has been a powerful tool for defining the epidemiology of RHD. The resulting increase in awareness and advocacy has reinvigorated the global health community to address this neglected

TABLE 13.5	
Considerations for Developing a New Echocardiographic Screening Program[a].	
1.	Partnership with Local Ministry of Health
2.	Partnership with schools and families; school visits for education of teachers, students, and families
3.	Program logistics
	Echocardiogram technology: handheld versus portable, power sources, batteries
	Scanning room, plinths, curtains, changing rooms, waiting areas, student flow
	Echocardiographer workforce and level of training
	Reporting clinicians (echocardiographers, cardiologists, physicians experienced in echocardiography of RHD)
4.	Protocols; abbreviated versus full scan. If abbreviated, pathways for full scan for those abnormal abbreviated scan
5.	Reporting in a timely manner. Release of reports to families
6.	Counseling of families with abnormal scans: RHD, congenital heart disease
7.	Agreed treatment threshold (including active surveillance of borderline RHD)
8.	Pathways linking to ongoing care for RHD and CHD patients
9.	Secondary prophylaxis pathways
10.	Treatment of advanced rheumatic and congenital heart disease

RHD, rheumatic heart disease; CHD, congenital heart disease.
[a] More extensive details are available in the Tools for Implementing RHD Control Programmes (TIPS) Handbook, developed by RHD Action.[102]

disease. Echocardiography has high sensitivity for latent RHD detection and is increasingly available in less-resourced settings. Criteria exist for the echocardiographic diagnosis of RHD, but with several limitations that impede their application to a screening context. Innovations in screening have included task shifting to scanning by nonexpert operators, the use of portable and handheld technology, and remote reporting. The natural history of latent RHD progression and the effectiveness of penicillin prophylaxis to improve outcomes are still being defined. Thus, there remains uncertainty as to whether screening is an effective RHD control strategy.

REFERENCES

1. Mirabel M, Fauchier T, Bacquelin R, et al. Echocardiography screening to detect rheumatic heart disease: a cohort study of schoolchildren in French Pacific Islands. *Int J Cardiol.* 2015;188:89−95.
2. Baroux N, Rouchon B, Huon B, Germain A, Meunier JM, D'Ortenzio E. High prevalence of rheumatic heart disease in schoolchildren detected by echocardiography screening in New Caledonia. *J Paediatr Child Health.* 2013;49:109−114.
3. Corsenac P, Heenan RC, Roth A, Rouchon B, Guillot N, Hoy D. An epidemiological study to assess the true incidence and prevalence of rheumatic heart disease and acute rheumatic fever in New Caledonian school children. *J Paediatr Child Health.* 2016;52:739−744.
4. Carapetis JR, Steer AC, Mulholland EK, Weber M. The global burden of group a streptococcal diseases. *Lancet Infect Dis.* 2005;5:685−694.
5. Marijon E, Ou P, Celermajer DS, et al. Prevalence of rheumatic heart disease detected by echocardiographic screening. *N Engl J Med.* 2007;357:470−476.
6. Tadele H, Mekonnen W, Tefera E. Rheumatic mitral stenosis in children: more accelerated course in sub-Saharan patients. *BMC Cardiovasc Disord.* 2013;13:95.
7. Zhang W, Okello E, Nyakoojo W, Lwabi P, Mondo CK. Proportion of patients in the Uganda rheumatic heart disease registry with advanced disease requiring urgent surgical interventions. *Afr Health Sci.* 2015;15:1182−1188.
8. Engelman D, Mataika RL, Ah Kee M, et al. Clinical outcomes for young people with screening-detected and clinically-diagnosed rheumatic heart disease in Fiji. *Int J Cardiol.* 2017;240:422−427.
9. Zuhlke L, Karthikeyan G, Engel ME, et al. Clinical outcomes in 3343 children and adults with rheumatic heart disease from 14 low- and middle-income countries: two-year follow-up of the global rheumatic heart disease registry (the REMEDY study). *Circulation.* 2016;134:1456−1466.
10. Tompkins DG, Boxerbaum B, Liebman J. Long-term prognosis of rheumatic fever patients receiving regular intramuscular benzathine penicillin. *Circulation.* 1972;45:543−551.
11. Carapetis JR, McDonald M, Wilson NJ. Acute rheumatic fever. *Lancet.* 2005;366:155−168.
12. Lawrence JG, Carapetis JR, Griffiths K, Edwards K, Condon JR. Acute rheumatic fever and rheumatic heart disease: incidence and progression in the Northern Territory of Australia, 1997 to 2010. *Circulation.* 2013;128:492−501.
13. Abbasi AS, Hashmi JA, Robinson Jr RD, Suraya S, Syed SA. Prevalence of heart disease in school children of Karachi. *Am J Cardiol.* 1966;18:544−547.
14. Maharaj B, Dyer RB, Leary WP, Arbuckle DD, Armstrong TG, Pudifin DJ. Screening for rheumatic heart disease amongst black schoolchildren in Inanda, South Africa. *J Trop Pediatr.* 1987;33:60−61.
15. Finau SA, Taylor L. Rheumatic heart disease and school screening: initiatives at an isolated hospital in Tonga. *Med J Aust.* 1988;148:563−567.
16. Thakur JS, Negi PC, Ahluwalia SK, Sharma R. Integrated community-based screening for cardiovascular diseases of childhood. *World Health Forum.* 1997;18:24−27.
17. Steer AC, Adams J, Carlin J, Nolan T, Shann F. Rheumatic heart disease in school children in Samoa. *Arch Dis Child.* 1999;81:372.
18. Talbot RG. Rheumatic fever and rheumatic heart disease in the Hamilton health district: II. Long term follow-up and secondary prophylaxis. *N Z Med J.* 1984;97:634−637.
19. WHO. *Rheumatic Fever and Rheumatic Herat Disease.* WHO Techincal Report Series; 2001.
20. Anabwani GM, Bonhoeffer P. Prevalence of heart disease in school children in rural Kenya using colour-flow echocardiography. *East Afr Med J.* 1996;73:215−217.
21. Paar JA, Berrios NM, Rose JD, et al. Prevalence of rheumatic heart disease in children and young adults in Nicaragua. *Am J Cardiol.* 2010;105:1809−1814.
22. Bhaya M, Panwar S, Beniwal R, Panwar RB. High prevalence of rheumatic heart disease detected by echocardiography in school children. *Echocardiogr.* 2010;27:448−453.
23. Carapetis JR. Pediatric rheumatic heart disease in the developing world: echocardiographic versus clinical screening. *Nat Clin Pract Cardiovasc Med.* 2008;5:74−75.
24. Beaton A, Aliku T, Dewyer A, et al. Latent rheumatic heart disease: identifying the children at highest risk of unfavorable outcome. *Circulation.* 2017;136:2233−2244.
25. Webb RH, Wilson NJ, Lennon DR, et al. Optimising echocardiographic screening for rheumatic heart disease in New Zealand: not all valve disease is rheumatic. *Cardiol Young.* 2011;21:436−443.
26. Carapetis J, Hardy M, Fakakovikaetau T, et al. Evaluation of a screening protocol using asculatation and portable echocardiography to detect asymptomatic rheumatic heart disease in Tongan schoolchildren. *Nat Clin Pract Cardiovasc Med.* 2008;7.
27. Godown J, Lu JC, Beaton A, et al. Handheld echocardiography versus auscultation for detection of rheumatic heart disease. *Pediatrics.* 2015.
28. Colquhoun SM, Kado JH, Remenyi B, Wilson NJ, Carapetis JR, Steer AC. Echocardiographic screening in a resource poor setting: borderline rheumatic heart disease could be a normal variant. *Int J Cardiol.* 2014;173:284−289.
29. Roberts KV, Brown AD, Maguire GP, Atkinson DN, Carapetis JR. Utility of auscultatory screening for detecting rheumatic heart disease in high-risk children in Australia's Northern Territory. *Med J Aust.* 2013;199:196−199.
30. Rothenbuhler M, O'Sullivan CJ, Stortecky S, et al. Active surveillance for rheumatic heart disease in endemic regions: a systematic review and meta-analysis of prevalence among children and adolescents. *Lancet Glob Health.* 2014;2:e717−e726.

31. Carapetis JR, Parr J, C T. *Standardization of Epidemiologic Protocols for Surveillance of Post-streptococcal Sequelae: Acute Rheumatic Fever, Rheumatic Heart Disease and Acute Post-streptococcal Glomerulonephritis.* 2006.

32. Remenyi B, Wilson N, Steer A, et al. World Heart Federation criteria for echocardiographic diagnosis of rheumatic heart disease–an evidence-based guideline. *Nat Rev Cardiol.* 2012;9:297–309.

33. Webb RH, Gentles TL, Stirling JW, Lee M, O'Donnell C, Wilson NJ. Valvular regurgitation using portable echocardiography in a healthy student population: implications for rheumatic heart disease screening. *J Am Soc Echocardiogr.* 2015;28:981–988.

34. Webb RH, Culliford-Semmens N, Sidhu K, Wilson NJ. Normal echocardiographic mitral and aortic valve thickness in children. *Heart Asia.* 2017;9:70–75.

35. Hunter LD, Monaghan M, Lloyd G, Pecoraro AJK, Doubell AF, Herbst PG. Prominent inter-scallop separations of the posterior leaflet of the mitral valve: an important cause of 'pathological' mitral regurgitation. *Echo Res Pract.* 2018.

36. Watkins DA, Johnson CO, Colquhoun SM, et al. Global, regional, and national burden of rheumatic heart disease, 1990–2015. *N Engl J Med.* 2017;377:713–722.

37. Zuhlke LJ, Steer AC. Estimates of the global burden of rheumatic heart disease. *Glob Heart.* 2013;8:189–195.

38. Saxena A, Zuhlke L, Wilson N. Echocardiographic screening for rheumatic heart disease: issues for the cardiology community. *Glob Heart.* 2013;8:197–202.

39. Mirabel M, Tafflet M, Noel B, et al. Prevalence of rheumatic heart disease in the Pacific: from subclinical to symptomatic heart valve disease. *J Am Coll Cardiol.* 2016;67:1500–1502.

40. Scheel A, Ssinabulya I, Aliku T, et al. Community study to uncover the full spectrum of rheumatic heart disease in Uganda. *Heart.* 2018.

41. Beaton A, Okello E, Scheel A, et al. Impact of heart disease on maternal, fetal and neonatal outcomes in a low-resource setting. *Heart.* 2018.

42. Popescu BA, Andrade MJ, Badano LP, et al. European Association of Echocardiography recommendations for training, competence, and quality improvement in echocardiography. *Eur J Echocardiogr.* 2009;10:893–905.

43. Ehler D, Carney DK, Dempsey AL, et al. Guidelines for cardiac sonographer education: recommendations of the American society of echocardiography sonographer training and education committee. *J Am Soc Echocardiogr.* 2001;14:77–84.

44. Via G, Hussain A, Wells M, et al. International evidence-based recommendations for focused cardiac ultrasound. *J Am Soc Echocardiogr.* 2014;27:683.e1–683.e33.

45. Neskovic AN, Edvardsen T, Galderisi M, et al. Focus cardiac ultrasound: the European association of cardiovascular imaging viewpoint. *Eur Heart J Cardiovasc Imaging.* 2014;15:956–960.

46. Galderisi M, Santoro A, Versiero M, et al. Improved cardiovascular diagnostic accuracy by pocket size imaging device in non-cardiologic outpatients: the NaUSiCa (Naples Ultrasound Stethoscope in Cardiology) study. *Cardiovasc Ultrasound.* 2010;8:51.

47. Colquhoun SM, Carapetis JR, Kado JH, et al. Pilot study of nurse-led rheumatic heart disease echocardiography screening in Fiji-a novel approach in a resource-poor setting. *Cardiol Young.* 2013;23:546–552.

48. Barnes SS, Sim J, Marrone JR, et al. Echocardiographic screening of schoolchildren in American Samoa to detect rheumatic heart disease: a feasibility study. *Pediatr Health Med Therapeut.* 2011;2:21.

49. Shmueli H, Burstein Y, Sagy I, et al. Briefly trained medical students can effectively identify rheumatic mitral valve injury using a hand-carried ultrasound. *Echocardiogr.* 2013;30:621–626.

50. Mirabel M, Bacquelin R, Tafflet M, et al. Screening for rheumatic heart disease: evaluation of a focused cardiac ultrasound approach. *Circ Cardiovasc Imaging.* 2015;8.

51. Ploutz M, Lu JC, Scheel J, et al. Handheld echocardiographic screening for rheumatic heart disease by non-experts. *Heart.* 2016;102:35–39.

52. Beaton A, Nascimento BR, Diamantino AC, et al. Efficacy of a standardized computer-based training curriculum to teach echocardiographic identification of rheumatic heart disease to nonexpert users. *Am J Cardiol.* 2016;117:1783–1789.

53. Engelman D, Kado JH, Remenyi B, et al. Focused cardiac ultrasound screening for rheumatic heart disease by briefly trained health workers: a study of diagnostic accuracy. *Lancet Glob Health.* 2016;4:e386–e394.

54. Sims Sanyahumbi A, Sable CA, Karlsten M, et al. Task shifting to clinical officer-led echocardiography screening for detecting rheumatic heart disease in Malawi, Africa. *Cardiol Young.* 2016:1–7.

55. Musuku J, Engel ME, Musonda P, et al. Prevalence of rheumatic heart disease in Zambian school children. *BMC Cardiovasc Disord.* 2018;18:135.

56. Beaton A, Aliku T, Okello E, et al. The utility of handheld echocardiography for early diagnosis of rheumatic heart disease. *J Am Soc Echocardiogr.* 2014;27:42–49.

57. Beaton A, Lu JC, Aliku T, et al. The utility of handheld echocardiography for early rheumatic heart disease diagnosis: a field study. *Eur Heart J Cardiovasc Imaging.* 2015;16:475–482.

58. Zuhlke LJ, Engel ME, Nkepu S, Mayosi BM. Evaluation of a focussed protocol for hand-held echocardiography and computer-assisted auscultation in detecting latent rheumatic heart disease in scholars. *Cardiol Young.* 2015:1–10.

59. Mirabel M, Celermajer D, Beraud AS, Jouven X, Marijon E, Hagege AA. Pocket-sized focused cardiac ultrasound: strengths and limitations. *Arch Cardiovasc Dis Suppl.* 2015;108:197–205.

60. Barrett PM, Topol EJ. To truly look inside. *Lancet.* 2016;387:1268–1269.

61. Nascimento BR, Beaton AZ, Nunes MC, et al. Echocardiographic prevalence of rheumatic heart disease in Brazilian schoolchildren: data from the PROVAR study. *Int J Cardiol.* 2016;219:439–445.

62. Lu JC, Sable C, Ensing GJ, et al. Simplified rheumatic heart disease screening criteria for handheld echocardiography. *J Am Soc Echocardiogr.* 2015;28:463−469.

63. Mirabel M, Celermajer DS, Ferreira B, et al. Screening for rheumatic heart disease: evaluation of a simplified echocardiography-based approach. *Eur Heart J Cardiovasc Imaging.* 2012;13:1024−1029.

64. WHO. *Task Shifting: Rational Redistribution of Tasks Amongst Health Workforce Teams: Global Recommendations and Guidelines.* 2008.

65. Saxena A. Task shifting rheumatic heart disease screening to non-experts. *Lancet Glob Health.* 2016;4:e349−e350.

66. Engelman D, Watson C, Remenyi B, Steer AC. *Echocardiographic Diagnosis of Rheumatic Heart Disease: Nurse Training Modules;* 2014. Available from: http://www.wiredhealthresources.net/EchoProject/.

67. Engelman D, Kado JH, Remenyi B, et al. Teaching focused echocardiography for rheumatic heart disease screening. *Ann Pediatr Cardiol.* 2015;8:118−121.

68. Engelman D, Okello E, Beaton A, et al. Evaluation of computer-based training for health workers in echocardiography for RHD. *Glob Heart.* 2017;12:17−23 e8.

69. Lopes EL, Beaton AZ, Nascimento BR, et al. Telehealth solutions to enable global collaboration in rheumatic heart disease screening. *J Telemed Telecare.* 2018;24:101−109.

70. Kotit S, Said K, ElFaramawy A, Mahmoud H, Phillips DIW, Yacoub MH. Prevalence and prognostic value of echocardiographic screening for rheumatic heart disease. *Open Heart.* 2017;4:e000702.

71. Remond M, Atkinson D, White A, et al. Are minor echocardiographic changes associated with an increased risk of acute rheumatic fever or progression to rheumatic heart disease? *Int J Cardiol.* 2015;198:117−122.

72. Zuhlke L, Engel ME, Lemmer CE, et al. The natural history of latent rheumatic heart disease in a 5 year follow-up study: a prospective observational study. *BMC Cardiovasc Disord.* 2016;16:46.

73. Bertaina G, Rouchon B, Huon B, et al. Outcomes of borderline rheumatic heart disease: a prospective cohort study. *Int J Cardiol.* 2017;228:661−665.

74. Engelman D, Wheaton GR, Mataika RL, et al. Screening-detected rheumatic heart disease can progress to severe disease. *Heart Asia.* 2016;8:67−73.

75. Saxena A, Ramakrishnan S, Roy A, et al. Prevalence and outcome of subclinical rheumatic heart disease in India: the RHEUMATIC (rheumatic heart echo utilisation and monitoring actuarial trends in Indian children) study. *Heart.* 2011;97:2018−2022.

76. Bhaya M, Beniwal R, Panwar S, Panwar RB. Two years of follow-up validates the echocardiographic criteria for the diagnosis and screening of rheumatic heart disease in asymptomatic populations. *Echocardiogr.* 2011;28:929−933.

77. Karthikeyan G. Measuring and reporting disease progression in subclinical rheumatic heart disease. *Heart Asia.* 2016;8:74−75.

78. Manji RA, Witt J, Tappia PS, Jung Y, Menkis AH, Ramjiawan B. Cost-effectiveness analysis of rheumatic heart disease prevention strategies. *Expert Rev Pharmacoecon Outcomes Res.* 2013;13:715−724.

79. Zachariah JP, Samnaliev M. Echo-based screening of rheumatic heart disease in children: a cost-effectiveness Markov model. *J Med Econ.* 2015;18:410−419.

80. Roberts K, Cannon J, Atkinson D, et al. Echocardiographic screening for rheumatic heart disease in indigenous Australian children: a cost-utility analysis. *J Am Heart Assoc.* 2017;6.

81. Wilson JMGJG. Principals and practices of screening for disease. *Public Health Pap.* 1968;34.

82. Roberts KV, Maguire GP, Brown A, et al. Rheumatic heart disease in Indigenous children in northern Australia: differences in prevalence and the challenges of screening. *Med J Aust.* 2015;203, 221.e1-7.

83. Santos JPA, Carmo GAL, Beaton AZ, et al. Challenges for the implementation of the first large-scale rheumatic heart disease screening program in Brazil: the PROVAR study experience. *Arq Bras Cardiol.* 2017.

84. Shung-King M, Zuhlke L, Engel ME, Mayosi BM. Asymptomatic rheumatic heart disease in South African schoolchildren: implications for addressing chronic health conditions through a school health service. *S Afr Med J.* 2016;106:761−762.

85. Gurney JK, Chong A, Culliford-Semmens N, Tilton E, Wilson NJ, Sarfati D. High levels of rheumatic fever and sore throat awareness among a high-risk population screened for rheumatic heart disease. *N Z Med J.* 2017;130:107−110.

86. Ploutz M, Aliku T, Bradley-Hewitt T, et al. Child and teacher acceptability of school-based echocardiographic screening for rheumatic heart disease in Uganda. *Cardiol Young.* 2017;27:82−89.

87. New Zealand National Health Committee. *Screening to Improve Health in New Zealand: Criteria to Assess Screening Programmes.* 2003.

88. Stacey D, Legare F, Lewis K, et al. Decision aids for people facing health treatment or screening decisions. *Cochrane Database Syst Rev.* 2017;4:Cd001431.

89. Gewitz MH, Baltimore RS, Tani LY, et al. American heart association committee on rheumatic fever E and kawasaki disease of the council on cardiovascular disease in the Y. Revision of the Jones criteria for the diagnosis of acute rheumatic fever in the era of Doppler echocardiography: a scientific statement from the American heart association. *Circulation.* 2015;131:1806−1818.

90. Perelini F, Blair N, Wilson N, Farrell A, Aitken A. Family acceptability of school-based echocardiographic screening for rheumatic heart disease in a high-risk population in New Zealand. *J Paediatr Child Health.* 2015;51:682−688.

91. Bradley-Hewitt T, Dantin A, Ploutz M, et al. The impact of echocardiographic screening for rheumatic heart disease on patient quality of life. *J Pediatr.* 2016;175:123−129.

92. Gurney J, Chong A, Culliford-Semmens N, Tilton E, Wilson NJ, Sarfati D. The benefits and harms of rheumatic heart disease screening from the perspective of

the screened population. *Int J Cardiol*. 2016;221: 734–740.

93. Wark EK, Hodder YC, Woods CE, Maguire GP. Patient and health-care impact of a pilot rheumatic heart disease screening program. *J Paediatr Child Health*. 2013;49: 297–302.

94. Scheel A, Beaton A, Okello E, et al. The impact of a peer support group for children with rheumatic heart disease in Uganda. *Patient Educ Couns*. 2018;101:119–123.

95. Perelini F, Blair N, Wilson N, Farrell A, Aitken A. Family acceptability of school-based echocardiographic screening for rheumatic heart disease in a high-risk population in New Zealand. *J Paediatr Child Health*. 2015.

96. Remond MG, Wark EK, Maguire GP. Screening for rheumatic heart disease in aboriginal and torres strait islander children. *J Paediatr Child Health*. 2013;49: 526–531.

97. Kane A, Mirabel M, Toure K, et al. Echocardiographic screening for rheumatic heart disease: age matters. *Int J Cardiol*. 2013;168:888–891.

98. Ledos P, Kamblock J, Bourgoin P, Eono P, Carapetis JR. Prevalence of rheumatic heart disease in young adults from New Caledonia. *Arch Cardiovasc Dis Suppl*. 2015; 108:16–22.

99. Gemechu T, Mahmoud H, Parry EH, Phillips DI, Yacoub MH. Community-based prevalence study of rheumatic heart disease in rural Ethiopia. *Eur J Prev Cardiol*. 2017;24:717–723.

100. Aliku T, Sable C, Scheel A, et al. Targeted echocardiographic screening for latent rheumatic heart disease in northern Uganda: evaluating familial risk following identification of an index case. *PLoS Neglected Trop Dis*. 2016; 10:e0004727.

101. Otto H, Saether SG, Banteyrga L, Haugen BO, Skjaerpe T. High prevalence of subclinical rheumatic heart disease in pregnant women in a developing country: an echocardiographic study. *Echocardiogr*. 2011;28:1049–1053.

102. Wyber RGG, Thompson A, Kennedy D, Johnson D, Taubert T, Carapetis JK. *Tools for Implementing RHD Control Programmes (TIPS) Handbook*. 2014.

CHAPTER 14

Group A *Streptococcus* Vaccines

JOSHUA OSOWICKI • JOHAN VEKEMANS • LUIZA GUILHERME • ANDREW C. STEER •
JEROME H. KIM

INTRODUCTION

Although a reinvigorated global vaccine development effort gives legitimate reason for cautious optimism, it is a sad reality that in 2019 the best introduction to a discussion on vaccines for group A *Streptococcus* (GAS) comes from 1967, by Professor Gene Stollerman:

> … one might have expected that the vast amount of biochemical and immunologic information about this organism would have led to the successful induction of artificial immunity in man against one of his major pathogens. The rewards for such an achievement remain great: the eradication of rheumatic fever and perhaps one major form of glomerulonephritis. The prospect of attaining the same goals by chemotherapy alone is limited … Why, then, have all but a few laboratories abandoned the direct pursuit of so worthy an objective? And what are the prospects for success for those who persist in this tantalizing search? [1]

By any of its multiple names: the anachronistic *Streptococcus haemolyticus*; the historical Lancefield Group A β-hemolytic *Streptococcus*; the microbiological *Streptococcus pyogenes*; or simply "Strep A," the scourge of GAS diseases has proven to be a remarkably potent and persistent problem. The global burden of GAS diseases spans mild to severe, local and systemic, acute and chronic, infectious and noninfectious syndromes.[2] Although the distribution of GAS diseases has changed with development and control efforts including antibiotics, and the greatest burden continues to fall upon low- and middle-income countries, morbidity and mortality from GAS diseases occur at all ages and in every social and geographic setting.[3,4]

Conservative global estimates of GAS diseases are of 615 million incident cases of GAS pharyngitis, 162 million prevalent cases of impetigo, 660,000 incident cases of invasive GAS infection, 470,000 incident cases of acute poststreptococcal glomerulonephritis (APSGN), and 470,000 incident cases of acute rheumatic fever (ARF), and over 33 million prevalent cases of rheumatic heart disease (RHD).[3–6] GAS is a major contributor to an estimated 61 million annual cases of cellulitis.[7,8] Despite retaining universal susceptibility to penicillin, GAS is associated with at least 500,000 annual deaths, including 320,000 from RHD alone.[4] Case-fatality rates are over 25% for the most severe invasive GAS infections. RHD and APSGN are important contributors to chronic noncommunicable disease states including heart failure, stroke, and chronic kidney disease. Pharyngitis and impetigo cause a less conspicuous but still major impact on healthcare utilization, absenteeism, and antibiotic use.[9,10] Inappropriate treatment of suspected GAS pharyngitis in an estimated 70% of cases has a direct cost of $200 million (USD) and a difficult-to-estimate indirect cost associated with antimicrobial resistance.[8,11,12] Despite this evidence of substantial morbidity, mortality, and cost due to GAS diseases, investment in GAS vaccine development has been miniscule and no current candidate vaccine has entered efficacy trials.[13,14]

The promise of vaccination to prevent ARF and RHD was recognized as the causal link with GAS infection was established. Before that, preceding even recognition and classification of the streptococci, there were active and passive vaccination efforts targeting scarlet fever, another GAS syndrome.[15,16] Despite the prodigious proliferation of GAS research continuing since Stollerman's prophetic words above, vaccine development has been impeded by scientific, regulatory, and commercial obstacles and this promise remains unrealized.[14,17,18] GAS vaccine development is now a stated priority of the World Health Organization (WHO), as the only healthcare intervention with a realistic prospect of achieving a sizable and sustainable reduction in the global burden of all GAS diseases.[14,19] The importance of vaccine development for RHD specifically was recognized in the 2018 WHO Global Resolution on Rheumatic Fever and Rheumatic Heart Disease. Only partial effects have been seen with

Acute Rheumatic Fever and Rheumatic Heart Disease. https://doi.org/10.1016/B978-0-323-63982-8.00014-3

major public investment in strategies for primary and secondary prevention of ARF and RHD,[20,21] and the management of patients with invasive GAS infections regularly stretches the capacities of even the most well-resourced high-technology hospitals.[22,23] There is now a coordinated global effort gathering momentum to overcome roadblocks to GAS vaccine development and carry candidate vaccines forward toward Phase 2b/3 trials to demonstrate vaccine safety and efficacy, initially against pharyngitis and possibly impetigo.[14,24]

ISSUES IN GAS VACCINE DEVELOPMENT

Strain Diversity. The pioneering streptococcal microbiologist professor Rebecca Lancefield initially segregated the streptococci pathogenic in humans on the basis of the serologic specificity of capsular polysaccharides.[25] Lancefield group A carbohydrate strains, the group A streptococci, were further characterized according to serologic specificity of surface-expressed M-proteins.[26] From approximately 50 M serotypes, molecular typing of the M-protein hypervariable region has now described more than 220 *emm* genotypes, which have subsequently been grouped by genetic and functional similarities into smaller *emm* "clusters." [27] Although the M serotypes, *emm* genotypes, and *emm* clusters are related, they are not fully compatible classification systems. Sequencing of the hypervariable *emm* region and whole genome sequencing has more recently given insight into even greater levels of complexity and strain diversity.[27,28]

The earliest vaccine studies employed relatively crude preparations of mixtures of killed GAS strains.[29] Mid-20th century research focused on the M-protein as the apparent immunodominant GAS antigen, finding that M-serotype-specific bactericidal immune responses correlated with protection against homologous infection but not against infection with heterologous strains.[26] It is largely unknown whether the conclusions reached by these studies finding type-specific bactericidal responses for some serotypes can be extrapolated across all ~50 M serotypes, or to the >220 *emm* genotypes, and the extent to which *emm* clusters correspond to cross-reactive functional antibody responses.

The initial promise of multivalent vaccines targeting strains belonging to *emm* types most prevalent in high-income countries has been undermined by evidence of extensive global GAS strain diversity, and the potential for rapid emergence of new strains, especially in the highest-burden settings.[30,31] The hope that cluster-based cross-reactivity might address this coverage challenge has been only partially substantiated.[32] An alternative but untested approach that has emerged is the notion that a novel synthetic protein vaccine could exploit conserved structural patterns lying beneath more superficial hypervariability of the most immunogenic M-protein regions.[33] A similar approach has also been discussed for vaccines based on the GAS T-antigen.[34] Other groups have shifted focus away from the M-protein hypervariable region to more conserved elements, or away from the M-protein entirely to other conserved antigens. Conserved "cryptic" epitopes from the C-repeat region of the M-protein that are not highly immunogenic after natural exposure have been developed as vaccine antigens, with promising preclinical and phase I results.[35–38] A growing list of conserved non-M-protein antigens have also shown promise in preclinical studies, some known for many decades (e.g., the group A carbohydrate, streptolysin O, T-antigen) and others more recently identified by reverse vaccinology methods.[39,40]

Protective immune responses. There is no established correlate of natural or vaccine-induced protection against GAS infection in humans and very few longitudinal data from which putative correlates may be inferred. It is a longstanding and widely propagated tenet that decreasing incidence of GAS pharyngitis with age is related to cumulative immunity following natural infections, although this does not offer lifelong protection and there is a spike in incidence of cellulitis and severe invasive GAS infections later in life. A study by Lancefield reporting that, "In 12 individuals type-specific antibodies against 11 different homologous types following 14 separate infections persisted for 4–32 years," has been widely referenced as indicative of long-lived type-specific protective immunity.[41] However, the sentence immediately following describes another 13 individuals without a type-specific bactericidal response 1–31 years after known GAS infections, including 3 who previously had a homologous type-specific response soon after infection. In 1970s controlled human infection studies with M1, M3, and M12 GAS strains, baseline serum type-specific bactericidal responses did not clearly correlate with protection against experimental pharyngitis caused by homologous strains applied by swab to the pharynx of healthy adult volunteers.[42–44] Others have demonstrated that antibody responses targeting the group A carbohydrate correlate with protection against GAS pharyngeal colonization, and in vitro responses against a number of other antigens do increase with age.[45]

Development of methods to measure relevant immune responses is central to vaccine development. For GAS, there are presently no widely available standardized high-throughput methods.[46] Widely used enzyme-linked immunosorbent assays to measure binding antibody suffer from a lack of standardization and reference GAS sera. Work continues on newer opsonophagocytic functional antibody assays to replace the laborious Lancefield serum bactericidal assay, which does not produce results that can be compared between assays or laboratories.[47,48] Qualification and validation of these newer assays, with availability of GAS reference serum, will be an important step forward.

Autoimmunity. The specter of autoimmune complications induced by vaccines against GAS has arguably been the greatest obstacle standing in the way of vaccine development.[1] ARF (with subsequent RHD) and APSGN are nonsuppurative immunological complications following GAS infections. The pediatric autoimmune neuropsychiatric disorders associated with streptococcal infections (PANDAS) hypothesis are also discussed in these terms. There have been extensive studies of humoral and cellular cross-reactivity and homology between human proteins and streptococcal antigens, focusing mostly on M-protein but also on non-M antigens including the group A carbohydrate (discussed in detail in Chapter 2).[49] Autoreactive T lymphocytes recognizing the N-terminal and midprotein domains of the M-protein have been described in ARF and cloned from the valves of RHD patients. Although many studies have found cross-reactivity and homology, particularly for some M-protein regions and the GlcNAc moiety of the group A carbohydrate, none has conclusively implicated an antigen or antigenic region in the causal pathway of ARF or APSGN in humans. Nonetheless, vaccine developers have been understandably cautious in avoiding the potentially cross-reactive antigens in their candidates.

Animal models. GAS is exquisitely adapted and restricted to its human host.[50] Professor Rebecca Lancefield illustrated this by recounting the difficulty she had experienced in attempts to infect mice, requiring multiple repeated passages, whereas accidental exposure of laboratory assistants to such a strain easily caused infection in humans, even when the strains had not seen a human host in many years.[26] It is possible to passage strains for adaption to some other species (typically mammalian) such as mice, or if nonhuman primates are inoculated with very high doses of bacteria.[51] Still, human host restriction for certain virulence factors may not be overcome, although humanized transgenic models can go some way to addressing this problem.[52] Importantly, even if every animal model was considered together, the diversity of human GAS disease syndromes has not been reproduced by animal models.

HISTORY OF GAS VACCINES

Recent reviews have suggested that the first clinical trial of a GAS vaccine was in 1923 by Bloomfeld et al. following an earlier finding by the same group that asymptomatic carriage of GAS prevented symptomatic pharyngitis.[17,29] However, there is also an important and latterly under-appreciated prehistory provided by publications describing vaccine studies targeting scarlet fever.[15,16] From 1833 to 1923, healthy adults and/or child participants in these studies were administered variously processed extracts of blood, serum, mucosal (pus, mucous) or cutaneous lesions (crusts) from scarlet fever cases, with the goal of inducing protective immune responses. The earliest of these studies explicitly hoped to emulate Edward Jenner's success in protecting against smallpox by inoculation of cowpox (*Variolae vaccinae*), an approach suggested in 1796 by Erasmus Darwin (Charles' grandfather):

> No one could do an act more beneficial to society, or glorious to himself, than by teaching humanity how to inoculate this fatal disease [scarlet fever]; and thus, to deprive it of its malignity. Matter might be taken from the ulcers in the throat, which would probably convey the contagion. Or warm water might be put on the eruption and scraped off again by the edge of a lancet. These experiments could be attended with no danger, and should be tried for the public benefit, and the honor of medical science.[15]

Although these scarlet fever inoculation experiments were of immense value in understanding the pathogenesis of scarlet fever, and more than one study led to brief and limited use of a product as an intended vaccine, none demonstrated sufficiently convincing protection to justify continued development.

In 1923, a heat-killed whole cell vaccine comprising 21 GAS strains isolated from recent cases of acute pharyngitis was administered by subcutaneous injection to female nursing student volunteers.[29] Across all 90 participants, over 4 months there were 3/35 (8.6%) cases of acute pharyngitis in vaccine recipients and 12/55 (21.8%) in those who received the placebo control (VE 61%; RR 0.39, 95% CI 0.12−1.29). There were zero cases of acute pharyngitis in vaccinated or control subjects who had asymptomatic GAS throat carriage at baseline. Considering only noncarriers, 3/18 (16.7%) vaccinated subjects developed pharyngitis compared to 12/39 (30.8%) controls (VE 46%; RR 0.54, 95% CI 0.17−1.69). For "severe" pharyngitis (fever ≥102°F; marked prostration, "violent pharyngeal reaction"), 0/18 of the vaccinated noncarriers were affected compared to 11/39 of the unvaccinated subjects (VE 100%; RR 0.09, 95% CI 0.006−1.47).

TABLE 14.1
Group A Streptococcal (GAS) Vaccines in Human Clinical Studies Before 1979[a].

Publication Year	Vaccine[b]	References
1923	Heat-killed whole-cell 21-strains	29
1930	Heat-killed whole-cell	95
1931	Heat-killed whole-cell	96
1932	Heat-killed whole-cell	97
1933–1943	"Toxin" and tannic acid-precipitated "toxin"	98–101
1937–1941	Tannic acid-precipitated "toxin"	102–104
1946	Heat-killed or ultraviolet-inactivated whole-cell M17 and M19	54
1949	Heat-killed whole-cell M3 and M17	105
1960	Partially purified M19	106
1962	M5 and M12 cell wall	107
1963	M14 cell wall	108
1968	Partially purified M3 protein	56
1969	Highly purified M12 protein	109
1973	Highly purified M1 protein	42
1975	Highly purified M1 protein (mucosal)	44
1978	Highly purified M3 protein (parenteral and mucosal vaccines) Highly purified M12 protein (parenteral and mucosal vaccines)	43
1979	Polypeptide fragment M24 protein	110

[a] Table adapted with permission from Steer et al.[111].
[b] Parenteral unless otherwise stated.

Subsequent to the promising study by Bloomfeld et al., a number of killed whole-cell vaccines were studied, and then partially purified M-protein vaccines (Table 14.1), with mixed results and/or unacceptable reactogenicity. During World War II, the US Navy tested a killed whole-cell vaccine (M17 and M19 serotypes) in recruits, with no protective efficacy observed even against M17 and M19—GAS pharyngitis persists as a problem in US military recruits to this day, and penicillin prophylaxis is still used.[53,54] Reactogenicity concerns were addressed by development of improved M-protein purification techniques.

Between 1973 and 1978, three important proof-of-concept human infection (controlled human infection, challenge) studies were published, including 172 participants in total. In each study, parenteral or mucosal M-protein vaccines were administered to healthy volunteers who were subsequently challenged with homologous serotype strains by direct application to the pharynx using a swab.[42–44] In the initial study of a parenteral highly purified monovalent M1-protein vaccine, protective efficacy against pharyngitis caused by a homologous M1 strain was 89% (95% CI 23–98).[42] This was followed by a study using a mucosal M1 vaccine, with vaccine efficacy of 68% (28–86).[44] Efficacy could not be demonstrated in the underpowered third study testing separate parenteral and mucosal M3 and M12 vaccines against challenge with homologous strains.[43] Across the three studies, colonization (positive throat cultures) was significantly reduced by mucosal but not parenteral vaccination, and vaccination (of any kind) was associated with statistically significant reductions in every symptom and sign of pharyngitis.[55] There were inconsistent quantitative (complement fixation, hemagglutination, radioimmune precipitation) and functional (bactericidal assay) antibody responses in serum and nasal secretions following vaccination and challenge, and none was predictive of protection against pharyngitis or colonization.

Unfortunately, a hiatus in GAS vaccine research and development occurred in the aftermath of a trial by Massell et al. administering between 18 and 33 weekly doses of a partially purified acid extract of M3 protein to 21 siblings of patients with ARF.[56] There were two definite cases and one probable case of ARF subsequently reported in study subjects after infection with heterologous GAS serotypes, with concerns raised in 1969 that the vaccine might be responsible as the rate appeared higher than expected compared to a historical cohort of siblings from the same facility.[57] Although the authors advised that the study design and small number of participants prevented firm conclusions from being made, the US Food and Drug Administration (FDA) responded in 1979 by issuing an embargo against further use of, "uncontrolled, poorly defined preparations presumed to contain antigens that have been demonstrated in earlier studies to produce local and systemic reactions." Although the 2006 revocation of this ruling suggests the intention was that this would not apply to highly purified well-characterized GAS antigens without demonstrable cross-reactivity with human tissues, the ruling did cast a pall on GAS vaccine research and development, with the practical effect of a ban.[58]

21ST CENTURY GAS VACCINE DEVELOPMENT

GAS vaccine research and development in the period following revocation of the FDA ruling can most easily be considered according to the various M-protein and non-M-protein targets of candidate vaccines (Table 14.2). Although there has been a steady increase in the number of preclinical vaccines since 2005, there has been a frustrating lack of progress in human clinical trials, with only four products tested in phase 1 and one vaccine reaching phase 2. None has entered efficacy trials, and major vaccine industry players have largely remained on the sidelines.

M-protein Vaccines

There have been two major approaches to modern development of M-protein vaccines: (1) multivalent polypeptide N-terminal vaccines (type-specific hypervariable region), and (2) use of relatively conserved epitopes from the C-repeat region. For both approaches, there have been careful steps taken to allay concerns of vaccine-induced immunity by avoiding cross-reactive epitopes.

Development of 6-, 26-, and 30-valent GAS vaccines comprising polypeptide strings (hybrid fusion proteins) of N-terminal M-protein fragments flows on from the work of Beachey et al. to define and separate type-specific N-terminal peptides from autoreactive M-protein epitopes, and then to prove the immunogenicity of these structurally defined antigens in animals and humans, first in isolation and then combined as polypeptides.[59] Three doses of the 6-valent vaccine were safe and immunogenic in human adults, with fourfold increases in binding antibody to vaccine strains in 95% of tested samples for 10 subjects vaccinated at the highest dose level (200 μg) and induction of opsonophagocytic and indirect bactericidal responses was observed for most participants against most of the vaccine strains.[60] Autoimmunity was not observed and postvaccination sera did not react with human tissue. Safety and immunogenicity results from initial human studies of a subsequent 26-valent vaccine including strain types most responsible for GAS disease in North America were similarly encouraging.[61,62] Concerns that global coverage of the 26-valent vaccine was 32%

−68% led to further development of a 30-valent formulation to increase global coverage toward 90%.[30,63] An initial observation that vaccination with these multivalent vaccines in rabbits (later replicated in humans) induced in vitro responses against nonvaccine GAS *emm* types (and *emm* type variants) has been understood to fit with the concept of cluster-based cross-reactivity, theoretically extending their coverage.[31,61,62,64,65] In the absence of human clinical data though, discussion of vaccine-induced cluster-based cross-protection should be considered still theoretical.[32] Addition of N-terminal fragments from M-related proteins to the 30-valent vaccine administered to rabbits further extended the strain coverage as measured by induction of opsonizing antibody.[66,67] The multivalent polypeptide string approach remains in active development, and investigation of the additive effect afforded by relatively conserved antigens such as M-related proteins continues. As understanding of natural and vaccine-induced immune responses has grown, the exciting prospect of a structure-based vaccine has emerged that would seek to recreate conserved broadly immunogenic structures underlying the genetically hypervariable type-specific M-protein N-terminal region.[33,68]

An alternative approach has been identification of conserved epitopes of the M-protein C-repeat region, described as "cryptic" because a humoral immune response to natural infections only occurs following repeated exposures.[37] The most advanced development programs have focused on (1) minimal B-cell epitope derivatives (J8, J14, P*17) of the p145 peptide,[38,69−71] and (2) a synthetic peptide vaccine (StreptInCor) comprising B- and T-cell epitopes derived from the C-repeat region of an M5 GAS strain.[35,36,72,73] J8 is a 12 amino acid minimal B-cell epitope and is part of a larger peptide, p145. Although immunity against p145, its subunits including J8, J14, and the related synthetic peptide P*17, is only variably induced following natural infection and appears to require repeated exposure, vaccination of mice with these cryptic epitopes protects against subsequent GAS infection, with J8 conjugated to diphtheria toxin (J8-DT) eliminating the need for a priming step. Anti-J8 responses in humans developed through natural exposure do not appear to correlate with risk of subsequent GAS infection, but J8-specific B cells may be important in vaccinated mice, highlighting the prospect that successful vaccine-derived immunity targeting conserved "cryptic" antigens might be substantively different from immunity developed through natural exposure.[37]

TABLE 14.2
21st Century Group A Streptococcal (GAS) Candidate Vaccines and Antigens[a].

Candidate Name/Identifier	STAGE OF DEVELOPMENT			Reference
	Preclinical	Phase I	Phase II	
M-protein: 6-valent N-terminal	X	X		60
M-protein: 26-valent N-terminal	X	X	X	61
M-protein: 30-valent N-terminal	X	X		64
M-related proteins	X			66,67
M-protein: minimal epitope J8	X	X		112
P*17: synthetic derivative of J8	X			69
M-protein: minimal epitope J14/p145	X			113
M-protein: five J14 variants (SV1)	X			114
M-protein: divalent N-terminal M1 + M12, with J14	X			115
M-protein: 10-valent N-terminal, expressed by live *Lactococcus lactis*	X			116
M-protein: C-repeat epitope (StreptInCor)	X			117
M-protein: C-repeat epitopes	X			118
Three conserved antigens (Combo): SLO, SpyAD, SpyCEP (currently in development with fourth antigen—group A carbohydrate)	X			39
Five conserved antigens (Combo5): arginine deiminase, C5a peptidase, streptolysin O, SpyCEP, trigger factor	X			51,52
Seven conserved antigens (Spy7): C5a peptidase, oligopeptide-binding protein, putative pullulanase, nucleoside-binding protein, hypothetical membrane associated protein, cell surface protein, SpyAD	X			88,89
Group A carbohydrate (GAC)	X			45
Group A carbohydrate (GAC) defective for GlcNAc side-chain	X			87
C5a peptidase (SCPA)	X			81
Sortase A (SrtA) + C5a peptidase (SCPA)	X			119
Fibronectin-binding protein (FBP)	X			120,121
Streptococcal protective antigen	X			61
Serum opacity factor (SOF)	X			122
Streptococcal pyrogenic exotoxin A/B/C (SpeA, SpeB, SpeC)	X			123–125
Streptococcal pyrogenic exotoxin (SpeAB) fusion protein	X			126
Streptococcal pili (T-antigen)	X			127,128
Serine protease (SpyCEP or S2 subunit)	X			74,129
Nine common antigens	X			130

[a] Table adapted with permission from Steer et al.[18] and updated.

J8-DT adjuvanted with alum (MJ8VAX) has been evaluated in humans and a single dose appeared to be safe (eight vaccinated subjects, two placebos).[38] The study was unfortunately placed on hold before a planned second dose, "because of a contractual issue that arose with a supplier of a component of the vaccine … [not] a safety concern for the participants, or for the integrity of the vaccine and its components." Peak immune responses to J8 were at day 28 after vaccination, decreasing to baseline by 180 days.[38] A proposed extension of this program to potentially increase immunogenicity and coverage of highly virulent strains is the combination of J8 (or the related "super immunogen" P*17) and a subunit ("S2") of the GAS IL-8 protease SpyCEP, each conjugated with DT or its nontoxic mutant CRM197.[69,74,75] In parallel to these efforts, the same group has been working on formulations for mucosal vaccines, including development of new adjuvants for mucosal and/or parenteral vaccine delivery, which have not yet entered human trials.

StreptInCor is a 55 amino acid peptide from the conserved C-repeat region of the M-protein of an M5 GAS, comprising B- and T-cell epitopes.[35,76,77] In vitro and in silico studies suggest relatively broad coverage for the diverse GAS strains prevalent in Brazil, and antibodies induced by StreptInCor are not cross-reactive with human tissues.[72,78] Vaccination in mice produces antibodies persisting for at least 12 months and protects against heterologous infection with M1 GAS.[73,79] A phase 1/2a study protocol is awaiting final approval by Brazilian regulatory authorities and the study is hoped to start in 2019.

Non-M-protein Vaccines

Increasing interest in non-M-protein antigens has led from a desire to avoid GAS vaccine targets possibly implicated in autoimmunity. Beginning with C5a peptidase (streptococcal C5a protease, SCPA) in the 1990s,[80–82] a variety of approaches have been used to identify at least 25 relatively highly conserved non-M-protein vaccine antigens immunogenic and protective alone or in combination after parenteral and/or mucosal administration in a range of GAS infection models (Table 14.2). Despite these encouraging findings, no vaccine including a non-M-protein antigen has reached human trials. Significant immune responses do occur to a number of non-M-protein antigens following natural GAS infection in humans, and adult humans show increased responses compared to children suggesting that immunity to these relatively conserved antigens builds through repeated exposure.[83–86] However, without human longitudinal clinical data, findings from experimental human infection (challenge) studies, or human vaccine trials, the

contribution of these responses to protection against GAS infection in humans is unknown.

The current leading non-M-protein candidate vaccine is the multiple-antigen "Combo" vaccine, under development by GSK Vaccines Institute for Global Health (formerly Novartis). This vaccine is the product of an early example of reverse vaccinology, using a multifaceted approach considering bacterial characteristics and human immune responses to identify conserved, highly expressed, surface-associated, and/or secreted protein antigens.[39] A combination ("Combo") vaccine including three protein antigens (SpyCEP, SpyAD, SLO) was shown to induce production of functional antibodies neutralizing the hemolytic activity of SLO, conferring complete protection in mice against injection of lethal doses of SLO, and inhibiting the proteolytic activity of SpyCEP against IL-8. Sera from mice immunized with the three-antigen Combo vaccine and whole blood from immunized rabbits demonstrated significant bactericidal and opsonophagocytic activity against GAS strains. Using immunization with adjuvant only as a negative control, and homologous M-protein as a positive control, mice vaccinated with Combo were protected from intranasal and intraperitoneal challenge with four GAS strains. Although development of this vaccine lay dormant for a number of years, the program has been reestablished with the group A carbohydrate[87] now included as a fourth conserved antigen and realistic prospects for phase 1 human trials in 2020.

Another project offering additional encouragement for the prospects of a non-M-protein is a multicomponent vaccine ("Spy7") reverse engineered from the antigenic targets of pooled human immunoglobin, including C5a peptidase and SpyAD, which was protective in a murine model of invasive GAS disease.[88,89] Separately, a vaccine combining five non-M-protein antigens ("Combo5"), including C5a peptidase, SLO, and SpyCEP, was tested in a nonhuman primate pharyngitis model and found to induce antibody responses against all its component antigens and to reduce clinical and microbiological markers of disease compared to controls.[51]

FUTURE DEVELOPMENT ACTIVITIES

Recognizing that clinical development of GAS vaccines had become impeded by technical, regulatory, and commercial obstacles, relevant stakeholders have recently engaged in a successful effort to reinvigorate and coordinate global efforts. Stakeholder meetings in 2016 (Seoul) and 2018 (London) supported by the WHO Initiative for Vaccine Research (IVR), International Vaccine Institute, and the Wellcome Trust have led to the development and publication of

WHO Preferred Product Characteristics and a Research and Development Roadmap for GAS vaccines in 2018 (Table 14.3), and formation of a global GAS vaccine consortium in 2019.[14,19,90,91] GAS vaccine has also been prioritized in recent years by the WHO Product Development for Vaccines Advisory Committee (PDVAC).[92] Development of a new controlled human infection model of GAS pharyngitis in healthy adults, identified as a priority activity in the WHO roadmap, will offer a platform for early proof-of-concept studies for vaccines, building the confidence of research groups, industry, funders, and regulators to pursue later phase development.[55,93] Together with national and regional initiatives, including the Australian and

TABLE 14.3

World Health Organization GAS Vaccines Research and Development Roadmap and Preferred Product Characteristics.[a]

Vision: A safe, globally effective, and affordable GAS vaccine is needed to prevent and potentially eliminate acute GAS infections (pharyngitis, skin infections, cellulitis, invasive disease) and associated antibiotic use, immune-mediated sequelae (kidney disease, rheumatic fever and rheumatic heart disease), and associated mortality.

Near-term strategic goal: To demonstrate favorable safety and proof of efficacy of a candidate vaccine against GAS pharyngitis and skin infections in children.	**Long-term strategic goal**: To develop a safe, globally effective, and affordable GAS vaccine for prevention of acute infections and associated antibiotic use, secondary immune-mediated sequelae, and associated mortality.

PREFERRED PRODUCT CHARACTERISTICS

Indication	Prevention of GAS-related pharyngitis, superficial skin infections, cellulitis, toxin-mediated disease, invasive infections and associated antibiotic use, secondary rheumatic fever, rheumatic heart disease, and poststreptococcal glomerulonephritis.
Target population for primary immunization	Primary schedule: infants and/or young children.
Schedule, primary immunization, and boosting	No more than three doses required for primary immunization
Efficacy targets	80% protection against nonsevere, noninvasive, confirmed GAS disease 70% protection against confirmed GAS cellulitis and invasive infections 50% protection against long-term immune-mediated sequelae
Strain and serotype coverage	A vaccine should cover the vast majority of current disease-causing isolates from the region targeted for use (at least 90%)
Safety	Safety and reactogenicity profile at least as favorable as current WHO-recommended routine vaccines
Adjuvant requirement	Evidence is required to justify adjuvant inclusion in the formulation
Immunogenicity	Established correlate/surrogate of protection based on a validated assay measuring immune effector levels/functionality
Noninterference	Favorable safety and immunologic noninterference upon coadministration with other vaccines recommended for target population(s)
Route of administration	Injectable (IM or SC) using standard volume
Registration, prequalification and programmatic suitability	Should be prequalified according to processes for assessing the acceptability of vaccines for purchase by UN agencies. WHO-defined criteria for programmatic suitability of vaccines should be met
Value proposition	Dosage, regimen, and cost of goods amenable to affordable supply. The vaccine should be cost-effective, and price should not be a barrier to access including in LMIC

VACCINE DEVELOPMENT TECHNOLOGY ROADMAP

Research priorities	- Improve global estimates of disease burden and better characterize the epidemiology of GAS infections - Further describe the spectrum of natural disease history - Drive improved understanding of GAS-related secondary immune-mediated diseases - Define the consequences of GAS-associated antibiotic use, and estimate the impact of vaccine use on antibiotic use and antimicrobial resistance—related morbidity and mortality
Priorities in vaccine development activities	- Pursue antigen discovery efforts, increasing the number of pipeline vaccine candidates - Develop consensus guidance about the appropriate use of safety monitoring tools in candidate vaccine trials - Characterize immunological surrogates/correlates of protection - Define appropriate pivotal clinical trial design for near-term and long-term strategic goals
Key capacities	- Define appropriate use of available and future animal models for GAS vaccine safety and efficacy evaluation - Develop clinically relevant human GAS experimental infection model(s) to support early vaccine proof-of-concept evaluation - Establish GAS expert research centers in LMICs with GCP trial research capacity and appropriate oversight; establish baseline rates of efficacy and safety outcomes - Access low-cost vaccine manufacturing under current GMP for late-stage development and commercial production - Develop standardized immunoassay platforms that meet quality requirements
Preparing for policy, commercialization and delivery	- Establish cost-effectiveness and develop research and implementation financial investment scenario(s) to support appropriate funding and policy decision making at the global and national levels, considering the full scope of costs and benefits - Ensure availability, affordability, and acceptability of a functional, cost-effective delivery platform for immunization - Develop effectiveness and safety vigilance platforms for postimplementation surveillance

GAS, Group A *Streptococcus*; *UN*, United Nations; *GCP*, Good clinical practice; *GMP*, Good manufacturing practice; *LMIC*, Low- and middle-income countries; *WHO*, World Health Organization; *IM*, intramuscular; *SC*, subcutaneous.
[a] Adapted with permission from the WHO Preferred Product Characteristics and Vaccine Development Technology Roadmap.[14,19,131,132] Refer to original publications for expanded details.

New Zealand Coalition to Advance Vaccines Against Group A *Streptococcus* (CANVAS)[94] and a major Australian Medical Research Future Fund (MRFF) $35 million Australian Dollar (AUD) investment in 2019, these initiatives have built consensus and momentum toward a clinical vaccine development pathway focused initially on demonstrating efficacy against pharyngitis and skin infection, precursors to development of the immune-mediated sequelae ARF, RHD, and APSGN. Simultaneously, there are growing efforts to address critical and persistent gaps in knowledge, advocacy, and understanding the full public health value proposition for a vaccine against GAS.[14,19,24]

REFERENCES

1. Stollerman GH. Prospects for a vaccine against group A streptococci: the problem of the immunology of M proteins. *Arthritis Rheum.* 1967;10:245–255.
2. Walker MJ, Barnett TC, McArthur JD, et al. Disease manifestations and pathogenic mechanisms of Group A *Streptococcus. Clin Microbiol Rev.* 2014;27:264–301.
3. Carapetis JR, Steer AC, Mulholland EK, Weber M. The global burden of group A streptococcal diseases. *Lancet Infect Dis.* 2005;5:685–694.
4. Watkins DA, Johnson CO, Colquhoun SM, et al. Global, regional, and national burden of rheumatic heart disease, 1990–2015. *N Engl J Med.* 2017;377:713–722.
5. Bowen AC, Mahe A, Hay RJ, et al. The global epidemiology of impetigo: a systematic review of the population prevalence of impetigo and pyoderma. *PLoS One.* 2015; 10:e0136789.
6. Zuhlke LJ, Beaton A, Engel ME, et al. Group A Streptococcus, acute rheumatic fever and rheumatic heart disease: epidemiology and clinical considerations. *Curr Treat Options Cardiovasc Med.* 2017;19:15.
7. Chira S, Miller LG. *Staphylococcus aureus* is the most common identified cause of cellulitis: a systematic review. *Epidemiol Infect.* 2010;138:313–317.
8. Cannon JW, Jack S, Wu Y, et al. An economic case for a vaccine to prevent group A streptococcus skin infections. *Vaccine.* 2018;36:6968–6978.
9. Hoy WE, White AV, Dowling A, et al. Post-streptococcal glomerulonephritis is a strong risk factor for chronic kidney disease in later life. *Kidney Int.* 2012;81: 1026–1032.
10. Katzenellenbogen JM, Ralph AP, Wyber R, Carapetis JR. Rheumatic heart disease: infectious disease origin, chronic care approach. *BMC Health Serv Res.* 2017;17: 793.
11. Pfoh E, Wessels MR, Goldmann D, Lee GM. Burden and economic cost of group A streptococcal pharyngitis. *Pediatrics.* 2008;121:229–234.
12. Barnett ML, Linder JA. Antibiotic prescribing to adults with sore throat in the United States, 1997–2010. *JAMA Intern Med.* 2014;174:138–140.
13. Macleod CK, Bright P, Steer AC, Kim J, Mabey D, Parks T. Neglecting the neglected: the objective evidence of underfunding in rheumatic heart disease. *Trans R Soc Trop Med Hyg.* 2019;113:287–290.
14. Vekemans J, Gouvea-Reis F, Kim JH, et al. The path to group A Streptococcus vaccines: WHO research and development technology roadmap and preferred product characteristics. *Clin Infect Dis.* 2019.
15. Hektoen L. The history of experimental scarlet fever in man. *J Am Med Assoc.* 1923;80:84–87.
16. Peterman MG. Immunization against scarlet fever. *Am J Dis Child.* 1937;54:89–95.
17. Dale JB, Batzloff MR, Cleary PP, et al. Current approaches to group A streptococcal vaccine development. In: Ferretti JJ, Stevens DL, Fischetti VA, eds. Streptococcus Pyogenes: *Basic Biology to Clinical Manifestations.* 2016. Oklahoma City (OK).
18. Steer AC, Carapetis JR, Dale JB, et al. Status of research and development of vaccines for *Streptococcus pyogenes. Vaccine.* 2016;34:2953–2958.
19. Osowicki J, Vekemans J, Kaslow DC, Friede MH, Kim JH, Steer AC. WHO/IVI global stakeholder consultation on group A Streptococcus vaccine development: report from a meeting held on 12-13 December 2016. *Vaccine.* 2018;36:3397–3405.
20. Ralph AP, Read C, Johnston V, et al. Improving delivery of secondary prophylaxis for rheumatic heart disease in remote Indigenous communities: study protocol for a stepped-wedge randomised trial. *Trials.* 2016;17:51.
21. Jack SJ, Williamson DA, Galloway Y, et al. Primary prevention of rheumatic fever in the 21st century: evaluation of a national programme. *Int J Epidemiol.* 2018;47:1585–1593.
22. Steer AC, Lamagni T, Curtis N, Carapetis JR. Invasive group a streptococcal disease: epidemiology, pathogenesis and management. *Drugs.* 2012;72:1213–1227.
23. Nelson GE, Pondo T, Toews KA, et al. Epidemiology of invasive group A streptococcal infections in the United States, 2005–2012. *Clin Infect Dis.* 2016;63:478–486.
24. Schodel F, Moreland NJ, Wittes JT, et al. Clinical development strategy for a candidate group A streptococcal vaccine. *Vaccine.* 2017;35:2007–2014.
25. Lancefield RC. A serological differentiation of human and other groups of hemolytic streptococci. *J Exp Med.* 1933; 57:571–595.
26. Lancefield RC. Current knowledge of type-specific M antigens of group A streptococci. *J Immunol.* 1962;89: 307–313.
27. Sanderson-Smith M, De Oliveira DM, Guglielmini J, et al. A systematic and functional classification of *Streptococcus pyogenes* that serves as a new tool for molecular typing and vaccine development. *J Infect Dis.* 2014;210: 1325–1338.
28. Davies MR, McIntyre L, Mutreja A, et al. Atlas of group A streptococcal vaccine candidates compiled using large-scale comparative genomics. *Nat Genet.* 2019;51: 1035–1043.
29. Bloomfield AL, Felty AR. Prophylactic vaccination against acute tonsillitis. *John Hopkins Hosp Bull.* 1923;34: 251–253.
30. Steer AC, Law I, Matatolu L, Beall BW, Carapetis JR. Global emm type distribution of group A streptococci: systematic review and implications for vaccine development. *Lancet Infect Dis.* 2009;9:611–616.
31. Dale JB, Penfound T, Chiang EY, Long V, Shulman ST, Beall B. Multivalent group A streptococcal vaccine elicits bactericidal antibodies against variant M subtypes. *Clin Diagn Lab Immunol.* 2005;12:833–836.
32. Frost HR, Laho D, Sanderson-Smith ML, et al. Immune cross-opsonization within emm clusters following group A Streptococcus skin infection: broadening the scope of type-specific immunity. *Clin Infect Dis.* 2017;65: 1523–1531.
33. Dale JB, Smeesters PR, Courtney HS, et al. Structure-based design of broadly protective group a streptococcal M protein-based vaccines. *Vaccine.* 2017;35:19–26.

34. Young PG, Raynes JM, Loh JM, Proft T, Baker EN, Moreland NJ. Group A Streptococcus T antigens have a highly conserved structure concealed under a heterogeneous surface that has implications for vaccine design. *Infect Immun.* 2019;87.
35. Guilherme L, Postol E, Ferreira FM, DeMarchi LM, Kalil J. StreptInCor: a model of anti-Streptococcus pyogenes vaccine reviewed. *Auto- immunity highlights.* 2013;4:81–85.
36. Guilherme L, Ferreira FM, Kohler KF, Postol E, Kalil J. A vaccine against *Streptococcus pyogenes*: the potential to prevent rheumatic fever and rheumatic heart disease. *Am J Cardiovasc Drugs.* 2013;13:1–4.
37. Ozberk V, Pandey M, Good MF. Contribution of cryptic epitopes in designing a group A streptococcal vaccine. *Hum Vaccines Immunother.* 2018;14:2034–2052.
38. Sekuloski S, Batzloff MR, Griffin P, et al. Evaluation of safety and immunogenicity of a group A streptococcus vaccine candidate (MJ8VAX) in a randomized clinical trial. *PLoS One.* 2018;13:e0198658.
39. Bensi G, Mora M, Tuscano G, et al. Multi high-throughput approach for highly selective identification of vaccine candidates: the Group A Streptococcus case. *Mol Cell Proteom.* 2012;11. M111 015693.
40. Loh JMS, Lorenz N, Tsai CJ, Khemlani AHJ, Proft T. Mucosal vaccination with pili from Group A Streptococcus expressed on *Lactococcus lactis* generates protective immune responses. *Sci Rep.* 2017;7:7174.
41. Lancefield RC. Persistence of type-specific antibodies in man following infection with group A streptococci. *J Exp Med.* 1959;110:271–292.
42. Fox EN, Waldman RH, Wittner MK, Mauceri AA, Dorfman A. Protective study with a group A streptococcal M protein vaccine. Infectivity challenge of human volunteers. *J Clin Investig.* 1973;52:1885–1892.
43. D'Alessandri R, Plotkin G, Kluge RM, et al. Protective studies with group A streptococcal M protein vaccine. III. Challenge of volunteers after systemic or intranasal immunization with Type 3 or Type 12 group A Streptococcus. *J Infect Dis.* 1978;138:712–718.
44. Polly SM, Waldman RH, High P, Wittner MK, Dorfman A. Protective studies with a group A streptococcal M protein vaccine. II. Challenge of volenteers after local immunization in the upper respiratory tract. *J Infect Dis.* 1975;131:217–224.
45. Sabharwal H, Michon F, Nelson D, et al. Group A streptococcus (GAS) carbohydrate as an immunogen for protection against GAS infection. *J Infect Dis.* 2006;193:129–135.
46. Tsoi SK, Smeesters PR, Frost HR, Licciardi P, Steer AC. Correlates of protection for M protein-based vaccines against group A Streptococcus. *J Immunol Res.* 2015;2015:167089.
47. Jones S, Moreland NJ, Zancolli M, et al. Development of an opsonophagocytic killing assay for group a streptococcus. *Vaccine.* 2018;36:3756–3763.
48. Salehi S, Hohn CM, Penfound TA, Dale JB. Development of an opsonophagocytic killing assay using HL-60 cells

for detection of functional antibodies against *Streptococcus pyogenes. mSphere.* 2018;3.
49. Bright PD, Mayosi BM, Martin WJ. An immunological perspective on rheumatic heart disease pathogenesis: more questions than answers. *Heart.* 2016;102:1527–1532.
50. Watson Jr ME, Neely MN, Caparon MG. Animal models of *Streptococcus pyogenes* infection. In: Ferretti JJ, Stevens DL, Fischetti VA, eds. Streptococcus pyogenes: *Basic Biology to Clinical Manifestations.* 2016. Oklahoma City (OK).
51. Rivera-Hernandez T, Carnathan DG, Jones S, et al. An experimental group A Streptococcus vaccine that reduces pharyngitis and tonsillitis in a nonhuman primate model. *MBio.* 2019;10.
52. Rivera-Hernandez T, Pandey M, Henningham A, et al. Differing efficacies of lead group A streptococcal vaccine candidates and full-length M protein in cutaneous and invasive disease models. *MBio.* 2016;7.
53. Webber BJ, Kieffer JW, White BK, Hawksworth AW, Graf PCF, Yun HC. Chemoprophylaxis against group A streptococcus during military training. *Prev Med.* 2019;118:142–149.
54. Young DC. Failure of type specific *Streptococcus pyogenes* vaccines to prevent respiratory infections. *Naval Med Bull.* 1946;46:709–718.
55. Osowicki J, Azzopardi KI, Baker C, et al. Controlled human infection for vaccination against *Streptococcus pyogenes* (CHIVAS): establishing a group A Streptococcus pharyngitis human infection study. *Vaccine.* 2019. https://doi.org/10.1016/j.vaccine.2019.03.059. PMID: 31101422.
56. Massell BF, Michael JG, Amezcua J, Siner M. Secondary and apparent primary antibody responses after group A streptococcal vaccination of 21 children. *Appl Microbiol.* 1968;16:509–518.
57. Massell BF, Honikman LH, Amezcua J. Rheumatic fever following streptococcal vaccination. Report of three cases. *JAMA.* 1969;207:1115–1119.
58. Revocation of status of specific products; Group A streptococcus. Direct final rule. *Fed Regist.* 2005;70:72197–72199.
59. Beachey EH, Bronze M, Dale JB, Kraus W, Poirier T, Sargent S. Protective and autoimmune epitopes of streptococcal M proteins. *Vaccine.* 1988;6:192–196.
60. Kotloff KL, Corretti M, Palmer K, et al. Safety and immunogenicity of a recombinant multivalent group a streptococcal vaccine in healthy adults: phase 1 trial. *J Am Med Assoc.* 2004;292:709–715.
61. McNeil SA, Halperin SA, Langley JM, et al. Safety and immunogenicity of 26-valent group a streptococcus vaccine in healthy adult volunteers. *Clin Infect Dis.* 2005;41:1114–1122.
62. Hu MC, Walls MA, Stroop SD, Reddish MA, Beall B, Dale JB. Immunogenicity of a 26-valent group A streptococcal vaccine. *Infect Immun.* 2002;70:2171–2177.
63. Dale JB, Penfound TA, Tamboura B, et al. Potential coverage of a multivalent M protein-based group A streptococcal vaccine. *Vaccine.* 2013;31:1576–1581.

64. Dale JB, Penfound TA, Chiang EY, Walton WJ. New 30-valent M protein-based vaccine evokes cross-opsonic antibodies against non-vaccine serotypes of group A streptococci. *Vaccine*. 2011;29:8175–8178.

65. Shulman ST, Tanz RR, Dale JB, Steer AC, Smeesters PR. Added value of the emm-cluster typing system to analyze group A Streptococcus epidemiology in high-income settings. *Clin Infect Dis*. 2014;59:1651–1652.

66. Dale JB, Niedermeyer SE, Agbaosi T, et al. Protective immunogenicity of group A streptococcal M-related proteins. *Clin Vaccine Immunol*. 2015;22:344–350.

67. Courtney HS, Niedermeyer SE, Penfound TA, Hohn CM, Greeley A, Dale JB. Trivalent M-related protein as a component of next generation group A streptococcal vaccines. *Clin Exp Vaccine Res*. 2017;6:45–49.

68. Buffalo CZ, Bahn-Suh AJ, Hirakis SP, et al. Conserved patterns hidden within group A Streptococcus M protein hypervariability recognize human C4b-binding protein. *Nat Microbiol*. 2016;1:16155.

69. Nordstrom T, Pandey M, Calcutt A, et al. Enhancing vaccine efficacy by engineering a complex synthetic peptide to become a super immunogen. *J Immunol*. 2017;199:2794–2802.

70. Steer AC, Magor G, Jenney AWJ, et al. Emm and C-repeat region molecular typing of beta-hemolytic streptococci in a tropical country: implications for vaccine development. *J Clin Microbiol*. 2009;47:2502–2509.

71. Batzloff M, Yan H, Davies M, Hartas J, Good M. Preclinical evaluation of a vaccine based on conserved region of M protein that prevents group A streptococcal infection. *Indian J Med Res*. 2004;119(Suppl):104–107.

72. De Amicis KM, Freschi de Barros S, Alencar RE, et al. Analysis of the coverage capacity of the StreptInCor candidate vaccine against *Streptococcus pyogenes*. *Vaccine*. 2014;32:4104–4110.

73. Postol E, Alencar R, Higa FT, et al. StreptInCor: a candidate vaccine epitope against *S. pyogenes* infections induces protection in outbred mice. *PLoS One*. 2013;8:e60969.

74. Pandey M, Mortensen R, Calcutt A, et al. Combinatorial synthetic peptide vaccine strategy protects against hypervirulent CovR/S mutant streptococci. *J Immunol*. 2016;196:3364–3374.

75. Pandey M, Langshaw E, Hartas J, Lam A, Batzloff MR, Good MF. A synthetic M protein peptide synergizes with a CXC chemokine protease to induce vaccine-mediated protection against virulent streptococcal pyoderma and bacteremia. *J Immunol*. 2015;194:5915–5925.

76. Guilherme L, Postol E, Freschi de Barros S, et al. A vaccine against *S. pyogenes*: design and experimental immune response. *Methods*. 2009;49:316–321.

77. Guilherme L, Alba MP, Ferreira FM, et al. Anti-group A streptococcal vaccine epitope: structure, stability, and its ability to interact with HLA class II molecules. *J Biol Chem*. 2011;286:6989–6998.

78. Freschi de Barros S, De Amicis KM, Alencar R, et al. *Streptococcus pyogenes* strains in Sao Paulo, Brazil: molecular characterization as a basis for StreptInCor coverage capacity analysis. *BMC Infect Dis*. 2015;15:308.

79. Guerino MT, Postol E, Demarchi LM, et al. HLA class II transgenic mice develop a safe and long lasting immune response against StreptInCor, an anti-group A streptococcus vaccine candidate. *Vaccine*. 2011;29:8250–8256.

80. Ji Y, Carlson B, Kondagunta A, Cleary PP. Intranasal immunization with C5a peptidase prevents nasopharyngeal colonization of mice by the group A Streptococcus. *Infect Immun*. 1997;65:2080–2087.

81. Cleary PP, Matsuka YV, Huynh T, Lam H, Olmsted SB. Immunization with C5a peptidase from either group A or B streptococci enhances clearance of group A streptococci from intranasally infected mice. *Vaccine*. 2004;22:4332–4341.

82. Park HS, Cleary PP. Active and passive intranasal immunizations with streptococcal surface protein C5a peptidase prevent infection of murine nasal mucosa-associated lymphoid tissue, a functional homologue of human tonsils. *Infect Immun*. 2005;73:7878–7886.

83. Mortensen R, Nissen TN, Blauenfeldt T, Christensen JP, Andersen P, Dietrich J. Adaptive immunity against *Streptococcus pyogenes* in adults involves increased IFN-gamma and IgG3 responses compared with children. *J Immunol*. 2015;195:1657–1664.

84. Mortensen R, Nissen TN, Fredslund S, et al. Identifying protective *Streptococcus pyogenes* vaccine antigens recognized by both B and T cells in human adults and children. *Sci Rep*. 2016;6:22030.

85. O'Connor SP, Darip D, Fraley K, Nelson CM, Kaplan EL, Cleary PP. The human antibody response to streptococcal C5a peptidase. *J Infect Dis*. 1991;163:109–116.

86. Shet A, Kaplan EL, Johnson DR, Cleary PP. Immune response to group A streptococcal C5a peptidase in children: implications for vaccine development. *J Infect Dis*. 2003;188:809–817.

87. van Sorge NM, Cole JN, Kuipers K, et al. The classical lancefield antigen of group a Streptococcus is a virulence determinant with implications for vaccine design. *Cell Host Microbe*. 2014;15:729–740.

88. Reglinski M, Lynskey NN, Choi YJ, Edwards RJ, Sriskandan S. Development of a multicomponent vaccine for *Streptococcus pyogenes* based on the antigenic targets of IVIG. *J Infect*. 2016;72:450–459.

89. Reglinski M, Gierula M, Lynskey NN, Edwards RJ, Sriskandan S. Identification of the *Streptococcus pyogenes* surface antigens recognised by pooled human immunoglobulin. *Sci Rep*. 2015;5:15825.

90. Stollerman GH. Rheumatogenic group A streptococci and the return of rheumatic fever. *Adv Intern Med*. 1990;35:1–25.

91. Markowitz M. Pioneers and modern ideas. Rheumatic fever–a half-century perspective. *Pediatrics*. 1998;102:272–274. discussion 88-9.

92. Kim JH, Steer AC. *Vaccines against Strep A [Internet]* Geneva. World Health Organization; 2018. Available from: https://www.who.int/immunization/research/meetings_workshops/pdvac_june18/en/.

93. Osowicki J, Azzopardi KI, McIntyre L, et al. A controlled human infection model of group A *Streptococcus pharyngitis*: which strain and why? *mSphere*. 2019;4.

94. Moreland NJ, Waddington CS, Williamson DA, et al. Working towards a group A streptococcal vaccine: report of a collaborative Trans-Tasman workshop. *Vaccine*. 2014;32:3713–3720.

95. Swift HF. Intravenous vaccination with streptococci in rheumatic fever. *J Assoc Am Phys*. 1930;45:181.

96. Wilson MG, Swift HF. Intravenous vaccination with hemolytic streptococci. *Amer J Dis Child*. 1931;42:42–51.

97. Collis WRF, Sheldon W. Intravenous vaccines of haemolytic streptococci in acute rheumatism in childhood. *Lancet*. 1932;220:1261–1264.

98. Wasson VP. Immunization against rheumatic fever with hemolytic streptococcus filtrate. *Am Heart J*. 1938;15:257–264.

99. Wasson VP. Immunization against rheumatic fever. *J Pediatr*. 1943;23:24–30.

100. Wasson VP, Brown EE. Immunization against rheumatic fever with hemolytic streptococcus filtrate. *Am Heart J*. 1940;20:1–11.

101. Wasson VP, Brown EE. Further studies in immunization against rheumatic fever. *Am Heart J*. 1942;23:291–305.

102. Veldee MV. Purification and precipitation of the erythrogenic factor of scarlet fever streptococcus toxin and its antigenic value. *Public Health Rep*. 1937;52:819–829.

103. Veldee MV. A further study of the purification and tannic acid precipitation of scarlet fever toxin. *Public Health Rep*. 1938;53:909–913.

104. Veldee MV. The Dick reaction and scarlet fever morbidity following injections of a purified and tannic acid precipitated erythrogenic toxin. *Public Health Rep*. 1941;56:957–974.

105. Rantz LA. Group A hemolytic streptococcus antibodies. A study of the simultaneous infection of a large number of men by a single type. *Arch Intern Med*. 1944;73:238–240.

106. Schmidt WC. Type-specific antibody formation in man following injection of streptococcal M protein. *J Infect Dis*. 1960;106:250–255.

107. Potter EV, Stollerman GH, Siegel AC. Recall of type specific antibodies in man by injections of streptococcal cell walls. *J Clin Invest*. 1962;14:301–310.

108. Wolfe CK, Hayashi JA, Walsh G, Barkulis SS. Type-specific antibody reponse in man to injections of cell walls and M protein from group A, type 14 streptococci. *J Lab Clin Med*. 1963;61:459–468.

109. Fox EN, Wittner MK, Dorfman A. Antigenicity of the M proteins of group A hemolytic streptococci III. Antibody responses and cutaneous hypersensitivity in humans. *J Exp Med*. 1966;124:1135–1151.

110. Beachey EH, Stollerman GH, Johnson RH, Ofek I, Bisno AL. Human immune response to immunization with a structurally defined polypeptide fragment of streptococcal M protein. *J Exp Med*. 1979;150:862–877.

111. Steer AC, Batzloff MR, Mulholland K, Carapetis JR. Group A streptococcal vaccines: facts versus fantasy. *Curr Opin Infect Dis*. 2009;22:544–552.

112. Batzloff MR, Hayman WA, Davies MR, Zeng M, Pruksakorn S, Brandt ER. Protection against group A streptococcus by immunization with J8-diptheria toxoid: contribution of J8-and diptheria toxoid-specific antibodies to protection. *J Infect Dis*. 2003;187:1598–1608.

113. Hayman WA, Toth I, Flinn N, Scanlon M, Good MF. Enhancing the immunogenicity and modulating the fine epitope recognition of antisera to a helical group A streptococcal peptide vaccine candidate from the M protein using lipid-core peptide technology. *Immunol Cell Biol*. 2002;80:178–187.

114. McNeilly C, Cosh S, Vu T, et al. Predicted coverage and immuno-safety of a recombinant C-repeat region based *Streptococcus pyogenes* vaccine candidate. *PLoS One*. 2016;11:e0156639.

115. Wu Y, Li S, Luo Y, et al. Immunogenicity and safety of a chemically synthesized divalent group A streptococcal vaccine. *Can J Infect Dis Med Microbiol*. 2018;2018:4702152.

116. Wozniak A, Scioscia N, Garcia PC, et al. Protective immunity induced by an intranasal multivalent vaccine comprising 10 *Lactococcus lactis* strains expressing highly prevalent M-protein antigens derived from group A *Streptococcus*. *Microbiol Immunol*. 2018;62:395–404.

117. Guilherme L, Faé KC, Higa F, et al. Towards a vaccine against rheumatic fever. *Clin Develop Immunol*. 2006;13:125–132.

118. Bessen D, Fischetti VA. Synthetic peptide vaccine against mucosal colonization by group A streptococci. I. Protection against a heterologous M serotype with shared C repeat region epitopes. *J Immunol*. 1990;145:1251–1256.

119. Chen X, Li N, Bi S, Wang X, Wang B. Co-activation of Th17 and antibody responses provides efficient protection against mucosal infection by group A Streptococcus. *PLoS One*. 2016;11:e0168861.

120. Kawabata S, Kunitomo E, Terao Y, et al. Systemic and mucosal immunizations with fibronectin-binding protein FBP54 induce protective immune responses against *Streptococcus pyogenes* challenge in mice. *Infect Immun*. 2001;69:924–930.

121. McArthur J, Medina E, Mueller A, et al. Intranasal vaccination with streptococcal fibronectin binding protein Sfb1 fails to prevent growth and dissemination of *Streptococcus pyogenes* in a murine skin infection model. *Infect Immun*. 2004;72:7342–7345.

122. Courtney HS, Hasty DL, Dale JB. Serum opacity factor (SOF) of *Streptococcus pyogenes* evokes antibodies that opsonize homologous and heterologous SOF-positive serotypes of group A streptococci. *Infect Immun*. 2003;71:5097–5103.

123. Roggiani M, Stoehr JA, Olmsted SB, et al. Toxoids of streptococcal pyrogenic exotoxin A are protective in rabbit models of streptococcal toxic shock syndrome. *Infect Immun*. 2000;68:5011–5017.

124. Kapur V, Maffei JT, Greer RS, Li LL, Adams GJ, Musser JM. Vaccination with streptococcal extracellular cysteine protease (interleukin-1 beta convertase) protects mice against challenge with heterologous group A streptococci. *Microb Pathog*. 1994;16:443–450.

125. McCormick JK, Tripp TJ, Olmsted SB, et al. Development of streptococcal pyrogenic exotoxin C vaccine toxoids that are protective in the rabbit model of toxic shock syndrome. *J Immunol.* 2000;165:2306–2312.

126. Burlet E, HogenEsch H, Dunham A, Morefield G. Evaluation of the potency, neutralizing antibody response, and stability of a recombinant fusion protein vaccine for *Streptococcus pyogenes. AAPS J.* 2017;19:875–881.

127. Mora M, Bensi G, Capo S, et al. Group A Streptococcus produce pilus-like structures containing protective antigens and Lancefield T antigens. *Proc Natl Acad Sci USA.* 2005;102:15641–15646.

128. Young PG, Moreland NJ, Loh JM, et al. Structural conservation, variability, and immunogenicity of the T6 backbone pilin of serotype M6 *Streptococcus pyogenes. Infect Immun.* 2014;82:2949–2957.

129. Turner CE, Kurupati P, Wiles S, Edwards RJ, Sriskandan S. Impact of immunization against SpyCEP during invasive disease with two streptococcal species: *Streptococcus pyogenes* and *Streptococcus equi. Vaccine.* 2009;27:4923–4929.

130. Fritzer A, Senn BM, Minh DB, et al. Novel conserved group A streptococcal proteins identified by the antigenome technology as vaccine candidates for a non-M protein-based vaccine. *Infect Immun.* 2010;78:4051–4067.

131. *Group A Streptococcus Vaccine Development Technology Roadmap: Priority Activities for Development, Testing, Licensure and Global Availability of Group A Streptococcus Vaccines.* Geneva: World Health Organization; 2018. Licence: CC BY-NC-SA 3.0 IGO.

132. *WHO Preferred Product Characteristics for Group A Streptococcus Vaccines.* Geneva: World Health Organization; 2018. Licence: CC BY-NC-SA 3.0 IGO.

CHAPTER 15

Awareness, Education, and Advocacy

ROSEMARY WYBER • JEREMIAH MWANGI • LIESL ZÜHLKE

INTRODUCTION

Health-seeking behavior is a critical determinant of success for rheumatic heart disease (RHD) control programs. If people at risk of RHD do not seek care for group A streptococcal (GAS) infections, primary prevention is impossible. If they do not present with symptoms of acute rheumatic fever (ARF), the window of opportunity for successful secondary prevention closes. Similarly, people with RHD will not benefit from advanced medical or surgical management if they do not know that care is available, or are not fully aware of all aspects of their care. Therefore, awareness of disease is a prerequisite to accessing and benefitting from care.[1]

BASELINE AWARENESS

Community and clinician awareness of RHD is low in almost all of the places where it has been explored. The protracted etiologic pathway of RHD and complex nomenclature are barriers to ready awareness. Equally, the autoimmune mechanism of ARF is not necessarily an intuitive concept in settings of low health literacy. In endemic settings with a high burden of RHD, access to formal education is low. For example, a small study in Iran reviewing 45 mothers whose children had been referred to local clinics for suspected pharyngitis showed that mother's knowledge of ARF prevention was significantly associated with her educational history.[2] Those with secondary school educational achievement had greater knowledge of ARF than those with primary school education, perhaps suggesting some exposure to this knowledge at different levels of education.

Community

Sporadic surveys among community members in various locations have largely found low levels of knowledge and awareness of sore throat, ARF, and RHD. In a 2010 Tanzanian study, most doctors surveyed reported that patients and families had no awareness of the consequences of untreated GAS infection.[3] This is supported by a study of 740 community members aged nine or above in the Kinondoni municipality in Tanzania, which found only 13% knew that sore throat is caused by an infection and only 14% were aware of the link between sore throat and ARF.[4] Furthermore, recruited in this study were 540 primary healthcare workers, who demonstrated improved awareness of ARF/RHD of 60%–89%. In the Haryana State in India in 1992, very few school children had ever heard of ARF.[5] In Kenya in 2008, 200 school children were surveyed about knowledge of sore throat, ARF and RHD before an education intervention. Baseline knowledge of the disease was poor.[6] A larger study in Iran in 2008 surveyed 443 mothers attending clinic with their children for immunization or primary care. Two thirds of mothers had poor or moderate knowledge about the epidemiology of ARF and over 90% had poor knowledge of symptoms and complications.[7] Similarly, in Samoa in 2011, 148 mothers surveyed about sore throat reported little knowledge about when to seek medical care.[8] In Nepal in 2016, 2245 people were interviewed in primary healthcare clinics and asked 30 yes/no questions about GAS, ARF, and RHD. Although 75% of people knew what throat infection was, less than 2% were aware of the link between throat infection and ARF or RHD.[9]

Although each of these studies used different designs and methodologies, and are therefore not directly comparable, results from different locations at different times generally support the idea of limited awareness of GAS infection, and in particular the link with ARF and RHD, within communities with a high burden of disease. In addition, many of these studies did not define the community members in detail nor the levels of healthcare workers, which does not allow for generalization or applicability to other contexts.

Teachers

School teachers are another group in the community who may benefit from an awareness of sore throat, ARF, and RHD. Theoretical roles for teachers to support

Acute Rheumatic Fever and Rheumatic Heart Disease. https://doi.org/10.1016/B978-0-323-63982-8.00015-5

care delivery may include understanding the need for timely access to care for sore throat, knowledge of some of the key symptoms of ARF (such as arthritis or severe exertional dyspnea), or facilitating time away from school to access secondary prophylaxis injections. However, very little has been published on the topic of school teacher awareness and these limited reports suggest limited baseline awareness. In Zambia, 53 teachers (some also acting as school health officers) from 45 schools participated in an educational workshop on RHD. At baseline, 55% of the teachers had heard of RHD but only half were aware of the association with sore throat.[10]

People and Families Living with Acute Rheumatic Fever and Rheumatic Heart Disease

People living with RHD could reasonably be expected to have a greater knowledge and understanding of the disease relative to the general population. However, qualitative research in a number of settings suggests that even people receiving treatment for the disease have limited knowledge, whether biomedical or based in belief systems, about the disease. In a study among Aboriginal people in a remote Australian setting, very few interviewees had a detailed understanding of RHD but agreed to secondary prophylaxis on the advice of trusted health practitioners.[11] Similarly, in Jamaica, 39 people receiving secondary prophylaxis injections knew that they had RHD but had a poor biomedical understanding of causality. These individuals also relied on recommendations from health professionals to help make decisions about persevering with secondary prophylaxis.[12] In South Africa, qualitative interviews of eight caregivers of children who had been diagnosed with ARF indicated that 6 of 8 did not know what caused ARF and 7 of 8 had not heard of the disease before diagnosis.[13] In Cameroon, RHD patients attending an out-patient facility demonstrated little knowledge of RHD. The concept was unknown to 82% of the participants and 95% of them did not know what caused RHD. Only 5.1% of the participants had what the authors considered to be an adequate knowledge of RHD.[14]

Clinicians

Limited community knowledge about sore throat, ARF, and RHD increases the need for health professionals to be able to provide high quality advice and education as well as clinical services. However, studies suggest that this knowledge is variable between settings. For example, in a survey of 395 primary care providers in Tanzania, 73% were aware of the association between

sore throat and ARF.[4] In Brazil, cardiologists' awareness of primary prevention was limited.[15] Among 242 Saudi Arabian emergency medicine physicians, only 67 (27%) adhered to guidelines for treating acute pharyngitis.[16] In South Africa in 2005, a survey showed that many doctors were not aware of national guidelines for primary and secondary prevention of ARF despite guidelines having been available for nearly a decade.[13]

Sudan demonstrated the ability to improve levels of awareness from poor to good with focused intervention and regular awareness and education programs for health workers.[17] The study focused on 87 pediatric doctors, 25 (29%) of whom were registrars, 14 (16%) were medical officers, and 48 (55%) were house officers. The doctors' awareness about the diagnosis of GAS pharyngitis was about 38%, which increased to 93% after lectures, as assessed by pre- and postquestionnaires. Intervention comprised of three lectures, manuals on primary and secondary prevention, teaching sessions, and practical workshops.

Policy Makers and Funders

GAS, ARF, and RHD have long been ignored by policy makers and funders in the fight against communicable and noncommunicable disease. Despite a burden, measured in DALYs, equivalent to breast cancer and leukemia, similar mortality numbers to rotavirus and about 50% of that of malaria, ARF, and RHD were reported in 2009 to have received only 0.07% of global funded toward research and development.[18] Although there has been a resurgence in research and policy interest in GAS, ARF, and RHD recently,[19–23] this has not translated into significant additional funding at community and policy level. Recently, a novel logarithmic disability neglect index (DNI), based on the Global Burden of Disease Study and funding from the G-FINDER database, described disease burden using disability-adjusted life years relative to funding for 16 major tropical diseases. Across a range of diseases, RHD received the least funding relative to disease burden with a DNI = 3.83 (similar to cysticercosis, DNI = 2.71 and soil transmitted helminths, DNI = 2.41). RHD thus remains severely underfunded relative to disease burden.[24]

INTERVENTIONS TO IMPROVE AWARENESS

Limited awareness of GAS, ARF, and RHD among all stakeholder groups means that education is needed to access the disease-altering benefits of care. Education and awareness activities have been recognized as a core element of RHD control initiatives by World

Health Organization (WHO), the ASAP program from South Africa (awareness, surveillance, advocacy, and prevention) to eradicate RHD in our lifetime, and initiatives form Australia and New Zealand.

Tools for Implementing RHD Control Programmes (TIPs) provides a framework for design, implementation and evaluation of RHD control programs (see Fig. 12.1, Chapter 12). Throughout the framework, education and increased awareness are highlighted as critical elements. As a consequence, Reach (to stop RHD) as part of RHD Action (incorporating the World Heart Federation (WHF)) has funded a series of small grants, resulting in an awareness and education program for health workers, communities, and patients.

In addition, it is important to note that programs that have managed to demonstrate a significant reduction in the incidence of ARF and prevalence of RHD, such as the French Caribbean islands of Guadeloupe and Martinique, Tunisia, Cuba, and regions of Brazil, have all included awareness raising and education as a key component of the RHD control programs.[25,26]

A large number of awareness-raising activities have been conducted around the world, though very few have been rigorously evaluated. Table 15.1 outlines a number of illustrative awareness-raising programs and Box 15.1 provides a case study of one of the best described awareness campaigns in a developed country setting.

A wide range of awareness-raising initiatives for ARF and RHD have been delivered around the world and community education is likely to be a prerequisite for programmatic success. With the passing of the World Health Assembly Resolution on ARF and RHD in May 2018, there is a clear need to formalize and scale-up these efforts to achieve global control of RHD. Increasing rigor is needed to ensure the best possible interventions are delivered most effectively, evaluated, and improved upon (Box 15.2).[40]

MOVING FROM ORGANIC TO STRATEGIC APPROACHES

Evidence for improving community awareness of ARF and RHD can be drawn from experience in other diseases. Overall, well-designed awareness-raising interventions have capacity to affect health changes in low- and middle-income countries. A meta-analysis of mass media campaigns directed at childhood survival in low-resource countries found evidence that media can be effective in influencing a range of behaviors including vasectomy, tuberculosis testing, bed net use, and vaccination uptake.[44] Similarly, a meta-analysis of mass media campaigns about HIV indicated an association with increased condom use, transmission, and prevention knowledge. Impacts on condom use were greatest in less developed settings and with more sustained information campaigns.[45]

Community education campaigns for noncommunicable diseases are also emerging and may present opportunities for improving RHD awareness. For example, the prevalence of Type II diabetes is increasing in settings with an endemic burden of RHD.[46] Diabetes also has a protracted causal period and may be asymptomatic for many years when people feel well but are at risk of complications. The International Diabetes Federation pioneered programs to raise awareness of diabetes in developing country settings, initially with the support of large pharmaceutical companies.[47] Large-scale projects have been delivered worldwide. For example, in India, the Prevention Awareness Counseling and Evaluation (PACE) project involved education systems and opportunistic blood glucose screening and formation of "PACE Diabetes Education Counters," which are estimated to have reached two million people in Chennai.[48] Evaluation of the project indicated a statistically significant increase in community awareness of diabetes, causes, and opportunities for prevention.[49]

Strategies to raise community awareness of GAS, ARF, and RHD must also account for the health beliefs of each community. These vary considerably in different settings. Beliefs about the causes of childhood fever are a good example of difference in health understanding because they have been explored in different settings across time. For example in Moshi, northern Tanzania, heads of households named a wide range of potential causes of childhood fever including malaria (76.3%), weather (62.1%), and witchcraft (2.5%).[50] In Kenya, caregivers identified potential causes of fever as infection (95.2%), change of weather (58.4%), and witchcraft (6.4%).[51] In Iraq, mothers named infection (96%), cold exposure (92%), and exposure to sunlight (78%) among other causes of fever.[52] Focus group conversations in Malawi included beliefs about maternal vaginal warts as a cause of childhood fever, along with malaria, playing in the dust and falling during play.[53] Childhood fever is a universal experience and the variety of beliefs about its cause demonstrate the broad interpretation of what fever is or what causes it in low-resource settings. Therefore, a robust understanding of baseline beliefs and attitudes is needed to plan and implement awareness campaigns.

Health communication programs that use an underlying theory of change or behavior model are more robust and more likely to be successful.[54] Use of

TABLE 15.1
Programs to Raise Awareness of Group A Streptococcus, Acute Rheumatic Fever, and Rheumatic Heart Disease.

	Schools/Teachers	Clinics/Clinicians	Written Materials	Audiovisual and Media	Other	Key Message	Impact
French Caribbean, 1980s[25]	Film shown	Newsletters and training workshops	Pamphlets to parents	Film shown in schools	Term for ARF simplified	Sore throat seems benign but can cause serious heart damage	Decline in ARF as part of comprehensive program
Cuba, 1980s[26]	Teachers and school children involved; details unspecified	Workshops, seminars or continuing health education courses	Thousands of pamphlets disseminated, and posters displayed in Spanish	Advertisements and programming on provincial radio and TV channels		"What to do if you have a sore throat" "Importance of adherence to secondary prophylaxis"	Decline in ARF as part of comprehensive program
India, 1992[5]	773 teachers trained in workshops	74 health workers trained in workshops	Posters, pamphlets, wall charts, and heart models	Not described	Case control study of the intervention	Rheumatic fever is a serious, life threatening disease that damages the heart (among others)	Statistically significant improvement in knowledge for health workers, teachers, and school children
India 2000–2010[27]	Leaflets and poster distributed at training sessions	Workshops and train-the-trainer events held	These included posters, pamphlets, and wall charts	Radio interviews and film about the project produced	Key messages disseminated through religious institutions	Not stated	Part of a broader program of RHD control
South Africa 2006–present[28]	Focus on school and learners	Training frontline health workers, especially school and community nurses	Posters, pamphlets, wall charts, and training material	TV, radio and YouTube, multiple messages, DVDs	Rheumatic fever week	A sore throat can break your heart	Decline in ARF as part of comprehensive program
Nepal, 2007 onwards[28]	RHD included in school curriculum	Training >1500 community health workers + 26 train-the-trainer workshops	Posters, calendars, hoarding boards.	TV documentary and radio jingles		Not stated	Part of a broader program of RHD control.

Zambia,[29] 2014 onwards	50 primary healthcare workers	Initially 7 workshops held across the capital	Posters, pamphlets, wall charts, and training materials disseminated to workers and provided to workers to train other workers at their own institutions.	TV, radio, and documentaries. Radio major medium of education with directed programming, discussions, and interviews.	RHD week	Seek skilled care for sore throat and anaphylaxis training "A sore throat can damage your heart|"	Uptake of awareness-raising activities by government
Fiji,[30] 2014 onwards	Teaching program for school children—distributed to all primary and secondary schools	Education program	Posters and pamphlets	https://www.health.gov.fj/wp-content/uploads/2019/03/Fiji-Guidelines-for-Acute-Rheumatic-Fever-and-Rheumatic-Heart-Disease-Diagnosis-Management-and-Prevention.pdf	Website and social media. Rheumatic fever week.	"A sore throat can kill you"	

ARF, acute rheumatic fever; *RHD*, rheumatic heart disease

BOX 15.1
Community Education and Awareness Activities, New Zealand

In 2011 New Zealand began the largest ever concerted effort to reduce the incidence of ARF, focusing on high risk Māori and Pacific Island populations.[31] The Rheumatic Fever Prevention Program had three main strategies:[32]
- Increase awareness of ARF, what it is and how to prevent it
- Reduce household crowding
- Improve access to timely and effective treatment for GAS infections
  The program cost $65 million NZD over 5 years.
  The first rheumatic fever awareness campaign was conducted in winter 2014 with the intention of "increasing awareness among parents and caregivers of at-risk children and young people about the cause and effects of rheumatic fever."[33] A number of key messages were developed and linked to "calls to action."[34] Delivery of these messages was intensive, including television advertising, radio, newspaper advertising, posters for health providers, and pamphlets in schools. Evaluation suggested that 60% of parents took health action as a direct result of the campaign.[34]
  The 2015 campaign built on this foundation and used a "chain of theorized outcomes" to underpin expected behavior change.[33] The 2015 Rheumatic Fever Awareness Campaign was independently evaluated using document review, interviews with policy makers, eight focus groups, and over 250 phone calls to the target audience. The results of the program were that population-based primary prevention of ARF through sore throat management may be effective in well-resourced settings where high-risk populations are geographically concentrated. However, where high-risk populations are dispersed, a school-based primary prevention approach appears ineffective and is expensive.
  The focus on ARF in New Zealand spurred communication innovations in some parts of the country: a wallet card to help empower families to show it to health providers and ask for their child's throat to be checked, stickers ("got a sore throat? Tell a grown up"), including messages about ARF embedded in telephone "on-hold" music for the hospitals.[35]
  In Auckland areas with a high burden of RHD, other strategies were developed by the Ministry of Youth Development, including a Rheumatic Fever Ambassadors Program, "Clear ya throat" spoken word stories and a "Dramatic Fever Edutainment Road show." Many of these elements were codesigned by young people from high-risk communities, including competitions to develop mobile phone applications and technology resources to share key messages.[36] A feature of the New Zealand communications programs was the use of young people living with ARF or RHD in communications material. Using relatable people and stories improved uptake and impact of key messages.[35]
  By 2017, a survey of caregivers conducted alongside an RHD echocardiography screening project found that over 90% had heard of ARF and most people were aware that it is caused by sore throat. Over 80% of participants indicated that children with a sore throat should see a doctor or a nurse straight away.[37]
  The scale of community education efforts in New Zealand is unprecedented and overwhelmingly positive in raising awareness of ARF. Synthesis of lessons from this New Zealand experience is ongoing. Emerging critiques include concerns that young people from high-risk communities received relatively didactic messages, some of which may have heightened stigma associated with ARF and RHD.[38,39] Although the New Zealand context has unique elements, unintended consequences of education campaigns should always be considered and, if possible, evaluated.

framework models helps people designing information campaigns to think about key messages, target audiences, and determinants of health-seeking behavior. Framework-based approaches have been used in Samoa and New Zealand but have not previously been a routine part of developing awareness-raising campaigns for ARF and RHD.[8,33]

In addition to strong theoretical frameworks, the best way to ensure education programs meet the needs of communities is for programs to be designed, delivered, and evaluated by end users.[54] This may also provide a vehicle for engaging communities at risk of ARF through employment and education—which may, in turn, improve the social determinants of health that drive RHD. Leadership in this area has come from

people living with RHD awareness initiatives in Zambia,[29] Namibia, and Uganda.[55] Participation in research projects also improves awareness and contributes to education among participants, their families, and health workers.[56] The pervasive lack of knowledge about GAS, ARF, and RHD in most endemic communities necessitates a whole-of-community approach to education. Global improvements in health awareness mean that key messages address target audiences (young people at risk of ARF/RHD, clinicians, community health workers, school teachers) in addition to people who might influence health-seeking behaviors (heads of households, parents-in-law, and people in positions of authority). Inclusive messaging that is supportive of action by all stakeholders is needed to have

> **BOX 15.2**
> **Listen to my Heart: A Patient and Community Education Initiative**
>
> The RHD community of researchers and healthcare workers at the University of Cape Town, under the banner of the Stop RHD ASAP program, have created a tradition of patient events, including recognizing and celebrating the RHD patient community. These events are held each year during Rheumatic Fever week, the first full week in August. The ASAP program has focused on the four pillars of awareness, surveillance, advocacy, and prevention in a grassroots approach to eradicate ARF and RHD in Africa.[41]
>
> A patient event held in Cape Town in 2014 established the need for a new, interactive approach to patient-level awareness and education. What became clear after a more didactic and unidirectional information session was that patients preferred hearing from each other, that messages of wellness, rather than illness, were better received and that a sense of empowerment was needed to then engage beyond the event with healthcare providers.
>
> In 2015, an educational demonstration component was added to the awareness event, with wellness booths, discussing elements of RHD care such as point-of-care INR management, height, weight, and blood pressure measurements, healthy cooking, heart models, and auscultation and an opportunity to share experiences and engage in fun community activities. These were actively demonstrated rather than discussed using lectures, patients were involved in the sessions and planning, and education materials were demonstrated that could be used and shown at home, such as DVDs.
>
> This "Listen to my heart" event was replicated in other centers, with some of the original organizing team traveling to Uganda and guiding similar activities in Namibia.
>
> Patient-centered and initiated research is growing in popularity and scope[42] with guidelines becoming available to provide information about how to partner with patients in conceptualizing research questions, conducting research, and disseminating findings.[43] A broadening of this approach may lead to totally patient-led education and awareness opportunities.

ARF, acute rheumatic fever; *RHD*, rheumatic heart disease; *ASAP*, awareness, surveillance, advocacy, and prevention; *INR*, internationalised normalised ratio

impact. Box 15.3 outlines the priorities that should be considered in designing campaigns to increase understanding and improve awareness of GAS, ARF, and RHD.

Finally, isolated disease-specific education activities are unlikely to be sustainable or desirable in the face of many competing health priorities and conditions. Integrating key messages about sore throat, ARF, and RHD into other campaigns offers improved efficiency, albeit at the risk of increased complexity and potential for confusion and message dilution.[57] We suggest that opportunities may include general health promotion information about respiratory hygiene and household crowding. However, focused education is also likely to be needed to address specific health-seeking behaviors for primary prevention.

LOCAL AND GLOBAL ADVOCACY EFFORTS

Defining Advocacy

We are all advocates. Every day we think about what we need, point out problems and things that need to be done, think of strategies to get what we want and achieve our objectives and talk to different people to make it possible. Sometimes we advocate on behalf of others—friends, family, colleagues—and often it is on behalf of ourselves. The process is the same. We see or

anticipate a problem or challenge, think about how it will affect us, present a solution to someone with the power to make a change either to avoid or fix the problem and then we monitor the progress to see if what we wanted happens. You as a healthcare worker may be advocating for yourself, your department, your family or community, your facility, or your patients.

When thinking about advocacy in more formal settings the process is similar but usually more structured. To be successful, advocates must have a sound, evidence-based argument (as far as this is possible; even limited or imperfect data can be a huge weapon for advocacy); understand the specific windows of opportunity for their cause; and build communication that fosters social awareness and a shared understanding of how to achieve measurable change. There has been a growing awareness of the expanded role of health practitioners in advocating for patients and families.[60]

What Can Be Achieved Through Successful Advocacy in Rheumatic Heart Disease?

Advocacy is a powerful tool that has contributed to positive change in the field of RHD. The successes have helped raise awareness of RHD at the global level, placing RHD on the global public health agenda in a way not seen before. It has supported regional activities

---

BOX 15.3
Priorities in Understanding and Improving Awareness of Group A Streptococcus, Acute Rheumatic Fever, and Rheumatic Heart Disease

- A validated, standardized survey tool is needed to quantify awareness of GAS, ARF, and RHD and to help assess the effects of any subsequent education. Knowledge and awareness assessment tools exist for a number of other diseases in low-resource settings, including hypertension and diabetes.[58,59]
- Standardized key messages are needed to minimize the burden of developing educational materials in low-resource settings. The RHD Action Resource Hub (http://rhdaction.org/resource-hub) currently provides a clearing house of health promotion and education resources. This should be amplified by adding resources that can be customized at a local level.
- People, families, and communities at risk of RHD or living with RHD should have a leadership role in shaping community education campaigns targeted at high-risk populations.
- Use of media and communication avenues should be designed to targetspecific communities: using mobile phones, e-messaging, and social media may direct messaging at a younger community.
- Integrated communication messages allow for a wider reach than only ARF/RHD approaches.
- Evaluation of mass media and awareness-raising campaigns should be designed before the campaign and use robust methodology including use of unbiased samples, multiple comparator groups, and advanced statistical methods. Campaign details including intensity and duration of exposure to messages should be clearly documented.[44]

GAS, group A streptococcus; *ARF*, acute rheumatic fever; *RHD*, rheumatic heart disease

---

and led to real impact at the national and local level.[61-] Some examples include:

- 2018 Global Resolution on RF and RHD[20]
- Government funding and support for comprehensive national RHD control programmes in Nepal and Fiji[62] (https://www.health.gov.fj/wp-content/uploads/2019/03/Fiji-Guidelines-for-AcuteRheumatic-Fever-and-Rheumatic-Heart-Disease-Diagnosis-Management-and-Prevention.pdf)
- African Union Communiqué supported by African Heads of State[18]
- Penicillin reestablished on the basic medicines list for the Non-Insured Health Benefits program[63]

Although there have been many successes, due to an increase in advocacy efforts in the last 10–15 years,[53] notably at the global, regional, and national level, these wins have not translated more widely, leaving us some way short of achieving the ambitious goal adopted by the World Heart Federation of a 25% reduction in premature deaths from ARF and RHD among individuals aged <25 years by the year 2025.[64] This is despite the strong evidence and cost-effective interventions at our disposal.

The necessary increase in resources to support these efforts is dependent on the prioritization of ARF and RHD by health systems, governments, and global health agencies. As RHD often affects those in limited-resource settings, many competing challenges exist. Moving RHD on to the list of priorities needs increased

advocacy on the part of all stakeholders.[19] Several successful programs were recently reviewed for key lessons and the role of local and regional advocates was a key element for a successful prevention and control program.[65,66]

Moving the Needle

When advocating for an increase in resources to tackle ARF/RHD, there are several essential steps to take. In a relatively unknown area where there is low awareness, such as for RHD, getting these steps correct from the outset will be the key to success. The following sections explore these in more detail.

1. **Conduct research**

Key decision makers may not be experts in RHD or even health matters and they will want to know salient data. "How many people are affected in my country? Which parts of the country have the highest burden? How many die annually? What is the annual cost of treating them?" It is critical to have the answer to these questions on hand when discussing RHD with policy makers and potential allies. Where investment of resources is required, numbers matter. Advocates need to be fully armed with as much information as possible on the cost of action and inaction, and the return on investment—lives and money saved.

2. **Define the problem and what needs to change**

Every death from RHD is a tragic failure of the health system, which often could have been prevented. As advocates, it is our responsibility to point out what went wrong, identify where the problems are, and offer solutions. In many cases, it makes sense to focus on a specific barrier. For example, until recently benzathine penicillin G (BPG) was on the Essential Medicines List in the Philippines but not covered by health insurance schemes. An advocacy campaign by the Philippines Heart Center identified this as a critical barrier that prevented poor patients from accessing the drugs they need. Targeted lobbying led to BPG being included in the universal health coverage benefit package, opening up access to a large number of patients who previously struggled to or could not meet the cost of BPG. A useful tool to help think through the barriers is the WHF Roadmap on RHD.[22] It identifies the different barriers facing countries around the world along the continuum of care from prevention to surgery.

3. **What needs to be done? What is the solution?**

We need to present a solution-driven answer. Politicians, policy makers, and managers within the health system often want a costed, tailor-made solution to a problem that they can use to make a case with their colleagues. As there are few experts in the RHD arena, the burden lies more heavily with advocates to offer suggestions for the solutions and to work in partnership with the relevant people to implement them. A useful tool for working through the solutions in addition to the WHF Roadmap is the TIPS RHD guide.[67] There are also organizations such as Reach (stoprhd.org) that can help provide guidance in making a case to the relevant parties.

4. **Identify who has the power to change things**

The institutions that can help change the reality on the ground vary widely in terms of who within those organizations would be an ideal ally or is standing in the way of you achieving your goal. It is important to identify supporters of your plan. In countries where ARF/RHD are endemic, you can often find people in government or the ministry of health who have come across RHD in their work or know someone living with or affected by the disease. They then can have a powerful voice to support wider advocacy activities and help build case for action. Action should not be restricted to ministries of health and governments. At each level of the health system, people have the power to make a difference in RHD. It could be the school nurse who agrees to run RHD awareness campaigns, the district manager who agrees to set up an RHD register, right up to the Minister of Health who appoints someone to be responsible for RHD within the Ministry.

5. **Persuade them to act**

It is individuals who will ultimately decide whether meaningful action on RHD will take place. Persuading them to act will rely on several things:

- *Being clear in the ask*. An advocacy message should not need interpreting. It should be straightforward and easy to act upon. The target of your advocacy should be able to explain what is being asked of them to their colleagues and peers.
- *Meets their individual objectives*. People have many responsibilities and commitments to fulfill. Tailoring an advocacy ask to the professional objectives a person has increases the chance that they will engage and act. Alternatively, if you can demonstrate that your plan helps them fulfill a commitment or aligns them with wider institutional objectives, it is easier for them to act on.
- *Demonstrating the support you can provide*. Demonstrating that you are a reliable partner and can provide capacity in knowledge and experience is key. Lack of knowledge of ARF and RHD is widespread; therefore, the people with the power to act often lack the tools and knowledge to do so. Be clear about what you can do and/or connect your advocacy target to the people who will be able to support their work.

6. **Find partners to help implement your strategy**

Partnerships can play a pivotal role in the success of RHD advocacy efforts. A wide range of voices from different stakeholders generates broader support for specific issues and increases the legitimacy and effectiveness of advocacy campaigns. A useful advocacy toolkit has been produced by UNICEF: https://www.unicef.org/evaluation/files/Advocacy_Toolkit.pdf.

Particularly effective in RHD has been the allying of those with a lived experience of RHD together with those who have technical expertise in treating or controlling the disease. Many organizations exist to support these groups, from patient support groups to health professional associations through to academic institutions. Government officials can similarly become strong advocacy partners; for example, a Ministry of Health official can be a key champion in securing funds from the treasury. Future RHD advocacy will rely on forming broad coalitions with different stakeholders to utilize the different experiences they bring. This will help strengthen the solutions and increase the pressure for change.

WHAT NEXT FOR ACUTE RHEUMATIC FEVER AND RHEUMATIC HEART DISEASE?

The 2018 World Health Assembly Resolution on ARF and RHD is a great starting point for future advocacy for RHD. However, taking that work a step further will require considerable effort on the part of the

RHD community to put forward relevant solutions at the national level. The ability for actors in RHD to translate the general asks of the Resolution to specific asks at the country and local level will determine how successful the efforts of the last few years will be. Several key questions will determine the response. Where no RHD program exists, what is the best starting point? Where there is a pilot program or some level of care, how can this be scaled up? What data/evidence can help persuade people to take the next step? What resources are needed?

In addition to national level activities, the broader RHD community has a role in supporting the monitoring of the global resolution. Building a picture of what is happening in countries will help the RHD community hold governments accountable to the instructions given and commitments made in the Resolution. Understanding how much progress is being made will help organizations like Reach push for increases in resources, where needed, and measure the progress of the resolution.

A FINAL WORD ON THE KEY ELEMENTS OF SUCCESS

Persistence and energy are perhaps the two elements most critical to advocacy success. To make change happen, it is important to be persistent, to cope with failure when things do not work out, to question, and to seek out potential allies and champions at every turn. Despite a relative lack of resources and political power, RHD advocates around the world have been able to improve the lives of the communities they live and work in through their ability to persuade others to act. Every voice matters and the more voices calling for action on RHD, the greater the chance we can achieve the vision of an RHD free generation by 2030.

REFERENCES

1. Saurman E. Improving access: modifying Penchansky and Thomas's theory of access. *J Health Serv Res Policy*. 2016; 21(1):36−39.
2. Zandiyeh Z. The effect of education on the knowledge of the mothers concerning prevention of rheumatic fever. *Early Hum Dev*. 2007;83(S1):S132.
3. Bergmark R, Bergmark B, Blander J, Fataki M, Janabi M. Burden of disease and barriers to the diagnosis and treatment of group a beta-hemolytic streptococcal pharyngitis for the prevention of rheumatic heart disease in Dar Es Salaam, Tanzania. *Pediatr Infect Dis J*. 2010;29(12):1135−1137.
4. Maria M. *Awareness of Rheumatid Heart Disease Prevention Among Primary Health Care Providers and People Aged Nine Years and above in Kinondoni Municipality Dar Es Salam.* Tanzania: Muhimbili University of Health and Allied Sciences; 2011.
5. Iyengar SD, Grover A, Kumar R, Ganguly NK, Wahi PL. Participation of health workers, school teachers and pupils in the control of rheumatic fever: evaluation of a training programme. *Indian Pediatr*. 1992;29(7):875−881.
6. Matheka D, Murgor M, Kibochi E, Nigel S, Nderitu J, Selnow G. Role of technology in creating rheumatic heart disease awareness among school-going children in Kenya. *Global Heart*. 2014;9(1S):e7.
7. Kasmaei P, Atrkar-Roushan Z, Majlesi F, Joukar F. Mothers' knowledge about acute rheumatic fever. *Paediatr Nurs*. 2008;20(9):32−34.
8. Allen LB, Allen M, Lesa RF, Richardson GE, Eggett DL. Rheumatic fever in Samoa: education as prevention. *Pac Health Dialog*. 2011;17(1):107−118.
9. Regmi P, Panthi L, Sanjel K. Level of knowledge among community people on acute rheumatic fever and rheumatic heart disease and their link with throat infection. *Global Heart*. 2016;11(2S):e65.
10. Musuku J, Chipili J, Long A, Tadmor B, Spector J. *Teachers' Knowledge and Attitudes Related to Rheumatic Heart Disease in Zambia.* Barcelona, Spain: European Society of Cardiology Congress; 2014.
11. Harrington Z, Thomas D, Currie B, Bulkanhawuy J. Challenging perceptions of non-compliance with rheumatic fever prophylaxis in a remote Aboriginal community. *Med J Aust*. 2006;184(10):514−517.
12. Thompson SB, Brown CH, Edwards AM, Lindo JL. Low adherence to secondary prophylaxis among clients diagnosed with rheumatic fever, Jamaica. *Pathog Glob Health*. 2014;108(5):229−234.
13. Robertson K, Volmink J, Mayosi B. Lack of adherence to the national guidelines on the prevention of rheumatic fever. *S Afr Med J*. 2005;95(1):52−56.
14. Nkoke C, Luchuo EB, Jingi AM, Makoge C, Hamadou B, Dzudie A. Rheumatic heart disease awareness in the South West region of Cameroon: a hospital based survey in a Sub-Saharan African setting. *PLoS One*. 2018;13(9): e0203864.
15. Rocha G, Ruffini V, Martin R, et al. Knowledge of cardiologists related to prophylaxis of rheumatic fever in Salvador-BA. *Braz J Med Biol Res*. 2014;2(2):69−74.
16. Alkhazi AA, Alessa KM, Almutairi AM, et al. Improving pediatric emergency department physicians' adherence to clinical practice guidelines on the diagnosis and management of group A beta-hemolytic streptococcal pharyngitis-a cross-sectional study. *Int J Emerg Med*. 2018;11:49.
17. Osman GM, Abdelrahman SM, Ali SK. Evaluation of physicians' knowledge about prevention of rheumatic fever and rheumatic heart disease before and after a teaching session. *Sudan J Paediatr*. 2015;15(2):37−42.
18. Watkins DA, Zuhlke LJ, Engel ME, Mayosi BM. Rheumatic fever: neglected again. *Science*. 2009;324(5923):37.
19. Watkins DA, Zuhlke LJ, Narula J. Moving forward the RHD agenda at global and national levels. *Glob Heart*. 2017; 12(1):1−2.

20. White A. WHO Resolution on rheumatic heart disease. *Eur Heart J.* 2018;39(48):4233.
21. Sliwa K, White A, Milan P, Olga Mocumbi A, Zilla P, Wood D. Momentum builds for a global response to rheumatic heart disease. *Eur Heart J.* 2018;39(48):4229−4232.
22. Palafox B, Mocumbi AO, Kumar RK, et al. The WHF Roadmap for reducing CV morbidity and mortality through prevention and control of RHD. *Glob Heart.* 2017;12(1):47−62.
23. Watkins D, Zuhlke L, Engel M, et al. Seven key actions to eradicate rheumatic heart disease in Africa: the Addis Ababa communique. *Cardiovasc J Afr.* 2016;27:1−5.
24. Macleod CK, Bright P, Steer AC, Kim J, Mabey D, Parks T. Neglecting the neglected: the objective evidence of underfunding in rheumatic heart disease. *Trans R Soc Trop Med Hyg.* 2019.
25. Bach JF, Chalons S, Forier E, et al. 10-year educational programme aimed at rheumatic fever in two French Caribbean islands. *Lancet.* 1996;347:644−648.
26. Nordet P, ed. *Rheumatic Fever/rheumatic Heart Disease Prevention:lessons Learned (Mm Ref 2142). 2nd Virtual Congress of Cardiology.* Argentine Federation of Cardiology; 2001.
27. Kumar R, Sharma M. reportJai Vigyan Mission Mode Project. Community Control of Rheumatic Fever and Rheumatic Heart Disease in India. Comprehensive Project Report 2000−2010. . Ansari Nagar, New Delhi: Indian Council of Medical Research; 201.
28. Regmi P. Comprehensive approach to rheumatic fever and rheumatic heart disease prevention and control: the Nepalese model. *Nepalse Heart J.* 2016;13(2):3−10.
29. Musuku J, Chipili J, Machila E, et al. Fostering public awareness for rheumatic heart disease in Zambia: progress and lessons learned. *Pediatrics.* 2018;141(1).
30. *National Rheuamtic Heart Disease Awareness Week: Medical Services Pacific;* 2014 [Available from: http://msp.org.fj/725/.
31. Jack SJ, Williamson DA, Galloway Y, Pierse N, Zhang J, Oliver J, et al. Primary Prevention of Rheumatic Fever in the 21st Century: Evaluation of a National Programme. (1464-3685 (Electronic)).
32. Jack S, Williamson D, Galloway Y, Pierse N, Milne R. *Interim Evaluation of the Sore Throat Management Component of the New Zealand Rheumatic Fever Prevention Program − Quantitative Findings.* Porirua, New Zealand: The Institue of Environmental Science and Research; 2015.
33. Vermillion P, Akroyd S, Tafuna P, et al. *Evaluation of the 2015 Rheumatic Fever Awareness Campaign.* Wellington, New Zealand: Allen + Clarke; 2015.
34. TNS New Zealand Limited. *Rheumatic Fever Campaign Evalutation.* Wellington, New Zealand: Health Promotion Agency; 2014.
35. Lowe L, Vipond R, Phillips D, Bunker S. *Evaluation of the 2014 Bay of Plenty Rheumatic Fever Awareness Campaign Toi Te Ora Public Health Service.* 2015.
36. *ADHB. Auckland District Health Board Rheumatic Fever Prevention Programme.* 2016. Auckland, New Zealand.
37. Gurney JK, Chong A, Culliford-Semmens N, Tilton E, Wilson NJ, Sarfati D. High levels of rheumatic fever and sore throat awareness among a high-risk population screened for rheumatic heart disease. *N Z Med J.* 2017; 130(1450):107−110.
38. Spray J. The value of anthropology in child health policy. *Anthropol Action.* 2018;25(1). https://doi.org/10.3167/aia.2018.250104.
39. Andrerson A, Leversha A, Ofanoa M, et al. *Māori and Pacific Whānau Experiences of Recurrent Rheumatic Fever and Unexpected Rheumatic Heart Disease in New Zealand.* Auckland, New Zealand: The University of Auckland; 2018.
40. Mayosi BM. National Rheumatic Fever Week: the status of rheumatic heart disease in South Africa. *S Afr Med J.* 2016; 106(8):740−741.
41. Engel M, Zühlke L, Robertson KA. ASAP programme: rheumatic fever and rheumatic heart disease: where are we now in South Africa? *SA Heart.* 2009;6:270−273.
42. Pushparajah DS. *Making Patient Engagement a Reality.* Patient; 2017.
43. Kirwan JR, de Wit M, Frank L, et al. Emerging guidelines for patient engagement in research. *Value Health.* 2017;20(3): 481−486.
44. Naugle DA, Hornik RC. Systematic review of the effectiveness of mass media interventions for child survival in low- and middle-income countries. *J Health Commun.* 2014; 19(Suppl 1):190−215.
45. LaCroix JM, Snyder LB, Huedo-Medina TB, Johnson BT. Effectiveness of mass media interventions for HIV prevention, 1986−2013: a meta-analysis. *J Acquir Immune Defic Syndr.* 2014;66(Suppl 3):S329−S340.
46. Shen J, Kondal D, Rubinstein A, et al. A multiethnic study of pre-diabetes and diabetes in LMIC. *Glob Heart.* 2016; 11(1):61−70.
47. Azevedo M, Alla S. Diabetes in sub-saharan Africa: Kenya, Mali, Mozambique, Nigeria, South Africa and Zambia. *Int J Diabetes Dev Ctries.* 2008;28(4):101−108.
48. Somannavar S, Lanthorn H, Pradeepa R, Narayanan V, Rema M, Mohan V. Prevention awareness counselling and evaluation (PACE) diabetes project: a mega multipronged program for diabetes awareness and prevention in South India (PACE- 5). *J Assoc Phys India.* 2008;56: 429−435.
49. Somannavar S, Lanthorn H, Deepa M, Pradeepa R, Rema M, Mohan V. Increased awareness about diabetes and its complications in a whole city: effectiveness of the "prevention, awareness, counselling and evaluation" [PACE] Diabetes Project [PACE-6]. *J Assoc Phys India.* 2008;56:497−502.
50. Hertz J, Munishi OM, Sharp J, Reddy E, Crump JA. Comparing actual and perceived causes of fever among community members in a low malaria transmission setting in northern Tanzania. *Trop Med Int Health.* 2013; 8(11):1406−1415.
51. Koech PJ, Onyango FE, Jowi C. Caregivers' knowledge and home management of fever in children. *East Afr Med J.* 2014;91(5):170−177.
52. Al-Nouri L, Basheer K. Mothers' perceptions of fever in children. *J Trop Pediatr.* 2006;52(2):113−116. discussion 7.

53. Chibwana AI, Mathanga DP, Chinkhumba J, Campbell Jr CH. Socio-cultural predictors of health-seeking behaviour for febrile under-five children in Mwanza-Neno district, Malawi. *Malar J.* 2009;8:219.

54. Sood S, Shefner-Rogers C, Skinner J. Health communication campaigns in developing countries. *J Creat Commun.* 2014;9(1):67–84.

55. Scheel A, Beaton A, Okello E, et al. The impact of a peer support group for children with rheumatic heart disease in Uganda. *Patient Educ Couns.* 2017.

56. Prendergast EA, Perkins S, Engel ME, et al. Participation in research improves overall patient management: insights from the Global Rheumatic Heart Disease registry (REMEDY). *Cardiovasc J Afr.* 2018;29(2):98–105.

57. Kabatereine NB, Malecela M, Lado M, Zaramba S, Amiel O, Kolaczinski JH. How to (or not to) integrate vertical programmes for the control of major neglected tropical diseases in sub-Saharan Africa. *PLoS Neglected Trop Dis.* 2010;4(6):e755.

58. Erkoc SB, Isikli B, Metintas S, Kalyoncu C. Hypertension Knowledge-Level Scale (HK-LS): a study on development, validity and reliability. *Int J Environ Res Public Health.* 2012;9(3):1018–1029.

59. Mohan D, Raj D, Shanthirani CS, et al. Awareness and knowledge of diabetes in Chennai–the Chennai urban rural epidemiology study [CURES-9]. *J Assoc Phys India.* 2005;53:283–287.

60. Kalaitzidis E, Jewell P. The concept of advocacy in nursing: a critical analysis. *Health Care Manag.* 2015;34(4):308–315.

61. Wyber R, Zuhlke L, Carapetis J. The case for global investment in rheumatic heart-disease control. *Bull World Health Organ.* 2014;92(10):768–770.

62. Regmi PR, Wyber R. Prevention of rheumatic Fever and heart disease: nepalese experience. *Glob Heart.* 2013;8(3):247–252.

63. Wyber R, Boyd BJ, Colquhoun S, et al. Preliminary consultation on preferred product characteristics of benzathine penicillin G for secondary prophylaxis of rheumatic fever. *Drug Deliv Transl Res.* 2016;6(5):572–578.

64. Remenyi B, Carapetis J, Wyber R, Taubert K, Mayosi BM. Position statement of the World Heart Federation on the prevention and control of rheumatic heart disease. *Nat Rev Cardiol.* 2013;10(5):284–292.

65. Dougherty S, Beaton A, Nascimento BR, Zuhlke LJ, Khorsandi M, Wilson N. Prevention and control of rheumatic heart disease: overcoming core challenges in resource-poor environments. *Ann Pediatr Cardiol.* 2018;11(1):68–78.

66. Abouzeid M, Wyber R, La Vincente S, et al. Time to tackle rheumatic heart disease: data needed to drive global policy dialogues. *Glob Public Health.* 2018:1–13.

67. Wyber RGG A, Thompson D, Kennedy D, Johnson T, Taubert K, Carapetis J. *Tools for Implementing RHD Control Programmes (TIPS) Handbook.* Perth, Australia; 2014 [Available from: http://www.rheach.org/resources/tips-(1)/.

CHAPTER 16

Complications of Rheumatic Heart Disease and Acute Emergencies

SCOTT DOUGHERTY • MOHAMMED R. ESSOP • RACHEL WEBB •
SUSANNA PRICE • NIGEL WILSON

INTRODUCTION

The clinical course of both acute rheumatic fever (ARF) and rheumatic heart disease (RHD) may be complicated by acute life-threatening conditions. This chapter will focus on: (1) the clinical evaluation, diagnosis, and management of acute heart failure (AHF); (2) infective endocarditis (IE); and (3) the management of overanticoagulation and bleeding in patients receiving oral anticoagulation. The etiology and pathophysiology of AHF in rheumatic carditis is discussed in Chapter 3. Chronic heart failure (HF) is discussed in detail in Chapters 5 and 6 and the management of RHD and HF in pregnancy is discussed in Chapter 9.

1: ACUTE HEART FAILURE

Definition and Classification

The main clinical syndrome resulting in death and disability in both ARF and RHD is HF, the natural history of which is characterized by episodes of acute decompensation (AHF). AHF is broadly defined as a potentially life-threatening syndrome, characterized by a rapid onset of new or worsening signs and symptoms of HF that typically requires urgent medical attention.[1]

The development of AHF as a consequence of ARF or RHD is challenging. Some patients develop an acute deterioration in valvular function, where the presentation is usually dramatic and potentially life threatening. In certain cases, however, clinical features suggesting a valvular cause of AHF may be subtle, for example, the regurgitant murmur in acute severe mitral or aortic regurgitation is often soft and difficult to hear. Successful management requires maintaining a high index of suspicion, appropriate hemodynamic assessment, and timely initiation of therapeutic options. In most cases, however, AHF results from chronic valvular disease with progressive deterioration in ventricular function, often culminating in repeated subacute presentations requiring hospitalization. Treatment may be challenging, particularly in resource-limited populations as patients are often deprived of access to valve surgery, the only intervention that improves outcomes. Despite this, optimal medical treatment will usually provide symptomatic improvement in the short term.

Although characterized by a common set of signs and symptoms, AHF is a syndrome rather than a single disease entity, and patients exhibit a wide spectrum of features (Box 16.1). Moreover, while our understanding of chronic HF has improved considerably over the last 20−30 years, the presentation and management of AHF is less well understood.[2] Nonetheless, admission to hospital with AHF is a significant prognostic event in the natural history of ARF or RHD, indicating that not only is the valve lesion important but also that an additional factor may have contributed to the clinical picture. For many patients, it also indicates a poor prognosis, with a high risk of readmission and death postdischarge.[3−6]

Epidemiology

A global epidemiological profile for AHF has emerged over the last 2 decades. Although most of the data originate from high-income countries (HICs), little is known about AHF in low- and middle-income countries (LMICs), where ARF and RHD are endemic.

In the landmark 1950s publication by Bland and Duckett Jones,[4] a 20-year analysis of 1000 patients

---

BOX 16.1
Classification of Acute Heart Failure[1,22]

AHF may present as a first occurrence (*de novo* AHF) or as a consequence of acute decompensation of chronic HF (ADHF).[1]

DE NOVO ACUTE HEART FAILURE
- Occurs in patients with advanced RHD
- Constitutes 70% of patients hospitalized for AHF in nonendemic populations[22]
- Causes: (1) primary cardiac dysfunction (usually worsening left ventricular function); (2) precipitated by extrinsic factors
- Typical presentation: with mild-to-moderate signs and symptoms of congestion and fluid retention
- Acuity: subacute over days to weeks (chronic neuro-hormonal compensatory mechanisms and preexisting medical therapy help ameliorate the severity of presentation)

ACUTE DECOMPENSATED HEART FAILURE
- In ARF:
  - Usually subacute presentation with some cardiac enlargement and compensation
  - Sometimes presents as fulminant carditis (see Chapters 3 and 4). In acute severe MR, the LA is noncompliant and acute pulmonary edema occurs within days
- In RHD: as a first presentation of chronic valve disease

---

showed HF to account for 80% of all deaths from RHD. Cardiac enlargement early in life (presumably during the phase of ARF) had the strongest correlate with mortality, suggesting that the development of HF during ARF carries an extremely poor prognosis. In the contemporary REMEDY study[5] (prospective registry, 3343 patients with RHD), congestive HF was the most frequent complication, and was seen in 33.4% of the patients. In addition, 25% of adults and 5.3% of children had reduced ejection fraction, and left ventricular (LV) dilatation occurred in 23% and 14.1%, respectively. Sixty percent of patients had multivalvular disease, and 66.7% of these were severely affected.

The sub-Saharan African Study of Heart Failure (THESUS-HF) was the first (and to date, only) prospective, observational survey that characterized the causes and short-term outcomes of African adult patients with AHF.[5] Here, 1006 patients with AHF (mean age 52 years) were recruited from 12 university hospitals in nine African countries between 2007 and 2010. In contrast to

data from HICs, the etiology of AHF in these patients was predominantly nonischemic, with hypertension (45.4%), idiopathic dilated cardiomyopathy (18.8%), and RHD (14.3%) accounting for 75.5% of cases. AHF presented around 2 decades earlier than in those patients from Europe and the United States. In-hospital mortality was 4.2% and estimated 180-day mortality was 17.8%, which were comparable to non-African registries. In a subanalysis of patients enrolled in THESUS-HF with RHD from South Africa, the 60-day mortality after admission with AHF due to RHD was 24.8% (95% CI 13.6%–42.5%) and 180-day mortality was 35.4% (95% CI 21.6%–54.4%).[6] The epidemiology of HF due to RHD is discussed further in Chapter 1.

Etiology of Acute Heart Failure
Acute rheumatic fever
A full discussion on the mechanisms of AHF in rheumatic carditis is presented in Chapter 3. In brief, acute severe mitral or mitral and aortic regurgitation (all secondary to valvulitis) are by far the most common causes of AHF in those who develop ARF. Rarely, chordae tendineae rupture (causing acute severe mitral regurgitation) or cardiac tamponade are the primary cause of AHF. Rheumatic myocarditis does not on its own cause significant myocardial dysfunction and AHF, unlike other forms of myocarditis (Table 16.1).

Rheumatic heart disease
In contrast to those with ARF, patients with established RHD have chronic valvular heart disease. When the valve disease is significant, this is often accompanied by varying degrees of LV dysfunction and remodeling similar to that seen in nonrheumatic disease. The valvular lesions in RHD patients also tend to be more complex than those seen in ARF, with mixed and multivalve disease being the most common phenotype.[5] RHD patients are also usually older and may suffer from significant comorbidities. They may require long-term medical therapy and have undergone mechanical or surgical valvular intervention.

The causes of AHF in those with RHD are therefore broad and are detailed in Box 16.2. In many patients, an episode of AHF is often the result of numerous interlinked factors but in 40%–50% of all admissions, no clear precipitant is found.[7]

Evaluation and Management of the Patient With Acute Heart Failure
The diagnostic work-up of AHF should start in the prehospital setting and continue in the emergency

TABLE 16.1
Key Differentiating Features Between Rheumatic Carditis and Viral Myocarditis.

	Acute Rheumatic Carditis	Acute Viral Myocarditis
Age (years)	Usually 5–15	Any age
Epidemiology	Usually in areas where ARF is endemic	Anywhere
Prodrome	Sore throat	Headache, myalgia, skin rash, gastroenteritis, coryza
Cardiac murmurs	Murmurs of MR, AR	Nil or flow murmur
Hypotension	Unusual	Common
ECG	Prolonged PR interval or advanced AV block Accelerated junctional tachycardia	Low-voltage QRS complexes Bundle branch block Tachyarrhythmias, including ventricular tachycardia Risk of sudden cardiac death
Echocardiography	Significant mitral and/or aortic regurgitation	Mild to moderate secondary mitral regurgitation
LV Ejection Fraction	Normal or increased	Decreased
Troponin T	Normal	Elevated
Serology or PCR	ASOT positive Anti-DNAse B positive	Parvovirus, Coxsackie, Echo, Herpes, adenovirus, influenza, parechovirus, enterovirus
Cardiac magnetic resonance	Minimal changes	Often abnormal especially on T2 mapping
Endomyocardial biopsy	Nonspecific. May have aschoff bodies	Myocarditis Lymphocytic inflammation, myocyte degeneration

AR, aortic regurgitation; ARF, acute rheumatic fever; ASOT, antistreptolysin O titer; AV, atrioventricular; ECG, electrocardiogram; LV, left ventricular; MR, mitral regurgitation; PCR, polymerase chain reaction.

department. Given the potentially life-threatening nature of AHF, establishing a definitive diagnosis of the underlying cause, with initiation of appropriate therapy as rapidly and efficiently as possible, are of key importance[1] as time to initiation of treatment is linked to outcome.[8,9]

In all acutely unwell patients, a systematic approach is essential. Fig. 16.1 presents an algorithmic approach to the initial evaluation of patients with suspected AHF from the latest HF guidelines of the European Society of Cardiology (ESC).[1] This algorithm highlights four phases, detailed later:
(1) early recognition, treatment, and triage of life-threatening conditions (i.e., respiratory failure and cardiogenic shock)
(2) early recognition and treatment of any acute etiology or relevant triggers requiring specific treatment (e.g., acute valvular regurgitation, arrhythmia, pericardial tamponade)

(3) completing the diagnostic work-up of AHF once the patient is stable
(4) defining the clinical profile of the patient to rapidly select the most appropriate therapy

Each of these phases will be discussed in order in the following sections. However, as stated in Box 16.1, most patients with ARF or RHD that develop AHF will present subacutely and many of the therapeutic strategies in phases I and II will not be necessary. Most patients will therefore enter the treatment algorithm at phase III.

Phase I: Early recognition, treatment, and triage of life-threatening conditions
Initial evaluation begins with an ABC assessment (airway, breathing, and circulation) while simultaneously taking a focused history and progressing toward diagnosis and treatment (Box 16.3).

The key elements of airway and breathing assessment are ensuring airway patency and determining

---

BOX 16.2
Factors Triggering Acute Heart Failure in Rheumatic Heart Disease

VALVE-RELATED
- Natural history of chronic, severe valve regurgitation causing myocardial (pump) failure
- Recurrent acute rheumatic fever
- Infective endocarditis
- Acute prosthetic valve syndrome
  - Dehiscence (e.g., infective endocarditis)
  - Thrombosis (most often causing stenosis)
  - Structural failure (e.g., tear or perforation of a bio-prosthetic valve)
- Iatrogenic mitral regurgitation following percutaneous mitral balloon commissurotomy

NONVALVULAR
- Tachyarrhythmia (e.g., atrial fibrillation, ventricular tachycardia)
- Acute rise in blood pressure or chronic hypertension
- Worsening renal failure
- Infection (e.g., pneumonia, sepsis, influenza)
- Anemia
- Pregnancy and peripartum-related disorders
- Nonadherence (e.g., medications, salt/fluid intake)
- Acute coronary syndrome
- Cerebrovascular insult
- Pulmonary embolism
- Heavy alcohol consumption
- Noncardiac surgery and perioperative complications

---

the need for supplemental oxygen and respiratory support (Table 16.2). Continuous pulse oximetry (S_pO_2) is mandatory. Although some degree of pulmonary edema is common in AHF, severe pulmonary edema only occurs in <3% of all AHF presentations.[10] Oxygen should not be used routinely in AHF as it may cause hyperoxia-induced vasoconstriction and reduced cardiac output.[1] Oxygen is a treatment for hypoxemia and not breathlessness and does not consistently alter the sensation of breathlessness in nonhypoxemic patients.[11] Intravenous (IV) morphine (for patients with severe anxiety or distress) should be used cautiously (if at all), particularly in those with hypotension, brady-cardia, advanced heart block, or hypercapnia.[1] Where concern arises, senior anesthetic/intensive care input is required.

If hypoxemia persists despite adequate oxygen therapy (F_iO_2 >40%), continuous positive airway pressure (CPAP) or noninvasive ventilation (NIV), delivered through tight-fitting face masks, should be given (Table 16.2). Both improve respiratory mechanics and unload the left ventricle (LV) by decreasing afterload. Because CPAP provides less inspiratory support (i.e., it is not a true ventilation modality) than NIV, the latter is more useful in the most severe patients (hypercapnic pulmonary edema, or respiratory fatigue). Meta-analyses and randomized controlled trials have shown that both CPAP and NIV decrease the need for intubation and improve physiological parameters (heart rate, dyspnea, hypercapnia, and acidemia),[12–15] although there is conflicting evidence regarding their impact on mortality.[13,14] Both should be used cautiously if the patient is hypotensive (systolic blood pressure (SBP) < 90 mmHg) and should be avoided in cardiogenic shock.

Assessment of the circulation is aimed at identifying hemodynamic instability and evidence of cardiogenic shock. Only a minority of adult patients with AHF present with an SBP <90 mmHg (<8%) or cardiogenic shock (<3%); most present with a preserved (90–140 mmHg) or elevated (≥140 mmHg) SBP.[1,10] ESC guidelines define cardiogenic shock in adults as an SBP <90 mmHg (with adequate volume) with clinical (cold extremities, oliguria, mental confusion, dizziness, and narrow pulse pressure) or laboratory (metabolic acidemia, elevated serum lactate, elevated serum creatinine) evidence of hypoperfusion.[1]

In children, the clinical diagnosis of shock can be challenging, particularly in resource-limited settings. The 2016 emergency triage, assessment, and treatment guidelines developed by the World Health Organization[16] (specifically for use in resource-limited settings) define shock as cold extremities *with* a capillary refill time >3 s *and* a weak, fast pulse (all signs must be present). When only one of these signs is present (i.e., capillary refill time >3 s *or* a weak, fast pulse *or* cold extremities), the patient meets the definition of "severely impaired circulation."[16] Patients with ARF (e.g., acute severe valvular regurgitation) or RHD (e.g., low output advanced end-stage chronic HF) may present with cardiogenic shock.

The initial management of adults and children with cardiogenic shock is summarized in Box 16.4. Fluid resuscitation in patients with cardiogenic shock should only be indicated in those without pulmonary edema. Isotonic crystalloids such as normal saline or Lactated Ringer's should be administered slowly to decrease the likelihood of exacerbating HF.

Vasoactive agents (Tables 16.3 and 16.4) represent "rescue therapy" in cardiogenic shock. They are used to stabilize and salvage, or as a bridge to nonpharmacological management such as mechanical circulatory

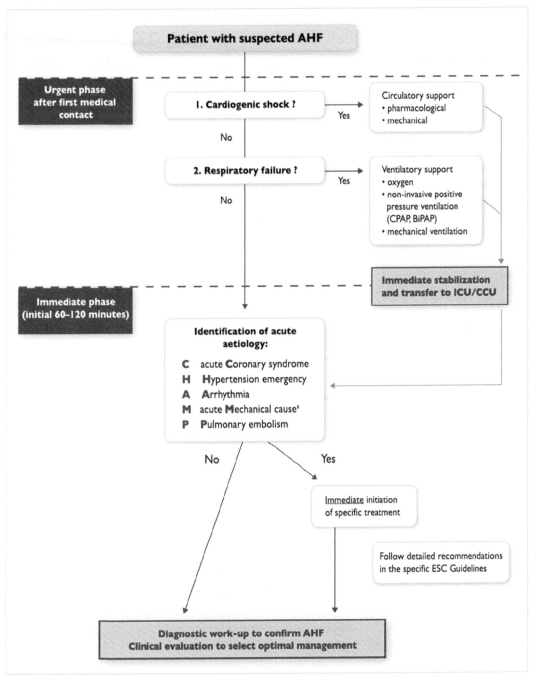

^aAcute mechanical cause: myocardial rupture complicating acute coronary syndrome (free wall rupture, ventricular septal defect, acute mitral regurgitation), chest trauma or cardiac intervention, acute native or prosthetic valve incompetence secondary to endocarditis, aortic dissection or thrombosis.

FIG. 16.1 Algorithm for initial evaluation and management of patients with suspected acute heart failure. AHF, acute heart failure; BiPAP, bi-level positive airway pressure; CCU, coronary care unit; CPAP, continuous positive airway pressure; ESC, European Society of Cardiology; ICU, intensive care unit. (Reproduced with permission from Ponikowski et al.[1])

BOX 16.3
ABC Assessment of the Unwell Patient

COMPLETE THE ABC ASSESSMENT WHILE TAKING A FOCUSED HISTORY:
- Any chest pain, dizziness, palpitations?
- Symptoms of AHF and duration
- Severity of breathlessness (NYHA class—see Chapter 5)
- Previous history of ARF/RHD/HF; previous cardiac surgery or hospitalizations
- Drug history, including any recent changes and adherence
- Any dietary change, including salt and water intake?
- Any change in urine output?

AIRWAY
- Look for and treat any evidence of airway obstruction (simple airway maneuvers, airway adjuncts, intubation)

BREATHING
- Look for signs of increased respiratory effort and/or ineffective respiration (e.g., inability to complete sentences, confusion)
- Tachypnea (>upper limit of normal for age of patient) is a sensitive and reliable marker of critical illness
- Give oxygen only if S_pO_2 is <90% (in all adults or children with respiratory distress) or if S_pO_2 is <94% in children with signs of shock ± respiratory distress[16]
- Examine the chest for signs of cardiac congestion (crackles, cardiac wheeze, pleural effusion)
- Order an urgent CXR (and ABG if unable to acquire a reliable S_pO_2 reading)
- Consider lung ultrasound (interstitial edema, pleural effusion)

CIRCULATION
- Assess the limbs for temperature (warm or cool) and check central capillary refill time in the sternal area (prolonged if >2 s in adults or >3 s in children)
- Palpate the pulse rate and rhythm, measure the blood pressure, and examine the JVP
- Listen to the heart sounds, record an ECG, and attach a cardiac monitor
- Assess for peripheral congestion (e.g., sacral and lower limb edema, hepatomegaly)
- Insert one or more wide-bore (depending on the age of the patient) cannulae and send urgent labs
- Monitor urine output, use catheter if necessary (aim >0.5 mL/kg/h)

ABC, airway, breathing, and circulation; ABG, arterial blood gas; AHF, acute heart failure; ARF, acute rheumatic fever; CXR, chest X-ray; ECG, electrocardiogram; HF, heart failure; NYHA, New York Heart Association; RHD, rheumatic heart disease; SpO2, peripheral oxygen saturation.

---

support (MCS), surgery, or transplantation. None of these agents improve outcomes and some may increase mortality. Because of these concerns, ESC guidelines restrict their use only in those who fulfill the definition of cardiogenic shock or in those who are symptomatically hypotensive.[1] Given that there is no robust evidence base, choice of vasoactive agent often differs between institutions.

Diuretics are relatively ineffective in cardiogenic shock and should generally be avoided. However, diuretics can be used in fluid-overloaded patients receiving vasoactive agents who demonstrate evidence of improved cardiac output (e.g., improved SBP >90 mmHg, mental state, skin perfusion). Vasodilators are also often contraindicated in cardiogenic shock, although can be considered if the SBP has improved

to ≥100 mmHg following treatment. The use of diuretics and vasodilators in AHF are discussed in detail in phase IV.

Immediate echocardiography is mandatory in patients with suspected cardiogenic shock (see also phase II). In addition to helping to confirm the underlying diagnosis, it can also help guide the need for IV fluids (preload insufficiency) and triage to more targeted medical therapy (Table 16.4) or surgical intervention (e.g., emergency surgery for chordal rupture with a flail leaflet). A standard 12-lead ECG and continuous telemetry are also essential and may reveal a tachy- or bradyarrhythmia or myocardial ischemia, warranting an early invasive approach such as electrical cardioversion, pacing, or primary percutaneous coronary intervention. ECG and blood pressure monitoring are also

TABLE 16.2
Oxygen and Ventilatory Support for Respiratory Failure due to Acute Heart Failure[1,11, 11a].[a]

Treatment	Indications	Comment
Oxygen	Hypoxemia: - S_pO_2 <90% or P_aO_2 <8 KPa (<60 mmHg) in all adults and children with respiratory distress - S_pO_2 <94% in children with shock	Target S_pO_2: 90%–96%: - If S_pO_2 <85%: use reservoir mask (15 L/min)[b]
Continuous positive airway pressure (CPAP)	Oxygenation failure: S_pO_2 <90% (or S_pO_2 <94% in shocked children), despite adequate oxygen therapy (F_iO_2 >40%)	Initiate at a PEEP of 5–7.5 cmH$_2$O and titrate to 10 cmH$_2$O as needed
Non-invasive ventilation (NIV)	Ventilatory failure: P_aCO_2 >6.1 KPa (>46 mmHg) and pH < 7.35	Initiate at an IPAP 8–10 cmH$_2$O and EPAP 4 cmH$_2$O. Increase IPEP in 2 –3 cmH$_2$O increments to a maximum of 25 cmH$_2$O
Endotracheal intubation and mechanical ventilation	Impending respiratory arrest (reduced GCS, pH <7.25, RR >35) or if oxygenation or ventilatory failure cannot be managed noninvasively	May not be appropriate if cardiac disorder is not remediable or patient is not a candidate for CPR

PEEP, positive end-expiratory pressure; IPAP, inspiratory positive airway pressure; EPAP, expiratory positive airway pressure; CPR cardiopulmonary resuscitation; GCS, Glasgow coma score.
[a] Settings need to be standardized according to weight and age of the patient. Close observation and repeated re-evaluation of the patient are important, with timely escalation or deescalation of therapy as appropriate.
[b] Severe heart failure in children should also be treated with high flow nasal prong therapy, either in the ward or intensive care setting.

BOX 16.4
Initial Management of Cardiogenic Shock in Adults and Children

ADULTS
1. IV fluid challenge only if no evidence of pulmonary edema
   - Give 500 mL isotonic crystalloid over 15 min
   - Repeat once if SBP remains <90 mmHg without evidence of pulmonary edema
2. IV vasoactive agents only if SBP remains <90 mmHg despite adequate filling and treatment of immediately reversible causes (see phase II)
   - See Tables 16.3 and 16.4 for type and indication of vasoactive agent
3. IV diuretics should be considered if evidence of fluid overload once cardiac input has improved
   - Give furosemide 40 mg IV bolus if the renal function is normal (consider higher doses if renal dysfunction)
   - Other patients that might benefit from diuretics are those who are "wet and cold" (see phase IV) and with a "normal" BP, that is, not meeting the definition of cardiogenic shock

CHILDREN
1. IV fluid challenge: same principles as for adults
   - Give 5–10 mL/kg over 10–20 min
   - Target Perfusion and SBP: 70 mmHg + [2 × age in years] in children 1 month–10 years; ≥90 mmHg in children ≥10 years old
2. IV vasoactive agents: same principles as for adults (with age-adjusted BP targets)
   - See Tables 16.3 and 16.4 for type and indication of vasoactive agent
3. IV diuretics: same principles as for adults
   - Give 1 mg/kg IV bolus

SBP, systolic blood pressure; IV, intravenous; BP, blood pressure.

TABLE 16.3

Mechanism of Action and Hemodynamic Effects of Common Vasoactive Medications Used in Cardiogenic Shock.

Medication	Usual Infusion Dose	RECEPTOR BINDING				Hemodynamic Effects
		α_1	β_1	β_2	Dopamine	
INOTROPES/VASOPRESSORS						
Dopamine	0.5–2 µg/kg/min	−	+	−	+++	↑ CO
	5–10 µg/kg/min	+	+++	+	++	↑↑ CO, ↑ SVR
	10–20 µg/kg/min	+++	++	−	++	↑↑ SVR, ↑ CO
Norepinephrine	0.05–0.4 µg/kg/min	++++	++	+	−	↑↑ SVR, ↑ CO
Epinephrine	0.01–0.5 µg/kg/min	++++	++++	+++	−	↑↑ CO, ↑↑ SVR
Phenylephrine	0.1–10 µg/kg/min	+++	−	−	−	↑↑ SVR
Vasopressin	0.02–0.04 U/min	Stimulates V_1 receptors in VSM				↑↑ SVR
INODILATORS (INOTROPE THAT REDUCES PERIPHERAL VASCULAR RESISTANCE)						
Dobutamine	2.5–20 µg/kg/min	+	++++	++	−	↑↑ CO, ↓ SVR, ↓ PVR
Isoproterenol	2–20 µg/min	−	++++	+++	−	↑↑ CO, ↓ SVR, ↓ PVR
Milrinone	0.125–0.75 µg/kg/min	PDE III inhibitor				↑ CO, ↓ SVR, ↓ PVR
Levosimendan	0.05–0.2 µg/kg/min	Myofilament Ca^{2+} sensitizer, PD-3 inhibitor				↑ CO, ↓ SVR, ↓ PVR

CO, cardiac output; SVR, systemic vascular resistance; PVR, pulmonary vascular resistance; PDE, phosphodiesterase III; VSM, vascular smooth muscle.

Reproduced with permission from van Diepen S et al.[127]

recommended during inotrope/vasopressor use as they can cause arrhythmias and myocardial ischemia. Urine output should always be measured because it provides an assessment of the effectiveness of therapy, and an indirect measure of cardiac and renal function.

Routine invasive hemodynamic evaluation, arterial line, or central venous line for diagnostic purposes are not indicated, but may be helpful in selected patients who are hemodynamically unstable with an unknown mechanism of deterioration.[1]

Early warning scores, for both adults and children, are used in many HICs and some LMICs to identify deranged physiology as early as possible, thus prompting review by senior medical staff and/or admission to an intensive care setting (Box 16.5). A combination of heart rate, respiratory rate, oxygen saturations, capillary refill time, and level of consciousness are more useful than a single parameter.[17,18] In units where high-flow respiratory therapy is restricted to ICU, this would also be an indication for earlier transfer.

In those who remain critically unwell despite respiratory and pharmacological intervention, MCS, if available, such as the intraaortic balloon pump (IABP),

extracorporeal membrane oxygenation (ECMO), or ventricular assist devices can help achieve temporary stabilization before emergency surgery for valve repair or replacement.[1,19] ECMO has been used successfully in the treatment of respiratory failure or cardiogenic shock resulting from fulminant rheumatic valvulitis.[20] IABP is contraindicated in those with significant (more than mild) aortic regurgitation (AR) because it augments aortic diastolic pressures and worsens the severity of the regurgitant volume.

In many resource-limited settings, access to most of these monitoring and treatment modalities is not available. Patients are also more likely to present late in their illness, thus requiring more intensive and specialized intervention early in the management course. Malnourishment, severe anemia, and an increased background prevalence of infectious agents, such as falciparum malaria and tuberculous, often complicate management. These factors must be taken into consideration when tailoring the administration of fluids, blood products, and vasoactive medications. First-line vasoactive agents in resource-limited settings will vary depending on local protocols and drug availability, although a useful

TABLE 16.4
Initial Vasoactive and Mechanical Management in Types of Cardiogenic Shock Most Relevant to Acute Rheumatic Fever or Rheumatic Heart Disease.[1,127]

Cause of Cardiogenic Shock	Vasoactive Management	Hemodynamic Rationale
Left Ventricular Dysfunction	Dobutamine or milrinone or other PDE III inhibitor Norepinephrine or higher dose dopamine (>5 µg/kg/min) Temporary MCS	Inodilator is used to increase cardiac output, increase BP, improve peripheral perfusion, and maintain end-organ perfusion Vasopressor added to inodilator if ongoing hypotension
Mitral Regurgitation	Norepinephrine or dopamine Dobutamine or milrinone Temporary MCS, including IABP	Vasopressor, although 1st line, may worsen degree of MR by increasing afterload If impaired LV contractility and ongoing hypotension, add inodilator IABP may reduce regurgitation fraction by reducing afterload and increasing CI
Mitral Stenosis	Phenylephrine or vasopressin Esmolol or amiodarone Electrical cardioversion PMBC	Shock resulting from MS is a preload-dependent state Aim to slow the HR and maintain atrioventricular synchrony Avoid agents that increase HR
Aortic Regurgitation	Dopamine Temporary pacing	Maintain an elevated HR (to shorten diastolic filling time and reduce LVEDP)
Aortic Stenosis	Phenylephrine or vasopressin If LVEF reduced, echo- or PAC-guided dobutamine titration	Shock caused by AS is an afterload-dependent state Inotropes may not improve hemodynamics if LVEF is preserved
Bradycardia	Chronotropic agents (atropine, isoproterenol, dopamine) Temporary pacing	Advanced heart block due to rheumatic carditis rarely (if ever) requires temporary pacing
Pericardial Tamponade	Fluid bolus Norepinephrine	Pericardiocentesis or surgical pericardial window required for definitive therapy

AS, aortic stenosis; CI, cardiac index; BP, blood pressure; HR, heart rate; IABP, intraaortic balloon pump; LV, left ventricular; LVEF, left ventricular ejection fraction; LVEDP, left ventricular end-diastolic pressure; MCS, mechanical circulatory support; MS, mitral stenosis; MR, mitral regurgitation; PAC, pulmonary artery catheter; PMBC, percutaneous mitral balloon commissurotomy; PDE III, phosphodiesterase III.
Adapted from van Diepen S et al.[127]

BOX 16.5
European Society of Cardiology Criteria for Admission to the Coronary Care or Intensive Care Unit in Adults[1a]

Need for intubation (or already intubated)
Signs and symptoms of hypoperfusion
S_pO_2 <90%, despite supplemental oxygen
Use of accessory muscles for breathing, respiratory rate >25 breaths/min
Heart rate <40 beats/min or >130 beats/min, systolic blood pressure <90 mmHg

[a]Similar criteria should be used for children but with pediatric cutoffs for physiological variables.

consideration is that dobutamine can be given through a peripheral line in settings where central line access is not available.

Phase II: Identification and treatment of acute etiologies or relevant triggers of AHF

As mentioned earlier, in patients presenting with suspected AHF secondary to ARF, it is important to consider acute valvular regurgitation. Factors that may trigger AHF in patients with RHD are summarized in Box 16.2. Immediate bedside echocardiography is necessary in patients who are either hemodynamically unstable or in patients with a suspected life-

BOX 16.6
Echocardiogram in a Patient With Acute Heart
Failure and Shock: Checklist

- Assess LV systolic function (and ideally LV size, presence of RWMAs)
- Valves
  - exclude MR, MS, or AR
  - exclude IE, flail leaflet
  - assess prosthetic valve function
- Exclude pericardial effusion
- Assess right ventricular size and function
- Estimate right atrial and pulmonary artery pressures

LV, left ventricle; RWMA, regional wall motion abnormality; MR, mitral regurgitation; MS, mitral stenosis; AR, aortic regurgitation; IE, infective endocarditis.

threatening mechanical pathology. Box 16.6 summarizes the key elements in the echocardiographic evaluation of the acutely unwell patient with suspected AHF. Transthoracic echocardiography is usually sufficient for diagnosis by demonstrating the underlying mechanism. If inconclusive, transesophageal echocardiography usually clarifies the diagnosis and underlying mechanism and may be used in the planning of operative repair.[19]

Acute valvular regurgitation. The medical management for organic causes of acute MR and acute AR leading to AHF is broadly similar. Diuretics and bed rest may be all that is required in patients with AHF secondary to severe valvular regurgitation as a consequence of acute rheumatic valvulitis.[21] Most of these patients will stabilise over hours to days. Some experts also recommend corticosteroids in these patients, despite the absence of high-quality evidence (see Chapter 4). Diuretics and vasodilators (discussed in phase IV, later) help reduce left-ventricular end-diastolic pressure and provide symptomatic relief. Vasodilators also reduce afterload and can improve forward cardiac output. Their use may be limited by systemic hypotension, and it may be necessary to commence inotropes first to achieve a satisfactory blood pressure.

Nitroprusside (see phase IV) is the vasodilator of choice in both acute MR and AR, although it is used in fewer than 1% of patients with AHF in Europe and the United States.[22] In acute MR, nitroprusside may reduce MR by up to 50%.[23] Because the determinants of the regurgitant volume in acute AR include the duration of diastole and the diastolic transvalvular gradient,

it is important to avoid bradycardia and arterial hypertension where possible.[24]

Acute presentation of chronic disease. These patients often have advanced RHD, and it is important to consider and correct/treat the etiologies or triggers summarized in Box 16.2. Otherwise, the mainstay of treatment is diuretics and vasodilators for the AHF episode, commencing/optimizing disease-modifying therapies for chronic HF once the patient is stable (discussed in Chapter 6), and, importantly, mechanical or surgical intervention of the valve lesion(s) (discussed in Chapters 7 and 8, respectively).

Prosthetic valve dysfunction (mechanical and bioprosthetic valves). The 2014 American Heart Association/American College of Cardiology (AHA/ACC) guidelines,[19] the 2017 AHA/ACC focused update,[25] and the 2017 European Society of Cardiology/European Association for Cardio-Thoracic Surgery (ESC/EACTS) valvular heart disease guidelines[26] provide detailed recommendations for assessment and management of prosthetic valves.

Mechanical valve dysfunction may be due to (1) valve thrombosis, (2) pannus formation, or (3) infective endocarditis. The presentation can vary from mild dyspnea to severe acute pulmonary edema. Urgent diagnosis, evaluation, and therapy are indicated because rapid deterioration can occur if there is thrombus causing malfunction of leaflet opening. The 2017 AHA/ACC focused update[25] recommends multimodality imaging with transthoracic echocardiography (TTE), transesophageal echocardiography (TEE), fluoroscopy, and/or computed tomography (CT). Combined imaging may be more effective than one imaging modality alone to diagnose and characterize valve thrombosis. TTE allows correct alignment of the Doppler beam with transvalvular flow for measurement of velocity, gradient, and valve area.[19]

Gradients should be compared to the baseline postoperative echocardiogram. Increasing valve gradients may indicate prosthetic valve dysfunction. However, the left atrial side of a prosthetic mitral valve is obscured by acoustic shadowing using TTE, so it is difficult to diagnose prosthetic mitral valve thrombus, pannus, or vegetation. TEE allows better images of the left atrial side of the mitral prosthesis. Fluoroscopy or CT imaging is very helpful to image aortic prosthetic leaflet motion. Differentiation of valve dysfunction due to thrombus versus fibrous tissue ingrowth (pannus) is challenging as the clinical presentations are similar. Thrombus is more likely when there is a history of inadequate anti-coagulation and with more acute onset of symptoms. Auscultation may reveal diminished or abolished mechanical prosthetic clicks together with a new systolic or diastolic murmur.

Prosthetic valve thrombosis management. Mechanical left-sided prosthetic valve obstruction is a serious complication and if left untreated has high mortality and morbidity. Urgent therapy with either fibrinolytic agents or surgical intervention is indicated. As of 2014, the weight of the evidence favored surgical intervention for left-sided prosthetic valve thrombosis unless the patient was asymptomatic and the thrombus burden was small.[19,25]

The 2017 ESC/EACTS guidelines favor urgent or emergency mechanical valve replacement in critically ill patients without serious comorbidity (class I recommendation) over fibrinolysis (class IIa).[26] Fibrinolysis regimens include recombinant tissue plasminogen activator 10 mg bolus plus 90 mg over 90 min with unfractionated heparin or streptokinase 1,500,000 units over 60 min without unfractionated heparin.[26] For bioprosthetic valve thrombosis, ESC/EACTS guidelines recommend anticoagulation using a vitamin K antagonist or unfractionated heparin before considering reintervention.[26]

However, new data were presented in the 2017 AHA/ACC guidelines.[25] The evidence indicates a 30-day surgical mortality rate of 10%–15%, with a lower mortality rate of <5% in patients with NYHA class I or II symptoms. Recent reports using an echocardiogram-guided slow-infusion low-dose fibrinolytic protocol has shown success rates >90%, with embolic event rates <2% and major bleeding rates <2%.[27,28] Moreover, fibrinolytic therapy regimens can be successful even in patients with advanced NYHA class and larger-sized thrombi. The 2017 AHA/ACC guidelines recommend urgent initial therapy for symptomatic prosthetic mechanical valve thrombosis. However, the decision for surgery versus fibrinolysis is dependent on individual patient characteristics and experience and capabilities of the institution.

These improved outcomes with fibrinolytic therapy are of great importance to those with RHD who may have had their surgery remote from where they live, or surgery undertaken by a fly-in fly-out team to the region. Fibrinolytic therapy may be the only realistic option for RHD patients who develop mechanical valve thrombosis.

Prosthetic valve stenosis. Bioprosthetic valve degeneration causes increasing stenosis, is not altered by medical treatment, and is treated by cardiac surgery. Chronic thrombus or pannus formation impinging on the leaflet motion of the valve can cause increasing stenosis of mechanical valves reflected by increased gradients detected by TTE.

Other prosthetic valve complications. Severe intravascular hemolysis may be due to paravalvular leak. This can be treated with surgery or complex catheter techniques. The latter have success rates of 80%–85% in specialized centers. Patient-prosthesis mismatch may require reoperation.

Indications for surgery in bioprosthetic valve regurgitation are the same as for native valve regurgitation. The technology of valve-in-valve transcatheter techniques is a rapidly evolving field. Outcomes are comparable or better for bioprosthetic aortic valve regurgitation/stenosis compared to revisional surgery.[19]

Pericardial tamponade. The signs and symptoms of pericarditis are a pericardial friction rub, positional chest pain, and sometimes reduced heart sounds (see also Chapter 3). Pericarditis is common in ARF with or without a small identifiable pericardial effusion but pericardial tamponade is rare.[29] Patients with HF and a pericardial effusion usually have severe valve regurgitation. In this setting, the relative contribution of a moderate effusion to the signs and symptoms of HF may be hard to judge. In particular, tachycardia is common to both. However, an adult patient with unequivocal signs of tamponade, that is, tachycardia greater than that would be expected for the degree of valve regurgitation, hypotension (SBP <100 mmHg), pulsus paradoxus (an abnormally large decrease in SBP (>10 mmHg) with inspiration), jugular venous distension, Kussmaul's sign (a paradoxical rise in jugular venous pressure with inspiration), muffled heart sounds, and echocardiographic signs of pericardial tamponade (Box 16.7) may benefit from pericardial drainage. The pericardial fluid will usually be hemorrhagic with potential for blockage of pigtail catheters left to drain. The reduction of symptoms and signs of tamponade (e.g., tachycardia) may be less dramatic than seen in pericardial tamponade due to viral pericarditis or postpericardiotomy syndrome. Rheumatic pericarditis only very rarely leads to constrictive pericarditis.

Tachyarrhythmia in chronic mitral stenosis. Patients with moderate or severe MS may deteriorate acutely, presenting with dyspnea and pulmonary edema or even cardiogenic shock. Some presentations may mimic

---

BOX 16.7
Echocardiographic Signs of Pericardial Tamponade

- Collapse of the free wall of the right ventricle during diastole
- Reduction in the left ventricular cavity size on inspiration
- A decease in mitral inflow velocity or aortic velocity by >25% on inspiration
- Enlarged inferior vena cava diameter with no inspiratory variation

---

acute respiratory distress syndrome, presenting with poor gas exchange and bilateral pulmonary infiltrates. Acute deterioration commonly occurs following an abrupt increase in heart rate or change in cardiac output, commonly seen with the onset of atrial fibrillation or immediately after delivery during labor. Subacute presentations due to increased cardiac output are more commonly seen with pregnancy, in the peripartum period or anemia. A thorough search for potential triggers is therefore important as it will often help guide the most appropriate therapy.

The management of unwell patients with MS who develop an acute tachyarrhythmia is broadly the same as patients who do not have MS, i.e. determining whether the patient is stable or unstable. Hemodynamically unstable tachycardia is usually defined as a heart rate ≥150 beats/min plus any of the following: hypotension (SBP <90 mmHg), acutely altered mental status, signs of shock, ischemic chest discomfort, or evidence of AHF. If any of these signs are present, an anesthetist should be called in preparation for synchronized DC cardioversion (the initial recommended doses varies depending on the guideline used). Conversely, in patients with hemodynamically stable tachycardias, cardioversion is usually not the first-line therapeutic option. Instead, a 12-lead ECG should be recorded to help guide targeted pharmacological management based on the type of tachyarrhythmia (Table 16.5).

The primary therapeutic aim is a reduction in heart rate. Diuretics and nitrates may also be considered as they will reduce LA pressures and provide symptomatic relief from pulmonary congestion, although should be used with caution as they can reduce LV filling and lead to a significant drop in stroke volume and cardiac output.[30] In those with sinus tachycardia, treatment should be targeted at the underlying cause, such as pain, anxiety, sepsis, hypoxemia, anemia, and thyrotoxicosis.

In patients with significant MS presenting with decompensated AHF, the threshold for percutaneous mitral balloon commissurotomy (PMBC) is lower than that for surgery, as surgical mortality in this context is very high (ranging from 20% to 50%). PMBC is also the treatment of choice as a "bridge to surgery" in those who are too unwell for immediate surgery or during pregnancy (best undertaken in the second trimester).[31−33]

Advanced heart block. Advanced atrioventricular (AV) block with second degree AV block, complete heart block, and accelerated junctional rhythm may occur in ARF, although are seldom associated with cardiac compromise and symptoms. Patients should be monitored with cardiac monitoring and frequent ECGs.[34−36] Monitoring will reveal return of AV synchrony for short periods, then permanently. Pacing should be avoided in most cases as return to sinus rhythm occurs spontaneously, although permanent pacemaker implantation has been reported, probably as the natural history was not understood. If pacing is decided upon, a temporary pacing lead rather than permanent pacemaker implantation is recommended. Paradoxically, advanced AV block has been associated with milder degrees of valvulitis (see Chapter 3).[34]

AV block with tachycardia is more common than bradycardia in ARF cases. The resulting accelerated junctional tachycardia[34−36] results in a junctional rate faster than the sinus rate. Cardiac monitoring may reveal sinus tachycardia (with first-degree block) alternating with the accelerated junctional tachycardia (with AV block by definition) at similar or slightly faster rates. Corticosteroids appear an intuitive treatment and are often given (for AV block with bradycardia or tachycardia) but this has not been tested in an randomized control trial (RCT). In conclusion, the presence of advanced AV block in a patient with suspected ARF is useful diagnostically, requires cardiac monitoring, but is expected to resolve spontaneously.

Phase III: Diagnostic work-up to confirm acute heart failure
Once the acute therapeutic processes in phases I and II have been completed (if required) and the patient hospitalized, an important next step is to complete the diagnostic work-up. Phase III also involves excluding alternative etiologies that might explain the

TABLE 16.5
Intravenous Rate-Control Therapy for Hemodynamically Stable Tachyarrhythmias.

Drug	Dose (intravenous)	Comment
ATRIAL FIBRILLATION, ATRIAL FLUTTER, OR ATRIAL TACHYCARDIA		
Esmolol	**Adult**: loading dose 500 mcg/kg over 1 min, followed by 50 mcg/kg over 4 min **Child**: loading dose 100–500 mcg/kg over 1 min, followed by 100–500 mcg/kg/min continuous infusion	Short half-life (8 min), useful if concerned about hypotension
Metoprolol	**Adult**: 5 mg over 5 min **Child**: not used	May cause hypotension Dose can be repeated after 5 min if required, up to maximum of 10–15 mg
Verapamil	**Adult**: 2.5–5 mg over 5 min, repeat every 15–30 min if required to max dose of 15 mg **Child** (1–15-year-old): 0.1–0.3 mg/kg IV −1, up to 5 mg 1st dose, 2nd dose up to 10 mg after 30 min	May cause hypotension Contraindicated if concomitant beta-blocker use or heart failure
Digoxin	**Adult**: 500–1000 mcg over 1 h **Child**: 15 mcg/kg stat and 5 mcg/kg after 6 h, then 3–5 mcg/kg. Rarely given as dose	Digoxin ± amiodarone are the preferred agents in patients with structural heart disease and reduced LVEF; however, both agents should be used with caution. Digoxin levels should be checked after 6 h
Amiodarone	**Adult**: loading dose 300 mg over 20 min via central line; maintenance 900–1200 mg over 24 h **Child**: Loading dose 25 mcg/kg/min for 4 h; maintenance 5–15 mcg/kg/min	
SUPRAVENTRICULAR TACHYCARDIA (AVNRT AND AVRT)		
Adenosine	**Adult**: 1st dose 6 mg, repeat dosing after 2 min if no response; 2nd dose 12 mg, 3rd dose 18 mg **Child**: <50 kg 0.05–0.1 mg/kg × 1, then increase by 0.05–0.1 mg/kg to max 0.3 mg/kg, up to 12 mg/dose **Child**: >50 kg 1st dose 6 mg IV, 2nd dose 12 mg	Vagal maneuvers are usually performed before adenosine Contraindicated in severe bronchospastic airways disease and coronary artery disease IV bolus should be given via wide-bore cannula followed by rapid saline flush
Verapamil	As discussed earlier	
Esmolol and metoprolol	As discussed earlier	
SUSTAINED MONOMORPHIC VENTRICULAR TACHYCARDIA		
Amiodarone	As discussed earlier	There is no consensus on which drug should be used first Lidocaine does not cause hypotension, unlike amiodarone and procainamide, and can also be given more quickly Amiodarone is slower in action than lidocaine and procainamide but has a major role in suppression of recurrent episodes
Lidocaine	**Adult**: loading dose 1.5 mg/kg over 2 min; maintenance 1–4 mg/min **Child**: 1 mg/kg × 1, can repeat dose after 10–15 min up to total dose of 3–5 mg/kg in 1st hour	
Procainamide	**Adult**: 20–50 mg/min until arrhythmia terminates or a max dose of 15–17 mg/kg is administered **Child**: 15 mg/kg ×1 or 3–6 mg/kg up to 100 mg every 5–10 min	

AVNRT, atrioventricular nodal re-entrant tachycardia; AVRT, atrioventricular re-entrant tachycardia.

presentation, such as acute renal failure, pneumonia, asthma, and anemia.

ESC guidelines[1] recommend that the diagnosis of AHF should be based on clinical history (Box 16.3 and Table 16.6) and examination (Table 16.6); prior cardiovascular history, including any potential cardiac and noncardiac precipitants (Box 16.2); and appropriate early investigations (Table 16.7).

Patients with AHF most often seek medical care because of worsening signs and symptoms of congestion. Dyspnea is the most common symptom of congestion, present in >90% of patients. Inspiratory crackles (found in 66%–87% of AHF patients) and peripheral edema (65%) are also commonly encountered, although most patients with chronic HF do not have inspiratory crackles due to compensation by pulmonary lymphatics.[37]

Because physical signs of congestion are based on detecting increased filling pressures, an elevated jugular venous pressure (JVP) is the single most useful finding on physical examination in AHF as it reflects right atrial pressure, which is usually an indirect measure of LV filling pressures[37,38] (exceptions may include significant mitral stenosis or tricuspid regurgitation). Any change in LV filling pressures because of therapy are usually paralleled by changes in JVP.[38]

An SBP <115 mmHg and low pulse pressure are independent predictors of in-hospital mortality in those admitted with AHF in adults.[37,39,40] The prognostic utility of other common clinical findings is less clear in AHF when compared to chronic HF, where an elevated JVP, presence of an S3 gallop, and elevated heart rate are

each associated with an increase in morbidity and mortality.[41,42] Elevated BUN is one of the strongest laboratory predictors for poor outcomes, particularly when ≥43 mg/dL, and is approximately proportional to the neurohormonal activation in AHF[39,43] (i.e., the higher the BUN, the more severe the AHF).

In patients that are hemodynamically stable, an echocardiogram within 48 h of admission is recommended if cardiac structure/function is unknown or may have changed since the last study.[1] Echocardiographic findings in ARF and RHD are discussed in Chapters 3 and 5, respectively. In comparison to a chest X-ray, which is normal in 20% of patients with congestion, lung ultrasound is superior at excluding interstitial edema and pleural effusion.[38]

Phase IV: Defining the clinical profile and optimal management strategy

Despite a lack of robust randomized data, the primary treatment of most patients with AHF is diuretics and vasodilators (Tables 16.8 and 16.9). Although regional differences exist in prescribing patterns,[44] there is little data on how patients with ARF or RHD who present with AHF are managed. Defining the hemodynamic profile of the patient however will help guide early therapy and also carries prognostic information. ESC guidelines[1] propose using the framework developed by Stevenson and colleagues (Fig. 16.2),[45] which is based on the severity of presentation rather than underlying etiology.

This simplistic approach can be completed at the bedside within 2 min by assessing for evidence of

---

TABLE 16.6
Clinical Features of Acute Heart Failure in Adults.

CONGESTION		HYPOPERFUSION	
Symptoms	**Signs**	**Symptoms**	**Signs**
Dyspnea	Inspiratory crackles	Chest pain	Tachycardia
Cough/wheeze	Pleural effusion	Dizziness	Hypotension (SBP <90 mmHg)
Orthopnea	Increasing S3, loud P2	Fatigue	Narrow pulse pressure
Bendopnea[a]	Weight gain	Altered mental status	Cool extremities (forearms and legs)
Paroxysmal nocturnal dyspnea	Elevated jugular venous pressure		Poor capillary refill
Peripheral edema	Hepatomegaly/splenomegaly		Confusion/drowsiness
Early satiety	Ascites		Oliguria
Abdominal fullness	Scleral icterus		Pulsus alternans (terminal)

SBP, systolic blood pressure.
[a] A recently defined symptom of heart failure. Instruct the patient to sit in a chair, then to bend forward at the waist and touch their feet. Bendopnea is considered present if dyspnoea develops within 30 s of bending.[37]

TABLE 16.7
Urgent Investigation of a Patient With Acute Heart Failure.

Electrocardiogram
- Rarely normal in AHF (high negative predictive value)
- Myocardial ischemia (ST-elevation, ST-depression, T wave inversion)
- Brady—or tachyarrhythmias
- Prolonged PR interval or accelerated junctional rhythm may suggest ARF

Chest X-ray
- Pulmonary edema
- Cardiomediastinal contours (e.g., cardiomegaly, exclude widened mediastinum)
- Exclude AHF triggers (pneumonia, chronic lung disease)

Echocardiogram
- Left ventricle (size, global and regional systolic function, diastolic function)
- Mitral, aortic, and tricuspid valves (morphology, function, evidence of IE, flail leaflet, prosthetic valve function)
- Right ventricular size and function
- Estimate right atrial and pulmonary artery pressures
- Pericardial effusion
- Help confirm or exclude the diagnosis of ARF or RHD

Natriuretic Peptides
- Have a high negative predictive value for ruling out AHF with congestion if:
  - BNP <100 pg/mL (29 pmol/L)
  - NT-pro-BNP <300 pg/mL (35 pmol/L)
- Obesity (BMI >30 kg/m^2) and HF treatment can lower natriuretic peptide levels
- LVH, PE, myocarditis, valvular heart disease, advanced age, ischemic stroke, renal dysfunction, COPD, liver cirrhosis can raise the level of natriuretic peptides

Other laboratory tests
- Plasma troponin (often raised in most patients with AHF; if the baseline level of troponin is raised, a >20% rise in 3 h is required for definition of an ACS)
- Na$^+$, K$^+$, urea/BUN, creatinine, glucose
- Full blood count
- Liver function, clotting studies, albumin, thyroid stimulating hormone
- Arterial blood gas (only if oxygenation cannot be readily assessed by pulse oximetry)
- Streptococcal serology/RADT/throat swab/ESR (only if ARF suspected)
- Blood cultures, procalcitonin, and CRP (only if infection or ARF suspected)

AHF, acute heart failure; ARF, acute rheumatic fever; IE, infective endocarditis; RHD, rheumatic heart disease; BNP, B-type natriuretic peptide; NT-pro-BNP, N-terminal-pro-B-type natriuretic peptide; BMI, body mass index; HF, heart failure; LVH, left-ventricular hypertrophy; PE, pulmonary embolism; COPD, chronic pulmonary obstructive disease; ACS, acute coronary syndrome; BUN, blood urea nitrogen; RADT, rapid antigen detection test; ESR, erythrocyte sedimentation rate; CRP, C-reactive protein.

hypoperfusion ("cold" indicating hypoperfusion; "warm" indicating well-perfused) and presence of congestion ("wet" indicating congestion; "dry" indicating not congested). Table 16.6 summarizes the features of hypoperfusion and congestion. Once complete, the patient is categorized into one of four distinct phenotypes, each with a defined treatment approach. An important point here is that although hypoperfusion is often accompanied by hypotension, they are not synonymous: normotensive patients may experience systemic hypoperfusion while those who are chronically hypotensive due to advanced HF may

not have associated acute hypoperfusion.[37] Those with a cold and wet profile have a 6-month mortality rate of 40%, compared with 11% for warm and dry patients.[45]

Most patients with AHF are wet and warm (95% of AHF patients are congested at presentation).[1] Accordingly, this section will focus on the management of these patients, which is likely also to reflect the presentation of most patients with AHF secondary to ARF or RHD.

Management goals in wet and warm patients consist of achieving thorough decongestion, ensuring adequate

TABLE 16.8
Diuretics and Vasodilators Used to Treat Acute Heart Failure in Adults.

Drug	Dosing
DIURETICS	
Furosemide[a] *Maximum total daily dose: 400–600mg*	**Moderate congestion**: 20–40 mg IV q12 h **Severe congestion**: 40–80 mg IV q12 h or bolus 60 mg IV + continuous infusion at 10–20 mg/h **Severe congestion and renal dysfunction (eGFR <30mL/min)**: 80–200 IV q12 h or bolus + continuous infusion at 20–40 mg/h
Bumetanide[a] *Maximum total daily dose: 10–15mg*	**Moderate congestion**: 0.5–1 mg IV q12 h **Severe congestion**: 1–2 mg IV q12 h or bolus of 2 mg IV + continuous infusion at 0.25–0.5 mg/h
Thiazide-like diuretics	Hydrochlorothiazide[b] 12.5–200 mg PO OD Metolazone[c] 2.5–20 mg PO OD Chlorothiazide 500–1000 mg PO/IV OD-BID
VASODILATORS[1]	
Nitroglycerine	Start with: 10–20 µg/min IV, increase up to 200 µg/min IV
Isosorbide dinitrate	Start with: 1 mg/h IV, increase up to 10 mg/h IV
Nitroprusside	Start with: 0.3 µg/kg/min IV, increase up to 5 µg/kg/min IV
Nesiritide	Bolus 2 µg/kg IV + infusion 0.01 µg/kg/min IV

BID, bis in die (twice daily); eGFR, estimated glomerular filtration rate; IV, intravenous; OD, omne in die (once daily); PO, per os (orally).

[a] Loop diuretics are more effective than other diuretics in patients with an eGFR <30 mL/min, although the natriuretic response is reduced in renal dysfunction. Thus, in order to achieve satisfactory diuresis, higher dosages or increased frequency are needed. Diuretics should be used with caution in renal dysfunction, however, and should be discontinued if increasing azotemia and oliguria.

[b] Caution advised if severe renal impairment; CrCl <10: avoid use

[c] Renal dysfunction: no adjustment if mild-moderate impairment; caution advised if severe impairment.

perfusion pressures to maintain organ perfusion, and continuing guideline-directed medical therapy for chronic HF, unless contraindicated.[38]

Diuretics. IV loop diuretics (furosemide, bumetanide) are usually the first-line therapy in the treatment of AHF (used in >90% of patients) and typically result in rapid symptom relief. They should be initiated in the emergency department without delay, although should be avoided if the patient is hypotensive (SBP <90 mmHg).[1] Diuretics promote the relief of symptoms caused by congestion by two mechanisms: venodilation, which reduces the left ventricular end-diastolic pressure (occurs at approximately 15 min following IV administration) and diuresis (occurs at approximately 30 min after IV administration, peaks at 1.5 h, and wears off by 6–8 h).[38,46]

The initial diuretic dose is dependent on the severity of congestion and renal function. Proposed initial doses of furosemide in those previously not on chronic diuretic therapy are provided in Tables 16.8 and 16.9. If the patient is on chronic diuretic therapy, the initial IV dose should be 1–2 times the 24-h oral home

dose.[38] There is no significant difference in safety or efficacy between a bolus and a continuous diuretic infusion.[47] However, it is essential that the patient is initially responsive to IV bolus therapy before commencement of a continuous infusion.

Urine spot sodium (>50–70 mEq/L) after 2 h and average urine output (>100–150 mL/h) after 6 h may be used to evaluate if there is an adequate diuretic response. If inadequate, the dose can be doubled within 6-hourly intervals as needed.[38] An evaluation of the 24-h urine output (UO) should be undertaken on the second day of admission: if UO is <3–4 L, then the diuretic dose should be increased further; if UO is >3–4 L then continue current dose until decongestion; but if the UO is >5 L then consider reducing the diuretic dose.[38] If the patient remains severely congested, vasodilators should also be considered (see later).

Reduced or inadequate diuresis that limits the ability to achieve euvolemia, despite sufficient dosages of diuretics, is indicative of loop diuretic resistance[38] and is associated with a poorer prognosis.[48] Loop diuretics are often combined with thiazide-like diuretics in an

TABLE 16.9
Diuretics and Vasodilators Used to Treat Acute Heart Failure in Children.

Drug	Dosing
DIURETICS	
Furosemide[a] *Maximum total daily dose: 6mg/kg*	Dose: 0.5–2 mg/kg IV q6–12 h (max 6 mg/kg/dose) or continuous infusion: <20 kg, 25 mg/kg in 50 mL 0.9% saline at 0.2–2 mL/h; >20 kg 10 mg/mL at 0.01–0.1 mL/kg/h (protect from light)
Bumetanide[a] *Maximum total daily dose: 10mg; no more than 2mg as an initial dose*	Dose: 0.015–0.1 mg IV q12–48 h; maximal diuretic effect is achieved at 0.035 –0.04/mg/kg/dose every 6–8 h
Thiazide-like diuretics	Hydrochlorothiazide[b] (2–12 years): 1–2 mg/kg/day PO divided OD-BID (max 100 mg/day) Metolazone[c] 0.2–0.4 mg/kg/day PO divided q12–24 h Chlorothiazide (6 months–12 years): 10–20 mg/kg/day PO divided q12–24 h (max 1 g/day); alternatively: 4 mg/kg/day IV divided q12–24 h
VASODILATORS	
Nitroglycerine	Start with: 0.25–0.5 µg/kg/min IV, increase by 0.5–1.0 µg/kg/min q3–5 min until response; max 20 µg/kg/min
Isosorbide dinitrate *Maximum daily dose: 40mg*	Sublingual: 0.1–0.2 mg/kg q2 hourly or as needed Oral: 0.5–1 mg/kg q6 hourly or as needed
Nitroprusside	If <30 kg: 3 mg/kg in 50 mL 5% DW @ 0.5–4 mL/h; >30 kg: 3 mg/kg in 100 mL 5% DW @ 1–8 mL/h. Use with caution, protect from light.
Nesiritide	Start with: 2 mcg/kg IV, then 0.01 mcg/kg/min

BID, bis in die (twice daily); DW dextrose in water; eGFR, estimated glomerular filtration rate; IV, intravenous; OD, omne in die (once daily); PO, per os (orally).
[a] Loop diuretics are more effective than other diuretics in patients with renal dysfunction, although the natriuretic response is reduced. Thus, in order to achieve satisfactory diuresis, higher dosages or increased frequency are needed. Diuretics should be used with caution in renal dysfunction, however, and should be discontinued if increasing azotemia and oliguria.
[b] Caution advised if severe renal impairment; CrCl <10: avoid use
[c] If mild-moderate renal impairment: no adjustment; caution advised in severe impairment.

attempt to overcome this problem and can result in significant diuretic synergy as the latter block the distal tubule, resulting in sequential nephron blockade. Combination drugs in lower doses are also more effective and safer than higher doses of a single drug. Acetazolamide or amiloride, sodium-glucose linked transporter two inhibitors (SGLT2-I), spironolactone, nitrates, or inotropes can also be combined with loop diuretics in an attempt to augment diuresis. Ultrafiltration (typically removing 3–4 L per session) should only be considered if substantial congestion persists despite optimal pharmacological therapy. No evidence supports its use as first-line therapy in AHF over loop diuretics.[38]

Vasodilators. The initial improvement in congestive symptoms can be accelerated by IV vasodilators and are recommended as an adjunct for patients whose initial response is inadequate to diuretics.[1] Routine use however does not improve outcomes and should be avoided.[47] Vasodilators should also be avoided if the SBP is <90 mmHg or if the patient has symptomatic hypotension.[1] They should be used with caution in patients who are preload or afterload dependent (mitral stenosis, aortic stenosis) as this may cause severe hypotension. Avoiding hypotension is particularly important due to its association with adverse effects, including myocardial ischemia. Conversely, in those presenting with hypertensive AHF (SBP >140 mmHg), which typically manifests as acute pulmonary edema, vasodilators should be considered as first-line therapy to improve the symptoms of congestion[1] (Fig. 16.2).

The organic nitrates (nitroglycerin and isosorbide dinitrate) are potent venodilators (reducing preload), thus providing rapid symptomatic improvement by reducing pulmonary venous and LV filling pressures. They can also act as arteriolar vasodilators at higher dosages, leading to afterload reduction and an increased

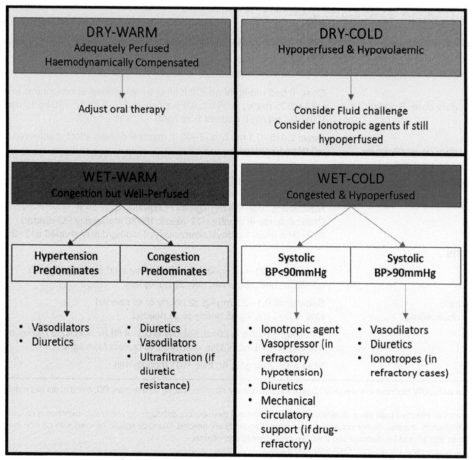

FIG. 16.2 Hemodynamic stratification and initial management of patients hospitalized with acute heart failure. BP, blood pressure. (Reproduced from Kurmani S et al.[2])

cardiac output. They may also reduce the severity of MR. Tolerance following continuous use is an important limitation, reducing their effectiveness to 16–24 h. Up-titrate dose for a rapid improvement in symptoms and aim for a reduction in mean arterial pressure of ≥10 mmHg while maintaining SBP >100 mmHg. The IV route is generally preferred (Tables 16.8 and 16.9) but in some resource-limited setting this may not be available. Sublingual nitrates (e.g., glyceryl trinitrate spray (onset: <5 min; duration <1 h)), oral nitrates (e.g., isosorbide dinitrate (onset: 15–40 min; duration: 4–6 h)), or glyceryl trinitrate patches (onset: 30–60 min; duration: prolonged), for example, may be used if no other options are available.

Sodium nitroprusside, which works by inducing a balanced arteriolar and venule dilation, is the vasodilator of choice for situations requiring acute, short-term afterload reduction. It is particularly useful in patients with ADHF, acute valvular regurgitation (where it may be used as a pharmacological bridge to surgery), or those with hypertensive AHF.[37] Up titrate dose for a rapid improvement in symptoms and maintain an SBP of 90–100 mmHg.

Ongoing management. Bed rest is important and should be enforced. Patients with AHF are at increased risk of venous thromboembolism and should be anticoagulated (e.g., with low molecular weight heparin), unless contraindicated.[1] Weight gain/loss, fluid input/output, vital signs (including orthostatic hypotension), symptoms and signs of HF, and electrolytes and renal function should be monitored on a daily basis.[37]

Particular care should be taken when using combinations of loop diuretics and thiazide-like diuretics, which may lead to profound hypotension, worsening renal function, and electrolyte abnormalities (in particular hypokalemia, which may precipitate arrhythmias).

Outpatient disease-modifying medications for chronic HF (e.g., ACE inhibitors/ARNIs/ARBS, β-blockers, and mineralocorticoid receptor antagonists) should be continued following hospitalization (and up-titrated as appropriate), unless there is a clear reason to either reduce the dose or stop the drug (symptomatic hypotension, hypoperfusion, bradycardia, hyperkalemia, severe renal impairment). β-Blockers in particular should be continued where possible as several trials have suggested continuation is associated with lower postdischarge mortality rates.[49−51] In previously unmedicated patients, these disease-modifying therapies should be initiated as an in-patient once the patient is stable (see Chapter 6). Due to the risk of severe electrolyte disturbances, avoid the concurrent use of thiazide diuretics with loop diuretics in the chronic ambulatory phase where possible.

Achieving euvolemia and determining when to stop decongestive therapy are important but significant challenges. More than 25% of patients treated for AHF in HICs are discharged with persistent congestion:[52,53] this is significant because clinical outcomes are extremely poor and readmission risk is higher in these patients, particularly if there is concomitant worsening renal function.[54] Relief of dyspnea and attaining a body weight when the patient was well are both poor markers of decongestion. Moreover, because it is yet to be determined exactly what euvolemia encompasses, no tests exist to determine euvolemia. Accordingly, the Heart Failure Association of the ESC recommends an integrative, multiparameter-based evaluation of congestion before discharge (Fig. 16.3).[38]

Finally, the patient should be included in a multidisciplinary disease-modifying program (including education on HF and ARF/RHD, as appropriate) and have early ambulatory clinical and laboratory follow-up (preferably within 2 weeks).[38] Discussion with a cardiosurgical team, if available, is important for many patients with AHF.

Conclusion

AHF is a common complication of RHD. Most patients present with hemodynamically stable, subacute disease without evidence of cardiogenic shock and/or acute respiratory failure. Echocardiography plays a central role in the diagnosis of AHF and in guiding appropriate management. Diuretics with or without vasodilators form the mainstay of treatment in the acute phase. Ensuring adequate decongestion and commencing disease-modifying HF therapies (discussed in Chapter 6) are of vital importance before discharge.

2: INFECTIVE ENDOCARDITIS

Introduction

IE is the microbial infection of the endothelial lining of the heart. Although IE usually occurs in those with a structurally abnormal heart or other underlying risk factors, it may occasionally occur in healthy individuals with structurally normal hearts. The presentation is usually acute, although can be indolent. Despite many advances in diagnostic tools and management, mortality remains high, around 25%−30% in contemporary multicenter studies.[55]

IE is a well-recognized complication of RHD and can occur in individuals with native rheumatic valves as well as following valve repair or replacement surgery. The specific characteristics of IE in RHD are not well described, with published literature consisting of small case series from high burden RHD settings.

In many LMICs, there is limited access to diagnostic microbiology, echocardiography, antibiotics, and cardiac surgery with resulting challenges for accurate diagnosis and management of this complex disease.

Pathophysiology of Infective Endocarditis in Rheumatic Heart Disease

Turbulent blood flow through a structurally abnormal heart can damage cardiac endothelium and lead to thrombus deposition.

Valvular dysfunction in RHD causes abnormal regurgitant jets and turbulent blood flow that damage the cardiac endothelium. Sterile mural thrombi may develop due to endothelial damage, cytokine release, and the activation of repair mechanisms such as extracellular matrix production, platelet adherence, and fibrin deposition.

During incidental bacteremia (rarely fungemia), circulating organisms may adhere to and infect the thrombus; infective vegetations then form in the thrombus and the cardiac valve endothelium. The resulting biofilms protect and aid the growth of bacteria leading to a source of persistent bacteremia, systemic illness, and infection of the valve. Depending

Variable		EUVOLEMIA			CONGESTED

	Variable					
Clinical congestion	Orthopnea	None		Mild	Moderate	Severe/worst
	JVP (cm)	<8 and no HJR	<8	8-10 or HJR+	11-15	>16
	Hepatomegaly		Absent	Liver edge	Moderate pulsatile enlargement	Massive enlargement and tender
	Edema		None	+1	+2	+3/+4
	6MWT	>400m	300-400m	200-300m	100-200m	<100m
Technical evaluation	NP (one of both): -BNP -NT-proBNP		<100 <400[a]	100-299 400-1500	300-500 1500-3000	>500 >3000
	Chest X-ray	clear	clear	cardiomegaly	- pulmonary venous congestion[b] - small pleural effusions[b]	- Interstitial or alveolar edema
	Vena Cava imaging	**none of two:** - Max diameter >2.2 cm - collapsibility <50%		**One of two:** - Max diameter >2.2 cm - collapsibility <50%		**Both:** - Max diameter >2.2 cm - collapsibility <50%
	Lung Ultrasound	<15 B-lines when scanning 28-sites		15-30 B-lines when scanning 28-sites		>30 B-lines when scanning 28-sites

[a]The cut-off for NT-proBNP to exclude congestion as endorsed by the Heart Failure Association position paper on grading congestion is higher than the cut-off endorsed by the European Society of Cardiology guidelines to exclude acute heart failure
[b]Chest X-ray can be clear but presence of abnormalities suggests higher degree of congestion

FIG. 16.3 Integrative, multiparametric evaluation of congestion at discharge. JVP, jugular venous pulse; HJR, hepatojugular reflux; 6MWT, 6 minute walk test; NP, natriuretic peptide; BNP, B-type natriuretic peptide; NT-proBNP, N-terminal-pro-B-type natriuretic peptide. (Reproduced with permission from Mullens W et al.[39])

on their location, vegetations can lead to valve deformity and dysfunction (valvular insufficiency or stenosis). Perivalvular extension of infection can lead to paravalvular abscess formation, fistulae, or occasionally conduction system abnormalities.[56]

Extracardiac manifestations result from peripheral embolization of thrombus material with subsequent infarction and/or infection of involved tissue. Bacterial embolization can also lead to mycotic aneurysm formation, characterized by infection and distension of the arterial wall. Mycotic aneurysms are most common in intracranial arteries but can also occur in abdominal vessels and the peripheral circulation.

Epidemiology of Infective Endocarditis and Rheumatic Heart Disease

In recent years, the global epidemiology of IE has changed, with rising incidence driven by increasing rates of healthcare-associated IE and *Staphylococcus aureus* infections.[55] The importance of RHD as a predisposing risk factor for IE varies considerably worldwide.

High income countries

The majority of recent global IE literature originates from high-income countries and consists of cohort studies. The International Collaboration on Endocarditis (ICE) prospective study and several pediatric studies found <5% of patients with IE had underlying RHD.[55,57−59]

Infective Endocarditis in Rheumatic Heart Disease-endemic countries

In LMICs, RHD is the most common predisposing cardiac condition for IE.[60,61] The majority of the literature consists of small, single-center case series, with few population-based studies on which to determine incidence. Table 16.10 summarizes reports of IE by where the proportion of patients with underlying RHD is described. Studies reported since the year 2000 or beyond, with >20 patients included. From Oceania, underlying RHD was present in 12%−37% of patients, with the dominant organism *S. aureus*. In contrast, a large study of 336 adults with IE from New Zealand, where data on the underlying prevalence of predisposing conditions was available for 274 patients, found only 4% (12/274) had underlying RHD and the predominant pathogens were Streptococci. In cohorts from Asia, underlying RHD has been reported in up to 50% of patients, with in-hospital mortality up to 35% in Pakistan and Lao PDR. Up to 65% of IE patients had underlying RHD in African cohorts.[62−64] Of interest, no cases of RHD were identified in a small Costa Rican case series, this being a relatively affluent (upper middle income) Latin American country.

Presenting Clinical Features

Patients with IE frequently appear acutely unwell with signs of sepsis and systemic toxicity. The diagnosis of acute IE should be considered in any person with RHD presenting with unexplained fever, bacteremia, acute neurological deficit, or other embolic phenomena. Subacute presentations of endocarditis can also occur. Features may be nonspecific and may include fever, anorexia, malaise, headache, abdominal pain, and arthralgia. A high degree of suspicion is required to identify these patients.

Systemic embolization occurs in up to 50% of patients with IE and is most frequently seen in the first 1−2 weeks postdiagnosis, occasionally weeks or months later.[81] Embolism can also be the presenting symptom of IE. Embolic events may cause infarction or abscess formation in the brain, lungs, kidneys, spleen, and extremities. Endocarditis may also present with acute heart failure secondary to acute valvular dysfunction, intracardiac abscess, fistulous tract formation, or destruction of indwelling prosthetic material.

Examination findings

The physical signs of endocarditis may be subtle and often vary across different patient groups. Data presented here are approximated from both older and more recent clinical series.[55,82−86] Fever is very common, found in 80%−90% of patents. Cardiac murmurs are found in 75%−85% of patients, although a new murmur is found in only 10%−50% and a changing murmur in 5%−20%. A new or changing murmur can be difficult to distinguish from an innocent "flow" murmur (infection tends to increase cardiac output) or preexisting rheumatic valvular pathology. Clinical findings secondary to acute heart failure (discussed earlier in this chapter) may also be evident.

Supportive signs for IE include central neurological abnormalities (20%−40%), which may arise from embolic infarcts, abscesses, or intracerebral hemorrhage, splenomegaly (10%−40%), and cutaneous manifestations. Petechiae are found in 20%−40% of patients and are the most common dermatological manifestation of IE. Evidence of peripheral embolization such as Janeway lesions (*nonpainful*, hemorrhagic areas of the palms or soles)—Fig. 16.4A, and splinter and subungual hemorrhages are unusual, particularly in children. In adults, splinter hemorrhages are seen in 5%−15% of cases. Immunological phenomenon may include glomerulonephritis (that can result in hematuria, proteinuria and renal impairment), Osler nodes (*tender*, red nodules on the finger pulps)—Fig. 16.4B, and Roth spots (retinal hemorrhages with a pale center)—Fig. 16.5, which are occasionally seen on fundoscopy. Roth spots are *not* pathognomonic for IE and can also be seen in diabetes, leukemia and HIV. New onset digital clubbing may also occur.

Investigations
Laboratory investigations

Blood cultures are the most useful laboratory investigation for IE, whereby identification of a causative organism will enable targeted antimicrobial treatment. Wherever feasible, at least three separate sets of blood cultures should be collected before antibiotic

TABLE 16.10
Reports of Infective Endocarditis Where Underlying Rheumatic Heart Disease is Described as a Predisposing Risk Factor.

Country	Underlying RHD	Ethnicity	Incidence Estimate	Age of Cohort	Study Period	Microbiology	Mortality
Oceania/Pacific region							
New Zealand[65]	11.8% (10/85)	54% polynesian (NZM/Pacific)	0.76 per 100,000-person years	Median 7.0 years (range 0–16 years)	1994–2012	88% (75/85) causative organism identified 31% S. aureus	4.7% (4/85) in-hospital mortality
Northern Australia[66]	13.5% (12/89)	33% (29/89) ATSI	6.5 per 100,000 person years (ATSI)	Median 45 years (36–61 years) 4 cases <18 years	2002–2007	92% (82/89) causative organism identified 44% S. aureus	20% (18/89) in-hospital mortality
New Caledonia[67]	37.3% (19/51)	84% (43/51) Oceanic (Polynesian/Melanesian)	6.7 per 100,000 person years (Oceanic)	Median age 54.4 years	2005–2010	31% (16/51) S. aureus	20% (11/51) in-hospital mortality 43% (21/51) late mortality
New Zealand[68]	4% (12/274)	Not specified	–	Median 59.5 years (IQR 41–73)	2000–2005	Viridans strep 32% S. aureus 24%	6% (20/336) in-hospital mortality 18 late deaths
Asia							
Lao PDR[69]	33.3% (12/36)	–	–	Median 25 years (IQR 18–42 years)	2006–2012	36% (13/36) positive BC 54% (7/13) Streptococcus spp.	25% (9/36) in-hospital mortality 5/36 late deaths
Pakistan[70]	40.5% (34/84)	–	–	Mean 42 ± 17 years	2002–2006	MRSA reported in 14.3%	32% (27/84) in-hospital mortality
Pakistan[71]	53% (24/45)	–	32 per 1000 admissions	Mean 7.9 ± 4 years (4 months–16 years)	1997–2000	47% (21/45) BC positive	13% (6/45) deaths
Pakistan[72]	4/36 (11%)	–	–	34.8 years mean age 15% <16 years	2015–2017	71% culture positivity 36% streptococci 17% staphylococci	19% mortality
Turkey[73]	28% (69/248)	–	–	Any	2005–2012	65% culture positivity S. aureus (29%)	33% in-hospital mortality

India[74]	47% (90/192)	—	Mean 27.2 ± 12.7 years	1992–2001	70% (134/192) culture positivity Streptococci 23% Staphylococci 19.7%	21% mortality during treatment
India[75]	31% (43/139)	—	Mean 47.9 ± 15.8 years	2007–2013	70% culture positive 31% alpha hemolytic Streptococci S. aureus 10.9%	17.3% in-hospital mortality
Africa						
Ethiopia[62]	49% (20/41)	—	Median 9 years (range 7 months–14 years)	2008–2013	4/31 positive	7% (3/41) CFR
Tunisia[76]	23% (17/73)	—	Mean 12 ± 4.8 years	1997–2013	23% S. aureus	13.6% 30-day mortality 19% 6-month mortality
Senegal[77]	65% (27/42)	—	Mean 27.5 years ±18years	2005–2014	Positive in 21%	31% in-hospital mortality
Americas						
USA[57]	4.7% (75/1588)	—	<21 years old	2000 and 2003	S. aureus(57%)	—
Brazil[78]	38% (78/203)	—	48.2 ± 16.6 years	2005–2017	18% (37/203) S. aureus 33% (68/203) culture negative	32% (65/203) in-hospital mortality
Costa Rica[79]	9% (0/38)	—	Mean 3.8 yrs (range 17d–11.8 years)	2000–2011	84% blood culture positivity S. aureus 18/38%	23% mortality
Brazil[80]	7% (2/28)	—	Mean 70.6 months ±59.2 months	1993–2001	36% (16/28) blood culture positivity S. aureus 56%	4% mortality

NZM, New Zealand Mori; ATSI, Aboriginal and Torres Strait Islanders; IQR, interquartile range; BC, blood culture; MRSA, methicillin-resistant Staphylococcus aureus; CFR, case fatality rate.

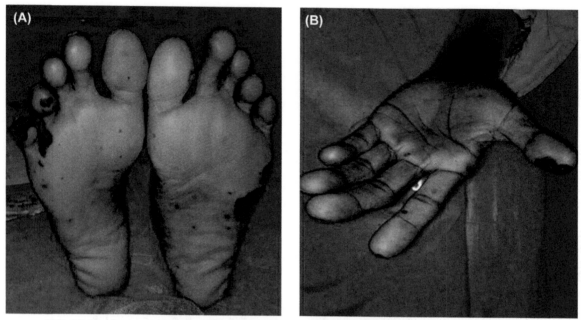

FIG. 16.4A Janeway lesions: multiple macular spots of varying sizes over both feet (A) and hand (B). These were nontender and noncompressible. (Reproduced with permission from Khanna N et al.[86a])

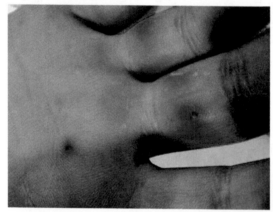

FIG. 16.4B Osler's nodes in the palm and finger. These were tender, erythematous lesions. (Reproduced with permission from Hirai T et al.[86b])

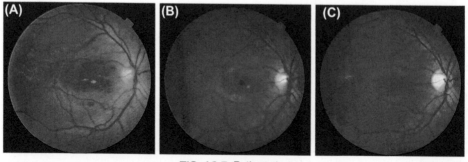

FIG. 16.5 Roth spots.

administration, with each set obtained several hours apart. In the subacute setting, when there is less clinical urgency to start antibiotics, additional blood cultures should be drawn if IE is suspected. Culture of explanted cardiac material can identify an etiologic agent, either by routine culture or in culture negative cases, by molecular testing such as polymerase chain reaction or 16s ribosomal RNA (16srRNA).[87,88] These techniques may only be available in reference laboratories.

Inflammatory markers such as white cell count, C-reactive protein, erythrocyte sedimentation rate, and rheumatoid factor may also be abnormal. Urinalysis may reveal features of associated immune nephritis (hematuria, proteinuria, dysmorphic red blood cells).

Bacterial pathogen/causative organisms. *Staphylococcus aureus* is now the leading global IE pathogen. In many parts of the world, a substantial proportion of *S. aureus* isolates are resistant to antistaphylococcal penicillins, known as methicillin-resistant *S. aureus* (MRSA). MRSA significantly complicates IE treatment and detailed susceptibility testing is required to guide treatment. Drugs such as vancomycin and daptomycin have significant associated dosing challenges and toxicities and may not be readily available in resource-limited settings.

Alpha hemolytic (viridans) streptococci are another important cause of IE. Other important etiological agents include enterococci, *Staphylococcus epidermidis* and HACEK group Gram-negative bacilli (*Haemophilus parainfluenzae, Aggregatibacter actinomycetemcomitans and Aggregatibacter aphrophilus, Cardiobacterium hominis, Eikenella corrodens* and *Kingella kingae*). HACEK organisms are fastidious, slow growing Gram-negative pathogens, thought to account for 1%–3% of all IE.[89,90]

Nontoxigenic *Corynebacterium diphtheriae* has also been described as an IE pathogen in young Polynesians with RHD in New Zealand.[65,91] Fungi such as Candida and Aspergillus species are rare causes of IE, most frequently occurring in neonates or immune compromised patients. Other agents such as *Streptococcus pneumoniae, Streptococcus pyogenes,* and *Listeria monocytogenes* are rare causes of endocarditis.

Up to 10%–20% of all cases of IE remain culture negative, the most common reason being that the patient has received prior antibiotic treatment. Other reasons include: presence of fastidious organisms (will only grow when specific nutrients are included in its dish, therefore difficult to culture), true culture-negative IE (see below), and obtaining insufficient blood cultures.[96] The importance of obtaining several blood cultures before commencing empiric antimicrobial therapy

is paramount, as failure to identify a causative pathogen can significantly complicate treatment.

Tropheryma whippelii (Whipples Disease), Bartonella sp., Coxiella burnetti, Chlamydia, and legionella and Brucella are all recognized causes of true culture-negative IE. Access to serologic and molecular investigations to confirm infection caused by one of these pathogens may be limited in many resource-limited settings.

Imaging

Chest X-ray (CXR) may reveal evidence of cardiac or pulmonary complications; however, these findings are nonspecific. Patchy pulmonary opacities can be due to infected emboli from a rheumatic tricuspid valve endocarditis lesion. CT, ultrasound, or magnetic resonance imaging (MRI) imaging of the abdomen and brain may be indicated. This may reveal symptomatic or asymptomatic emboli.

Echocardiography and newer imaging modalities

Echocardiography is essential, but while echocardiography may confirm a diagnosis, it cannot exclude IE. Transthoracic image quality is adequate in most pediatric patients,[93,94] but transesophageal echocardiography has a higher accuracy in adults[95,96] and is indicated when transthoracic views are inadequate, particularly in right-sided IE, suspected IE involving prosthetic valves or an indwelling cardiac device, or if a paraaortic abscess or other complications are suspected. In situations where there is high clinical suspicion of IE but the initial echocardiogram is negative or inconclusive, repeat echocardiogram in 5–7 days is recommended.

Newer imaging modalities for IE include multislice CT, which can be particularly useful in defining aortic IE and complications such as aortic root abscess, pseudoaneurysm, and fistulae. Contrast-enhanced CT may be useful in defining embolic complications and abscesses of solid abdominal organs. MRI is particularly useful at evaluation of intracerebral complications including abscess, cerebral mycotic aneurysms, and microbleeds, which are found in as many as 60% of patients and in most cases are asymptomatic.[97]

The diagnostic utility of nuclear imaging techniques including single photon emission CT (SPECT) and positron emission tomography CT (PET/CT) in suspected IE is currently under evaluation.

Diagnostic Criteria

There is no single gold standard clinical sign or laboratory test to confirm the diagnosis of IE. Although a variety of diagnostic criteria for IE exist, including Von Reyn[98] and Beth Israel,[99] the modified Duke criteria for diagnosis of IE are the most accepted diagnostic criteria and these have been validated for use in both adults and children[101] (see later). There are three diagnostic categories within the modified Duke criteria: definite endocarditis, possible endocarditis, and rejected cases. Definite IE, using clinical criteria, requires the presence of two major, one major with three minor, or five minor criteria (Table 16.11). Possible endocarditis is defined by one major with one minor, or three minor criteria. Rejected cases are those where manifestations are explained by a clear alternate diagnosis or resolve after antibiotic therapy for 4 days or less. Definite IE may also be established using pathological criteria, either through examination of pathological lesions (vegetation or intracardiac abscess demonstrates active endocarditis histologically) or if microorganisms are demonstrated by culture or histology of a vegetation or intracardiac abscess.

Differential Diagnosis

The modified Duke criteria are very useful when there is diagnostic uncertainty; however, it is uncertain in clinical practice how frequently the Duke criteria are utilized when the diagnosis of IE is unequivocal. The presentation of IE is similar to many systemic inflammatory conditions. A high index of suspicion for IE is required among individuals with underlying RHD and bacteremia. In situations when blood cultures remain negative and the Duke criteria are not fulfilled, alternative diagnoses must be considered. Recurrent ARF,

---

TABLE 16.11
Modified Duke Criteria for the Diagnosis of Infective Endocarditis.

MAJOR CRITERIA

Blood Culture Positive for infective endocarditis (one of the following)

- Typical microorganisms consistent with IE from at least two separate blood cultures (viridans Streptococci, *Streptococcus gallolyticus (formerly S bovis)*, HACEK group, *Staphylococcus aureus*, or community-acquired enterococci, in the absence of a primary focus)

- Microorganisms consistent with IE from persistently positive blood cultures, defined as:
  - ≥ 2 positive cultures of blood samples drawn >12 h apart; **or**
  - All 3 or a majority of ≥ 4 separate cultures of blood (with first and last samples drawn at least 1 h apart)

- Single positive blood culture for *Coxiella burnetii* or phase I IgG antibody titer >1:800

Evidence of Endocardial Involvement (one of the following)

- Echocardiogram positive for IE[a], defined as follows:
  - Vegetation (oscillating intracardiac mass on valve or supporting structures, in the path of regurgitant jets, or on implanted material in the absence of an alternative anatomic explanation); **or**
  - Abscess; **or**
  - New partial dehiscence of prosthetic valve

- New valvular regurgitation (worsening or changing of preexisting murmur not sufficient)

MINOR CRITERIA

Predisposition: presence of a predisposing heart condition or intravenous drug use

Fever: temperature >38°C (100.4°F)

Vascular phenomenon: major arterial emboli, septic pulmonary infarcts, mycotic aneurysm, intracranial hemorrhage, conjunctival hemorrhage, Janeway lesions

Immunological phenomenon: glomerulonephritis, Osler nodes, Roth spots, or rheumatoid factor

Microbiological evidence: positive blood culture but does not meet a major criterion as noted earlier[b] or serological evidence of active infection with organism consistent with IE

IE, infective endocarditis; HACEK, Haemophilus parainfluenzae, Aggregatibacter actinomycetemcomitans and Aggregatibacter aphrophilus, Cardiobacterium hominis, Eikenella corrodens, and Kingella kingae.
[a] Transesophageal echocardiography recommended in patients with prosthetic valves, rated at least "possible IE" by clinical criteria, or complicated IE (paravalvular abscess); transthoracic echocardiography as first test in other patients.
[b] Excludes single positive cultures for coagulase-negative staphylococci and organisms that do not cause infective endocarditis.
Reproduced with permission from Li JS et al.[128]

Kawasaki disease, systemic lupus erythematosus, and leukemia can all have similar presenting features to IE.

Medical Management

Immediate management priorities include (1) control of sepsis (2) treatment of acute cardiac features, and (3) management of end-organ involvement. Careful consideration of patient characteristics (comorbidities, valve involvement, acute complications) and pathogen factors (pathogen characteristics and susceptibility profile) is needed to formulate a treatment plan.[100] Comprehensive guidelines describing the approach to investigation and management of IE have been published by the American Heart Association (AHA),[92] the European Society of Cardiology (ESC),[85] and the British Society for Antimicrobial Chemotherapy (BSAC).[101] Emerging data supports the use of a multidisciplinary team-based approach including cardiology, cardiosurgical, and infectious diseases expertise to improve outcomes.[102,103]

Principles of antibiotic therapy for infective endocarditis

As bacteria in vegetations are embedded in a dense fibrin matrix, and heart valves are poorly vascularized, eradication of infection requires prolonged high-dose parenteral therapy, preferably with bactericidal rather than bacteriostatic agent(s).

The causative organism is usually unknown at presentation, and therefore the choice of empiric treatment should take into consideration the patient's clinical presentation and background history (including whether immune compromised, underlying heart disease, native valve or indwelling prosthetic material, healthcare-associated or community onset, colonization with MRSA or other multiresistant organisms, local antimicrobial susceptibility patterns, kidney function, and β-lactam allergy). Initial and definitive antibiotic combinations for various scenarios are described in the AHA[92,104] and ESC guidelines[85]. Pediatric treatment recommendations are extrapolated from adult recommendations.

General principles include the use of bactericidal agents at high doses via the intravenous route. Oral antibiotics are not suitable for IE treatment (with the exception of some cases of true blood culture negative IE) due to their unpredictable absorption and bioavailability.

For acutely unwell patients, an antistaphylococcal agent should be included in the initial combination. Vancomycin should be used if there is a prosthetic valve, penicillin allergy, healthcare-associated infection or risk of MRSA. An aminoglycoside (usually gentamicin) is usually included in the initial regimen for synergistic killing. Targeted therapy varies according to patient characteristics and pathogen susceptibility profiles, and detailed antimicrobial treatment approaches are described in AHA[92] and ESC guidelines.[85]

Tables 16.12 and 16.13 provide initial antibiotic choices and doses, respectively, for IE in acutely unwell patients. Clinical judgment and individualized decision-making may be required, particularly in resource-limited settings where availability of certain antibiotics may be limited and there may be high rates of antimicrobial resistance.

The duration of parenteral therapy is usually 4–6 weeks, but longer courses may be required in prosthetic valve IE, recurrent IE, fungal IE, and complicated multifocal infection. Early consultation with infectious diseases specialists/microbiologists should be undertaken to optimize antimicrobial therapy and ensure appropriate laboratory investigations have been performed. In adequately-resourced settings, treatment can be offered via home IV therapy for clinically stable patients who are deemed to be at low risk of complications. Therapeutic drug monitoring should be undertaken for patients receiving aminoglycosides or vancomycin, along with careful monitoring for nephrotoxicity, ototoxicity, and hematologic toxicity.

Blood culture negative IE presents numerous challenges regarding ongoing treatment. Administration of antibiotics before obtaining blood cultures and in some circumstances limited access to diagnostic microbiology services may mean that no pathogen is identified and a prolonged course of empiric antibiotics is required. Consultation with an infectious disease specialist is recommended wherever possible.

Clinical Course and Complications

Stroke/intracranial hemorrhage/neurologic events

A spectrum of neurologic complications can occur including ruptured mycotic aneurysm, intracranial hemorrhage, embolism and brain abscess. Risk of stroke is greatest in the first 1–2 weeks after diagnosis, and decreases after initiation of effective antimicrobial therapy.[81,105–107] Stroke can complicate decisions regarding surgery for IE, due to the anticoagulation required for cardiac bypass and concern that cardiac bypass may exacerbate intracranial hemorrhage. Neurologic consultation and individualized decision-making are required.

TABLE 16.12
Suggested Empiric Antibiotic Therapy for Infective Endocarditis in Adults and Children.[85,104]

1. COMMUNITY-ACQUIRED ENDOCARDITIS IN PATIENTS WITH NATIVE VALVES OR LATE PROSTHETIC VALVE ENDOCARDITIS (≥12 MONTHS POSTSURGERY) AND LOW SUSPICION OF MRSA OR OTHER MULTIRESISTANT ORGANISM

- Ampicillin or amoxicillin or penicillin **PLUS**
- Flucloxacillin or oxacillin **PLUS**
- Gentamicin

OR (also suitable for β-lactam allergy)
- Vancomycin **PLUS**
- Gentamicin

OR (in subacute presentations when HACEK organisms are suspected)
- Cefotaxime **PLUS**
- Gentamicin

2. NOSOCOMIAL ENDOCARDITIS[a] OR OTHER HEALTHCARE-ASSOCIATED ENDOCARDITIS[b] OR EARLY PROSTHETIC VALVE ENDOCARDITIS (<12 MONTHS POSTSURGERY) AND/OR HIGH SUSPICION OF MRSA

- Vancomycin **PLUS**
- Gentamicin **PLUS**
- Rifampicin *if prosthetic valve endocarditis and/or high suspicion MRSA*

CONSIDER ADDING
- Third or fourth generation cephalosporin if risk factors for gram-negative IE **OR**
- Meropenem if risk factors for multiresistant Gram-negative IE

HACEK, Haemophilus parainfluenzae, Aggregatibacter actinomycetemcomitans and Aggregatibacter aphrophilus, Cardiobacterium hominis, Eikenella corrodens and Kingella kingae; MRSA, methicillin-resistant Staphylococcus aureus; IE, infective endocarditis
[a] Nosocomial infective endocarditis has been defined as a diagnosis of infective endocarditis made >72 h following admission in patients with no evidence of infective endocarditis on admission or infective endocarditis that develops within 60 days of a previous hospital admission.[128]
[b] Nonnosocomial healthcare-associated infective endocarditis is defined as infective endocarditis occurring in out-patients who had extensive exposure to medical care.[55,84,129]

Other vascular complications

Patients with IE should be carefully monitored for embolic and vascular complications outside the central nervous system. Any suggestion of acute limb ischemia or intraabdominal complications should prompt urgent radiologic investigations to search for acute embolism and/or mycotic aneurysm formation.

Uncontrolled sepsis and persistent bacteremia

Failure to clear positive blood cultures and/or ongoing signs of sepsis indicate progressive infection and may signal suboptimal antibiotic therapy. In these situations, repeat echocardiography to look for evolving intracardiac abscess or other surgically drainable infection is indicated. Careful evaluation should also be undertaken to look for metastatic foci of infection outside the heart. Antimicrobial therapy should be reviewed to ensure that dose, route, and choice are optimized.

Cardiac surgical management. The need for surgical management of IE depends primarily on the response to initial antimicrobial therapy and medical treatment. The

presence of embolic features may also be a key indicator for surgery. Perivalvular abscesses, obstructive vegetations, cardiac fistulae, and prosthetic dehiscence often require surgery. Other indications include persistent bacteremia, recurrent embolization, and fungal endocarditis.[85,92]

Decision-making regarding timing of surgery can be challenging and an individualized peroperative assessment, taking into account all potential risks/benefit, is needed (Box 16.8).[108]

The role of routine neuroimaging preoperatively is uncertain. In adults, earlier surgery for *S. aureus* IE is associated with improved outcomes.[109]

Prognosis

In the preantibiotic era, IE was a uniformly fatal condition. In current times, the overall mortality of IE remains high[65,104] at around 25%, and morbidity is also considerable. Poor prognosis is associated with *Staphylococcus aureus* infection and fungal IE, prosthetic IE, significant embolic complications, and intracardiac abscess formation. Limited access to cardiac surgery is a significant barrier to optimal management of IE in LMICs.

TABLE 16.13

Doses of Commonly Used Intravenous Antibiotics for Endocarditis.[85,104, a]

Agent	TOTAL DAILY DOSE		Usual Dose Interval	Notes and Monitoring Recommendations
	Adults	Children[b]		
Penicillin G sodium (also known as benzylpenicillin)[c]	12–24 million IU/ 24 h	200–300,000 IU/kg/24 h	Q4 hrly	Higher doses for nosocomial IE, prosthetic valve, high MIC/ relative penicillin-resistance
Amoxicillin	12 g/24 h	200–300 mg/kg/ 24 h	Q4 hrly	—
Ampicillin	12 g/24 h	200–300 mg/kg/ 24 h	200– 300 mg/kg/ 24 h	—
Flucloxacillin/oxacillin	12 g/24 h	200–300 mg/kg/ 24 h	Q4 hrly	Delayed neutropenia
Gentamicin	3–6 mg/kg/24 h	3–6 mg/kg/24 h	Q8 hrly OR Q24 hrly	Q8 hrly dosing is used in enterococcal and streptococcal IE as it may improve synergistic killing Monitor drug levels Monitor for ototoxicity and nephrotoxicity Optional in *S. aureus* IE
Vancomycin	30–60 mg/kg/24 h	60 mg/kg/24 h	Q6–8 hrly (children) Q8–12 hrly (adults)	Monitor drug levels Target trough usually 10–15 µg/ mL although higher levels (15–20 µg/mL) are recommended for MRSA isolates with vancomycin MIC >1 µg/mL Monitor for nephrotoxicity
Rifampicin	900–1200 mg/24 h	20 mg/kg/24 h	Q12 hrly	Monitor liver function
Ceftriaxone	2–4 g/24 h	100 mg/kg/24 h	Q12–24 hrly	If dose ≥2 g, divide dose q12 hrly
Cefipime	6 g/24 h	150 mg/kg/24 h	Q8 hrly	Only for suspected/confirmed Gram-negative IE Preferred agent for ESBL cover is meropenem
Ceftazidime	6 g/24 h	200 mg/kg/24 h	Q8 hrly	Only for suspected/confirmed Gram-negative IE Preferred agent for ESBL cover is meropenem
Cefazolin	6 g/24 h	150 mg/kg/24 h	Q8 hrly	-
Meropenem	2 g	60–120 mg/kg/ 24 h	Q8 hrly	Only for suspected/confirmed multiresistant Gram-negative IE including ESBL producers

IE, infective endocarditis; MIC, minimal inhibitory concentration; MRSA, meticillin-resistant Staphylococcus aureus; ESBL, extended spectrum beta-lactamase.

[a] Doses for neonates and infants not included.

[b] Maximum daily dose or adult dose should not be exceeded on a per kilogram basis when treating children.

[c] Benzylpenicillin should NOT be confused with benzathine penicillin G (the latter of which, if given intravenously, can cause fatal reactions).

BOX 16.8
List of (Relative) Surgical Indications in Infective Endocarditis.

- Uncontrolled sepsis/bacteremia
- Uncontrolled local infection—IE abscess, false aneurysm, fistula, enlarging vegetations
- Uncontrolled valvular regurgitation/acute heart failure
- Fungal or multiresistant organism
- Large vegetation >10 mm despite appropriate antiinfective treatment
- Enlarging or ruptured mycotic aneurysm[a]

---

[a]mycotic aneurysms may be extracardiac and require treatment by a vascular surgeon.

Prevention and Antibiotic Prophylaxis

Recommendations regarding antibiotic prophylaxis for IE vary across the world[110,111] Australasian guidelines adopt recommendations from the AHA but differ by specifically including RHD as a significant risk factor for IE.[112–114] In the UK, the National Institute for Clinical Excellence (NICE) does not routinely recommend antibiotic prophylaxis against IE before dental procedures.[115]

Conditions where prophylaxis is recommended in Australasia include:

- Rheumatic heart disease
- Prosthetic cardiac valves;
- Cardiac transplant with subsequent valvulopathy;
- Rheumatic heart disease with previous infective endocarditis;
- Congenital heart disease if:
  - unrepaired cyanotic defect;
  - completely repaired defect with prosthetic material up to 6 months postprocedure;
  - repaired defects with residual defect at prosthetic part.

Chemoprophylaxis depends on the procedure being performed and current guidelines should be consulted to optimize management in each case. Australasian guidelines suggest dental (e.g. reimplantation of avulsed tooth) and upper respiratory tract procedures receive amoxicillin (50 mg/kg orally, maximum 2000 mg/dose) as a single dose 1 h before the procedure. Cephalexin, clarithromycin or clindamycin are alternatives for penicillin sensitivity and for individuals with RHD on benzathine penicillin G prophylaxis. Genitourinary and gastrointestinal procedures require ampicillin just before the procedure, or vancomycin if penicillin allergic. Endotracheal intubation and urinary catheterization do not require antibiotic prophylaxis.[112]

It is of note that there is no published evidence to show that antibiotic prophylaxis prevents IE. Endocarditis is thought more likely to result from random bacteremia than from bacteremia associated with dental, GI, or GU procedures.

Conclusions

IE is a well-recognized complication of RHD; however, there is limited contemporary data on the epidemiological, clinical, and laboratory characteristics of IE among patients with RHD. Essential components of diagnosis and treatment include access to echocardiography, obtaining several sets of blood cultures before antibiotic initiation and access to cardiac surgery, which may all be limited in high-burden RHD populations.

3: OVERANTICOAGULATION AND BLEEDING

Introduction

Oral anticoagulants (OACs), such as vitamin K antagonists (VKAs) and nonvitamin K antagonist oral anticoagulants (NOACs), are often indicated in the management of patients with RHD (e.g., mechanical heart valves, atrial fibrillation, previous thromboembolism—see Chapter 6).

The use of OACs is associated with an increased risk of bleeding, which may be life threatening or disabling. For example, 90% of warfarin-related deaths are due to intracerebral hemorrhage and most of those who survive are left with permanent disability.[116] In the REMEDY study,[5] OAC-associated major bleeding affected 1.9% of children and adults with RHD from low-income countries, rising to 2.8% in lower-middle-income countries and 3.5% in upper-middle-income countries.

In patients receiving VKAs, the risk of major bleeding increases substantially when the INR exceeds 4.5 and rises exponentially when the INR exceeds 6.0.[26] Some patients may experience bleeding at therapeutic or subtherapeutic INR levels. In patients receiving NOACs, routine coagulation testing cannot be used to accurately determine the anticoagulation status of the patient. In these patients, the specific drug used, dose, time since last dose, and renal function can all be used instead.[117]

Management

The management of warfarin-associated bleeding and/or overanticoagulation is summarized in Table 16.14. Clinical judgment is vital when assessing the severity of bleeding and the degree and urgency of OAC reversal. Ideally, management should also be discussed with a hematologist. As a general rule, patients with major bleeding require rapid, full reversal of any OAC effect.

TABLE 16.14
Summary of the Management of Warfarin-Associated Bleeding and/or Overanticoagulation.

Clinical Setting	Management
Major bleeding • INR >1.1[19,26,123–125]	Hold warfarin Administer 4-factor PCC[a] FFP or thawed plasma if PCC not available IV vitamin K (over 20–60 min): • Adult: 10 mg • Children: 250–300 mcg/kg (max 10 mg)
Minor bleeding • Supratherapeutic INR[123]	Hold warfarin Vitamin K 1–2.5 mg oral or IV
No bleeding • INR >10[19,123,124 b]	Hold warfarin Vitamin K 1–2.5 mg oral or IV
No bleeding • INR 5–10[19,124 c]	Hold warfarin Consider vitamin K 1–2.5 mg oral

INR, international normalized ratio; PCC, prothrombin complex concentrate; FFP, fresh frozen plasma; IV, intravenous; SIGN, Scottish Intercollegiate Guidelines Network; ACCP, American College of Chest Physicians.
[a] Contains factors II, VII, IX, and X in inactive forms. PCC is dose-adjusted according to INR and should be discussed with a hematologist where possible. A typical dose for INR >6 is 50 IU/kg.
[b] SIGN guidelines suggest a cut-off INR of >8.
[c] ACCP guidelines use a lower cut-off INR of 4.5.

The definition of major bleeding includes that which is not amenable to local control, is life threatening, threatens vital organ function, or occurs within a critical closed space[118] (e.g., intracranial bleeding, compartment syndrome). In these patients, prothrombin complex concentrate (PCC) or, if not available, fresh frozen plasma (FFP) should be used. Vitamin K should also be given (by slow intravenous infusion (no faster than 1 mg/min) to minimize the risk of anaphylaxis).[119,120]

The INR should have normalized (usually <1.4 in most laboratories) within 30 min of administration of PCC or FFP. Additional dosing of these agents may be required if the INR remains elevated.[120,121] Vitamin K dosing can be repeated every 12 h if the INR remains elevated.[122]

Minor bleeding, which is still clinically significant and may require treatment, includes slow gastrointestinal bleeding, epistaxis, ecchymosis, and severe menorrhagia. In these patients, rapid correction of the INR is not usually required. Patients with minor bleeding

with a supratherapeutic INR or those with no bleeding but INR >10 should receive low-dose vitamin K.[19,123,124] Oral vitamin K is usually preferred over the intravenous route as it results in a more gradual decrease in the INR, minimizing the chances of a subtherapeutic INR and subsequent thromboembolism, and it removes the small risk of anaphylaxis associated with IV administration.

For patients who are not bleeding and have an INR 5–10, often holding the VKA and allowing the INR to fall naturally is all that is required.[19,124] Low-dose vitamin K should however be considered in those who are at greater risk of bleeding (e.g., major bleeding in the previous month, major surgery in the last 2 weeks, thrombocytopenia (platelet count $<50 \times 10^9$/L), known liver disease, or concurrent antiplatelet therapy), and at a lower risk of thromboembolism.

The management of NOAC-associated bleeding is beyond the scope of this book.

REFERENCES

1. Ponikowski P, Voors AA, Anker SD, et al. ESC guidelines for the diagnosis and treatment of acute and chronic heart failure: the task force for the diagnosis and treatment of acute and chronic heart failure of the European society of cardiology (ESC) developed with the special contribution of the heart failure association (HFA) of the ESC. *Eur Heart J*. 2016;37(27):2129–2200.
2. Kurmani S, Squire I. Acute heart failure: definition, classification and epidemiology. *Curr Heart Fail Rep*. 2017; 14(5):385–392.
3. Damasceno A, Mayosi BM, Sani M, et al. The causes, treatment, and outcome of acute heart failure in 1006 Africans from 9 countries. *Arch Intern Med*. 2012;172(18): 1386–1394.
4. Bland EF, Duckett Jones T. Rheumatic fever and rheumatic heart disease; a twenty year report on 1000 patients followed since childhood. *Circulation*. 1951;4(6): 836–843.
5. Zuhlke L, Engel ME, Karthikeyan G, et al. Characteristics, complications, and gaps in evidence-based interventions in rheumatic heart disease: the global rheumatic heart disease registry (the REMEDY study). *Eur Heart J*. 2015; 36(18), 1115-22a.
6. Zühlke L, Watkins D, Engel ME. Incidence, prevalence and outcomes of rheumatic heart disease in South Africa: a systematic review protocol. *BMJ Open*. 2014;4(6). e004844-e.
7. Opasich C, Rapezzi C, Lucci D, et al. Precipitating factors and decision-making processes of short-term worsening heart failure despite "optimal" treatment (from the IN-CHF Registry). *Am J Cardiol*. 2001;88(4):382–387.

8. Felker GM, Januzzi Jr JL. Time is muscle" in acute heart failure: critical concept or fake news? *JACC Heart Fail.* 2018;6(4):295–297.

9. Cosentino N, Campodonico J. Acute heart failure: diagnosis first and then treatment. *Int J Cardiol.* 2018;269: 224–225.

10. Gheorghiade M, Zannad F, Sopko G, et al. Acute heart failure syndromes: current state and framework for future research. *Circulation.* 2005;112(25):3958–3968.

11. O'Driscoll BR, Howard LS, Earis J, Mak V, British Thoracic Society Emergency Oxygen Guideline Group, BTS Emergency Oxygen Guideline Development Group. BTS guideline for oxygen use in adults in healthcare and emergency settings. *Thorax.* 2017;72(Suppl 1):ii1–ii90.

11a. Siemieniuk RAC, Chu DK, Kim LH, Guell-Rous MR, Alhazzani W, Soccal PM, et al. Oxygen therapy for acutely ill medical patients: a clinical practice guideline. *BMJ.* 2018;363. k4169.

12. Rochwerg B, Brochard L, Elliott MW, et al. Official ERS/ATS clinical practice guidelines: noninvasive ventilation for acute respiratory failure. *Eur Respir J.* 2017;50(2):1–20.

13. Vital FM, Ladeira MT, Atallah AN. Non-invasive positive pressure ventilation (CPAP or bilevel NPPV) for cardiogenic pulmonary oedema. *Cochrane Database Syst Rev.* 2013;(5):CD005351.

14. Weng CL, Zhao YT, Liu QH, et al. Meta-analysis: noninvasive ventilation in acute cardiogenic pulmonary edema. *Ann Intern Med.* 2010;152(9):590–600.

15. Gray A, Goodacre S, Newby DE, et al. Noninvasive ventilation in acute cardiogenic pulmonary edema. *N Engl J Med.* 2008;359(2):142–151.

16. *Updated Guideline: Paediatric Emergency Triage WHO;* 2016. Available at: http://www.who.int/maternal_child_adolescent/documents/paediatric-emergency-triage-update/en/.

17. Chapman SM, Maconochie IK. Early warning scores in paediatrics: an overview. *Arch Dis Child.* 2019;104(4):395–399.

18. Royal College of Physicians. *National Early Warning Score (NEWS) 2: Standardising the Assessment of Acute-Illness Severity in the NHS.* Updated Report of a Working Party. London: RCP.

19. Nishimura RA, Otto CM, Bonow RO, et al. AHA/ACC guideline for the management of patients with valvular heart disease: a report of the American College of cardiology/American heart association task force on practice guidelines. *J Am Coll Cardiol.* 2014;63(22):e57–185.

20. Crain FE, Pham N, Wagoner SF, Rycus PT, Maher KO, Fortenberry JD. Fulminant valvulitis from acute rheumatic fever: successful use of extracorporeal support. *Pediatr Crit Care Med.* 2011;12(3):e155–e158.

21. Anderson YWN, Nicholson R, Finucane K. Fulminant mitral regurgitation due to ruptured chordae tendinae in acute rheumatic fever. *J Paediatr Child Health.* 2007; 44(3):134–137.

22. Nieminen MS, Brutsaert D, Dickstein K, et al. EuroHeart Failure Survey II (EHFS II): a survey on hospitalized acute heart failure patients: description of population. *Eur Heart J.* 2006;27(22):2725–2736.

23. Stevenson LW. Clinical use of inotropic therapy for heart failure: looking backward or forward? Part I: inotropic infusions during hospitalization. *Circulation.* 2003;108(3): 367–372.

24. Levine HJ, Gaasch WH. Vasoactive drugs in chronic regurgitant lesions of the mitral and aortic valves. *J Am Coll Cardiol.* 1996;28(5):1083–1091.

25. Nishimura RA, Otto CM, Bonow RO, et al. AHA/ACC focused update of the 2014 AHA/ACC guideline for the management of patients with valvular heart disease: a report of the American College of cardiology/American heart association task force on clinical practice guidelines. *J Am Coll Cardiol.* 2017;70(2):252–289.

26. Baumgartner H, Falk V, Bax JJ, et al. ESC/EACTS guidelines for the management of valvular heart disease. *Eur Heart J.* 2017;38(36):2739–2791.

27. Ozkan M, Cakal B, Karakoyun S, et al. Thrombolytic therapy for the treatment of prosthetic heart valve thrombosis in pregnancy with low-dose, slow infusion of tissue-type plasminogen activator. *Circulation.* 2013;128(5): 532–540.

28. Ozkan M, Gunduz S, Gursoy OM, et al. Ultraslow thrombolytic therapy: a novel strategy in the management of PROsthetic MEchanical valve Thrombosis and the prEdictors of outcomE: the Ultra-slow PROMETEE trial. *Am Heart J.* 2015;170(2):409–418.

29. Unal N, Kosecik M, Saylam GS, Kir M, Paytoncu S, Kumtepe S. Cardiac tamponade in acute rheumatic fever. *Int J Cardiol.* 2005;103(2):217–218.

30. Boon NA, Bloomfield P. The medical management of valvar heart disease. *Heart.* 2002;87(4):395–400.

31. Patel JJ, Munclinger MJ, Mitha AS, Patel N. Percutaneous balloon dilatation of the mitral valve in critically ill young patients with intractable heart failure. *Br Heart J.* 1995;73(6):555–558.

32. Goldman JH, Slade A, Clague J. Cardiogenic shock secondary to mitral stenosis treated by balloon mitral valvuloplasty. *Cathet Cardiovasc Diagn.* 1998;43(2): 195–197.

33. Lokhandwala YY, Banker D, Vora AM, et al. Emergent balloon mitral valvotomy in patients presenting with cardiac arrest, cardiogenic shock or refractory pulmonary edema. *J Am Coll Cardiol.* 1998;32(1):154–158.

34. Agnew R, Wilson N, Skinner J, Nicholson R. Beyond first degree heart block in acute rheumatic fever. *Cardiol Young.* 2019 (in press).

35. Balli S, Oflaz MB, Kibar AE, Ece I. Rhythm and conduction analysis of patients with acute rheumatic fever. *Pediatr Cardiol.* 2013;34(2):383–389.

36. Zalzstein E, Maor R, Zucker N, Katz A. Advanced atrioventricular conduction block in acute rheumatic fever. *Cardiol Young.* 2003;13(6):506–508.

37. Thibodeau JT, Drazner MH. The role of the clinical examination in patients with heart failure. *JACC Heart Fail.* 2018;6(7):543–551.

38. Felker GM, Teerlink JR. Diagnosis and management of acute heart failure. In: Zipes DP, Libby P, Bonow RO, Mann DL, Tomaselli GF, eds. *Braunwald's Heart Disease*

A Textbook of Cardiovascular Medicine. 11th ed. Philadelphia: Elsevier; 2018:462–489.

39. Mullens W, Damman K, Harjola VP, et al. The use of diuretics in heart failure with congestion – a position statement from the heart failure association of the European society of cardiology. *Eur J Heart Fail*. 2019;21(2):137–155.

40. Fonarow GC, Adams Jr KF, Abraham WT, et al. Risk stratification for in-hospital mortality in acutely decompensated heart failure: classification and regression tree analysis. *JAMA*. 2005;293(5):572–580.

41. Yancy CW, Lopatin M, Stevenson LW, et al. Clinical presentation, management, and in-hospital outcomes of patients admitted with acute decompensated heart failure with preserved systolic function: a report from the Acute decompensated heart failure national registry (ADHERE) database. *J Am Coll Cardiol*. 2006;47(1):76–84.

42. Drazner MH, Rame JE, Stevenson LW, Dries DL. Prognostic importance of elevated jugular venous pressure and a third heart sound in patients with heart failure. *N Engl J Med*. 2001;345(8):574–581.

43. Bohm M, Swedberg K, Komajda M, et al. Heart rate as a risk factor in chronic heart failure (SHIFT): the association between heart rate and outcomes in a randomised placebo-controlled trial. *Lancet*. 2010;376(9744):886–894.

44. O'Connor CM, Mentz RJ, Cotter G, et al. The PROTECT in-hospital risk model: 7-day outcome in patients hospitalized with acute heart failure and renal dysfunction. *Eur J Heart Fail*. 2012;14(6):605–612.

45. Mentz RJ, O'Connor CM. Pathophysiology and clinical evaluation of acute heart failure. *Nat Rev Cardiol*. 2016;13(1):28–35.

46. Nohria A, Tsang SW, Fang JC, et al. Clinical assessment identifies hemodynamic profiles that predict outcomes in patients admitted with heart failure. *J Am Coll Cardiol*. 2003;41(10):1797–1804.

47. Nelson GI, Silke B, Ahuja RC, Hussain M, Taylor SH. Haemodynamic advantages of isosorbide dinitrate over frusemide in acute heart-failure following myocardial infarction. *Lancet*. 1983;1(8327):730–733.

48. Dworzynski K, Roberts E, Ludman A, Mant J, Guideline Development Group of the National Institute for Health Care Excellence. Diagnosing and managing acute heart failure in adults: summary of NICE guidance. *BMJ*. 2014;349:g5695.

49. Paul S. Balancing diuretic therapy in heart failure: loop diuretics, thiazides, and aldosterone antagonists. *Congest Heart Fail*. 2002;8(6):307–312.

50. Fonarow GC, Abraham WT, Albert NM, et al. Influence of beta-blocker continuation or withdrawal on outcomes in patients hospitalized with heart failure: findings from the OPTIMIZE-HF program. *J Am Coll Cardiol*. 2008;52(3):190–199.

51. Metra M, Torp-Pedersen C, Cleland JG, et al. Should beta-blocker therapy be reduced or withdrawn after an episode of decompensated heart failure? Results from COMET. *Eur J Heart Fail*. 2007;9(9):901–909.

52. Butler J, Young JB, Abraham WT, et al. Beta-blocker use and outcomes among hospitalized heart failure patients. *J Am Coll Cardiol*. 2006;47(12):2462–2469.

53. Gheorghiade M, Filippatos G, De Luca L, Burnett J. Congestion in acute heart failure syndromes: an essential target of evaluation and treatment. *Am J Med*. 2006;119(12 Suppl 1):S3–S10.

54. Fonarow GC, Committee ASA. The acute decompensated heart failure national registry (ADHERE): opportunities to improve care of patients hospitalized with acute decompensated heart failure. *Rev Cardiovasc Med*. 2003;4(Suppl 7):S21–S30.

55. Ambrosy AP, Pang PS, Khan S, et al. Clinical course and predictive value of congestion during hospitalization in patients admitted for worsening signs and symptoms of heart failure with reduced ejection fraction: findings from the EVEREST trial. *Eur Heart J*. 2013;34(11):835–843.

56. Murdoch DR, Corey GR, Hoen B, et al. Clinical presentation, etiology, and outcome of infective endocarditis in the 21st century: the international collaboration on endocarditis-prospective cohort study. *Arch Intern Med*. 2009;169(5):463–473.

57. Pettersson GB, Hussain ST, Shrestha NK, et al. Infective endocarditis: an atlas of disease progression for describing, staging, coding, and understanding the pathology. *J Thorac Cardiovasc Surg*. 2014;147(4), 1142-1149.e2.

58. Day MD, Gauvreau K, Shulman S, Newburger JW. Characteristics of children hospitalized with infective endocarditis. *Circulation*. 2009;119(6):865–870.

59. Marom D, Levy I, Gutwein O, Birk E, Ashkenazi S. Healthcare-associated versus community-associated infective endocarditis in children. *Pediatr Infect Dis J*. 2011;30(7):585–588.

60. Thornhill MH, Jones S, Prendergast B, et al. Quantifying infective endocarditis risk in patients with predisposing cardiac conditions. *Eur Heart J*. 2018;39(7):586–595.

61. Watt G, Lacroix A, Pachirat O, et al. Prospective comparison of infective endocarditis in Khon Kaen, Thailand and Rennes, France. *Am J Trop Med Hyg*. 2015;92(4):871–874.

62. Holland TL, Baddour LM, Bayer AS, Hoen B, Miro JM, Fowler Jr VG. Infective endocarditis. *Nat Rev Dis Primers*. 2016;2:16059.

63. Moges T, Gedlu E, Isaakidis P, et al. Infective endocarditis in Ethiopian children: a hospital based review of cases in Addis Ababa. *Pan Afr Med J*. 2015;20:75.

64. Wilson SE, Chinyere UC, Queennette D. Childhood acquired heart disease in Nigeria: an echocardiographic study from three centres. *Afr Health Sci*. 2014;14(3):609–616.

65. Kingue S, Ba SA, Balde D, et al. The VALVAFRIC study: a registry of rheumatic heart disease in Western and Central Africa. *Arch Cardiovasc Dis*. 2016;109(5):321–329.

66. Webb R, Voss L, Roberts S, Hornung T, Rumball E, Lennon D. Infective endocarditis in New Zealand children 1994–2012. *Pediatr Infect Dis J*. 2014;33(5):437–442.

67. Baskerville CA, Hanrahan BB, Burke AJ, Holwell AJ, Remond MG, Maguire GP. Infective endocarditis and rheumatic heart disease in the north of Australia. *Heart Lung Circ.* 2012;21(1):36–41.

68. Mirabel M, Andre R, Barsoum P, et al. Ethnic disparities in the incidence of infective endocarditis in the Pacific. *Int J Cardiol.* 2015;186:43–44.

69. Walls G, McBride S, Raymond N, et al. Infective endocarditis in New Zealand: data from the international collaboration on endocarditis prospective cohort study. *N Z Med J.* 2014;127(1391):38–51.

70. Mirabel M, Rattanavong S, Frichitthavong K, et al. Infective endocarditis in the Lao PDR: clinical characteristics and outcomes in a developing country. *Int J Cardiol.* 2015;180:270–273.

71. Arshad S, Awan S, Bokhari SS, Tariq M. Clinical predictors of mortality in hospitalized patients with infective endocarditis at a tertiary care center in Pakistan. *J Pak Med Assoc.* 2015;65(1):3–8.

72. Sadiq M, Nazir M, Sheikh SA. Infective endocarditis in children–incidence, pattern, diagnosis and management in a developing country. *Int J Cardiol.* 2001;78(2):175–182.

73. Shahid U, Sharif H, Farooqi J, Jamil B, Khan E. Microbiological and clinical profile of infective endocarditis patients: an observational study experience from tertiary care center Karachi Pakistan. *J Cardiothorac Surg.* 2018;13(1):94.

74. Elbey MA, Akdag S, Kalkan ME, et al. A multicenter study on experience of 13 tertiary hospitals in Turkey in patients with infective endocarditis. *Anadolu Kardiyoloji Dergisi.* 2013;13(6):523–527.

75. Garg N, Kandpal B, Garg N, et al. Characteristics of infective endocarditis in a developing country-clinical profile and outcome in 192 Indian patients, 1992–2001. *Int J Cardiol.* 2005;98(2):253–260.

76. Subbaraju P, Rai S, Morakhia J, Midha G, Kamath A, Saravu K. Clinical – microbiological characterization and risk factors of mortality in infective endocarditis from a tertiary care academic hospital in Southern India. *Indian Heart J.* 2018;70(2):259–265.

77. Jomaa W, Ben Ali I, Abid D, et al. Clinical features and prognosis of infective endocarditis in children: insights from a Tunisian multicentre registry. *Arch Cardiovasc Dis.* 2017;110(12):676–681.

78. Ba DM, Mboup MC, Zeba N, et al. Infective endocarditis in principal hospital of Dakar: a retrospective study of 42 cases over 10 years. *Pan Afr Med J.* 2017;26:40.

79. Nunes MCP, Guimaraes-Junior MH, Murta Pinto PHO, et al. Outcomes of infective endocarditis in the current era: early predictors of a poor prognosis. *Int J Infect Dis.* 2018;68:102–107.

80. Yock-Corrales A, Segreda-Constenla A, Ulloa-Gutierrez R. Infective endocarditis at Costa Rica's children's hospital, 2000–2011. *Pediatr Infect Dis J.* 2014;33(1):104–106.

81. Pereira CA, Rocio SC, Ceolin MF, et al. Clinical and laboratory findings in a series of cases of infective endocarditis. *J Pediatr.* 2003;79(5):423–428.

82. Dickerman SA, Abrutyn E, Barsic B, et al. The relationship between the initiation of antimicrobial therapy and the incidence of stroke in infective endocarditis: an analysis from the ICE prospective cohort study (ICE-PCS). *Am Heart J.* 2007;154(6):1086–1094.

83. Lopez J, Revilla A, Vilacosta I, et al. Age-dependent profile of left-sided infective endocarditis: a 3-center experience. *Circulation.* 2010;121(7):892–897.

84. Lopez J, Fernandez-Hidalgo N, Revilla A, et al. Internal and external validation of a model to predict adverse outcomes in patients with left-sided infective endocarditis. *Heart.* 2011;97(14):1138–1142.

85. Benito N, Miro JM, de Lazzari E, et al. Health care-associated native valve endocarditis: importance of non-nosocomial acquisition. *Ann Intern Med.* 2009;150(9):586–594.

86. Habib G, Lancellotti P, Antunes MJ, et al. ESC guidelines for the management of infective endocarditis: the task force for the management of infective endocarditis of the European society of cardiology (ESC). Endorsed by: European association for cardio-thoracic surgery (EACTS), the European association of nuclear medicine (EANM). *Eur Heart J.* 2015;36(44):3075–3128.

86a. Khanna N, Roy A, Bahl VK. Janeway lesions: an old sign revisited. *Circulation.* 2013;127(7):861.

86b. Hirai T, Koster M. Osler's nodes, Janeway lesions and splinter haemorrhages. *BMJ Case Rep.* 2013;2013.

87. Nadji G, Rusinaru D, Remadi JP, Jeu A, Sorel C, Tribouilloy C. Heart failure in left-sided native valve infective endocarditis: characteristics, prognosis, and results of surgical treatment. *Eur J Heart Fail.* 2009;11(7):668–675.

88. Harris KA, Yam T, Jalili S, et al. Service evaluation to establish the sensitivity, specificity and additional value of broad-range 16S rDNA PCR for the diagnosis of infective endocarditis from resected endocardial material in patients from eight UK and Ireland hospitals. *Eur J Clin Microbiol Infect Dis.* 2014;33(11):2061–2066.

89. Kumar NV, Menon T, Pathipati P, Cherian KM. 16S rRNA sequencing as a diagnostic tool in the identification of culture-negative endocarditis in surgically treated patients. *J Heart Valve Dis.* 2013;22(6):846–849.

90. Chambers ST, Murdoch D, Morris A, et al. HACEK infective endocarditis: characteristics and outcomes from a large, multi-national cohort. *PLoS One.* 2013;8(5):e63181.

91. Sharara SL, Tayyar R, Kanafani ZA, Kanj SS. HACEK endocarditis: a review. *Expert Review of Anti-infective Therapy.* 2016;14(6):539–545.

92. Muttaiyah S, Best EJ, Freeman JT, Taylor SL, Morris AJ, Roberts SA. Corynebacterium diphtheriae endocarditis: a case series and review of the treatment approach. *Int J Infect Dis.* 2011;15(9):e584–e588.

93. Baddour LM, Wilson WR, Bayer AS, et al. Infective endocarditis in adults: diagnosis, antimicrobial therapy, and management of complications: a scientific statement for healthcare professionals from the American heart association. *Circulation.* 2015;132(15):1435–1486.

94. Penk JS, Webb CL, Shulman ST, Anderson EJ. Echocardiography in pediatric infective endocarditis. *Pediatr Infect Dis J.* 2011;30(12):1109−1111.

95. Humpl T, McCrindle BW, Smallhorn JF. The relative roles of transthoracic compared with transesophageal echocardiography in children with suspected infective endocarditis. *J Am Coll Cardiol.* 2003;41(11):2068−2071.

96. Bai AD, Steinberg M, Showler A, et al. Diagnostic accuracy of transthoracic echocardiography for infective endocarditis findings using transesophageal echocardiography as the reference standard: a meta-analysis. *J Am Soc Echocardiogr.* 2017;30(7), 639-646 e8.

97. Flachskampf FA, Wouters PF, Edvardsen T, et al. Recommendations for transoesophageal echocardiography: EACVI update 2014. *Eur Heart J Cardiovasc Imaging.* 2014;15(4):353−365.

98. Duval X, Iung B, Klein I, et al. Effect of early cerebral magnetic resonance imaging on clinical decisions in infective endocarditis: a prospective study. *Ann Intern Med.* 2010; 152(8), 497−504, W175.

99. Tissieres P, Gervaix A, Beghetti M, Jaeggi ET. Value and limitations of the von Reyn, Duke, and modified Duke criteria for the diagnosis of infective endocarditis in children. *Pediatrics.* 2003;112(6 Pt 1):e467.

100. Stockheim JA, Chadwick EG, Kessler S, et al. Are the Duke criteria superior to the Beth Israel criteria for the diagnosis of infective endocarditis in children? *Clin Infect Dis.* 1998;27(6):1451−1456.

101. Wang A, Gaca JG, Chu VH. Management considerations in infective endocarditis: a review. *JAMA.* 2018;320(1):72−83.

102. Gould FK, Denning DW, Elliott TS, et al. Guidelines for the diagnosis and antibiotic treatment of endocarditis in adults: a report of the working party of the British society for antimicrobial chemotherapy. *J Antimicrob Chemother.* 2012;67(2):269−289.

103. Erba PA, Habib G, Glaudemans A, Miro JM, Slart R. The round table approach in infective endocarditis & cardiovascular implantable electronic devices infections: make your e-Team come true. *Eur J Nucl Med Mol Imaging.* 2017;44(7):1107−1108.

104. Kaura A, Byrne J, Fife A, et al. Inception of the 'endocarditis team' is associated with improved survival in patients with infective endocarditis who are managed medically: findings from a before-and-after study. *Open Heart.* 2017;4(2):e000699.

105. Baltimore RS, Gewitz M, Baddour LM, et al. Infective endocarditis in childhood: 2015 update: a scientific statement from the American heart association. *Circulation.* 2015;132(15):1487−1515.

106. Derex L, Bonnefoy E, Delahaye F. Impact of stroke on therapeutic decision making in infective endocarditis. *J Neurol.* 2010;257(3):315−321.

107. Merkler AE, Chu SY, Lerario MP, Navi BB, Kamel H. Temporal relationship between infective endocarditis and stroke. *Neurology.* 2015;85(6):512−516.

108. Salaun E, Touil A, Hubert S, et al. Intracranial haemorrhage in infective endocarditis. *Arch Cardiovasc Dis.* 2018;111(12):712−721.

109. Yanagawa B, Pettersson GB, Habib G, et al. Surgical management of infective endocarditis complicated by embolic stroke: practical recommendations for clinicians. *Circulation.* 2016;134(17):1280−1292.

110. Lalani T, Cabell CH, Benjamin DK, et al. Analysis of the impact of early surgery on in-hospital mortality of native valve endocarditis: use of propensity score and instrumental variable methods to adjust for treatment-selection bias. *Circulation.* 2010;121(8):1005−1013.

111. Wilson W, Taubert KA, Gewitz M, et al. Prevention of infective endocarditis: guidelines from the American heart association: a guideline from the American heart association rheumatic fever, endocarditis, and Kawasaki disease committee, council on cardiovascular disease in the young, and the council on clinical cardiology, council on cardiovascular surgery and anesthesia, and the quality of care and outcomes research interdisciplinary working group. *Circulation.* 2007;116(15):1736−1754.

112. Thornhill MH, Lockhart PB, Prendergast B, Chambers JB, Shanson D. NICE and antibiotic prophylaxis to prevent endocarditis. *Br Dent J.* 2015;218(11):619−621.

113. Infective Endocarditis Prophylaxis Expert Group. *Prevention of Endocarditis. 2008 Update from Therapeutic Guidelines: Antibiotic Version 13, and Therapeutic Guidelines: Oral and Dental Verison 1;* 2008:16. Available from: https://www.csanz.edu.au/wp-content/uploads/2014/12/Prevention_of_Endocarditis_2008.pdf.

114. New Zealand Heart Foundation. *New Zealand Heart Foundation. New Zealand Guidelines for Rheumatic Fever: Diagnosis, Management and Secondary Prevention of Acute Rheumatic Fever and Rheumatic Heart Disease: 2014 Update.* 2014. Auckland. https://www.heartfoundation.org.nz.

115. RHD Australia (ARF/RHD writing group), National Heart Foundation of Australia, Cardiac Society of Australia and New Zealand. *The Australian guideline for prevention, diagnosis and management of acute rheumatic fever and rheumatic heart disease.* 2nd ed. Full Guidelines 2012:1−136 pp. Available from: https://www.rhdaustralia.org.au/arf-rhd-guideline.

116. Chambers JB, Thornhill MH, Dyer M, Shanson D. A change in the NICE guidelines on antibiotic prophylaxis: British Heart Valve Society update. *BJGP Open.* 2017;1(1). bjgpopen17X100593.

117. Fang MC, Go AS, Chang Y, et al. Death and disability from warfarin-associated intracranial and extracranial hemorrhages. *Am J Med.* 2007;120(8):700−705.

118. Scaglione F. New oral anticoagulants: comparative pharmacology with vitamin K antagonists. *Clin Pharmacokinet.* 2013;52(2):69−82.

119. Pernod G, Godier A, Gozalo C, Tremey B, Sie P, French National Authority for H. French clinical practice guidelines on the management of patients on vitamin K antagonists in at-risk situations (overdose, risk of bleeding, and active bleeding). *Thromb Res.* 2010;126(3):e167−e174.

120. Fredriksson K, Norrving B, Stromblad LG. Emergency reversal of anticoagulation after intracerebral hemorrhage. *Stroke.* 1992;23(7):972−977.

121. Yasaka M, Sakata T, Minematsu K, Naritomi H. Correction of INR by prothrombin complex concentrate and vitamin K in patients with warfarin related hemorrhagic complication. *Thromb Res.* 2002;108(1): 25–30.
122. Evans SJ, Biss TT, Wells RH, Hanley JP. Emergency warfarin reversal with prothrombin complex concentrates: UK wide study. *Br J Haematol.* 2008;141(2): 268–269.
123. Ansell J, Hirsh J, Hylek E, Jacobson A, Crowther M, Palareti G. Pharmacology and management of the vitamin K antagonists: American College of chest Physicians evidence-based clinical practice guidelines (8th Edition). *Chest.* 2008;133(6 suppl l), 160S-98S.
124. http://www.sign.ac.uk. SIGNSAiamESSpnAAfU.
125. Holbrook A, Schulman S, Witt DM, et al. Evidence-based management of anticoagulant therapy: antithrombotic therapy and prevention of thrombosis, 9th ed: American college of chest Physicians evidence-based clinical practice guidelines. *Chest.* 2012;141(2 suppl l). e152S-e84S.
126. Witt DM, Nieuwlaat R, Clark NP, et al. American society of hematology 2018 guidelines for management of venous thromboembolism: optimal management of anticoagulation therapy. *Blood Adv.* 2018;2(22):3257–3291.
127. van Diepen S, Katz JN, Albert NM, et al. Contemporary management of cardiogenic shock: a scientific statement from the American heart association. *Circulation.* 2017; 136(16):e232–e268.
128. Li JS, Sexton DJ, Mick N, et al. Proposed modifications to the Duke criteria for the diagnosis of infective endocarditis. *Clin Infect Dis.* 2000;30(4):633–638.
129. Martin-Davila P, Fortun J, Navas E, et al. Nosocomial endocarditis in a tertiary hospital: an increasing trend in native valve cases. *Chest.* 2005;128(2):772–779.
130. Fowler Jr VG, Miro JM, Hoen B, et al. *Staphylococcus aureus* endocarditis: a consequence of medical progress. *JAMA.* 2005;293(24):3012–3021.

Index

Note: Page numbers followed by "f" indicate figures, "t" indicates tables and "b" indicate boxes

Printed and bound by CPI Group (UK) Ltd, Croydon, CR0 4YY

03/10/2024

01040383-0002